Atlas of
Ultrasound
Measurements

Atlas of
Ultrasound
Measurements

Barry B. Goldberg, M.D.
John P. McGahan, M.D.

Second Edition

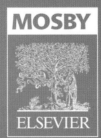

MOSBY

ELSEVIER

1600 John F. Kennedy Blvd.
Ste 1800
Philadelphia, PA 19103-2899

ATLAS OF ULTRASOUND MEASUREMENTS,
SECOND EDITION

ISBN-13: 978-0-323-03229-2
ISBN-10: 0-323-03229-X

Some material was previously published.

Library of Congress Cataloging-in-Publication Data

Goldberg, Barry B., 1937–
    Atlas of ultrasound measurements / Barry B. Goldberg, John P. McGahan.–2nd ed.
        p. cm.
Includes bibliographical references and index.
ISBN 0-323-03229-X
    1. Diagnosis, Ultrasonic–Atlases.   2. Ultrasonic imaging–Atlases.
I. McGahan, John P.   II. Title.
    RC78.7.U4G65 1990
    616.07'540223–dc22

                                                                2005054404

Senior Acquisitions Editor: Meghan McAteer
Editorial Assistant: Ryan Creed
Project Manager: Mary Stermel
Marketing Manager: Emily Christie

Printed in China

Last digit is the print number: 9 8 7 6 5 4 3 2 1

*To all our colleagues, support staff, and
especially our families, who have given
unselfishly of themselves to support
us and the work we love.
This text is dedicated to you.*

JPM/BBG

Contributors

Ronald S. Adler, M.D., Ph.D.
Professor of Radiology
Weill Medical College
Cornell University
Chief, Division of Ultrasound and Body
    Imaging
Hospital for Special Surgery
New York, New York

Elizabeth L. Affel, M.S.
Director, Diagnostic Testing Services
Wills Eye Ophthalmology
Wills Eye Hospital
Philadelphia, Pennsylvania

Diane Babcock, M.D.
Professor of Radiology and Pediatrics
College of Medicine
University of Cincinnati
Department of Radiology
Cincinnati Children's Hospital Medical Center
Cincinnati, Ohio

Aparna Balachandran, M.D.
Assistant Professor of Radiology
Department of Diagnostic Radiology
M.D. Anderson Cancer Center
University of Texas
Houston, Texas

Lincoln L. Berland, M.D., F.A.C.R.
Professor of Radiology
Department of Radiology
University of Alabama at Birmingham
University of Alabama Hospital
Birmingham, Alabama

Bijan Bijan, M.B.A., M.D.
Assistant Professor of Radiology and Nuclear
    Medicine
Divisions of Cross-sectional Body Imaging/
    MRI and Nuclear Medicine PET
Davis Medical Center
University of California
Director of MRI and PET
Stockton MRI and Molecular Imaging Medical
    Center
Stockton, California

Sam Chao, M.S., M.D.
Resident, Diagnostic Radiology
University of Texas Southwestern Medical
    Center
Dallas, Texas

Michael S. Cronan, R.T., R.D.M.S.
Professor
University of California, Davis
Chief Sonographer
Department of Diagnostic Ultrasound
University of California, Davis
Sacramento, California

Greggory R. DeVore, M.D.
Fetal Diagnostic Center
Pasadena, California

Hedieh Eslamy, M.D.
Resident, Nuclear Medicine
Department of Radiology
Division of Nuclear Medicine
Johns Hopkins University
Baltimore, Maryland

Maria Fogata, M.D.
Assistant Professor of Clinical Radiology
Department of Radiology
Davis Medical Center
University of California
Sacramento, California

Eugenio Gerscovich, M.D.
Professor of Radiology
Department of Radiology
Davis Medical Center
University of California
Sacramento, California

Marijo A. Gillen, M.D., Ph.D.
Assistant Professor of Radiology
Department of Radiology
Davis Medical Center
University of California
Sacramento, California

Edward Grant, M.D.
Professor of Radiology
University of Southern California
Chairman, Department of Radiology
University of Southern California
Chief, Imaging Services
USC University Hospital
Los Angeles, California

Ethan J. Halpern, M.S., M.D.
Professor of Radiology and Urology
Thomas Jefferson University
Philadelphia, Pennsylvania

Lyndon Hill, M.D.
Professor of Obstetrics and Gynecology
University of Pittsburgh School of Medicine
Medical Director
Department of Ultrasound
Magee-Womens Hospital
Pittsburgh, Pennsylvania

Mira L. Katz, M.P.H., Ph.D.
Assistant Professor
Division of Health Behavior and Health
  Promotion
School of Public Health
Ohio State University
Columbus, Ohio

Mark E. Lockhart, M.P.H., M.D.
Assistant Professor
Department of Diagnostic Radiology
University of Alabama at Birmingham
Birmingham, Alabama

Jonathan S. Luchs, M.D.
Assistant Professor of Clinical Radiology
State University of New York at Stony Brook
Director of Musculskeletal Imaging
Medical Director, Winthrop Radiology
  Associates, P.C.
Department of Radiology
Winthrop-University Hospital
Mineola, New York

Anita J. Moon-Grady, M.D.
Assistant Professor
Department of Pediatrics
University of California, Davis
University of California, San Francisco
Sacramento, California

Laurence Needleman, M.D.
Associate Professor of Radiology
Jefferson Medical College
Attending Radiologist
Radiology Director, Noninvasive Vascular
  Laboratory
Thomas Jefferson University Hospital
Philadelphia, PA

Suhas G. Parulekar, M.D.
Professor of Radiology
Department of Diagnostic Radiology
M.D. Anderson Cancer Center
University of Texas
Houston, Texas

Philip W. Ralls, M.D.
Professor of Radiology
Keck School of Medicine
University of Southern California
Los Angeles, California

Henry Sebata, M.D.
Resident Physician
Los Angeles County Medical Center
University of Southern California
Los Angeles, California

Rebecca Stein-Wexler, M.D.
Assistant Professor of Radiology
University of California, Davis Medical Center
U.C. Davis Children's Hospital
Shriner Hospital
Sacramento, California

Hisham Tchelepi, M.D.
Instructor of Radiology
Keck's School of Medicine
University of Southern California
Radiologist
Department of Radiology
Division of Body Imaging
Los Angeles County–University of Southern
  California Hospital
Los Angeles, California

Preface

In the second edition of the *Atlas of Ultrasound Measurements* we have provided numerous updates, as well as changes in the basic format. The previous edition had extensive discussion with minimal tabular data for the readers. We have tried to make this second edition of the atlas more user-friendly. We hope this allows readers to easily find the information or table needed, which will be helpful in their daily practice of ultrasound. Toward this end, we have kept the discussion portion of each section to a minimum and placed more emphasis on tabular data with minimal but pertinent illustrations or sonograms that illustrate how different measurements should be used. Furthermore, we have made every effort to organize this atlas with a straightforward approach with a table of contents that we hope is user-friendly. We hope this format is useful to our readers and helps them quickly find information that they need, thus providing a reference to be used in their daily practice.

The contributors to this atlas are all experts in ultrasound, and each section is compiled according to specialties or subspecialties. These individuals include sonologists, radiologists, obstetricians, and cardiologists, as well as other specialists.

We are proud of this second edition of the *Atlas of Ultrasound Measurements* and hope you find the data and information within this text valuable in your daily practice of sonography.

Acknowledgments

We would like to express our deepest appreciation to the outstanding group of international experts in the field of ultrasound who have contributed their time and effort to this project. Without them, this text and atlas would not be possible. These individuals have outstanding reputations in their areas of expertise and their contributions to this project reflect their knowledge and experience. Because of their hard work and dedication this atlas will be an important reference text to be used by those who perform and interpret clinical ultrasound.

We also thank those individuals who worked directly with these contributors and helped both in typing and editing the chapters. These individuals include our coworkers and administrative assistants: Elisa Valenton; Julie Ostoich; Marilyn Lin-Kempster; Daniel A. Merton, B.S., R.D.M.S.; Ji-Bin Liu, M.D.; and Rosemarie Boccella-Costantino, who have devoted their time and effort to this project.

In addition, we would like to thank our coworkers, both sonographers and sonologists, who supplied some of the materials for this atlas, helping make it a success. They deserve our sincere gratitude for their help.

Contributors from Elsevier Mosby who have helped, including Meghan McAteer, Andy Pellegrini, Allan Ross, and Mary Stermel, as well as Bruce Siebert and his associates at Graphic World Publishing Services have also helped to make this project a success.

Contents

Contents—continued

Contents—continued

First Trimester Obstetrical Measurements

CHAPTER 1

John P. McGahan

Amniotic Fluid in the First Trimester

Introduction

Amniotic fluid volume is a useful predictor of fetal well-being. Most studies calculate amniotic fluid volume in the second and third trimester. However, adequate volume of amniotic fluid is important in the first trimester of pregnancy.

Materials

The three dimensions of the amniotic sac (A, B, C) are obtained for these measurements. Amniotic sac volume is then calculated using the ellipsoid shape formula as follows.

$$4/3p(A/2 \times B/2 \times C/2) \text{ or } (A \times B \times C)/2$$

The fetal embryonic volume would then be calculated and subtracted from the amniotic sac volume to obtain the amniotic fluid volume. However, Weissman et al[1] found that the fetus occupied only 5% to 16% of the total amniotic sac volume in early pregnancy. Therefore for a simplified calculation, the amniotic sac volume was used as the amniotic fluid volume in early pregnancy. The amniotic fluid volume is presented for gestational age and for crown-rump length in Tables 1-1 and 1-2.

DISCUSSION

It is known that either poly- or oligohydramnios are prognostic indicators of poor embryonic/fetal outcomes.[2,3] This tabular data allows an objective measurement of amniotic fluid volume in the first trimester of pregnancy.

As amniotic fluid volume increases from approximately 2 mL at 7 weeks to approximately 100 mL at 13 weeks, early amniocentesis may remove a large portion of the amniotic fluid. If 1 mL of amniotic fluid were removed per week of gestation between 9 and 12 weeks, this would in effect remove 72% of the total amniotic fluid volume at 9 weeks and 20% of the total amniotic fluid volume at 12 weeks.[1,4]

Table 1-1 Estimated amniotic fluid volume by gestational age

Week of gestation	n	Mean (95% CI) (mL)	Range (mL)
7	8	1.5 (0.7)	0.8-3.4
8	18	3.9 (0.9)	0.9-11.2
9	19	12.5 (3.0)	5.2-28.6
10	15	24.2 (5.8)	9.3-37.8
11	13	48.4 (6.8)	23.8-86
12	12	57.8 (8.8)	27.4-80
13	10	99.6 (13.5)	67-158

From Weissman A, Itskovitz-Eldor J, Jakobi P: Sonographic measurement of amniotic fluid volume in the first trimester of pregnancy. J Ultrasound Med 1996;15:771-774.

Table 1-2 Estimated amniotic fluid quantity by crown-rum length (CRL)

CRL (cm)	n	Mean (95% CI) (mL)	Range (mL)
1-1.9	18	2.5 (0.8)	0.9-7
2-2.9	21	9.2 (2.3)	3.2-18
3-3.9	14	27.7 (5.5)	15-51
4-4.9	17	54 (9.7)	33-99
5-5.9	12	59 (11.4)	27-82
6-6.9	8	90 (22.2)	56-134
7-7.9	5	101 (45.3)	67-158

From Weissman A, Itskovitz-Eldor J, Jakobi P: Sonographic measurement of amniotic fluid volume in the first trimester of pregnancy. J Ultrasound Med 1996;15:771-774.

References

1. Weissman A, Itskovitz-Eldor J, Jakobi P: Sonographic measurement of amniotic fluid volume in the first trimester of pregnancy. J Ultrasound Med 1996;15:771-774.
2. Bronshtein M, Zimmer EZ: First and early second trimester oligohydramnios: a predictor of poor fetal outcome except in iatrogenic oligohydramnios post chorionic villus biopsy. Ultrasound Obstet Gynecol 1991; 1:245.
3. Harrow MM: Enlarged amniotic cavity: a new sonographic sign of early embryonic death. Am J Roentgenol 1992;158:359.
4. Elejalde BR, Elejalde MM, Acuna JM, et al: Prospective study of amniocentesis performed between weeks 9 and 16 of gestation: its feasibility, risks, complications and use in early genetic prenatal diagnosis. Am J Med Genet 1990;35:188.

CHAPTER 2

John P. McGahan

Crown-Rump Length

Introduction

There have been a number of measurements of the crown-rump length using both the transabdominal and transvaginal scanning to establish gestational age. These are among the more reliable, if not the most reliable, methods of gestational dating.

Materials/Methods

Most methods used to obtain the crown-rump length are similar and measure the embryo or fetus from frozen images. For the embryo, measurement cursors are placed from the cephalic to the caudal ends (Fig. 2-1). In the fetus, calipers are placed from cranium to the buttocks.

Four different equations for prediction of crown-rump length are listed in Table 2-1.[1-4] Crown-rump length measurements in millime-

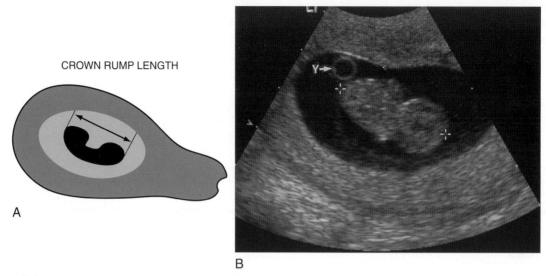

CROWN RUMP LENGTH

A

B

Figure 2-1
A, Cursors are placed from the cephalic to through caudal end of the long axis of the embryo or fetus to obtain the crown-rump length. **B,** Cursors are placed from the cephalic to caudal end of the long axis of the embryo to obtain the crown-rump length. Y = Yolk sac.

Table 2-1	Equations for gestational age prediction using crown-rump length	
Study	**Equation Units**	**Equation**
Robinson	GA = weeks CRL = mm	MA = 5.3066 + (2.0943 x CRL) – (0.21264 x CRL^2) + (0.011206 × CRL^3)
Daya	GA = days CRL = mm^2	GA = 40.447 + 1.125 (CRL) – 0.0058 (CRL)
Hadlock	MA = weeks CRL = cm	In(MA) = 1.684969 + 0.315646 (CRL) – 0.049306 (CRL)^2 + 0.004057 (CRL)^3 – 0.000120456 (CRL)^4
Goldstein	GA = days CRL = mm	GA = 42 + CRL

From references 1, 2, 3, 4 (modified by Peter Doubilet, MD, Boston).

ters are related to menstrual age in weeks. A combination of data sets for predicted gestational ages by crown-rump length are listed in Table 2-2.[1-4] The table is a combination of four different studies that originally used transabdominal scanning and later used endovaginal scanning. There is fairly close approximation of the data points among the four studies, accessing to the reproducibility of the crown-rump length in determining gestational age. These data present the crown-rump length in millimeters, with correlation of the gestational age in weeks. This is tabulated from 6 to 12 weeks (see Tables 2-1 and 2-2).

DISCUSSION

Robinson[4] originally proposed a method for establishing gestational age on the basis of measurements of crown-rump length using transabdominal scanning in 1973. They found with a 95% probability, the error in the crown-rump length with one measurement was plus or minus 4.7 days. Others have shown the crown-rump length to reliably establish the menstrual age within 1 week.[5-6]

A number of articles have shown that a crown-rump length in the first trimester and a biparietal diameter obtained from 20 to 24

Table 2-2 Mean predicted MA (weeks)

CRL (mm)	A	B	C	D	CRL (mm)	A	B	C	D
1	—	—	—	6.1	29	9.9	9.7	9.7	—
2	5.7	6.1	5.7	6.3	30	10	9.9	9.9	—
3	5.9	6.3	5.9	6.4	31	10.1	10	10	—
4	6.1	6.4	6.1	6.6	32	10.2	10.1	10.1	—
5	6.3	6.6	6.2	6.7	33	10.3	10.1	10.2	—
6	6.5	6.7	6.4	6.9	34	10.4	10.3	10.3	—
7	6.7	6.9	6.6	7	35	10.5	10.4	10.4	—
8	6.9	7	6.7	7.1	36	10.6	10.4	10.5	—
9	7	7.1	6.9	7.3	37	10.7	10.6	10.6	—
10	7.2	7.3	7.1	7.4	38	10.8	10.7	10.7	—
11	7.4	7.4	7.2	7.6	39	10.9	10.7	10.8	—
12	7.5	7.6	7.4	7.7	40	11	10.9	10.9	—
13	7.7	7.7	7.5	7.9	41	11.1	11	11	—
14	7.9	7.9	7.7	8	42	11.2	11	11.1	—
15	8	8	7.9	8.1	43	11.3	11.2	11.2	—
16	8.2	8.1	8	8.3	44	11.4	11.3	11.2	—
17	8.3	8.3	8.1	8.4	45	11.4	11.3	11.3	—
18	8.5	8.4	8.3	8.6	46	11.5	11.4	11.4	—
19	8.6	8.6	8.4	8.7	47	11.6	11.4	11.5	—
20	8.7	8.7	8.6	8.9	48	11.7	11.6	11.6	—
21	8.9	8.9	8.7	9	49	11.8	11.7	11.7	—
22	9	8.9	8.9	9.1	50	11.9	11.7	11.7	—
23	9.1	9	9	9.3	51	11.9	11.8	11.8	—
24	9.3	9.1	9.1	9.4	52	12	11.8	11.9	—
25	9.4	9.3	9.2	9.6	53	12.1	12	12	—
26	9.5	9.4	9.4	—	54	12.2	12	12	—
27	9.6	9.6	9.5	—	55	12.3	12.1	12.1	—
28	9.7	9.6	9.6	—					

CRL = Crown-rump length.
From references 1(B), 2(D), 3(C), 4(A).

weeks are equally accurate in predicting gestational age.[7,8] After 12 weeks the fetus is likely to flex and extend, making the crown-rump length less accurate. Therefore Table 2-2 is limited to 12 weeks. The differences from four different studies using both the transabdominal and endovaginal technique are small. The largest difference is no more than 4 days among the different studies.[1-3] Most ultrasound equipment currently utilizes the formula and tables published by Hadlock et al[3] for determining gestational age by crown-rump length.

References

1. Daya S: Accuracy of gestational age estimation by means of fetal crown-rump length measurement. Am J Obstet Gynecol 1993; 168:903-908.

2. Goldstein SR, Wolfson R: Endovaginal ultrasonographic measurement of early embryonic size as a means of assessing gestational age. J Ultrasound Med 1994;13: 27-31.

3. Hadlock FP, Shah YP, Kanon DJ, et al: Fetal crown-rump length: reevaluation of the relation to menstrual age (5-18 weeks) with high resolution real-time ultrasound. Radiology 1992;182:501-505.

4. Robinson HP: Sonar measurement of fetal crown-rump length as means of assessing maturity of first trimester of pregnancy. Br Med J 1973;4:28-31.

5. Drumm JE: The prediction of delivery date by ultrasonic measurement of fetal crown-rump length. Br J Obstet Gynaecol 1997; 84:1-5.

6. Parker AJ: Assessment of gestational age of the Asian fetus by the sonar measurement

of crown-rump length and biparietal diameter. Br J Obstet Gynaecol 1982;89:836-838.

7. Kopta MM, May RR, Crane JP: A comparison of the reliability of the estimated data of confinement predicted by crown-rump length

and biparietal diameter. Am J Obstet Gynecol 1983;145:562-565.

8. Smazal SF, Weisman LE, Hoppler KD, et al: Comparative analysis of ultrasonographic methods of gestational age assessment. J Ultrasound Med 1983;2:147-150.

CHAPTER 3

Henry Sabata
John P. McGahan

Embryonic Heart Rate

Introduction

Embryonic cardiac activity can be detected as early as the sixth week of gestational age with the use of endovaginal sonography.[1,2] Although the presence of embryonic cardiac activity confirms viability, it cannot differentiate the embryos at higher risk for poor pregnancy outcome. Determining early first trimester embryonic heart rate (EHR) provides additional prognostic information in viable embryos.

Materials/Methods

Most studies utilize endovaginal sonography to measure early first trimester EHR.

The transvaginal approach allows earlier detection of EHR compared with transabdominal sonography.[3] However, transabdominal measurements are still used for later gestational ages. Embryonic cardiac activity is identified with real-time B-mode imaging, and cardiac cycles are recorded in M-mode display. Heart rates are calculated from cardiac cycle intervals measured by electronic calipers.

Estimated gestational age is calculated by crown-rump length measurements and/or on the basis of reliable reporting of the first day of the last menstrual period. Some studies included patients that conceived via in vitro fertilization. In these cases, 2 weeks were added to the time elapsed since embryo transfer.

DISCUSSION

EHR normally increases progressively during the early embryonic period.[1,2,4-7] Doubilet and Benson[7] documented a progressive increase in EHR from 6 to 8 weeks' gestation. This study utilizes a large sample size, and the association between gestational age and heart rate is statistically significant. Several studies have shown the peak EHR occurs at 9 weeks of gestational age.[1,4-6] Rempen[1] evaluated EHR in 363 single-ton pregnancies with normal outcomes.[1] The mean EHR increased from 110 ± 8 beats per minute (bpm) at 5 weeks to 170 ± 6 bpm at 9 weeks. Thereafter EHR gradually decreased to 159 ± 3 bpm at 13 weeks (Fig. 3-1). Robinson and Shaw-Dunn[4] and van Heeswijk et al[6] reported a similar trend. These characteristic changes in heart rate may reflect anatomic differentiation and conduction system maturation.[4] However,

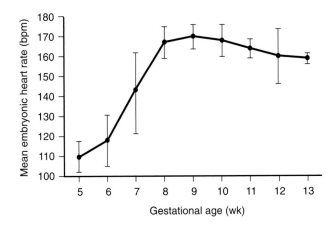

Gestational age (wk)	Mean EHR (bpm)	Standard deviation
5	110	8
6	118	13
7	143	19
8	167	8
9	170	6
10	168	8
11	164	5
12	160	14
13	159	3

Figure 3-1
Embryonic heart rate (mean ± standard deviation) in relation to gestational age. (From Rempen A: Diagnosis of viability in early pregnancy with vaginal sonography. J Ultrasound Med 1990;9:711-716.)

Hertzberg et al[5] have shown the EHR to plateau after 9 weeks at around 137 to 144 bpm.

A slow EHR is associated with an increased risk for first trimester spontaneous abortion.[7-10] Doubilet and Benson[7] established the lower limit of normal EHR for different age groups on the basis of first trimester mortality rates. For embryos = 6.2 weeks, a slow EHR was defined as heart rate less than 100 bpm. EHRs less than 100 bpm are associated with increased first trimester mortality. The risk increases as the EHR drops below 90 bpm, and the risk decreases with heart rates above 110 bpm (Table 3-1). For embryos 6.3 to 7 weeks, they defined a slow EHR as heart rate less than 120 bpm. Although a slow EHR increases the risk of poor first trimester outcome, embryos that survive beyond the first trimester have survival rates similar to those with normal heart rates.[10] However, the embryos with slow heart rates are at twice the risk of having cardiac, chromosomal, and other anomalies.[10]

Doubilet et al[11] examined the effects of rapid EHR on pregnancy outcome.[11] The upper limit of normal heart rate was 134 bpm for embryos = 6.2 weeks and 154 bpm for embryos 6.3 to 7 weeks. Heart rates faster than this are not associated with poor short-term outcome. Although an increase in frequency of major anomalies was observed in the rapid EHR group, the increase was not significant.

Table 3-1	Relationship between embryonic heart rate and first trimester mortality rate	
Embryonic heart rate (bpm)	**First trimester mortality rate ≤6.2 weeks**	**First trimester mortality rate 6.3-7.0 weeks**
<80	100%	100%
80-89	64%	100%
90-99	32%	100%
100-109	16%	43%
110-119	11%	18%
120-129	4%	5%
≥130	20%	10%

From Doubilet PM, Benson CB: Embryonic heart rate in the early first trimester: what rate is normal? J Ultrasound Med 1995;14: 431-434.

References

1. Rempen A: Diagnosis of viability in early pregnancy with vaginal sonography. J Ultrasound Med 1990;9:711-716.
2. Howe RS, Isaacson KJ, Albert JL, et al: Embryonic heart rate in human pregnancy. J Ultrasound Med 1991;10:367-371.
3. Pennell RG, Needleman L, Pajak T, et al: Prospective comparison of vaginal and abdominal sonography in normal early pregnancy. J Ultrasound Med 1991;10:63-67.
4. Robinson HP, Shaw-Dunn J: Fetal heart rates as determined by sonar in early pregnancy. J Obstet Gynaecol Br Commonw 1973;80:805-809.
5. Hertzberg BS, Mahony BS, Bowie JD: First trimester fetal cardiac activity. Sonographic documentation of a progressive early rise in heart rate. J Ultrasound Med 1988;7:573-575.
6. van Heeswijk M, Nijhuis JG, Hollanders HM: Fetal heart rate in early pregnancy. Early Hum Dev 1990;22:151-156.
7. Doubilet PM, Benson CB: Embryonic heart rate in the early first trimester: what rate is normal? J Ultrasound Med 1995;14:431-434.
8. Laboda LA, Estroff JA, Benacerraf BR: First trimester bradycardia. A sign of impending fetal loss. J Ultrasound Med 1989;8:561-563.
9. Benson CB, Doubilet PM: Slow embryonic heart rate in early first trimester: indicator of poor pregnancy outcome. Radiology 1994;192:343-344.
10. Doubilet PM, Benson CB, Chow JS: Long-term prognosis of pregnancies complicated by slow embryonic heart rates in the early first trimester. J Ultrasound Med 1999;18:537-541.
11. Doubilet PM, Benson CB, Chow JS: Outcome of pregnancies with rapid embryonic heart rates in the early first trimester. AJR Am J Roentgenol 2000;175:67-69.

CHAPTER 4

John P. McGahan

Gestational Sac Size–Crown-Rump Length Difference

Introduction

In early pregnancy the gestational sac size is due to the additive size of the embryo, the amniotic cavity and its content, and the chorionic cavity and its content. A small gestational sac size relative to the size of the crown-rump length may have certain prognostic indicators.

Materials/Methods

A number of studies have evaluated the differences in the mean sac diameter (MSD) and the crown-rump length and its prognostic significance.[1-3] In these studies the mean sac diameter was obtained by taking the three measurements of the sac and dividing it by three to obtain a mean. Bromley et al[1] found that a difference in the mean sac size (MSS) and crown-

Table 4-1	Pregnancy outcome according to gestational sac diameter–crown-rump length difference determined by vaginal ultrasound		
GSD-CRL difference (mm)		**Births**	**Abortions**
<5		2 (20.0%)	8 (80.0%)
5-7.9		50 (73.5%)	18 (26.5%)
≥8		412 (89.4%)	49 (10.6%)

GSD-CRL = gestational sac diameter–crown-rump length.
Modified from Dickey RP, Olar TT, Taylor SN, et al: Relationship of small gestational sac–crown-rump length differences to abortion and abortus karyotypes. Obstet Gynecol 1992;79: 554-557.

Table 4-2	Difference in mean sac diameter (MSD) and the crown-rump length (CRL) versus menstrual age from 5 to 12 weeks in a normal population
Menstrual Age (weeks)	**MSD-CRL (mm)**
5	11
6	12
7	13
8	14
9	13
10	11
11	5
12	1

From Rowling SE, Coleman BG, Langer JE, et al: First-trimester US parameters of failed pregnancy. Radiology 1997;203: 211-217.

rump length of less than 5 mm occurred in 1.9% of pregnancies between 5.5 and 9 weeks in their study. They found that 94% of these first trimester pregnancies had a spontaneous abortion. Dickey et al[2] found that MSD minus crown-rump length (CRL) of less than 5 mm occurred in 1.9% of pregnancies scanned 37 days (5.3 weeks) to 65 days (9.3 weeks) after their last menstrual period. They found an embryonic death rate of 80%. They further stratified their patients and found a 26% abor-tion rate when this difference was 5 to 7.9 mm and an abortion rate of only 11% when the difference was greater than 8 mm (Table 4-1). However, Rowling et al[3] had differing results in that 0.74% of their study had an MSD minus CRL of less than 5 mm. Although they had fairly poor follow-up, they had 17 patients in the group with the difference of 5 mm or less. Six (35%) had a normal follow-up, two (12%) had a spon-taneous abortion, and 53% were lost to follow-up.

DISCUSSION

There seems little doubt that the differences in mean sac diameter and the crown-rump length of less than 5 mm may be associated with a poor fetal outcome.[1,2] However, more recent data show that the prognosis is not as unfavorable as once thought. Also, indeterminate difference, 5 to 7.9 mm, may have a poorer prognosis than pregnancies with a difference greater than 8 mm.

Although we may wish to attribute the decrease in sac size to oligohydramnios, it may be the loss of the chorionic fluid rather than the amniotic fluid that is the etiology of the difference.

Finally, the difference in MSS and CRL in normal pregnancies is 14.4 mm at 8 weeks, which decreases to 1 mm by 12 weeks[3] (Table 4-2). Therefore differences in MSS and CRL should not be calculated for pregnancies longer than 9 weeks.[3]

References

1. Bromley B, Harlow BL, Laboda LA, et al: Small sac size in the first trimester: a predic-tor of poor fetal outcome. Radiology 1991;178: 375-377.
2. Dickey RP, Olar TT, Taylor SN, et al: Relation-ship of small gestational sac-crown rump length differences to abortion and abortus karyotypes. Obstet Gynecol 1992;79:554-557.
3. Rowling SE, Coleman BG, Langer JE, et al: First-trimester US parameters of failed preg-nancy. Radiology 1997;203:211-217.

CHAPTER 5

John P. McGahan

Human Chorionic Gonadotropin Values Correlated with Sonography

Introduction

Human chorionic gonadotropin (hCG) values rise in early pregnancy. There has been an attempt to correlate these values with findings on transvaginal sonography.

Materials/Methods

Probably one of the most quoted studies regarding correlation of hCG values with findings on transvaginal sonography was a study published by Bree et al[1] in 1989. In his study Bree et al[1] correlated the sonographic findings in early pregnancy with hCG values. He performed endovaginal sonography 75 times in 53 patients using a 7-MHz probe. He established discriminatory levels where certain findings could always be identified. His findings are summarized in Table 5-1. At 1000 mIU/mL, using the First Interpretation Reference Preparation (IRP), a gestational sac was always seen. At 7200 mIU/mL a yolk sac was always seen, and at 10,800 mIU/mL a visible embryo with a heartbeat was seen.

DISCUSSION

There has been considerable confusion within the literature concerning correlation of early ultrasound findings with hCG values. This confusion has occurred because of the different standards used. For instance, Nyberg et al[2] used the older Second International Standard in establishing a discriminatory value of 1800 mIU/mL for visualization of a gestational sac using the transabdominal approach. Most authors agree that these Second International Standard values need to be roughly doubled to correlate with the values of the first IRP. Thus the value of 1800 mIU/mL, using the older standard, would correlate with a value of 3600 mIU/mL using the first IRP; this is with transabdominal scanning. To further confuse the issue, there are now other standards. For instance, the newer Third International Reference Preparation roughly corresponds to the first IRP. An individual must further check in regards to which commercial assay of a particular standard is utilized. Numerous manufacturers may have different established values for use of hCG. As such, my preference is to use no absolute cut-off. When we use hCG values in early pregnancy, we are trying to establish one of three possibilities (Table 5-2). In normal pregnancies, we can follow quantitative hCG values that double every 48 hours. However, values

Table 5-1	Discriminatory values for HCG correlated with transvaginal ultrasound findings using the First International Reference Preparation
Values	**Ultrasound Findings**
1000 mIU/mL	Gestational sac
7200 mIU/mL	Yolk sac
10,800 mIU/mL	Live embryo

From Bree RL, Edwards M, Bohm-Velez M, et al: Transvaginal sonography in the evaluation of normal early pregnancy: correlation with HCG level. Am J Roentgenol 1989;153:75-79.

Table 5-2	Three most common possibilities for early elevation of hCG values

Normal intrauterine pregnancy (IUP)
Abnormal IUP (including spontaneous abortion)
Ectopic pregnancy

Table 5-3	Representative hCG ranges during pregnancy

Week from the Last Menstrual Period	Approximate Amount of hCG (mIU/mL, IU/L)
3	5-50
4	4-426
5	19-7340
6	1080-56,500
7-8	7650-229,000
9-12	25,700-288,000
13-16	13,300-254,000
17-24	4060-165,400
25-40	3640-117,100

From The International Council on Infertility Information Dissemination, Inc. Arlington, VA, 2001.

only hCG and are called intact-hCG test. Still further confusing is that other hCG tests check hCG, its free β-subunit, and possibly other hCG fragments. Adding to this confusion, there are more than 40 different professional laboratory serum hCG tests that are sold in the United States for quantifying serum β-hCG. A representative hCG range during normal pregnancy is summarized in Table 5-3.[5] However, because other clinical references may show different values, each laboratory should establish its own reference range. These tables are for β-specific hCG, as used in the World Health Organization Reference for the Third International Standard.[6]

References

1. Bree RL, Edwards M, Bohm-Velez M, et al: Transvaginal sonography in the evaluation of normal early pregnancy: correlation with HCG level. Am J Roentgenol 1989;153: 75-79.
2. Nyberg DA, Filly RA, Mahony BS, et al: Early gestation: correlation of HCG levels and sonographic identification. Am J Roentgenol 1985; 144:951-954.
3. Borrelli PT, Butler SA, Docherty SM, et al: Human chorionic gonadotropin isoforms in the diagnosis of ectopic pregnancy. Clin Chem 2003;49:2045-2049.
4. Cole LA: Use of hCG test for evaluating trophoblastic disease: choosing an appropriate hCG assay, false detection of hCG, unexplained elevated hCG and quiescent trophoblastic disease. In Hancock, Newland, Berkowitz, Cole: Gestational Trophoblastic Disease, 2nd ed. Web Publication (in press), 2002.
5. The International Council on Infertility Information Dissemination, Inc. Arlington, VA, 2001.
6. Standardization of protein immunoprocedures. Scand J Clin Lab Invest 1993;53(suppl 216):42-78.

actually double every 1.5 days up to the fifth week and then every 3.5 days from the seventh week.[1,3] In ectopic pregnancy values may increase in a similar fashion, but more often these values plateau or decrease. For a spontaneous abortion, values will precipitously drop. Therefore a safe approach is to be cautious in correlation of absolute values of hCG with ultrasound findings in early pregnancy.

In addition to regular hCG, there are at least five major variants of hCG that are present in serum samples.[4] Commercial hCG tests use at least one antibody directed against the β-subunit. This has led to the commonly used term "β-hCG test." However, some tests detect

CHAPTER 6

John P. McGahan

Mean Sac Diameter

Introduction

A number of different authors have correlated gestational sac size with early gestational dating. These measurements have been used for more than a quarter of a century in establishing early gestational dating.[1]

Materials/Methods

Either the transabdominal or endovaginal technique may be utilized. Whenever possible the endovaginal technique is preferred, as the sac may be identified earlier. Other important landmarks such as the yolk sac, embryo, or embryonic cardiac activity may be visualized earlier with the endovaginal technique compared with the transabdominal techniques.

Early articles did not define the exact site used for the measurements of the gestational sac or whether the average diameter or longest diameter of the sac was used. It is now well established that the mean sac diameter (MSD) be used in all measurements. The cursors should be placed from the inner edge to the opposite inner edge of the gestational sac. The width, length, and anterior-posterior measurement should be obtained (Fig. 6-1). Most equipment will enter these measurements automatically to obtain a mean sac diameter.

The initial gestational sac measurements, using the transabdominal route, are from Hellman et al[1] in 1969 and are reproduced in Table 6-1. A more recent chart was produced from Daya et al[2] using endovaginal scanning, reproduced in Table 6-2.[2]

DISCUSSION

It is important to recognize differences and similarities in data obtained for estimating gestational age using sac diameter. Single sac measurements may have been used in early data, but MSD is the current accepted method to obtain sac measurements to account for sac distortion (see Fig. 6-1).

Endovaginal sonography will allow earlier visualization of the gestational sac. In data from Hellman et al, the smallest sac diameter measured by transabdominal scanning was 10 mm. Daya et al[2] measured sac diameters as small as 2 mm. Also, there are discrepancies among different tables. For instance, in an article published by Hellman et al[1] in 1969, using the transabdominal approach, at a gestational age of 5 weeks, the sac diameter was 10 mm, while at 6 weeks it was 17 mm. More recent data using the endovaginal approach from Daya

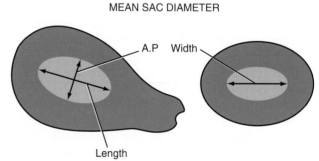

MEAN SAC DIAMETER

Figure 6-1
Mean sac diameter is obtained by taking the length, width, and anterior-posterior dimension and dividing it by three, demonstrated in this drawing of early gestational sac.

Table 6-1	Gestational sac measurement		
Mean predicted gestational sac (mm)	**Gestational age (wks)**	**Mean predicted gestational sac (mm)**	**Gestational age (wks)**
10	5.0	36	8.8
11	5.2	37	8.9
12	5.3	38	9.0
13	5.5	39	9.2
14	5.6	40	9.3
15	5.8	41	9.5
16	5.9	42	9.6
17	6.0	43	9.7
18	6.2	44	9.9
19	6.3	45	10.0
20	6.5	46	10.2
21	6.6	47	10.3
22	6.8	48	10.5
23	6.9	49	10.6
24	7.0	50	10.7
25	7.2	51	10.9
26	7.3	52	11.0
27	7.5	53	11.2
28	7.6	54	11.3
29	7.8	55	11.5
30	7.9	56	11.6
31	8.0	57	11.7
32	8.2	58	11.9
33	8.3	59	12.0
34	8.5	60	12.2
35	8.6		

Formula: GA (wks) = (GS (mm) + 25.43)/7.02, where GA is gestational age and GS is gestational sac.
From Hellman LM, Kobayashi M, Fillisti L, et al: Growth and development of the human fetus prior to the twentieth week of gestation. Am J Obstet Gynecol 1969;103(6):789-800.

et al[2] in 1991 showed that the sac diameter at 5 weeks was 2 mm and at 6 weeks was 10 mm. A publication in 1984 using transabdominal scanning by Cadkin and McAlpin[3] showed the sac diameter at 5 weeks to be 5 mm and at 6 weeks to be 12 mm. The exact reason for these differences is uncertain. Many equipment manufacturers use the Hellman tables as the standard for determination of gestational age.

Robinson[4] described a method of determining gestational sac volumes in early pregnancy with ultrasound. Scans of this gestational sac were obtained in parallel sections a certain distance apart, such as 1 cm. The area of each section, determined by plainmetry, was multiplied by 1 cm. This is the distance between individual scans and is used to determine an individual volume. Each parallel sac volume is summated to determine the gestational sac volume. Although accurate, this method is complex and not routinely used.

Table 6-2 Mean diameter of gestational sac and corresponding estimates of gestational age

Mean sac diameter (mm)	Mean gestational age (wks)	Gestational age (days)	
		Mean	95% confidence interval
2	5.0	34.9	34.3-35.5
3	5.1	35.8	35.2-36.3
4	5.2	36.6	36.1-37.2
5	5.4	37.5	37.0-38.0
6	5.5	38.4	37.9-38.9
7	5.6	39.4	38.9-39.7
8	5.7	40.2	39.8-40.6
9	5.9	41.1	40.7-41.4
10	6.0	41.9	41.6-42.3
11	6.1	42.8	42.5-43.2
12	6.2	43.7	43.4-44.0
13	6.4	44.6	44.3-44.9
14	6.5	45.5	45.2-45.8
15	6.6	46.3	46.0-46.6
16	6.7	47.2	46.9-47.5
17	6.9	48.1	47.8-48.4
18	7.0	49.0	48.6-49.4
19	7.1	49.9	49.5-50.3
20	7.3	50.8	50.3-51.2
21	7.4	51.6	51.2-52.1
22	7.5	52.5	52.0-53.0
23	7.6	53.4	52.9-53.9
24	7.8	54.3	53.7-54.8
25	7.9	55.2	54.6-55.7
26	8.0	56.0	55.4-56.7
27	8.1	56.9	56.3-57.6
28	8.3	57.8	57.1-58.5
29	8.4	58.7	58.0-59.4
30	8.5	59.6	58.8-60.4

From Daya S, Woods S, Ward S, et al: Early pregnancy assessment with transvaginal ultrasound scanning. Can Med Assoc J 1991;144(4):441-446.

References

1. Hellman LM, Kobayashi M, Fillisti L, et al: Growth and development of the human fetus prior to the twentieth week of gestation. Am J Obstet Gynecol 1969;103:789-800.
2. Daya S, Wood S, Ward S, et al: Early pregnancy assessment with transvaginal ultrasound scanning. Can Med Assoc J 1991; 144:441-446.
3. Cadkin AV, McAlpin J: The deciduas-chorionic sac: a reliable sonographic indicator of intrauterine pregnancy prior to detection of a fetal pole. J Ultrasound Med 1984;3:539-548.
4. Robinson HP: "Gestation sac" volumes as determined by sonar in the first trimester of pregnancy. Br J Obstet Gynaecol 1975;82: 100-107.

Sam Chao
John P. McGahan

CHAPTER 7

Yolk Sac

Introduction

Mantoni and Pederson[1] were the first to document visualization of the secondary yolk sac by sonography. The yolk sac is the first extraembryonic structure that can be detected with transvaginal sonography in the chorionic cavity and can be seen from the 5th to 12th week of menstrual age[2] (Table 7-1). A number of articles have investigated the utility of yolk sac presence, size, and shape in the prediction of poor pregnancy outcomes.[3-17]

Yolk sac size is conventionally measured by recording the mean yolk sac diameter.[3,9]

However, more recent studies have used volumetry to correlate size with first trimester pregnancy outcomes. Yolk sac volumetry is more complex than measuring the mean yolk sac diameter and, to date, has little clinical benefit.[5,6]

Results are still conflicting regarding the prognostic significance of either the absence or abnormalities in size and shape of the yolk sac as potential predictors of poor pregnancy outcome.[7-17]

Materials/Measurements

Both the transabdominal and endovaginal techniques can be used to measure the yolk sac. However, the endovaginal technique is the preferred method because it can detect the yolk sac earlier and has better axial and lateral resolution.[7,11-13,15] Transvesicular ultrasonography is rarely employed due to distortion of uterine contents.

The yolk sac is normally round or oval and has a uniformly thick, echogenic wall surrounding an echo-free core (Fig. 7-1). It floats within the lumen of the gestational sac and is connected to the inner wall of the gestational sac

by the vitelline duct. It is often found near the periphery of the gestational sac. Manual compression of the abdomen, the use of linear transducers, and increased gain settings may assist visualization of the yolk sac.

The cursor of the electronic calipers should be placed from one inner edge to the opposite inner edge of the yolk sac. The longitudinal and transverse internal diameters should be measured. Most equipment will automatically enter these measurements to obtain a mean yolk sac diameter.

DISCUSSION

BACKGROUND

The yolk sac can often be demonstrated by endovaginal ultrasound when the mean sac diameter (MSD) is 5 to 6 mm, and it is usually seen before the embryo. Yolk sac grows at about 0.1 mm per millimeter of MSD growth before 15 mm MSD, after which it grows at a rate of 0.03 mm per millimeter of MSD growth (Table 7-2).[12] Levi and Nyberg report that normal yolk sacs can usually be demonstrated in normal

pregnancies when the mean sac diameter is greater than or equal to 8 mm using endovaginal sonography or 20 mm using transabdominal sonography.[10-13] Its growth throughout the first trimester of normal gestation has often been reported: the yolk sac reaches a diameter of 5 to 6 mm in the 10th week.[12] After 10 or 11 weeks of menstrual age, it shows a decrease in size[12] (see Table 7-1). However, its remnant may be seen for up to 20 weeks' gestation.

Table 7-1	Normal values for yolk sac (YS) diameter versus menstrual age (MA) in days	
MA	**Mean YS diameter (mm)**	**95% CI**
31	0.4	0-2
32	0.7	0-2.2
33	1	0-2.5
34	1.2	0-2.7
35	1.4	0-2.9
36	1.6	0.1-3.1
37	1.7	0.2-3.2
38	1.9	0.4-3.4
39	2	0.5-3.6
40	2.2	0.7-3.7
41	2.3	0.8-3.8
42	2.4	0.9-3.9
43	2.5	1.0-4.0
44	2.6	1.1-4.1
45	2.7	1.2-4.2
46	2.7	1.2-4.2
47	2.8	1.3-4.3
48	2.8	1.3-4.3
49	2.9	1.4-4.4
50	2.9	1.4-4.4
51	3	1.5-4.5
52	3	1.5-4.5
53	3	1.5-4.5
54	3.1	1.6-4.6
55	3.1	1.6-4.6
56	3.1	1.6-4.6
57	3.2	1.7-4.7
58	3.2	1.7-4.7
59	3.2	1.7-4.7
60	3.3	1.8-4.8
61	3.3	1.8-4.8
62	3.4	1.8-4.9
63	3.4	1.9-4.9
64	3.5	1.9-5.0
65	3.5	2.0-5.0
66	3.6	2.1-5.1
67	3.7	2.1-5.2
68	3.8	2.2-5.3

From Lindsay DJ, Lovett IS, Lyons EA, et al: Yolk sac diameter and shape at endovaginal US: predictors of pregnancy outcome in the first trimester. Radiology 1992;183:115-118.

Table 7-2	Normal values for yolk sac (YS) diameter versus mean sac diameter (MSD)	
MSD	**Mean YS diameter (mm)**	**95% CI**
2	0.4	0-1.8
3	0.6	0-2.1
4	0.9	0-2.4
5	1.2	0-2.7
6	1.5	0-2.9
7	1.7	0.3-3.2
8	1.9	0.5-3.4
9	2.1	0.7-3.6
10	2.3	0.8-3.7
11	2.4	1.0-3.9
12	2.6	1.1-4.0
13	2.7	1.2-4.1
14	2.8	1.3-4.2
15	2.9	1.4-4.3
16	3	1.5-4.3
17	3	1.5-4.4
18	3	1.6-4.4
19	3.1	1.6-4.5
20	3.1	1.6-4.5
21	3.1	1.6-4.5
22	3.1	1.6-4.5
23	3.1	1.6-4.5
24	3.1	1.6-4.5
25	3.1	1.6-4.5
26	3.1	1.6-4.5
27	3.1	1.6-4.5
28	3.1	1.6-4.5
29	3.1	1.6-4.5
30	3.1	1.7-4.6
31	3.1	1.7-4.6
32	3.1	1.7-4.6
33	3.2	1.7-4.6
34	3.2	1.8-4.7
35	3.3	1.8-4.7
36	3.3	1.9-4.8
37	3.4	1.9-4.9
38	3.5	2.0-5.0
39	3.6	2.1-5.1
40	3.7	2.2-5.2
41	3.9	2.3-5.4
42	4.1	2.5-5.6
43	4.2	2.6-5.8
44	4.4	2.7-6.0
45	4.5	2.8-6.1

From Lindsay DJ, Lovett IS, Lyons EA, et al: Yolk sac diameter and shape at endovaginal US: predictors of pregnancy outcome in the first trimester. Radiology 1992;183:115-118.

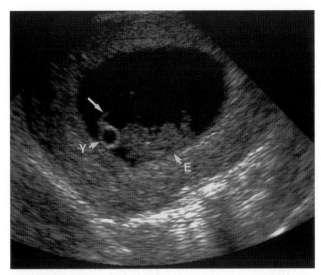

Figure 7-1
The ringlike yolk sac (*Y*) floats within the gestational sac and is connected to the gestational sac by the vitelline duct (*long arrow*). E = Embryo.

YOLK SAC PRESENCE

The presence of the yolk sac is important in a number of situations, including defining normal first trimester anatomy, determining the existence of an intrauterine pregnancy, and identifying the number and type of multiple gestations.[3-5] Nyberg et al[13] believed that the identification of the yolk sac is as reliable as demonstrating a living embryo for confirming an intrauterine pregnancy. Levi observed that the absence of a yolk sac in a gestational sac of greater or equal to 8mm almost always led to a nonviable pregnancy.[10,11] In the first trimester, the absence of the yolk sac in the presence of an embryo is always abnormal and usually is associated with embryonic death.[10,11]

YOLK SAC SIZE

Numerous studies have found that the yolk sac size is a sensitive predictor for abnormal outcome in the first trimester.[12] Nevertheless, a few authors observed that the yolk size has no prognostic value for embryonic demise and pregnancy outcome.[4]

An abnormal change in yolk sac size may reflect abnormal metabolic function in the yolk sac. This may lead to an increase or decrease in secretive substances and, therefore, alterations in yolk sac size. Some authors have sug-

gested that alterations in size of the yolk sac in spontaneous abortions may be a consequence of embryonic death rather than the primary cause of pregnancy failure. Stampone et al[15] observed that yolk sac size (below or above two standard deviations of the regression) was predictive of spontaneous abortion in 91.6% of cases, with a sensitivity of 68.7% and a specificity of 99%. Lindsay et al[12] and Rempen et al[14] found that a yolk sac diameter greater than 5.6 to 6 mm was associated with spontaneous abortions. Further, Zalel et al[17] observed that extremely large yolk sacs with diameters of 11 mm were associated with partial moles.

YOLK SAC SHAPE

A persistently abnormal yolk sac shape is also a predictor of abnormal outcome. Lindsay et al[12] observed that if an abnormal yolk sac shape persists at 1-week follow-up, embryos were at increased risk for demise or fetal anomaly. However, if the shape reverted to normal, then the outcome was normal. Lindsay et al[12] recommends the measurement of yolk sac diameter and assessment of yolk sac shape in all pregnancies less than 10 weeks' menstrual age.

References

1. Mantoni M, Pedersen JF: Ultrasound visualization of the human yolk sac. J Clin Ultrasound 1979;7:459-460.
2. Ferrazzi E, Brambati B, Lanzani A, et al: The yolk sac in early pregnancy failure. Am J Obstet Gynecol 1988;158:137-142.
3. Nyberg DA, Mack LA, Harvey D, et al: Value of the yolk sac in evaluating early pregnancies. J Ultrasound Med 1988;7:129-135.
4. Kurtz AB, Needleman L, Pennell RG, et al: Can detection of the yolk sac in the first trimester be used to predict the outcome of pregnancy? A prospective sonographic study. Am J Roentgenol 1992;158:843-847.
5. Babinszki A, Nyari T, Jordan S, et al: Three-dimensional measurement of gestation and yolk sac volumes as predictors of pregnancy outcome in the first trimester. Am J Perinatology 2001;18:203-211.
6. Figueras F, Torrents M, Munoz A, et al: Three-dimensional yolk and gestational sac volume. J Reprod Medicine 2003;48:252-256.

7. Cepni I, Bese T, Ocal P, et al: Significance of yolk sac measurements with vaginal sonography in first trimester in the prediction of pregnancy outcome. Acta Obstet Gyn Scand 1997:76:969-972.

8. Crooij MJ, Westhuis J, Schoemaker J, et al: Ultrasonographic measurement of the yolk sac. Br J Obstet Gynaecol 1982;89:931.

9. Kucuk T, Duru NK, Yenen MC: Yolk sac size and shape as predictors of poor pregnancy outcome. J Perinatal Med 1999;27:316-320.

10. Levi CS, Dashefsky SM, Lyons EA, et al: First trimester ultrasound in McGahan JP, Goldberg BB, eds. Diagnostic ultrasound – a logical approach. Lippincott-Raven Press, 1998, pp. 127-154.

11. Levi CS, Lyons EA, Lindsay DJ: Early diagnosis of nonviable pregnancy with endovaginal US. Radiology 1988;167:383.

12. Lindsay DJ, Lovett IS, Lyons EA, et al: Yolk sac diameter and shape at endovaginal US: predictors of pregnancy outcome in the first trimester. Radiology 1992;183:115-118.

13. Nyberg DA, Mack LA, Laing FC, Datter RM: Distinguishing normal from abnormal gestational sac growth in early pregnancy. J Ultrasound Med 1987;1:23-27.

14. Rempen A: The embryonal yolk sac in disordered early pregnancy. Geburt Frauen 1988;48:804.

15. Stampone C, Nicotra M, Muttinelli C, et al: Transvaginal sonography of the yolk sac in normal and abnormal pregnancy. J Clin Ultrasound 1996;24:3-9.

16. Timor-Tritsch IE, Farine D, Rosen MG: A close look at early embryonic development with high-frequency transvaginal transducer. Am J Obstet Gynecol 1988;159:676.

17. Zalel Y, Shalev E, Yanay N, et al: A large yolk sac: a possible clue to early diagnosis of partial hydatiform mole. J Clin Ultrasound 1994;22:519-521.

Second and Third Trimester Obstetrical Measurements

Amniotic Fluid Index

Introduction

Adequate amniotic fluid is important for fetal well-being. Original estimates were based on a qualitative assessment of amount of amniotic fluid, while more recent publications have used semi-quantitative measurements of amniotic fluid.

Materials/Methods

Dye-dilution techniques and the direct measurement of amniotic fluid at hysterotomy have determined amniotic fluid volume at various menstrual ages. The mean amniotic fluid volume at 30 weeks' menstrual age is 817 ml with a range of 318 to 2100 ml. Hence, an amniotic fluid volume less than 318 ml indicates oligohydramnios and includes 2.5% of pregnancies.[1]

Historically, a visual assessment of amniotic fluid was graded as decreased (Fig. 8-1), adequate (Fig. 8-2), or increased (Fig. 8-3).

Semi-quantitative criteria for the sonographic diagnosis of oligo- and polyhydramnios have been reported by a number of authors. Manning[2] popularized a maximum vertical pocket measurement of amniotic fluid volume. Oligohydramnios was defined as a single deepest pocket of amniotic fluid less than 2 × 2 cm (Fig. 8-4). A

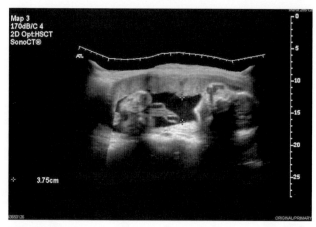

Figure 8-2
A panoramic view of normal amount of amniotic fluid.

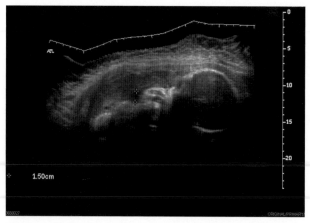

Figure 8-1
A panoramic view of oligohydramnios.

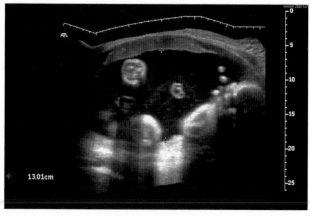

Figure 8-3
A panoramic view of polyhydramnios.

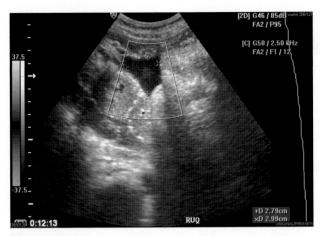

Figure 8-4
A 2.79 × 2.99 cm pocket of amniotic fluid that would be sufficient for the biophysical profile score.

Table 8-1	Definitions of polyhydramnios	
Definition		**Author**
AFI		
>20 cm		Phelan[19]
>24 cm		Jeng[13]
>25 cm		Phelan[7]
>95th percentile		
(21.4–24.9 cm)		Moore[11]
Single Deepest Pocket		
>8 cm (mild)		
>12 cm (moderate)		Hill[18]
>16 cm (severe)		

maximum vertical pocket greater than 8 cm was considered polyhydramnios.[3]

Phelan et al[4] described a method of assessing amniotic fluid in the four quadrants of the uterus using the linea nigra and umbilicus as landmarks. The deepest pocket of amniotic fluid in each quadrant is measured. The original method described the transducer as parallel to the maternal sagittal plane. However, holding the transducer perpendicular to the sagittal plane in each quadrant can also be employed. Only pockets of amniotic fluid free of umbilical cord and extremities should be measured.[5] The sum of the four measurements is the amniotic fluid index (AFI). With this method, an AFI of less than 5 cm is considered oligohydramnios.[6] Some commonly accepted definitions of polyhydramnios are in Table 8-1. Since an AFI of more than 25 cm is associated with a higher incidence of macrosomia, prematurity, and congenital anomalies,[7] it would seem to be the preferable AFI definition of polyhydramnios. The intraobserver and interobserver variation in the measurement of the AFI is between 0.5 and 1 cm and 1 and 2 cm, respectively.[8]

DISCUSSION

The single deepest pocket assessment of amniotic fluid volume and the AFI are both sensitive to abdominal pressure. There is a 21% decrease in the AFI with high pressure (p < 0.001). Measurement of amniotic fluid with either technique should therefore be made with the lowest possible abdominal pressure that prevents image fallout. This technique will result in the highest possible values and lowest intra- and interobserver variation.[9]

The single deepest pocket method of amniotic fluid volume assessment has been compared with the AFI in 1400 normal pregnancies.[6] In this study oligohydramnios was defined as a single deepest pocket of less than 2 cm × 2 cm or an AFI of more than 5 cm. The prevalence of oligohydramnios utilizing these definitions was 1% and 8% (p < 0.0001), respectively. Polyhydramnios was defined as a single deepest pocket greater than 8 cm or an AFI greater than 24 cm.

Hydramnios occurred in 0.7% of patients utilizing a single deepest pocket definition; none of the patients had an AFI of more than 24 cm (p < 0.0001). It is not surprising that the prevalence of oligo- and polyhydramnios will be different with the two techniques. Sonographic estimates of amniotic fluid volume performed best at identifying normal amniotic fluid (accuracy 83% to 94%).[10]

Table 8-2 provides the percentile values for the single deepest pocket of amniotic fluid throughout normal pregnancy.

Tables 8-3 and 8-4 are the percentile values for AFI throughout pregnancy from two different institutions. Gestational age-specific percentiles do not predict oligo- and polyhydramnios any better than the fixed cut-off values mentioned earlier.[10] The percentile values for the two studies are significantly different. At less than 37 weeks' menstrual age, the fifth percentile for

| Table 8-2 | Single deepest pocket values of amniotic fluid during normal pregnancy, from the 5th through to the 95th percentile | | | | | | |

Menstrual age (wks)	No.	Single deepest pocket (cm)					
		5th Percentile	10th Percentile	50th Percentile	Mean	90th Percentile	95th Percentile
14	50	1.7	1.9	2.9	3.1	4.7	5.0
15	50	2.0	2.2	3.4	3.5	5.1	5.5
16	50	2.3	2.5	3.6	3.8	5.4	5.9
17	50	2.5	2.7	3.9	4.0	5.7	6.2
18	50	2.7	2.9	4.1	4.2	5.9	6.4
19	50	2.8	3.1	4.3	4.4	6.1	6.6
20	50	2.9	3.2	4.4	4.5	6.2	6.7
21	50	2.9	3.3	4.5	4.6	6.3	6.8
22	50	3.0	3.3	4.6	4.7	6.3	6.8
23	50	3.0	3.4	4.6	4.7	6.3	6.8
24	50	3.1	3.4	4.7	4.8	6.3	6.8
25	50	3.0	3.3	4.7	4.8	6.3	6.8
26	50	3.0	3.3	4.8	4.8	6.4	6.8
27	50	3.0	3.3	4.8	4.8	6.4	6.9
28	50	3.0	3.3	4.8	4.8	6.4	6.9
29	50	2.9	3.3	4.8	4.8	6.4	6.9
30	50	2.9	3.3	4.8	4.8	6.4	6.9
31	50	2.9	3.2	4.8	4.9	6.5	7.0
32	50	2.9	3.2	4.8	4.9	6.6	7.1
33	50	2.9	3.2	4.82	4.9	6.6	7.2
34	50	2.8	3.2	4.8	4.8	6.6	7.2
35	50	2.8	3.1	4.7	4.8	6.6	7.2
36	50	2.7	3.1	4.7	4.7	6.6	7.1
37	50	2.6	2.9	4.5	4.6	6.5	7.0
38	50	2.4	2.8	4.4	4.5	6.3	6.8
39	50	2.3	2.7	4.2	4.3	6.1	6.6
40	50	2.1	2.5	3.9	4.0	5.8	6.2
41	50	1.9	2.2	3.7	3.7	5.4	5.7

From Magann EF, Sanderson M, Martin JN Jr, et al: The amniotic fluid index, single deepest pocket and two diameter pocket in normal pregnancy. Am J Obstet Gynecol 2000;182:1581-1588.

AFI varies between 8.8[11] and 6.9 cm,[6] and the 95th percentile between 14.2[11] and 10.6 cm.[6] If the data of Moore and Cayle[11] are used to evaluate the data of Magann et al,[6] 36% of patients beyond 16 weeks' menstrual age would be categorized as abnormal. The study group of Moore and Cayle[11] was not evenly distributed; there were between 11 and 162 patients at each menstrual age week. Although a regression curve can be fitted to the data, the derived relationship is not as accurate as when the data are evenly distributed by menstrual age. In the study by Magann et al,[6] there were 50 patients for each menstrual week. Unlike Magann et al,[6] Moore and Cayle[11] did not superimpose the percentiles on a scatter diagram of the observations as a check of their fit.[12] These methodologic differences may explain some of the variation in the data reported between the two facilities. Most institutions define oligohydramnios as an AFI of less than 5 cm[6] and polyhydramnios as an AFI of more than 24[13] or 25 cm.[7] As long as these fixed definitions of an abnormal amniotic fluid volume are used, the difference in the

Table 8-3	Amniotic fluid index values in normal pregnancy, from the 2.5th through to the 97.5th percentile					
	Amniotic fluid index (mm) percentile values					
Week	**2.5th**	**5th**	**50th**	**95th**	**97.5th**	**n**
16	73	79	121	185	201	32
17	77	83	127	194	211	26
18	80	87	133	202	220	17
19	83	90	137	207	225	14
20	86	93	141	212	230	25
21	88	95	143	214	233	14
22	89	97	145	216	235	14
23	90	98	146	218	237	14
24	90	98	147	219	238	23
25	89	97	147	221	240	12
26	89	97	147	223	242	11
27	85	95	146	226	245	17
28	86	94	146	228	249	25
29	84	92	145	231	254	12
30	82	90	145	234	258	17
31	79	88	144	238	263	26
32	77	86	144	242	269	25
33	74	83	143	245	274	30
34	72	81	142	248	278	31
35	70	79	140	249	279	27
36	68	77	138	249	279	39
37	66	75	135	244	275	36
38	65	73	132	239	269	27
39	64	72	127	226	255	12
40	63	71	123	214	240	64
41	63	70	116	194	216	162
42	63	69	110	175	192	30

From Moore TR, Cayle JE: The amniotic fluid index in normal human pregnancy. Am J Obstet Gynecol 1990;162:1168-1173.

centile values between these reports is not clinically relevant.

Three-dimensional determinations of amniotic fluid volume have shown that the four-quadrant technique accounts for approximately 50% of the total amniotic fluid volume.[14] The fact that the ultrasonic assessment of amniotic fluid volume is a poor reflection of actual volume may explain the differences in the values obtained between institutions.

Several groups have measured amniotic fluid in twins. A single vertical pocket[15] or a two-diameter pocket[15] in each gestational sac, as well as a four-quadrant AFI[16] of the entire uterus, have been reported. Individual AFI indices for each gestational sac are reported in Table 8-5.[17] The AFI for individual twins are similar. The intra- and interobserver variations in the ascertainment of twin AFI values is 7.4% and 12.2%, respectively. The confidence intervals for singleton AFIs[11] and twin AFIs overlap; there is no statistical evidence that the median values are different.[17]

Table 8-4 Amniotic fluid index values during normal pregnancy, from the 5th through to the 95th percentile

| Menstrual age (wks) | No. | Amniotic fluid index (cm) | | | | | |
		5th Percentile	10th Percentile	50th Percentile	Mean	90th Percentile	95th Percentile
14	50	2.8	3.1	5.0	5.4	8.0	8.6
15	50	3.2	3.6	5.4	5.7	8.2	9.1
16	50	3.6	4.1	5.8	6.1	8.5	9.6
17	50	4.1	4.0	6.3	6.6	9.0	10.3
18	50	4.6	5.1	6.8	7.1	9.7	11.1
19	50	5.1	5.6	7.4	7.7	10.4	12.0
20	50	5.5	6.1	8.0	8.3	11.3	12.9
21	50	5.9	6.6	8.7	8.9	12.2	13.9
22	50	6.3	7.1	9.3	9.6	13.2	14.9
23	50	6.7	7.5	10.0	10.3	14.2	15.9
24	50	7.0	7.9	10.7	11.0	15.2	16.9
25	50	7.3	8.2	11.4	11.7	16.1	17.8
26	50	7.5	8.4	12.0	12.3	17.0	18.7
27	50	7.6	8.6	12.6	12.8	17.8	19.4
28	50	7.6	8.6	13.0	13.3	18.4	19.9
29	50	7.6	8.6	13.4	13.6	18.8	20.4
30	50	7.5	8.5	13.6	13.8	18.9	20.6
31	50	7.3	8.4	13.6	13.8	18.9	20.6
32	50	7.1	8.1	13.6	13.7	18.7	20.4
33	50	6.8	7.8	13.3	13.4	18.2	20.0
34	50	6.4	7.4	12.9	13.0	17.7	19.4
35	50	6.0	7.0	12.4	12.5	16.9	18.7
36	50	5.6	6.5	11.8	11.8	16.2	17.9
37	50	5.1	6.0	11.1	11.1	15.3	16.9
38	50	4.7	5.5	10.3	10.3	14.4	15.9
39	50	4.2	5.0	9.4	9.4	13.7	14.9
40	50	3.7	4.5	8.6	8.6	12.9	13.9
41	50	3.3	4.0	7.8	7.7	12.3	12.9

From Magann EF, Sanderson M, Martin JN Jr, et al: The amniotic fluid index, single deepest pocket and two diameter pocket in normal pregnancy. Am J Obstet Gynecol 2000;182:1581-1588.

Table 8-5 Amniotic fluid index percentile values for normal twin pregnancies

| Gestation (wks) | Percentile | | | | | | | No. |
	2.5th	5th	10th	50th	90th	95th	97.5th	
14-16	83.2	85.2	87.5	103.0	128.1	148.5	153.8	42
17-19	85.1	92.4	94.7	14.0	158.6	170.7	176.0	106
20-22	81.9	89.9	99.8	134.0	183.9	198.6	215.7	46
23-25	89.7	95.5	110.5	150.0	182.6	191.3	211.0	46
26-28	91.3	104.4	110.0	149.0	205.0	229.3	236.4	57
29-31	85.1	91.5	101.0	139.0	189.0	194.5	202.1	54
32-34	70.5	97.0	106.0	140.0	190.0	200.0	216.0	59
35-37	71.5	85.0	92.0	132.0	185.0	219.0	265.0	59
38-40	92.0	92.0	96.0	131.0	190.0	191.0	191.0	19
Total	85.2	92.0	97.0	131.0	180.0	193.0	205.0	488

All measurements are in millimeters.
From Hill LM, Krohn M, Lazechnik N, et al: The Amniotic Fluid Index in normal twin pregnancies. Am J Obstet Gynecol 2000;182:950-954.

References

1. Brace RA, Wolff EF: Normal amniotic fluid volume changes throughout pregnancy. Am J Obstet Gynecol 1989;161:382-388.
2. Manning FA: Dynamic ultrasound based fetal assessment: the fetal biophysical score. Clin Obstet Gynecol 1995;38:26-44.
3. Chamberlain PF, Manning FA, Morrison I, et al: Ultrasound evaluation of amniotic fluid volume II. The relationship of increased amniotic fluid volume to perinatal outcome. Am J Obstet Gynecol 1984;150:250-254.
4. Phelan JP, Ahn MO, Smith CV, et al: Amniotic fluid index measurement during pregnancy. J Reprod Med 1987;32:601-604.
5. Moore TR: Superiority of the four-quadrant sum over the single-deepest pocket technique in ultrasonographic identification of abnormal amniotic fluid volumes. Am J Obstet Gynecol 1990;163:762-767.
6. Magann EF, Sanderson M, Martin JN Jr, et al: The amniotic fluid index, single deepest pocket and two diameter pocket in normal pregnancy. Am J Obstet Gynecol 2000;182:1581-1588.
7. Phelan JP, Park YW, Ahn MO, et al: Polyhydramnios and perinatal outcomes. J Perinatol 1990;12:347-350.
8. Rutherford SE, Smith CV, Phelan JP, et al: Four-quadrant assessment of amniotic fluid volume. Interobserver and intraobserver variation. J Reprod Med 1987;32:587-589.
9. Flack NJ, Doré C, Southwell D, et al: The influence of operator transducer pressure on ultrasonographic measurements of amniotic fluid volume. Am J Obstet Gynecol 1994;171:218-222.
10. Magann EF, Doherty DA, Chauhan SP, et al: How well do the amniotic fluid index and single deepest pocket indices (below the 3rd and 5th and above the 95th and 97th percentiles) predict oligohydramnios and hydramnnios? Am J Obstet Gynecol 2004;190:164-169.
11. Moore TR, Cayle J: The amniotic fluid index in normal human pregnancy. Am J Obstet Gynecol 1990;162:1168-1173.
12. Altman DG, Chitty LS: Charts of fetal size: 1. methodology. Br J Obstet Gynaecol 1994;101:29-34.
13. Jeng CJ, Jou TJ, Wang Y-C, et al: Amnniotic fluid index measurement with the four-quadrant technique during pregnancy. J Reprod Med 1990;35:674-677.
14. Grover J, Mentakis A, Ross MG: Three-dimensional method for determination of amniotic fluid volume in intrauterine pockets. Obstet Gynecol 1997;90:1009-1010.
15. Chau AC, Kjos S, Kovacs BW: Ultrasonic measurement of amniotic fluid in normal diamniotic twin pregnancies. Am J Obstet Gynecol 1990;174:1003-1007.
16. Porter TF, Dildy GA, Blanchard JR, et al: Normal values for amniotic fluid index during uncomplicated twin pregnancy. Obstet Gynecol 1995;87:699-702.
17. Hill LM, Krohn M, Lazechnik N, et al: The Amniotic Fluid Index in normal twin pregnancies. Am J Obstet Gynecol 2000;182:950-954.
18. Hill LM, Breckle R, Thomas ML, et al: Polyhydramnios: ultrasonically detected prevalence and neonatal outcome. Obstet Gynecol 1987;69:21-25.
19. Phelan JP, Smith CV, Small M: Amniotic fluid volume assessment with the four-quadrant technique at 36-42 weeks' gestation. J Reprod Med 1987;32:540-542.

Lyndon Hill

CHAPTER 9

Biophysical Profile Score

Introduction

Although most fetal measurements are used to evaluate fetal growth, the biophysical profile is used to assess fetal well-being.

Materials/Methods

Since its original description, there has been some variation in the scores given for each parameter of the biophysical profile. Current components of the biophysical profile score, their definition, and the score for the presence or absence of each variable are outlined in Table 9-1. The description, distribution, and perinatal mortality of each biophysical profile score is outlined in Table 9-2. During a 30 minute testing interval, 97.5% of biophysical profiles will receive a normal score.

DISCUSSION

The presence of a normal biophysical activity suggests that the segment of the central nervous system that controls that activity is not suppressed. Although there are potentially multiple causes of central nervous system suppression, the obstetrician is primarily concerned with discriminating the final common pathway of hypoxia/asphyxia from the normal variation of the sleep-wake cycle. Different anatomic sites within the brain control the biologic variables evaluated with the biophysical profile score. The biophysical activities that develop first are the last to disappear with the onset of asphyxia. This graded response to asphyxia permits an estimation of the severity of fetal compromise. Fetal heart rate reactivity and breathing movements are compromised when the pH is below 7.2. At a pH less than 7.1, movement and fetal tone are abolished.[1] When the umbilical vein pH is used as the "gold standard," the biophysical profile score has been shown to accurately predict the presence or absence of acidosis as early as 17.5 weeks' gestation.[2]

Table 9-1	30 Minute biophysical profile score	
Activity	**Definition**	**Score**
Body movements	≥3 body/limb movements	2
	<3 body/limb movements	0
Tone	One episode extension/flexion	2
	No episodes extension/flexion	0
Breathing movements	Any breathing movements or hiccups	2
	Absent	0
Amniotic fluid volume	One pocket ≥ 2 cm in 2 perpendicular planes	2
	<2 × 2 cm pocket	0
Nonstress test	≥2 accelerations > 15 bpm lasting ≥ 15 sec	2
	<2 accelerations	0

Table 9-2	Description, distribution, and perinatal mortality of the biophysical profile score		
Score	Description	Percent	Perinatal Mortality/ 1000
8-10	Normal	97.52	1.86[+]
6	Equivocal	1.72	9.76
4	Abnormal	0.52	26.3
2	Abnormal	0.18	94.0
0	Abnormal	0.06	285.7

[+]*0.6/1000 within 1 week.*
From:
Manning FA, Morrison I, Lange IR, et al: Fetal assessment based on fetal biophysical profile scoring: experience in 12,620 referred high-risk pregnancies. I. Perinatal mortality by frequency and etiology. Am J Obstet Gynecol 1985;151: 343-350.
Manning FA, Harman CR, Morrison I, et al: Fetal assessment based on fetal biophysical profile scoring. IV. An analysis of perinatal morbidity and mortality. Am J Obstet Gynecol 1990;162:703-709.
Manning FA: Fetal biophysical profile scoring: theoretical considerations and clinical applications, chapter 6. In Manning FA (ed): Fetal Medicine: Principles and Practice. Norwalk, CT, Appleton and Lange, 1995.

There have not been any randomized controlled trials comparing patients managed with biophysical profile scores versus controls that do not have any antepartum surveillance. However, when compared with an untested population, composed of primarily lower-risk patients with a perinatal mortality of 7.69 per 1000, high-risk patients managed with the biophysical profile score had a perinatal mortality of 1.86 per 1000.[3]

The false-negative rate within 1 week of the biophysical profile score of 0.6 per 1000 has remained stable in Manitoba, Canada, for more than 15 years.[3] The false-negative rate reflects the underlying perinatal mortality at a given institution—as the perinatal mortality increases, so does the false-negative rate. The false-negative rate is approximately 10% of the perinatal mortality. At Columbia-Presbyterian, the gross perinatal mortality is 22.1/1000 live births.

The false-negative rate of the biophysical profile score at this institution is 2.3/1000.[4]

Nearly all false-negative biophysical profile scores (i.e., fetal death within 1 week of testing) are because of an acute lethal insult after the test. Because these events (e.g., placental abruption, fetomaternal hemorrhage) cannot be predicted, increasing the testing interval would not have a significant impact on the false-negative rate. Manning et al[5] have reported that timely intervention for an abnormal biophysical score may reduce the presence of asphyxia-related diseases (i.e., cerebral palsy).

The negative predictive value of a normal biophysical profile score is not as high when a congenital anomaly is present. Sudden fetal death has been reported with a normal biophysical profile score in fetuses with gastroschisis, omphalocele, and diaphragmatic hernia.[3]

References

1. Vintzileos AM, Gaffney SE, Salinger LM, et al: The relationship between fetal biophysical profile and cord pH in patients undergoing caesarean section before the onset of labor. Obstet Gynecol 1987;70:196-201.
2. Manning FA, Snijders R, Harman CR, et al: Fetal biophysical profile score. VI. Correlation with antepartum umbilical venous fetal pH. Am J Obstet Cynecol 1993;169:755-763.
3. Manning FA: Fetal biophysical profile scoring: theoretical considerations and clinical applications, Chapter 6. In Fetal Medicine: Principles and Practice. Norwalk, CT, Appleton and Lange, 1995.
4. Dayal AK, Manning FA, Berck DJ, et al: Fetal death after normal biophysical profile score: An eighteen-year experience. Am J Obstet Gynecol 1999;181:1231-1236.
5. Manning FA, Bondaji N, Harman CR, et al: Fetal assessment based on fetal biophysical profile scoring. VIII. The incidence of cerebral palsy in tested and untested perinates. Am J Obstet Gynecol 1998;178:696-706.

CHAPTER 10

Cervical Length

Introduction

Cervical length is a continuous variable relative to preterm delivery. Because it is not a categorical variable (all-or-none), there is no single value that can distinguish between preterm and term delivery.[1]

Materials/Methods

Although the cervical length has been measured both transabdominally and trans labially, the endovaginal technique is preferred. Some of the cervical measurements (Figs. 10-1 and 10-2) that are used include the following[2]:

1. Remaining cervical length
2. Cervical funnel (length and width)
3. Percent funnel (funnel ÷ funnel + cervical length)
4. Rate of change in cervical length over time

DISCUSSION

Observational studies suggest that the transvaginal evaluation of cervical length between 18 and 22 weeks' menstrual age can identify patients at increased risk for preterm delivery. However, the low prevalence of preterm delivery in a low-risk population prohibits utilizing cervical length as a screening tool (sensitivity 14.7% to 37.3%; positive predictive value 6% to 31.6%).[3-5] The sensitivities and positive predictive values of cervical length are much higher in high-risk patients (sensitivity 74%; positive predictive value 37%).[6] Some reasons for preterm labor are not associated with a shortened cervical length.

The percentiles for cervical length in singleton and multiple gestations are outlined in Table 10-1. The cervical length percentiles for the general population of women with singleton pregnancies are remarkably consistent among studies. The relative risk of delivery at less than

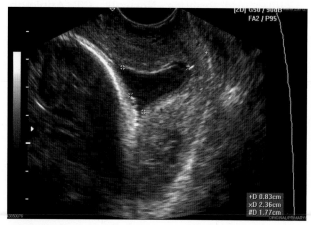

Figure 10-1
There is a cervical funnel with a length of 2.36 cm and a width of 1.77 cm; the remaining cervix measures 0.83 cm. Funneling % = B/A + B, where B = funnel and A = cervical length (2.36/3.19 = 74%)

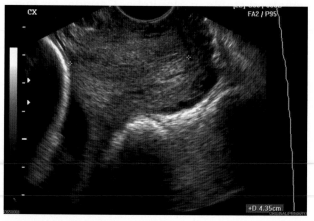

Figure 10-2
A normal cervical length of 4.35 cm.

Table 10-1 Percentiles of cervical length (mm) from 1% through 75%, expressed for single, twin, and triplet pregnancies

Percentile	N	1	5	10	25	50	75
Singletons—General Population							
Iams[3]	2915	13	22	26	30	35	40
To[12]	6819	11	22	—	—	36	—
Heath [13]	2567	11	23	—	—	38	—
Twins							
Souka[11]	215	7	19	—	—	38	—
Vayassiere[14]	251		22	27	—	40.6	—
Skentou[10]	464	7	16	—	—	36	—
Triplets							
To[15]	43	—	15	—	—	34	—

Table 10-2 Relative risk in the general population of delivering at less than 35 weeks' menstrual age with a specific cervical length

Cervical Length at 24 Weeks (cm)	Relative Risk of Delivery < 35 Weeks
≤4.0	1.98
≤3.5	2.35
≤3.0	3.79
≤2.6	6.19
≤2.2	9.49
≤1.3	13.99

From Iams JD, Goldenberg RL, Meis PJ, et al: The length of the cervix and the risk of spontaneous premature delivery. National Institute of Child Health and Human Development Maternal Fetal Medicine Unit Network. N Engl J Med 1996;334:567-572.

35 weeks' menstrual age based on cervical length is provided in Table 10-2. In the general population the sensitivity and specificity of a cervical length equalling or less than 1.5 cm for predicting preterm delivery is 8.2% and 99.7%, respectively.[7] In a high-risk population, receiver operating characteristic curves indicate that a cervical length equal to or less than 2.5 cm is the best "cut-off" between 15 and 24 weeks' gestation to predict preterm birth.[8]

The recurrence risk of spontaneous preterm birth varies widely according to cervical length and fetal fibronectin. The probability of delivering at less than 35 weeks' gestation with a cervical length equalling or less than 2.5 cm varies from 25% with a negative fibronectin to 64% when the fibronectin is positive.[9]

A cervical length equal to or less than 2 cm occurs in 8% of twins; this subgroup contains 40% of women delivering prior to 33 weeks.[10]

The optimal cut-off cervical length predicting preterm labor may vary with the obstetric risk factor. The positive predictive value of a cervical length measurement increases with high-risk status and decreasing cervical length. Funneling does not improve the prediction of preterm labor over a cervical length equal to or less than 1.5 cm.[11]

References

1. Iams JD, Johnson F, Sonek J, et al: Cervical competence as a continuum: a study of sonographic cervical length and obstetrical performance. Am J Obstet Gynecol 1995; 172:1097-1103.

2. Guzman ER, Ananth CV: Cervical length and spontaneous prematurity: laying the foundation for future interventional randomized trials for the short cervix (opinion). Ultrasound Obstet Gynecol 2001;18:195-199.

3. Iams JD, Goldenberg RL, Meis PJ, et al: The length of the cervix and the risk of spontaneous delivery. N Engl J Med 1996;334:567-572.

4. Taipale P, Hiilesmea V: Sonographic measurement of uterine cervix at 18-22 weeks' gestation and the risk of preterm delivery. Obstet Gynecol 1998;92:902-907.

5. Hassan SS, Romero R, Barry SM, et al: Patients with an ultrasonographic cervical length ≤ 15mm have nearly a 50% risk of early spontaneous preterm delivery. Am J Obstet Gynecol 2000;182:1458-1467.

6. Berghella V, Tolosa JE, Kuhlman K, et al: Cervical ultrasonography compared with manual examination as a predictor of preterm delivery. Am J Obstet Gynecol 1997; 177:723-730.

7. Hassan SS, Romero R, Berry SM, et al: Patients with an ultrasonographic cervical length = 15 mm having nearly a 50% risk of early spontaneous preterm delivery. Am J Obstet Gynecol 2000;182:1458-1467.

8. Guzman ER, Walters C, Ananth CV, et al: A comparison of sonographic cervical parameters in predicting spontaneous preterm birth in high-risk singleton gestations. Ultrasound Obstet Gynecol 2001;18:204-210.

9. Iams JD, Goldenberg RL, Mercer BM, et al: The Preterm Prediction Study: recurrence risk of spontaneous preterm birth. Am J Obstet Gynecol 1998;178:1035-1040.

10. Skentou C, Souka AP, To MS, et al: Prediction of preterm delivery in twins by cervical assessment at 23 weeks. Ultrasound Obstet Gynecol 2001;17:7-10.

11. Souka AP, Heath V, Flint S, et al: Cervical length at 23 weeks in twins in predicting spontaneous preterm delivery. Obstet Gynecol 1999;94:450-454.

12. To MS, Skentou C, Liao AW, et al: Cervical length and funneling at 23 weeks of gestation in the prediction of spontaneous early preterm delivery. Ultrasound Obstet Gynecol 2001;18:200-203.

13. Heath VCF, Southall TR, Souka AP, et al: Cervical length at 23 weeks of gestation: prediction of spontaneous preterm delivery. Ultrasound Obstet Gynecol 1998;12:312-317.

14. Vayssière C, Favre R, Audibert F, et al: Cervical length and funneling at 22 and 27 weeks to predict spontaneous birth before 32 weeks in twin pregnancies: a French prospective multicenter study. Am J Obstet Gynecol 2002;187:1596-1604.

15. To MS, Skentou C, Cicero S, et al: Cervical length at 23 weeks in triplets: prediction of spontaneous preterm delivery. Ultrasound Obstet Gynecol 2000;16:515-518.

C H A P T E R 11

Lyndon Hill

Fetal Abdominal Circumference

Introduction

The abdominal circumference can be used to determine menstrual age. It is also the essential measurement in assessing abnormalities of fetal growth.

Materials/Methods

Careful scanning technique is required to properly measure the abdominal circumference.

The following landmarks define an accurate abdominal circumference (Fig. 11-1):

1. A 90-degree transverse view of the spine at 3 or 9 o'clock.
2. The stomach is appropriately positioned in the left fetal abdomen.
3. The ribs are symmetric on either side of the abdomen.
4. The junction of the left and right portal vein is present on the image.

If a long segment of the left portal vein is visualized, rather than the junction of the left and right portal veins, the plane of section is too tangential and the abdomen will have an ellipti-

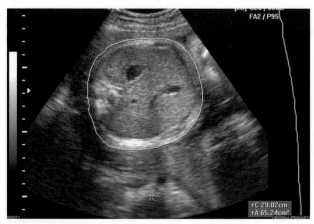

Figure 11-1
An abdominal circumference at 32 weeks' menstrual age. The circumference around the fetal abdomen has been traced.

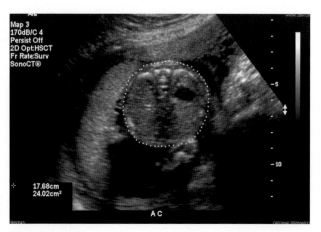

Figure 11-3
Incorrect orientation of the abdominal circumference at 21 weeks' menstrual age with the spine up positioned.

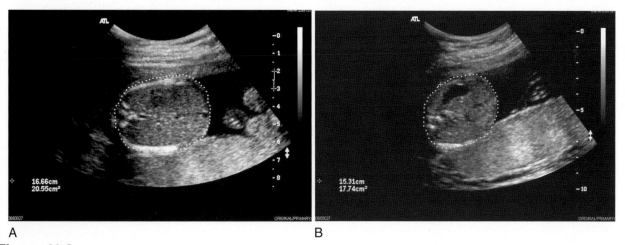

A   B

Figure 11-2
20 weeks' menstrual age. **A,** The incorrect abdomen circumference has an elliptical shape. **B,** Normal abdominal circumference taken 2 minutes later.

cal rather than a spherical shape (Fig. 11-2). An elliptical shape will erroneously increase the size of the abdominal circumference. When the spine is at 12 o'clock, the junction of the right and left portal vein cannot be visualized (Fig. 11-3). An abdominal circumference measure-ment should therefore not be taken when the fetus is in this position. Because of the multiple landmarks required, the abdominal circumfer-ence is generally the most difficult measure-ment to obtain in the assessment of gestational age.

DISCUSSION

Campbell and Wilkin[1] originally described the abdominal circumference measurement to esti-mate fetal weight. In the 1980s, several authors[2-4] used the abdominal circumference to estimate gestational age (Table 11-1). Table 11-2 com-pares the fitted 50th percentile of abdominal circumference from four studies. The derived technique uses the two axes of the abdominal circumference to calculate the circumference. The ellipse function in current ultrasound units uses this technique (Fig. 11-4). When the cir-cumference is traced (see Fig. 11-1), the values

Table 11-1   Predicted menstrual age for abdominal circumference measurements (10 to 36 cm)

Abdominal Circumference (cm)	Menstrual Age (wks)	Abdominal Circumference (cm)	Menstrual Age (wks)
10.0	15.6	23.5	27.7
10.5	16.1	24.0	28.2
11.0	16.5	24.5	28.7
11.5	16.9	25.0	29.2
12.0	17.3	25.5	29.7
12.5	17.8	26.0	30.1
13.0	18.2	26.5	30.6
13.5	18.6	27.0	31.1
14.0	19.1	27.5	31.6
14.5	19.5	28.0	32.1
15.0	20.0	28.5	32.6
15.5	20.4	29.0	33.1
16.0	20.8	29.5	33.6
16.5	21.3	30.0	34.1
17.0	21.7	30.5	34.6
17.5	22.2	31.0	35.1
18.0	22.6	31.5	35.6
18.5	23.1	32.0	36.1
19.0	23.6	32.5	36.6
19.5	24.0	33.0	37.1
20.0	24.5	33.5	37.6
20.5	24.9	34.0	38.1
21.0	25.4	34.5	38.7
21.5	25.9	35.0	39.2
22.0	26.3	35.5	39.7
22.5	26.8	36.0	40.2
23.0	27.3		

From Callen PW (ed): Ultrasonography in Obstetrics and Gynecology, 3rd ed. Philadelphia, WB Saunders, 1994. Modified from Hadlock FP, Deter RL, Harrist RB, Park SK: Fetal abdominal circumference as a predictor of menstrual age. AJR Am J Roentgenol 1982;139: 367-370.

Table 11-2   Fitted 50th centile (cm) of abdominal circumference

Gestational Age (weeks)	Hadlock[7]	Smulian[8]	Kumanavicius[9]	Chitty[5]	Chitty[5]
14		8.3	8.0	8.3	7.9
16	9.9	10.5	10.3	10.6	10.2
18	12.5	12.8	12.5	12.9	12.4
20	15.0	15.0	14.8	15.2	14.6
22	17.4	17.2	16.9	17.5	16.8
24	19.7	19.3	19.1	19.7	18.9
26	21.9	21.5	21.2	21.8	21.0
28	24.0	23.6	23.2	23.9	23.1
30	26.1	25.7	25.2	26.0	25.0
32	28.1	27.8	27.1	28.0	27.0
34	30.0	29.9	28.9	29.9	28.8
36	31.8	31.9	30.7	31.7	30.6
38	33.6	33.9	32.4	33.5	32.4
40	35.3	35.9	34.0	35.3	34.0
42		37.9	35.5	36.9	35.6
N	400	10,070	5807	425	425
Technique	Measured	Derived	Derived	Measured	Derived
Country	USA	USA	Switzerland	UK	UK

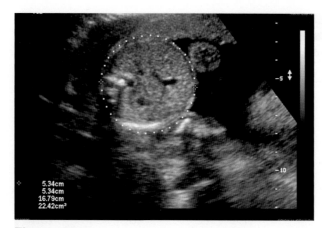

Figure 11-4
An abdominal circumference measurement at 21 weeks' menstrual age using the ellipse function.

Table 11-4	Estimation of variability in predicting menstrual age from the abdominal circumference	
Gestational age (wks)	**Variability (± 2SD) (wks)**	
	Benson[16]	**Hadlock[2]**
12-18	—	1.9
14-20	2.1	—
18-24	—	2.0
20-26	3.7	—
24-30	—	2.2
26-32	3.0	—
30-36	—	3.0
32-42	4.5	—
36-42	—	2.5

Table 11-3	Evaluation of race as a factor in abdominal circumference assessment of menstrual age				
Author	**Ref**	**N**	**Study Design**	**Race**	**Significant Difference**
Arenson	10	126	Longitudinal; comparison to published charts	Oriental	No
Jacquemyn	11	524	Cross-sectional; populations compared in study	Belgian Moroccan Turkish	Yes
Humphrey	12	192	Longitudinal; populations compared in study	Australian Aborigines; Caucasian	No
Westerway	13	300	Cross-sectional; compared with published charts	Australian, no Aborigines	Yes
Spencer	14	20	Longitudinal; compared with prior study	Bangladeshi	Yes
Meire	15	349	Longitudinal; populations compared in study	Asian, Caucasian	Yes

obtained are consistently 3.5% larger than from the derived technique.[5] One should therefore use the same technique as the authors who developed the data used to assess gestational age.

The majority of studies outlined in Table 11-3 indicate that ethnicity has a significant effect on the abdominal circumference measurement obtained at a specific gestational age. Gardosi et al[6] have shown that ethnicity has an effect on birth weight (and by implication abdominal circumference) that is independent of maternal stature.

The variability in estimating gestational age from the abdominal circumference in two different studies is outlined in Table 11-4. Both studies indicated that the accuracy of gestational age prediction worsens as gestational age advances.

The percentile values of the abdominal circumference by gestational age[7] have been derived from the original data of Hadlock et al[2] (Table 11-5).

Table 11-5 Percentile values for fetal abdominal circumference

Menstrual Week	Abdominal Circumference (cm)				
	3rd	**10th**	**50th**	**90th**	**97th**
14	6.4	6.7	7.3	7.9	8.3
15	7.5	7.9	8.6	9.3	9.7
16	8.6	9.1	9.9	10.7	11.2
17	9.7	10.3	11.2	12.1	12.7
18	10.9	11.5	12.5	13.5	14.1
19	11.9	12.6	13.7	14.8	15.5
20	13.1	13.8	15.0	16.3	17.0
21	14.1	14.9	16.2	17.6	18.3
22	15.1	16.0	17.4	18.8	19.7
23	16.1	17.0	18.5	20.0	20.9
24	17.1	18.1	19.7	21.3	22.3
25	18.1	19.1	20.8	22.5	23.5
26	19.1	20.1	21.9	23.7	24.8
27	20.0	21.1	23.0	24.9	26.0
28	20.9	22.0	24.0	26.0	27.1
29	21.8	23.0	25.1	27.2	28.4
30	22.7	23.9	26.1	28.3	29.5
31	23.6	24.9	27.1	29.4	30.6
32	24.5	25.8	28.1	30.4	31.8
33	25.3	26.7	29.1	31.5	32.9
34	26.1	27.5	30.0	32.5	33.9
35	26.9	28.3	30.9	33.5	34.9
36	27.7	29.2	31.8	34.4	35.9
37	28.5	30.0	32.7	35.4	37.0
38	29.2	30.8	33.6	36.4	38.0
39	29.9	31.6	34.4	37.3	38.9
40	30.7	32.4	35.3	38.2	39.9

From Callen PW (ed): Ultrasonography in Obstetrics and Gynecology, 3rd ed. Philadelphia, WB Saunders, 1994. Modified from Hadlock FP, Deter RL, Harrist RB, Park SK: Estimating fetal age: computer-assisted analysis of multiple fetal growth parameters. Radiology 1984;152:497-501.

References

1. Campbell S, Wilkin D: Ultrasonic measurement of fetal abdominal circumference in the estimation of fetal weight. Br J Obstet Gynaecol 1975;82:689-697.
2. Hadlock FP, Deter RL, Harrist RB, et al: Fetal abdominal circumference as a predictor of menstrual age. Am J Roentgenol 1982;139:367-370.
3. Tamura RK, Sabbagha RE: Percentile ranks of sonar fetal abdominal circumference measurement. Am J Obstet Gynecol 1980;138:475-479.
4. Hoffbauer H, Arabin PB, Baumann ML: Control of fetal development with multiple ultrasonic body measures. Contrib Gynecol Obstet 1979;6:147-156.
5. Chitty LS, Altman DG, Henderson A, et al: Charts of fetal size: 3. Abdominal measurements. Br J Obstet Gynaecol 1994;101:125-131.
6. Gardosi J, Mongelli M, Wilcox M, et al: An adjustable fetal weight standard. Ultrasound Obstet Gynecol 1995;6:168-174.
7. Callen PW (ed): Ultrasonography in Obstetrics and Gynecology, 3rd ed. Philadelphia, WB Saunders, 1994. Modified from Hadlock FP, Deter RL, Harrist RB, et al: Fetal abdominal circumference as a predictor of menstrual age. Am J Roentgenol 1982;139:367-370.

8. Smulian JC, Ananth CV, Vintzileos AM, et al: Revisiting sonographic abdominal circumference measurements: a comparison of outer centiles with established nomograms. Ultrasound Obstet Gynecol 2001; 18:237-243.
9. Kurmanavicius J, Wright EM, Royston P, et al: Fetal ultrasound biometry: 2. Abdomen and femur length reference values. Br J Obstet Gynaecol 1999;106:136-143.
10. Arenson AM, Chan P-L, Withers C, et al: Value of standardized gestational age charts for fetuses of first-generation Oriental immigrants to Canada. Can Assoc Radiol J 1995;46:111-113.
11. Jacquemyn Y, Sys SU, Verdonk P: Fetal biometry in different ethnic groups. Early Hum Devel 2000;57:1-13.
12. Humphrey M, Holzheimer D: Fetal growth charts for Aboriginal fetuses. Aust NZ J Obstet Gynaecol 2000;40:388-393.
13. Westerway SC, Davison A, Cowell S: Ultrasonic fetal measurements: new Australian standards for the new millennium. Aust NZ J Obstet Gynaecol 2000;40:297-302.
14. Spencer JAD, Chang TC, Robson SC, et al: Fetal size and growth in Bangladeshi pregnancies. Ultrasound Obstet Gynecol 1995;5:313-317.
15. Meire HB, Farrant P: Ultrasound demonstration of an unusual fetal growth pattern in Indians. Br J Obstet Gynaecol 1981;88:260-263.
16. Benson CB, Doubilet PM: Sonographic prediction of gestational age: accuracy of second and third trimester fetal measurements. Am J Roentgenol 1991;157:1275-1277.

CHAPTER 12

Fetal Adrenal Gland

Marijo A. Gillen

Introduction

The adrenal glands are paired retroperitoneal organs located superiorly, medially, and slightly anterior to the kidneys. The right adrenal is posterior to the IVC and lateral to the right crus of the diaphragm. The left adrenal gland is located lateral to the left crus of the diaphragm and the aorta. The adrenal glands are enclosed in tough connective tissue and surrounded by fat. They are confined within the perirenal fascia along with the kidneys but are affixed to the top of the perirenal fascia, unlike the kidneys.

Materials/Measurements

LINEAR DIMENSIONS

Lewis et al[1] evaluated 34 women with normal pregnancies and found the fetal adrenal lengths (maximum longitudinal length or cranial-caudal dimension) in normal pregnancies ranged from 14 to 22 mm in fetuses from 30 to 39 weeks. Ratios of the lengths of the fetal adrenal to the fetal kidney ranged from 0.48 to 0.66, similar to the ratio of adrenal length to kidney length for newborn autopsies found in the *Report of the Task Group on Reference Man*,[2] which was 0.38 to 0.7. The ratio of the maximum AP diameter of the fetal adrenal to the AP diameter of the fetal kidney was approximately 1:1 at 30 to 39 weeks.[1]

Jeanty et al[3] studied 40 consecutive normal OB patients and found the measurements shown in Table 12-1.

Table 12-1	Size of the fetal adrenal glands (mm)			
	Fetal age in weeks			
Measurement	**20-25**	**26-29**	**30-35**	**36-40**
Mean length (AP)	10	13	16	19
Range	7-12	12-17	14-18	16-24
Mean thickness	3	5	5	6
Range	2-5	2-8	3-7	4-9

Length = AP diameter; Thickness = diameter perpendicular to the length.
Modified from Jeanty P, Chervenak F, Grannum P, Hobbins JC: Normal ultrasonic size and characteristics of the fetal adrenal glands. Prenat Diagn 1984;4:21-28.

Table 12-2	Value of FAGA, FAGC, FAGL, and gestational age		
Gestational Age (weeks)	**FAGA (mm²)**	**FAGC (mm)**	**FAGL (mm)**
28 (n = 20)	168 ± 26	54 ± 10	16 ± 4
29 (n = 20)	182 ± 34	56 ± 8	17 ± 4
30 (n = 24)	202 ± 30	60 ± 8	17 ± 4
31 (n = 20)	205 ± 28	63 ± 8	17 ± 6
32 (n = 27)	225 ± 46	64 ± 10	17 ± 4
33 (n = 25)	236 ± 50	66 ± 10	19 ± 4
34 (n = 28)	255 ± 44	69 ± 10	20 ± 4
35 (n = 25)	301 ± 44	72 ± 8	21 ± 6
36 (n = 35)	318 ± 40	76 ± 12	22 ± 4
37 (n = 40)	326 ± 42	77 ± 10	23 ± 10
38 (n = 27)	355 ± 42	78 ± 12	22 ± 4
39 (n = 29)	358 ± 36	80 ± 10	22 ± 4
40 (n = 26)	377 ± 38	81 ± 10	24 ± 6

FAGA, fetal adrenal gland area; FAGC, fetal adrenal gland circumference; FAGL, fetal adrenal gland length.
From Hata K, Hata T, Kitao M: Ultrasonographic identification and measurement of the human fetal adrenal gland in utero: clinical application. Gynecol Obstet Invest 1988;25:16-22.

Hata et al[4] measured the fetal adrenal gland area (FAGA), fetal adrenal gland circumference (FAGC), and fetal adrenal gland length (FAGL) in 346 pregnant Japanese women and found the average measurements shown in Table 12-2.

VOLUME

Chang et al[5] measured fetal adrenal gland volume in 150 Taiwanese fetuses from 21 to 40 weeks using a 3-D ultrasound transducer. He calculated an equation between the fetal adrenal gland volume and the gestational age (GA):

Fetal adrenal gland volume (mL) = $-0.2683 \times$ GA $+ 0.0082 \times$ GA$^2 + 3.1927$ (r = 0.93, n = 119, $p < 0.0001$)

SD (mL) = $1.2533 \times (-019559 + 0.0198 \times$ GA)

Chang et al[5] also calculated percentiles for adrenal gland volume and gestational age as shown in Table 12-3.

WEIGHT

From the *Report of the Task Group on Reference Man*,[2] the total weight of each adrenal gland in male and female fetuses (from autopsy specimens) as a function of gestational age is given in Table 12-4.

Table 12-3	Predicted values of adrenal gland volume using gestational age (GA) as the independent variable and adrenal gland volume as the dependent variable							
	Fetal adrenal gland volume (mL)							
GA (weeks)	**5th**	**10th**	**25th**	**50th**	**75th**	**90th**	**95th**	**SD**
21	0.70	0.80	0.97	1.16	1.34	1.51	1.61	0.28
22	0.74	0.86	1.04	1.24	1.44	1.63	1.74	0.30
23	0.80	0.92	1.12	1.34	1.56	1.79	1.88	0.33
24	0.88	1.01	1.22	1.45	1.69	1.90	2.06	0.35
25	0.97	1.11	1.33	1.59	1.84	2.07	2.21	0.38
26	1.07	1.22	1.46	1.73	2.00	2.25	2.39	0.40
27	1.20	1.35	1.61	1.90	2.19	2.44	2.60	0.42
28	1.34	1.50	1.78	2.08	2.38	2.65	2.82	0.45
29	1.49	1.67	1.96	2.28	2.60	2.88	3.06	0.47
30	1.67	1.85	2.15	2.49	2.83	3.13	3.31	0.50
31	1.85	2.05	2.37	2.72	3.07	3.39	3.58	0.52
32	2.06	2.26	2.59	2.96	3.34	3.67	3.87	0.55
33	2.28	2.49	2.84	3.23	3.61	3.96	4.17	0.57
34	2.52	2.74	3.10	3.51	3.91	4.27	4.49	0.60
35	2.77	3.00	3.38	3.80	4.22	4.60	4.83	0.62
36	3.04	3.28	3.67	4.11	4.55	4.94	5.18	0.65
37	3.33	3.58	3.98	4.44	4.89	5.30	5.55	0.67
38	3.63	3.89	4.31	4.78	5.25	5.68	5.93	0.70
39	3.95	4.22	4.66	5.14	5.63	6.07	6.34	0.72
40	4.29	4.56	5.02	5.52	6.02	6.48	6.75	0.75

From Chang CH, Yu CH, Chang FM, et al: Assessment of fetal adrenal gland volume using three-dimensional ultrasound. *Ultrasound Med Biol* 2002;28:1383-1387.

Table 12-4	Total weight of both adrenal glands in males and females as a function of gestational age					
Gestational Age (days)	**N**	**Male Mean wt. (g)**	**SD**	**n**	**Female Mean wt. (g)**	**SD**
140	5	2.5		4	2.2	
168	14	3.2	2.4	17	3.8	2.3
196	47	4.1	1.7	39	3.9	2.1
224	70	4.9	2.4	45	4.8	2.2
252	62	6.2	2.8	53	6.9	3.0
280[a]	64	8.5	3.5	72	8.0	3.2
280[b]	91	7.0	2.8	55	6.9	3.1

[a] Stillborn.
[b] Liveborn to 1 week.
From International Commission on Radiological Protection. Task Group on Reference Man. Report of the Task Group on Reference Man. Prepared by the Task Group Committee. No. 2. International Commission on Radiologic Protection, New York, Pergamon Press, 1975, pp 202-206.

DISCUSSION

EMBRYOLOGY

At approximately 5 to 6 weeks of gestational age, the fetal adrenal cortex is derived from peritoneal mesothethial cells near the cranial end of the mesonephros. At approximately 7 weeks of development, chromaffin cells from primitive sympathetic ganglia migrate into the primitive adrenal cortex and invade the medial aspect to form the adrenal medulla. At approximately 8 weeks, more cells arise from the peritoneal mesothelium; these cells engulf the fetal cortex and will become the adult cortex. By about 8 weeks the cortical mass separates from the peritoneum and is enveloped in the retroperitoneum. By the 18th week the chromaffin cells of the medulla have become totally embedded in the central portion of the fetal cortex. After birth the fetal cortex involutes and disappears by 1 year. Full differentiation of the remaining cortex into the three zones of the adult cortex is not completed until age 3.[6]

SONOGRAPHY

The adrenal glands are proportionally much larger in the fetus and neonate with respect to other organs than in adults.[1] The adrenal glands are not routinely screened as a part of the normal fetal anatomic survey. However, Lewis et al[1] found that in normal pregnancies, the adrenal glands were routinely seen at 30 weeks but could be seen as early as 25 weeks. The preferred technique is to locate the fetal kidneys and scan superiorly and anteriorly. Lewis et al[1] found that the fetal adrenals were visualized in 91% of the 34 pregnant patients who were observed at 30 to 39 weeks. Both adrenals were visualized in 41% of his patients; in these the fetuses had their back to the transducer. In 50% only the more anterior of the adrenals was visualized; in these patients the fetus was on its side and the posterior adrenal was obscured by the fetal spine. Lewis found that the adrenals were isoechoic to the fetal kidney with a hypoechoic periphery, corresponding to the cortex. Sixty-two percent of the fetal adrenals had a hyperechoic central portion corresponding to the medulla. He found the adrenals to be ovoid (Fig. 12-1) or triangular (Fig. 12-2).

In 1984 Jeanty et al[3] identified three layers in the fetal adrenal gland; these were the hypoechoic anterior aspect, a hyperechoic middle aspect, and a hypoechoic posterior aspect (Fig. 12-3). Each layer was approximately one third of the thickness of the adrenal in fetuses younger than 35 weeks old, but in fetuses older than 35 weeks old the hyperechoic central area increased to one half of the thickness. Jeanty et al[3] scanned 40 consecutive normal OB patients and demonstrated the fetal adrenals in 71% to 94% of fetuses after 20 weeks. Chang et al[5] studied 150 Taiwanese fetuses from 20 to 40 weeks and successfully visualized the fetal adrenal in 79.3% of cases.

Visualization of the fetal adrenal and distinguishing its appearance from the fetal kidney

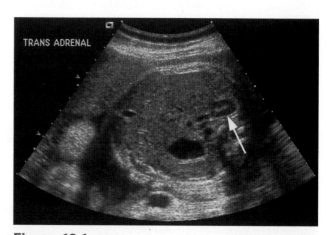

Figure 12-1
Transverse image of fetal abdomen with a tri-layered ovoid adrenal gland (*arrow*).

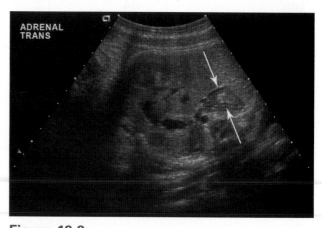

Figure 12-2
Transverse image of fetal abdomen with a tri-layered triangular adrenal gland (*arrows*).

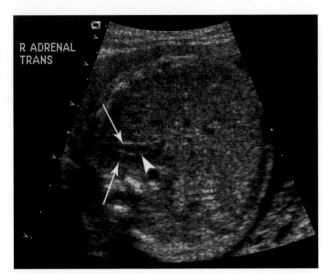

Figure 12-3
Transverse image of fetal abdomen showing three layers of right adrenal gland: the hypoechoic anterior and posterior aspects (*arrows*), corresponding to the adrenal cortex and the hyperechoic middle aspect (*arrowhead*), corresponding to the adrenal medulla.

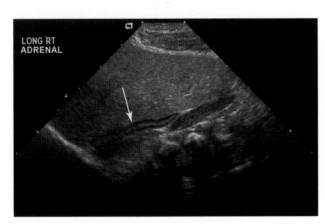

Figure 12-4
Longitudinal image of newborn with right renal agenesis showing "lying down" or flattened tri-layered right adrenal gland (*arrow*).

is important in excluding renal agenesis or ectopia. In most cases of renal agenesis or ectopia, the adrenal gland is flat rather than ovoid or triangular (Fig. 12-4); it is the so-called flattened or "lying down" adrenal[7] and is probably secondary to the lack of pressure on the fetal adrenal by the fetal kidney. This flattened adrenal can be mistaken for a fetal kidney but can be recognized by its tri-layered appearance.

References

1. Lewis E, Kurtz A, Dubbins P, et al: Real-time ultrasonogaphic evaluation of normal fetal adrenal glands. J Ultrasound Med 1982;1: 265-270.
2. International Commission on Radiological Protection. Task Group on Reference Man. Report of the Task Group on Reference Man. Prepared by the Task Group Committee. No. 2. International Commission on Radiologic Protection. New York, Pergamon Press, 1975, pp 202-206.
3. Jeanty P, Chervenak F, Grannum P, Hobbins JC: Normal ultrasonic size and characteristics of the fetal adrenal glands. Prenat Diagn 1984;4:21-28.
4. Hata K, Hata T, Kitao M: Ultrasonographic identification and measurement of the human fetal adrenal gland in utero: clinical application. Gynecol Obstet Invest 1988;25:16-22.
5. Chang CH, Yu CH, Chang FM, et al: Assessment of fetal adrenal gland volume using three-dimensional ultrasound. Ultrasound Med Biol 2002;28:1383-1387.
6. Moore KL, Persaud TVN: The Developing Human: Clincially Oriented Embryology. Philadelphia, Saunders, 1988.
7. Hoffman CK, Filly RA, Callen PW: The "lying down" adrenal sign: a sonographic indicator of renal agenesis or ectopia in fetuses and neonates. J Ultrasound Med 1992;11: 533-536.

Fetal Biparietal Diameter

Introduction

The biparietal diameter (BPD) was one of the earliest measurements used to assess menstrual age. The BPD soon became the gold standard against which other measurements were compared.

Materials/Methods

The anatomic landmarks used to obtain the biparietal diameter (BPD) include symmetrically positioned thalami and third ventricle, as well as visualization of the septum pellucidum at one third the fronto-occipital distance from the frontal bone. If these landmarks are obtained, the head circumference can also be measured with the same image. A leading edge–to–leading edge measurement (outer-to-inner) is used in the United States (Fig. 13-1); Switzerland and Germany measure from the proximal to the distal outer skull table (outer-to-outer).[1] Several groups in the United States and abroad have reported their experience with predicting menstrual age from the BPD (Tables 13-1 and 13-2).

DISCUSSION

The fetal head is quite malleable. Breech presentation, oligohydramnios, or a large leiomyoma compressing the uterus are but a few of the factors that may affect head shape and consequently the BPD.

The cephalic index (CI) should be used to evaluate the validity of the biparietal diameter. Hadlock et al[2] obtained the CI by measuring the widest transverse and longitudinal dimensions of the skull (outer-to-outer) at the level of the BPD (CI = short axis/long axis × 100). The mean CI (78.3: SD 4.4) did not change with menstrual age. A cephalic index greater than 1 SD from the mean (< 74 [dolichocephaly]; > 83 [brachicepahly]) (Fig. 13-2; Fig. 13-3) may be associated with a significant alteration of the expected BPD for a given menstrual age. Jeanty et al[3] derived the cephalic index using the BPD as the short axis (Fig. 13-4). With this formula the mean CI is 80.64 ± 4.97. Hence dolichocephaly would be defined by a CI < 75.67 and brachicephaly by a CI > 85.61.

The variability in estimating menstrual age from the biparietal diameter increases progressively throughout gestation. The ±250 interval of the biparietal diameter measurement in five menstrual age periods is outlined in Table 13-3.

Ethnicity (Table 13-4) does not appear to affect the biparietal diameter.

The biparietal diameter is highly correlated with the head circumference. In a multivariate analysis, the BPD did not add additional significant information to menstrual age assessment when the head circumference was included.[4]

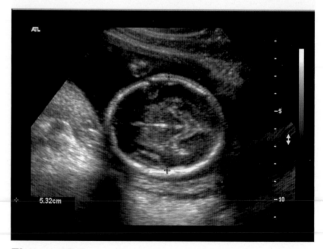

Figure 13-1
An outer-to-inner BPD consistent with a 21.5 weeks' menstrual age.

Table 13-1   Predicted menstrual age for biparietal diameter (BPD) measurements (2.6-9.7 cm)

BPD (cm)	Menstrual Age (wks)	BPD (cm)	Menstrual Age (wks)	BPD (cm)	Menstrual Age (wks)	BPD (cm)	Menstrual Age (wks)
2.6	13.9	4.5	19.5	6.4	26.1	8.3	33.8
2.7	14.2	4.6	19.9	6.5	26.4	8.4	34.2
2.8	14.5	4.7	20.2	6.6	26.8	8.5	34.7
2.9	14.7	4.8	20.5	6.7	27.2	8.6	35.1
3.0	15.0	4.9	20.8	6.8	27.6	8.7	35.6
3.1	15.3	5.0	21.2	6.9	28.0	8.8	36.1
3.2	15.6	5.1	21.5	7.0	28.3	8.9	36.5
3.3	15.9	5.2	21.8	7.1	28.7	9.0	37.0
3.4	16.2	5.3	22.2	7.2	29.1	9.1	37.5
3.5	16.5	5.4	22.5	7.3	29.5	9.2	38.0
3.6	16.8	5.5	22.8	7.4	29.9	9.3	38.5
3.7	17.1	5.6	23.2	7.5	30.4	9.4	38.9
3.8	17.4	5.7	23.5	7.6	30.8	9.5	39.4
3.9	17.7	5.8	23.9	7.7	31.2	9.6	39.9
4.0	18.0	5.9	24.2	7.8	31.6	9.7	40.5
4.1	18.3	6.0	24.6	7.9	32.0		
4.2	18.6	6.1	25.0	8.0	32.5		
4.3	18.9	6.2	25.3	8.1	32.9		
4.4	19.2	6.3	25.7	8.2	33.3		

From Callen PW (ed): Ultrasonography in Obstetrics and Gynecology, 3rd ed. Philadelphia, WB Saunders, 1994. Modified from Hadlock FP, Deter RL, Harrist RB, Park SK: Estimating fetal age: computer-assisted analysis of multiple fetal growth parameters. Radiology 1984;152:497-501.

Table 13-2   Mean biparietal diameter (mm) from 14 to 42 weeks' menstrual age

Menstrual Age (wks)	Chitty[5]	Sabbagha[6]	Hadlock[7]	Kurmanavicius[1]
14	27.3	—	27.0	28.7
16	33.6	37.0	33.0	36.2
18	40.5	43.0	40.0	43.5
20	45.2	47.0	46.0	50.4
22	52.1	53.0	53.0	57.1
24	58.4	59.0	58.0	63.4
26	63.8	66.0	64.0	69.4
28	71.8	72.0	70.0	74.9
30	77.0	78.0	75.0	80.1
32	81.3	83.0	79.0	84.7
34	84.8	87.0	84.0	88.9
36	88.5	90.0	88.0	92.6
38	91.9	93.0	91.0	95.7
40	94.9	95.0	95.0	98.2
42	96.7	—	—	100.1
N	594	198	533	6217
Technique	Outer-inner	Outer-inner	Outer-inner	Outer-outer
Study design	Cross-sectional	Longitudinal	Cross-sectional	Cross-sectional
Country	UK	USA	USA	Variable, primarily Switzerland

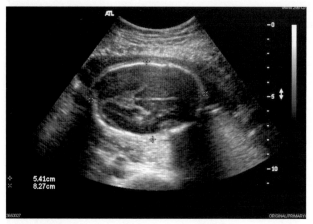

Figure 13-2

The cephalic index using an outer-to-outer BPD as the short axis is 65.1%, indicating dolichocephaly.

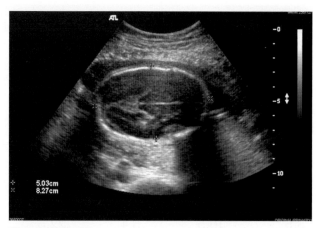

Figure 13-4

The same image as in Figure 13-2. However, the cephalic index is calculated using an outer-to-inner BPD as the short axis and is 60.5%, indicating dolichocephaly.

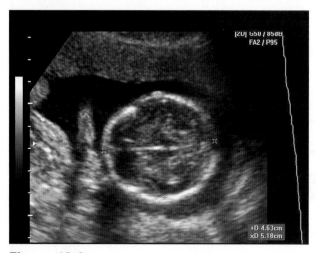

Figure 13-3

At 19.4 weeks, the cephalic index derived from the BPD as the short axis (88.5%) indicates brachycephaly.

Table 13-3	Estimated variability associated with determining menstrual age from the biparietal diameter	
Menstrual Age (wks)	**Variability (±2 SD) (wks)**	
	Hadlock[7]	**Benson[8]**
12-18	1.2	1.4
18-24	1.7	2.1
24-30	2.2	3.8
30-36	3.1	4.1
36-42	3.2	4.1

Table 13-4	Evaluation of race as a factor in the biparietal diameter assessment of menstrual age				
Author	**Ref**	**N**	**Study Design**	**Race**	**Significant Difference**
Kurmanavicius	1	6217	Cross-sectional; comparison with published charts	Switzerland; mixed	No
Jacquemyn	9	524	Cross-sectional; populations compared in study	Belgian, Moroccan, Turkish	No
Arenson	10	126	Longitudinal; comparison to published charts	Oriental	No
Westerway	11	300	Cross-sectional; compared with published charts	Australian; no Aborigines	No
Humphrey	12	192	Longitudinal; populations compared in study	Australian Aborigines, Caucasian	No

References

1. Kurmanavicius J, Wright EM, Royston P, et al: Fetal ultrasound biometry: 1. Head reference values. Br J Obstet Gynaecol 1999;106:126-135.
2. Hadlock FP, Deter RL, Carpenter RJ, et al: Estimating fetal age: effect of head shape on BPD. Am J Roentgenol 1981;137:83-85.
3. Jeanty P, Cousaert E, Hobbins JC, et al: A longitudinal study of fetal head biometry. Am J Perinatol 1984;1:118-128.
4. Chervenak FA, Skupski DW, Romero R, et al: How accurate is fetal biometry in the assessment of fetal age? Am J Obstet Gynecol 1998;178:678-687.
5. Chitty LS, Altman DG, Henderson A, et al: Charts of fetal size: 2. Head measurements. Br J Obstet Gynaecol 1994;101:35-43.
6. Sabbagha RE, Hughey M: Standardization of sonar cephalometry and gestational age. Obstet Gynecol 1978;52:402-406.
7. Hadlock FP, Deter LR, Harrist RD, et al: Fetal biparietal diameter: a critical re-evaluation of the relation to menstrual age by means of real-time ultrasound. J Ultrasound Med 1982;1:97-104.
8. Benson CB, Doubilet PM: Sonographic prediction of gestational age: accuracy of second- and third-trimester fetal measurements. Am J Roentgenol 1991;157:1275-1277.
9. Jacquemyn Y, Sys SU, Vendonk P: Fetal biometry in different ethnic groups. Early Hum Devel 2000;57:1-13.
10. Arenson AM, Chan P-L, Withers C, et al: Value of standardized gestational age charts for fetuses of first-generation Oriental immigrants to Canada. Can Assoc Radiol J 1995;46:111-113.
11. Westerway SC, Davison A, Cowell S: Ultrasonic fetal measurements: new Australian standards for the new millennium. Aust NZ J Obstet Gynaecol 2000;40:297-302.
12. Humphrey M, Holzheimer D: Fetal growth charts for Aboriginal fetuses. Aust NZ J Obstet Gynaecol 2000;40:388-393.

CHAPTER 14

Lyndon Hill

Fetal Clavicular Length

Introduction

Although fetal clavicular length correlates with gestational age,[1] its coefficient of correlation (0.81) is significantly less than that of the biparietal diameter (0.967).[2]

Materials/Methods

The upper chest is scanned transversely in order to obtain the maximal length of the clavicle (Fig. 14-1).

DISCUSSION

Yarkoni et al[1] studied 85 patients between 15 and 40 weeks' gestation. The menstrual age in weeks was approximately equal to the length of the clavicle in millimeters (Table 14-1). Congenital syndromes in which the clavicular length may be affected include cleinocranial dysplasia

Table 14-1	Menstrual age as obtained from clavicle length		
Clavicle Length (mm)	**Menstrual Age (weeks and days) Percentile**		
	5th	**50th**	**95th**
11	8 + 3	13 + 6	17 + 2
12	9 + 1	14 + 4	18 + 1
13	10 + 0	14 + 3	19 + 6
14	11 + 6	15 + 2	20 + 5
15	12 + 5	16 + 1	21 + 4
16	12 + 3	18 + 0	21 + 3
17	13 + 2	18 + 5	22 + 2
18	14 + 1	19 + 4	23 + 0
19	16 + 0	19 + 3	24 + 6
20	16 + 6	20 + 2	25 + 5
21	17 + 4	21 + 1	26 + 4
22	17 + 3	22 + 6	26 + 2
23	18 + 2	23 + 5	27 + 1
24	19 + 1	24 + 4	28 + 0
25	21 + 0	24 + 3	29 + 6
26	21 + 5	25 + 1	30 + 5
27	22 + 4	26 + 0	30 + 3
28	22 + 3	27 + 6	31 + 2
29	23 + 2	28 + 5	32 + 1
30	24 + 0	29 + 4	34 + 0
31	25 + 6	29 + 2	34 + 6
32	26 + 5	30 + 1	35 + 4
33	27 + 4	31 + 0	35 + 3
34	27 + 3	32 + 6	36 + 2
35	28 + 1	33 + 5	37 + 1
36	29 + 0	33 + 3	39 + 0
37	30 + 6	34 + 2	39 + 5
38	31 + 5	35 + 1	40 + 4
39	32 + 4	37 + 0	40 + 3
40	32 + 2	37 + 6	41 + 2
41	33 + 1	38 + 4	42 + 0
42	35 + 0	38 + 3	43 + 6
43	35 + 6	39 + 2	44 + 5
44	36 + 5	40 + 1	45 + 4
45	36 + 3	41 + 6	45 + 3

From Yarkoni S, Schmidt W, Jeanty P, et al: Clavicular measurement: a new biometric parameter for fetal evaluation. J Ultrasound Med 1985;4:467-470, Table 4, p. 469.

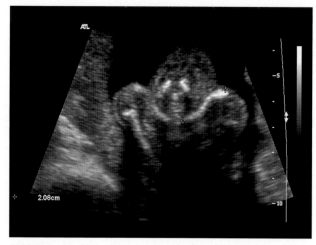

Figure 14-1
Clavicular length at 19 weeks' menstrual age.

with aplasia of the clavicle; in the Holt-Orem syndrome, the clavicle is shortened.

Although this measurement may be helpful in certain syndromes, its large confidence intervals prohibit its use as a standard measurement of menstrual age assessment.

References

1. Yarkoni S, Schmidt W, Jeanty P, et al: Clavicular measurement: a new biometric parameter for fetal evaluation. J Ultrasound Med 1985;4:467-470.
2. Hadlock FP, Deter RL, Harrist RB, et al: Computer assisted analysis of fetal age in the third trimester using multiple fetal growth parameters. J Clin Ultrasound 1983;11: 313-316.

Lyndon Hill

CHAPTER 15

Fetal Ear Length

Introduction

The mean ear length for newborns with Down's syndrome is 21% less than the mean value for controls.[1] Hence this nonspecific sign has been evaluated as a sonographic marker for Down's syndrome in the second trimester.

Materials/Methods

The ear is measured as the maximal distance from the helix to the end of the lobe in a coronal view (Fig. 15-1). A parasagittal view can also be obtained (Fig. 15-2).

DISCUSSION

There is a linear relationship between ear length and menstrual age.[2,3] The correlation coefficient between ear length and menstrual age is between 0.84[2] and 0.96.[3] In the second trimester the intra- and interobserver variation in ear length are 3.6 ± 1.9% and 3 ± 1.5%, respectively.[2] Table 15-1 provides a nomogram of fetal ear length (in millimeters) according to percentile distribution. Table 15-2 shows 50th percentile ear length (mm) by menstrual age.

A short ear length in the second and third trimesters has generally been defined as a measurement less than the 10th percentile for menstrual age.[4] In one study[4] of 1311 high-risk patients, 11 of 34 (32.4%) fetuses with a significant chromosomal abnormality had a short ear length. When the 34 cases were divided into subgroups, 5 of 19 (26.3%) trisomy 21 fetuses and 3 of 4 (75%) trisomy 18 fetuses had a short ear length.

Between 11 and 14 weeks' menstrual age, ear length also increases linearly with menstrual age.[5] Although the median ear length of trisomy 21 fetuses is significantly below the normal mean, only 2 of 32 (6.3%) trisomy 21 fetuses had an ear length less than the fifth percentile.

Recently, three-dimensional ultrasound has been used to better examine the fetal ear.[6] As a

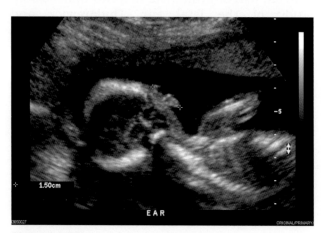

Figure 15-1
Coronal view of a fetal ear at 21 weeks' menstrual age.

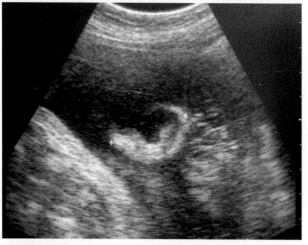

Figure 15-2
Parasagittal view of a fetal ear in the third trimester.

Table 15-1 Nomogram of fetal ear length (mm) according to percentile distribution

Weeks' Gestation	No. of Fetuses	5%	10%	50%	90%	95%
15	34	6.7	7.0	8.5	10.4	10.4
16	464	8.2	8.5	10.0	11.2	11.6
17	387	8.6	9.0	10.6	12.3	12.9
18	258	9.0	9.8	11.7	13.7	14.3
19	248	10.6	11.2	12.9	15.1	15.5
20	217	11.5	12.3	14.3	16.4	17.3
21	142	12.2	13.2	15.3	17.4	18.1
22	101	13.2	14.2	16.7	18.6	18.9
23	68	14.0	14.9	18.1	20.6	21.6
24	44	15.3	15.8	19.7	21.9	22.3
25	39	15.7	16.8	21.4	24.2	24.5
26	37	16.6	16.8	21.2	23.8	24.2
27	29	19.4	19.6	22.5	26.4	27.8
28	28	17.6	19.9	24.4	30.1	31.9
29	43	18.7	20.0	25.3	28.2	28.5
30	22	18.3	20.7	25.1	27.9	31.6
31	41	21.4	21.9	26.7	29.8	31.2
32	40	25.3	25.8	28.1	31.1	33.0
33	53	21.4	23.5	28.6	32.4	32.9
34	48	22.7	26.9	29.2	33.3	34.0
35	57	23.0	26.7	31.2	33.7	35.0
36	47	23.9	27.5	31.1	33.3	34.5
37	63	27.3	28.1	31.9	35.6	36.4
38	34	24.8	25.6	32.2	36.9	38.7
39	23	26.2	27.7	33.3	36.2	37.5
40	16	28.1	29.3	32.6	35.7	37.6

From Chitkara U, Lee L, El-Sayed YY, et al: Ultrasonographic ear length measurement in normal second- and third-trimester fetuses. Am J Obstet Gynecol 2000;183:230-234.

Table 15-2 50th percentile ear length (mm) by menstrual age

Menstrual Age (wks)	Lettieri[2]	Chitkara[3]
15	8	8.5
16	9	10.0
17	11	10.6
18	12	11.7
19	13	12.9
20	14	14.3
21	16	15.3
22	17	16.7
23	18	18.1
24	19	19.7
25	21	21.4

result, not only size but shape (see Fig. 15-2), ridge pattern, axis, and orientation of the fetal ear can be evaluated. In a two-dimensional study of the fetal ear, Dudarewicz and Kaluzewski[7] found that abnormal ear shape increased the clinical value of fetal ear length in the prenatal screening for chromosomal abnormalities.

References

1. Aase JM, Wilson AC, Smith DW: Small ears in Down's syndrome: a helpful diagnostic aid. J Pediatr 1973;82:845-847.
2. Lettieri LA, Rodis JF, Vintzileos AM, et al: Ear length in second trimester aneuploid fetuses. Obstet Gynecol 1993;81:57-60.

3. Chitkara U, Lee L, El-Sayed YY, et al: Ultrasonographic ear length measurement in normal second- and third-trimester fetuses. Am J Obstet Gynecol 2000;183:230-234.
4. Chitkara U, Lee L, Oehler JW, et al: Fetal ear length measurement: a useful prediction of aneuploidy? Ultrasound Obstet Gynecol 2002;19:131-135.
5. Sacchini C, El-Sheikhah A, Cicero S, et al: Ear length in trisomy 21 fetuses at 11-14 weeks of gestation. Ultrasound Obstet Gynecol 2003;22:460-463.
6. Shih J-C, Shyu M-K, Lee C-N, et al: Antenatal depiction of the fetal ear with three-dimensional ultrasonography. Obstet Gynecol 1998;91:500-505.
7. Dudarewicz L, Kaluzewski B: Prenatal screening for fetal chromosomal abnormalities using ear length and shape as an ultrasound marker. Med Sci Monit 2000;6:801-806.

CHAPTER 16

Lyndon Hill

Fetal Weight

Introduction

Abnormalities of fetal growth, either macrosomia or growth restriction, are associated with increased perinatal mortality and morbidity. An estimation of fetal size is, therefore, the starting point for any evaluation of a suspected fetal growth disturbance.

Materials/Methods

Campbell and Wilkin[1] initially reported use of the fetal abdominal circumference to estimate fetal weight in 1975. There are now more than 2 dozen equations[2] (Table 16-1) that use:

1. Abdominal circumference
2. Abdominal circumference, biparietal diameter
3. Abdominal circumference, head circumference
4. Abdominal circumference, femur length
5. Abdominal circumference, biparietal diameter, femur length
6. Abdominal circumference, head circumference, biparietal diameter, femur length

DISCUSSION

The accuracy of the same equation to predict neonatal weight varies among centers. As a result, each center must select the equation that is most appropriate for its patient population.[3] The wide interobserver variations in measuring the biparietal diameter, head circumference, and abdominal circumference affect the clinical applicability of an estimated fetal weight.[4] Some examiners tend to overestimate, and others tend to underestimate fetal weight.[5]

Most studies comparing sonographic estimated fetal weight and birth weight report a high correlation (0.775 to 0.96).[6-8] However, from a clinical perspective the range of values about the mean significantly reduces the applicability of an estimated fetal weight in patient management. Hadlock et al[7] report a two standard deviation error of ±15% to 18.2%, depending on the fetal parameters incorporated in the estimation of fetal weight. Some authors have

Table 16-1 | Equations for the estimation of fetal weight

Source	Year	Equation
AC equations		
Campbell and Wilkin*	1975	$\text{Ln EFW} = -4.564 + 0.282\,(AC) - 0.00331\,(AC)^2$
Hadlock et al	1984	$\text{Ln EFW} = 2.695 + 0.253\,(AC) - 0.00275\,(AC)^2$
Jordaan	1983	$\text{Log}_{10}\,\text{EFW} = 0.6328 + 0.1881\,(AC) - 0.0043\,(AC)^2$ $+ 0.000036239\,(AC)^3$
Warsof et al*	1977	$\text{Log}_{10}\,\text{EFW} = -1.8367 + 0.092\,(AC) - 0.000019\,(AC)^3$
Higginbottom et al	1975	$\text{EFW} = 0.0816\,(AC)^3$
FL equation		
Warsof et al	1986	$\text{Ln EFW} = 4.6914 + 0.151\,(FL)^2 - 0.0119\,(FL)^3$
AC/FL equations		
Hadlock et al	1985	$\text{Log}_{10}\,\text{EFW} = 1.304 + 0.05281\,(AC) + 0.1938\,(FL)$ $- 0.004\,(AC)(FL)$
Warsof et al	1986	$\text{Ln EFW} = 2.792 + 1.08\,(FL) + 0.0036\,(AC)^2 - 0.027\,(FL)\,(AC)$
Woo et al	1985	$\text{Log}_{10}\,\text{EFW} = 0.59 + 0.08\,(AC) + 0.28\,(FL) - 0.00716\,(AC)\,(FL)$
AC/BPD equations		
Warsof et al*	1977	$\text{Log}_{10}\,\text{EFW} = 1.599 + 0.144\,(BPD) + 0.032\,(AC) - 0.000111$ $(BPD)^2\,(AC)$
Hadlock et al	1984	$\text{Log}_{10}\,\text{EFW} = 1.1134 + 0.05845\,(AC) - 0.000604\,(AC)^2$ $- 0.007365\,(BPD)^2 + 0.000595\,(BPD)\,(AC) + 0.1694\,(BPD)$
Jordaan*	1983	$\text{Log}_{10}\,\text{EFW} = -1.1683 + 0.0377\,(AC) + 0.0950\,(BPD) - 0.0015$ $(BPD)\,(AC)$
Hsieh et al	1987	$\text{Log}_{10}\,\text{EFW} = 2.1315 + 0.0056541\,(AC)\,(BPD)$ $- 0.00015515\,(BPD)\,(AC)^2 + 0.000019782\,(AC)^3$ $+ 0.052594\,(BPD)$
Woo et al	1985	$\text{Log}_{10}\,\text{EFW} = 1.63 + 0.16\,(BPD) + 0.00111\,(AC)^2$ $- 0.0000859\,(BPD)\,(AC)^2$
Vintzileos et al	1987	$\text{Log}_{10}\,\text{EFW} = 1.879 + 0.084\,(BPD) + 0.026\,(AC)$
Shepard et al*	1982	$\text{Log}_{10}\,\text{EFW} = -1.7492 + 0.166\,(BPD) + 0.046\,(AC)$ $- 0.002546\,(BPD)$
AC/BPD/FL equations		
Woo et al	1985	$\textbf{Log}_{10}\,\textbf{EFW} = \textbf{1.54} + \textbf{0.15}\,\textbf{(BPD)} + \textbf{0.00111}\,\textbf{(AC)}^2 -$ $0.0000764\,(BPD)\,(AC)^2 + 0.05\,(FL) - 0.000992\,(FL)\,(AC)$
Shinozuka et al†	1987	$\textbf{EFW} = \textbf{0.23966}\,\textbf{(AC)}^2\,\textbf{(FL)} + \textbf{1.6230}\,\textbf{(BPD)}^3$
Hadlock et al	1985	$\textbf{Log}_{10}\,\textbf{EFW} = \textbf{1.335} - \textbf{0.0034}\,\textbf{(AC)}\,\textbf{(FL)} + \textbf{0.0316}\,\textbf{(BPD)}$ $+ 0.0457\,(AC) + 0.1623\,(FL)$
Hsieh et al	1987	$\textbf{Log}_{10}\,\textbf{EFW} = \textbf{2.7193} + \textbf{0.0094962}\,\textbf{(AC)}\,\textbf{(BPD)} - \textbf{0.1432}$ $(FL) - 0.00076742\,(AC)\,(BPD)^2 + 0.001745\,(FL)\,(BPD)^2$
AC/HC/FL equations		
Hadlock et al	1984	$\textbf{Log}_{10}\,\textbf{EFW} = \textbf{1.326} - \textbf{0.00326}\,\textbf{(AC)}\,\textbf{(FL)} + \textbf{0.0107}\,\textbf{(HC)}$ $+ 0.0438\,(AC) + 0.158\,(FL)$
Ott et al*	1986	$\textbf{Log}_{10}\,\textbf{EFW} = \textbf{2.0661} + \textbf{0.04355}\,\textbf{(HC)} + \textbf{0.05394}\,\textbf{(AC)}$ $0.0008582\,(HC)\,(AC) + 1.2594\,(FL/AC)$
Combs et al	1993	$\textbf{EFW} - \textbf{0.23718}\,\textbf{(AC)}^2\,\textbf{(FL)} + \textbf{0.03312}\,\textbf{(HC)}^3$
AC/HC/BPD/ ± FL equations		
Jordaan	1983	$\text{Log}_{10}\,\text{EFW} = 2.3231 + 0.02904\,(AC) + 0.0079\,(HC)\,0.0058\,(BPD)$
Hadlock et al	1985	$\textbf{Log}_{10}\,\textbf{EFW} = \textbf{1.3596} + \textbf{0.0064}\,\textbf{(HC)} + \textbf{0.0424}\,\textbf{(AC)}$ $+ 0.174\,(FL) + 0.00061\,(BPD)\,(AC) - 0.00386\,(AC)\,(FL)$

Table 16-1	Equations for the estimation of fetal weight—cont'd		
Source		**Year**	**Equation**
Maternal characteristics equation			
Nahum et al‡		2002	**EFW = Gestational age (d) × (9.38 + 0.264 × fetal sex**§ + 0.000233 x maternal height [cm] × maternal weight at 26.0 wks [kg] + 4.62 × third-trimester maternal weight gain rate [kg/d] × [parity + 1])‖

AC, FL, BPD, and HC are expressed in centimeters.

*The estimated fetal weight for these six algorithms is expressed in kilograms rather than grams.

†The equation of Shinozuka et al has been modified from its original form to include the fetal AC instead of the fetal transverse and anteroposterior abdominal diameters, as were described in the original equation. (Shinozuka N, et al: J Obstet Gynecol 1987;157:1140 and Combs CA, et al: Obstet Gynecol 1993;82:365).

‡This equation applies only to healthy white mothers who carry term singleton pregnancies. Fetal weight estimates that use this equation should be adjusted systematically for (1) black maternal race (decrement by 161 g), (2) East Asian maternal race (decrement by 291 g), (3) chronic hypertension (decrement by 161 g), (4) pregnancy-induced hypertension/preeclampsia (decrement by 105 g), (5) maternal cigarette smoking (decrement by 17 g per cigarette smoked per day), and (6) high altitude (decrement by 102 g for every 1000 meters in altitude above sea level).

§Fetal sex independently explains approximately 1% of the variance in term fetal weight. It is a significant predictor of birth weight (F test, P < 0.001), but it has little overall impact on birth weight predictions. When 0 is entered for fetal sex so that sex is ignored, the mean absolute prediction error does not change, and the median absolute prediction error increases only slightly by 10 g (0.2%). Thus fetal sex, although potentially useful if available, is nonessential for use of the maternal characteristics equation.

‖ Where fetal sex = +1 for male, –1 for female, and 0 when sex is not known; gestational age = days since the onset of the last normal period = the conception age (in days) plus 14.

Ln, Natural logarithm; EFW, estimated fetal weight (expressed in grams).

Wahum GG and Stanislaw H. Ultrasonographic prediction of term birth weight: How accurate is it? Am J Obstet Gynecol 2003; 188:566-574.

proposed that the 10th and 90th percentiles be provided to assist the clinician in the interpretation of an estimated fetal weight.[9]

The estimated fetal weight tends to be overestimated when the fetus is large for gestational age and underestimated with intrauterine growth restriction and preterm premature rupture of membranes.[6]

There are primarily three factors that significantly affect the accuracy of estimating fetal weight:

1. Errors in assigning gestational age
2. Measurement errors
3. The inability to accurately assess fetal density. Unfortunately, density varies considerably between fetuses/neonates (0.833 to 1.012 g/ml).[10] The error in estimating weight given these discrepancies in density is between 8% and 21%.[11]

A sonographic estimation of fetal weight does not add significantly to the routine clinical evaluation of fetal size.[12-14] When used to detect macrosomia, an ultrasonically estimated fetal weight has a low sensitivity, a low positive predictive value, and a high negative predictive value. Because Hadlock et al[7] optimized the accuracy of an estimated fetal weight for the majority of fetuses rather than the "outliers," this should not be surprising. The likelihood ratio of an ultrasonic estimated fetal weight for the detection of macrosomia does not exceed the critical threshold for clinical usefulness of 5.[8] The true value of an estimated fetal weight may, therefore, be to rule out rather than to predict macrosomia.[15]

References

1. Campbell S, Wilkin D: Ultrasonic measurement of fetal abdomen circumference in the estimation of fetal weight. Br J Obstet Gynaecol 1975;82:689-697.

2. David C, Tagliavini G, Pilu G, et al: Receiver-operator characteristic curves for the ultrasonographic prediction of small-for-gestational-age fetuses in low risk pregnancies. Am J Obstet Gynecol 1996;174:1037-1042.

3. Chauhan SP, Charania SF, McLaren RA, et al: Ultrasonographic estimate of birth weight at 24 to 34 weeks: a multicenter study. Am J Obstet Gynecol 1998;178:909-916.

4. Sarmandal P, Bailey SM, Grant JM: A comparison of three methods of assessing interobserver variation applied to ultrasonic fetal measurement in the third trimester. Br J Obstet Gynaecol 1989;96:1261-1265.

5. Kurmanavicius J, Burkhardt T, Wisser J, et al: Ultrasonographic fetal weight estimation: accuracy of formulas and accuracy of examiners by birth weight from 500 to 5000 g. J Perinat Med 2004;32:155-161.

6. Ben-Haroush A, Yogev Y, Bar J, et al: Accuracy of sonographically estimated fetal weight in 840 women with different pregnancy complications prior to induction of labor. Ultrasound Obstet Gynecol 2004;23: 172-176.

7. Hadlock FP, Harrist RB, Carpenter RJ, et al: Sonographic estimation of fetal weight. The value of femur length in addition to head and abdomen measurements. Radiology 1984;150:535-540.

8. Nahum G, Stanislow H: Ultrasonographic prediction of term birth weight: how accurate is it? Am J Obstet Gynecol 2003;188: 566-574.

9. Smith GCS, Smith MFS, McNay MB, et al: The relation between fetal abdominal circumference and birth weight: findings in 3512 pregnancies. Br J Obstet Gynaecol 1997;104:186-190.

10. Thompson TE, Manning FA, Morrison I: Determination of fetal volume in utero by an ultrasound method: correlation with neonatal birth weight. J Ultrasound Med 1983;2:113-116.

11. Manning FA: Intrauterine Growth Retardation–Etiology, Petrophysiology, Diagnosis, and Treatment. In Fetal Medicine Principles and Practice, Chap 7. Stamford, Conn, Appleton and Lang, 1995.

12. Sherman DJ, Arieli S, Tovbin J, et al: A comparison of clinical and ultrasonic estimation of fetal weight. Obstet Gynecol 1998;91:212-217.

13. Hendrix NW, Grady CS, Chauhan S: Clinical vs. sonographic estimate of birth weight in term participants. A randomized clinical trial. J Reprod Med 2000;45:317-322.

14. Weiner Z, Ben-Shlomo I, Beck-Fruchter R, et al: Clinical and ultrasonographic weight estimation in large for gestational age fetus. Eur J Obstet Gynecol 2002;105:20-24.

15. Ben-Harousch A, Yogev Y, Hod M: Fetal weight estimation in diabetic pregnancies and suspected fetal macrosomia. J Perinat Med 2004;32:113-121.

CHAPTER 17

Lyndon Hill

Estimates and Ratios of Menstrual Age and Fetal Weight

Introduction

Originally, only the biparietal diameter (BPD) was used to evaluate menstrual age. However, it soon became apparent that the shape of the fetal head could markedly affect the BPD and, therefore, menstrual age assessment. Use of multiple biometric parameters improves the accuracy of menstrual age assessment.

Materials/Methods

The data set used for each biometric parameter is outlined in the appropriate chapter.

DISCUSSION

There is a constant pattern of fetal growth over the first 20 weeks of gestation that crosses ethnic and socioeconomic lines. Sonographic measurements during this time period, therefore, reflect the inherent genetic drive of the embryo/fetus. Between 14 and 21 weeks' menstrual age, a model using all four menstrual age parameters [biparietal diameter (BPD, head circumference (HC), abdominal circumference (AC), and femur length (FL)] is statistically superior to any individual parameter for menstrual age assessment and to all combinations of two parameters, except HC and FL.[1,2] Chervenak et al[3] also found that the addition of one parameter (AC or FL) or two parameters (AC and FL) to HC improved the accuracy of predicting menstrual age between 14 and 22 weeks' gestation. A statistically significant difference is not always clinically relevant—the improvement in accuracy was less than 1 day.[3,4]

As the fetus enters the third trimester, biologic variability, as well as multiple outside influences, may affect fetal growth. If multiple parameters are utilized to assess menstrual age, equal weight is given to each parameter. Agreement between different independent measurements strengthens the assignment of menstrual age. It therefore follows that individual measurements that differ significantly from a number of concordant values should not be incorporated into menstrual age assessment. Specific age-independent ratios, (e.g., cephalic index,[5] see section on biparietal diameter), FL/BPD,[6] and FL/AC[7] are helpful in determining the reason for the discrepancy in menstrual age assessment by different parameters. The FL/BPD ratio between 23 and 40 weeks' menstrual age is 79% ± 8% (90% confidence interval). If the FL/BPD ratio is above normal, the FL is overestimated, the BPD is underestimated, or the possibility of microcephaly should be considered. The FL/AC ratio[7] after 21 weeks' gestation is 22 ± 2 (mean ± SD). The normal biometric ratios of HC/AC, AC/FL and BPD/FL are outlined in Table 17-1.[8]

When compared with individual parameters, statistically significant improvement in the variability of the estimation of menstrual age during the third trimester occurs with all combinations of two, three, or four parameters (i.e., BPD, HC, AC, and FL). The results of multiple linear regression analysis are similar to the results obtained from simple averaging of the menstrual age estimates obtained from each parameter. For example, between 28 weeks and term the biparietal diameter alone has a 95% confidence interval of ± 3.6 weeks, while the BPD/AC/FL has a confidence interval of 2.6 weeks.[1,2] Hadlock et al[4] also reported a significant reduction in variability with four measurements to assess menstrual age. Regression equations from this publication are presented in Table 17-2.[4] Also, the subgroup variability using equations in Table 17-2 are presented in Table 17-3.[4] The two standard deviation range in estimating menstrual age is approximately 7%. Hence the variability is 1.4 weeks at 20 weeks' gestation and 2.1 weeks at 30 weeks.[9] Hill et al[10] found a slight increase in R^2 when two fetal parameters, rather than one, were used to determine menstrual age; the addition of other fetal biometric parameters to the HC and FL did not improve menstrual age assessment.

By completing the standard fetal growth profile (BPD, HC, AC, FL) along with the appropriate ratios, the sonologist will be more likely to detect not only abnormalities of fetal growth but also certain congenital anomalies.

Estimating Fetal Weight

Biometry has also been utilized to estimate fetal weight. Initially, neonatal weights were used to establish weight percentiles for a given menstrual age.[11] However, it has been shown that preterm neonates tend to have a lower weight at delivery when compared with the weight that a full-term infant would have had at the same menstrual age.[12,13] As a result, Hadlock et al[12] (Table 17-4) developed menstrual age-specific weight percentiles on the basis of the estimated fetal weight of accurately dated pregnancies that delivered at term. However, this technique merely substitutes the variation in estimated fetal weight for the growth-inhibiting effects of preterm delivery.

Doubilet et al[13] used first trimester ultrasound to determine gestational age; their weight percentiles are based on the delivery weight. Doubilet et al[13] (Table 17-5), therefore, provide a weight percentile if delivery occurred immediately after the ultrasound examination. This group also published gender-specific neonatal birth weights from the 5th through the 95th percentiles (Table 17-6).

Text continued on p. 56

Table 17-1	Normal biometric ratios of head circumference (HC)/abdominal circumference (AC), AC/femur length (FL), and biparietal diameter (BPD)/FL

	HC/AC[a]			AC/FL[b]			BPD/FL[c]		
GA (wks)	5th	50th	95th	5th	50th	95th	5th	50th	95th
14	1.13	1.23	1.34	4.93	5.51	6.16	1.75	1.92	2.11
15	1.12	1.22	1.33	4.73	5.29	5.92	1.66	1.82	2.00
16	1.11	1.21	1.32	4.57	5.11	5.71	1.58	1.74	1.91
17	1.10	1.20	1.31	4.43	4.95	5.54	1.52	1.67	1.83
18	1.09	1.19	130	4.32	4.83	5.40	1.47	1.61	1.77
19	1.08	1.18	1.29	4.23	4.73	5.29	1.42	1.56	1.71
20	1.07	1.17	1.28	4.16	4.65	5.20	1.39	1.52	1.67
21	1.06	1.17	1.28	4.11	4.59	5.13	1.36	1.49	1.64
22	1.05	1.16	1.26	4.07	4.55	5.08	1.34	1.47	1.61
23	1.04	1.15	1.25	4.04	4.52	5.05	1.32	1.45	1.59
34	1.03	1.14	1.24	4.03	4.50	5.03	1.30	1.43	1.57
35	1.02	1.13	1.23	4.02	4.50	5.03	1.29	1.42	1.56
36	1.01	1.12	1.22	4.03	4.50	5.03	1.29	1.41	1.55
37	1.00	1.11	1.21	4.04	4.51	5.04	1.28	1.41	1.54
38	0.99	1.10	1.20	4.05	4.53	5.06	1.28	1.40	1.54
39	0.98	1.09	1.19	4.07	4.55	5.09	1.28	1.40	1.54
30	0.97	1.08	1.18	4.10	4.58	5.12	1.27	1.40	1.53
31	0.96	1.07	1.17	4.12	4.61	5.15	1.27	1.40	1.53
32	0.95	1.06	1.16	4.15	4.64	5.18	1.27	1.39	1.53
33	0.94	1.05	1.16	4.17	4.67	5.22	1.27	1.39	1.52
34	0.94	1.04	1.15	4.20	4.69	5.24	1.26	1.38	1.52
35	0.93	1.03	1.14	4.21	4.71	5.27	1.25	1.37	1.51
36	0.92	1.02	1.13	4.23	4.73	5.28	1.24	1.36	1.20
37	0.91	1.01	1.12	4.23	4.73	5.29	1.23	1.35	1.48
38	0.90	1.00	1.11	4.23	4.73	5.29	1.21	1.33	1.46
39	0.89	0.99	1.10	4.22	4.71	5.27	1.19	1.30	1.43
40	0.88	0.98	1.09	4.19	4.69	5.24	1.16	1.28	1.40

[a]$HC/AC = 0.3668952 − 0.0096 \times GA$ (SD = 0.064) Modified formula to fit published tabular data.
[b]$Log\ (AC/FL) = 1.3260806 − 0.0693157 \times GA + 0.0023154 \times GA^2\ 0.0000248 \times GA^3$ (SD 0.02458).
[c]$Log\ (BPD/FL) = 1.0205449 − 0.0865895 \times GA + 0.0028771 \times GA^2 − 0.0000321 \times GA^3$ (SD 0.02458).
GA, gestational age.
From Snijders RJ, Nicolaides KH: Fetal biometry at 14-40 weeks' gestation. Ultrasound Obstet Gynecol 1994;4:34-48.

Table 17-2 Regression equations for predicting menstrual age

Parameters Used	Regression Equation for Menstrual Age	SD (wks)	Max ERR (wks)	R Squared
BPD	$09.54 + 1.482 \, (BPD) + 0.1676 \, (BPD)^2$	1.36	5.1	0.967
HC	$08.96 + 0.540 \, (HC) + 0.0003 \, (HC)^3$	1.23	4.1	0.973
AC	$08.14 + 0.753 \, (AC) + 0.0036 \, (AC)^2$	1.31	4.6	0.969
FL	$10.35 + 2.460 \, (FL) + 0.170 \, (FL)^2$	1.28	4.9	0.971
BPD, AC	$09.57 + 0.524 \, (AC) + 0.1220 \, (BPD)^2$	1.18	3.8	0.975
BPD, HC	$10.32 + 0.009 \, (HC)^2 + 1.3200 \, (BPD) + 0.00012 \, (HC)^3$	1.21	3.5	0.974
BPD, FL	$10.50 + 0.197 \, (BPD) \, (FL) + 0.9500 \, (FL) + 0.7300 \, (BPD)$	1.10	3.6	0.978
HC, AC	$10.31 + 0.012 \, (HC)^2 + 0.3850 \, (AC)$	1.15	4.3	0.976
HC, FL*	$11.19 + 0.070 \, (HC) \, (FL) + 0.2630 \, (HC)$	1.04	3.3	0.980
AC, FL	$10.47 + 0.442 \, (AC) + 0.3140 \, (FL)^2 - 00121 \, (FL)^3$	1.11	3.8	0.978
BPD, AC, FL*	$10.61 + 0.175 \, (BPD) \, (FL) + 0.2970 \, (AC) + 0.7100 \, (FL)$	1.06	3.4	0.980
BPD, HC, FL*	$11.38 + 0.070 \, (HC) \, (FL) + 0.9800 \, (BPD)$	1.04	3.2	0.981
HC, AC, FL*	$10.33 + 0.031 \, (HC) \, (FL) + 0.3610 \, (HC) + 0.0298 \, (AC) \, (FL)$	1.03	3.4	0.981
HC, AC, BPD	$10.58 + 0.005 \, (HC)^2 + 0.3635 \, (AC) + 0.02864 \, (BPD) \, (AC)$	1.14	4.0	0.977
BPD, HC, AC, FL*	$10.85 + 0.060 \, (HC) \, (FL) + 0.6700 \, (BPD) + 0.1680 \, (AC)$	1.02	3.2	0.981

Equations that provided best estimates. From Hadlock FP, Deter RL, Harrist RB, Park SK: Estimating fetal age: computer-assisted analysis of multiple fetal growth parameters. Radiology 1984; 152:497–501.
AC, abdominal circumference; BPD, biparietal diameter; FL, femur length; HC, head circumference; Max Err, maximum error; SD, Standard deviation.

Table 17-3 Subgroup variability in predicting menstrual age, using equations in Table 17-1

	Subgroup Variability (±2 SD)				
Parameters Used	12-18 wks $n = 43$	18-24 wks $n = 69$	24-30 wks $n = 76$	30-36 wks $n = 95$	36-40 wks $n = 78$
BPD	1.19	1.73	2.18	3.08	3.20
HC	1.19	1.48	2.06	2.98	2.70
AC	1.66	2.06	2.18	2.96	3.04
FL	1.38	1.80	2.08	2.96	3.12
BPD, AC	1.26	1.68	1.92	2.60	2.88
BPD, HC	1.08	1.49	1.99	2.86	2.64
BPD, FL	1.12	1.46	1.84	0.60	2.62
HC, AC	1.20	1.52	1.98	2.68	2.52
HC, FL*	1.08	1.34	1.86	2.52	2.28
AC, FL	1.32	1.64	1.88	2.66	2.60
BPD, AC, FL*	1.20	1.52	1.82	2.50	2.52
BPD, HC, FL*	1.04	1.35	1.81	2.52	2.34
HC, AC, FL*	1.14	1.46	1.86	2.52	2.34
HC, AC, BPD	1.21	1.58	1.94	2.60	2.52
BPD, HC, AC, FL*	1.08	1.40	1.80	2.44	2.30

Equations that provided best estimates. From Hadlock FP, Deter RL, Harrist RB, Park SK: Estimating fetal age: computer-assisted analysis of multiple fetal growth parameters. Radiology 1984; 152:497–501.
AC, abdominal circumference; BPD, biparietal diameter; FL, femur length; HC, head circumference; SD, Standard deviation.

Table 17-4 In utero fetal weight standards for normal singleton pregnancies

Weeks	Percentiles of Fetal Weight (g)					Weeks	Percentiles of Fetal Weight (g)				
	3rd	10th	50th	90th	97th		3rd	10th	50th	90th	97th
10	26	29	35	41	44	26	685	758	913	1068	1141
11	34	37	45	53	56	27	791	876	1055	1234	1319
12	43	48	58	68	73	28	908	1004	1210	1416	1513
13	55	61	73	85	91	29	1034	1145	1379	1613	1724
14	70	77	93	109	116	30	1169	1294	1559	1824	1649
15	88	97	117	137	146	31	1313	1453	1751	2049	2189
16	110	121	146	171	183	32	1465	1621	1953	2285	2441
17	136	150	181	212	226	33	1622	1794	2162	2530	2703
18	167	185	223	261	279	34	1783	1973	2377	2781	2971
19	205	227	273	319	341	35	1946	2154	2595	3036	3244
20	248	275	331	387	414	36	2110	2335	2813	3291	3516
21	299	331	399	467	499	37	2271	2513	3028	3543	3785
22	359	398	478	559	598	38	2427	2686	3226	3786	4045
23	426	471	568	665	710	39	2576	2851	3435	4019	4291
24	503	556	670	784	838	40	2714	3004	3619	4234	4524
25	589	652	785	918	981						

From Hadlock FP, Harrist RB, Martinez-Poyer J: In utero analysis of fetal growth: sonographic weight standard. Radiology 1991; 181:129-133.

Table 17-5 Neonatal birth weights and percentiles based on gestational age (GA) derived by first-trimester ultrasound (males and females combined)

GA (wks)	Neonatal Weight Percentiles (g)						
	5th	10th	25th	50th	75th	90th	95th
25	450	489	564	660	772	890	968
26	523	568	652	760	885	1016	1103
27	609	659	754	875	1015	1160	1257
28	707	764	870	1005	1161	1323	1430
29	820	884	1003	1153	1327	1505	1623
30	947	1019	1152	1319	1511	1707	1836
31	1090	1170	1317	1502	1713	1928	2070
32	1249	1337	1499	1702	1933	2167	2321
33	1422	1519	1696	1918	2168	2422	2588
34	1607	1713	1906	2146	2416	2688	2865
35	1804	1918	2126	2383	2671	2960	3148
36	2006	2128	2350	2622	2927	3231	3428
37	2210	2339	2572	2859	3177	3493	3698
38	2409	2544	2786	3083	3412	3737	3947
39	2595	2734	2984	3288	3622	3952	4164
40	2762	2903	3156	3462	3798	4128	4340
41	2900	3041	3293	3597	3929	4255	4462
42	3002	3141	3388	3685	4008	4323	4523
43	3060	3195	3433	3717	4026	4325	4515

Note: Ln(Wt) = 5.5952 − 0.16626 × GA² + 0.0001555 × GA³; and SD of Ln(Wt) = 0.39269 − 0.0063838 × GA.
Ln, Natural log; wt, weight.
From Doubilet PM, Benson CB, Nadel AS, Ringer SA: Improved birth weight table for neonates developed from gestations dated by early ultrasonography. J Ultrasound Med 1997;16:241-249.

Table 17-6 Gender-specific reference values for neonatal birth weights based on gestational age (GA) derived by first-trimester ultrasound

Birth Weights (g)

GA (wks)	Male[a] Percentiles							Female[b] Percentiles						
	5th	10th	25th	50th	75th	90th	95th	5th	10th	25th	50th	75th	90th	95th
25	460	501	577	676	791	911	992	450	487	557	646	749	856	927
26	533	578	664	773	901	1034	1123	526	568	647	748	864	984	1064
27	617	668	764	886	1028	1175	1273	613	662	751	865	995	1130	1219
28	715	772	879	1015	1173	1335	1443	713	768	869	997	1144	1294	1393
29	827	891	1011	1162	1336	1515	1634	827	889	1002	1146	1309	1477	1587
30	955	1027	1160	1327	1519	1716	1846	955	1024	1151	1311	1493	1678	1800
31	1099	1179	1326	1511	1722	1937	2078	1097	1174	1316	1493	1694	1898	2032
32	1259	1348	1510	1713	1943	2177	2331	1253	1339	1496	1691	1911	2135	2281
33	1435	1532	1710	1931	2181	2434	2599	1423	1517	1689	1902	2143	2385	2543
34	1625	1731	1924	2164	2433	2704	2881	1603	1706	1893	2125	2384	2646	2815
35	1827	1941	2149	2406	2693	2982	3169	1792	1904	2105	2354	2632	2911	3092
36	2036	2159	2380	2653	2957	3260	3456	1986	2105	2321	2586	2881	3176	3366
37	2248	2377	2611	2897	3215	3530	3734	2180	2306	2534	2813	3123	3431	3630
38	2455	2591	2834	3130	3458	3783	3991	2368	2500	2738	3029	3350	3669	3874
39	2651	2790	3040	3343	3677	4006	4217	2544	2681	2926	3225	3554	6880	4088
40	2826	2967	3220	3525	3860	4189	4398	2701	2841	3091	3394	3727	4054	4261
41	2971	3112	3364	3667	3997	4320	4525	2831	2972	3223	3526	3858	4184	4391
42	3078	3216	3462	3757	4078	4389	4587	2928	3068	3316	3615	3941	4259	4462
43	3138	3271	3507	3790	4094	4390	4577	2986	3122	3364	3654	3968	4275	4470

Males: $Ln(Wt) = 6.5464 - 0.24681 \times GA + 0.014222 \times GA^2 - 0.00017596 \times GA^3$; SD of $Ln(Wt) = 0.39791 - 0.0065856 \times GA$

Females: $Ln(Wt) = 4.4807 - 0.0689 \times GA + 0.0091683 \times GA^2 - 0.00012913 \times GA^2$; SD of $Ln(Wt) = 0.35439 - 0.0053902 \times GA$

Ln, Natural log; wt, weight.

From Doubilet PM, Benson CB, Nadel AS, Ringer SA: Improved birth weight table for neonates developed from gestations dated by early ultrasonography. J Ultrasound Med 1997;16: 241-249.

Table 17-7	Tenth percentile estimated fetal weights		
Menstrual Age (wks)	**Hadlock[12]**	**Doubilet[13]**	**Difference**
25	652	489	+163
26	758	568	+190
27	876	659	+217
28	1004	764	+240
29	1145	884	+261
30	1294	1019	+275
31	1453	1170	+283
32	1621	1337	+284
33	1794	1519	+275
34	1973	1713	+260
35	2154	1918	+236
36	2335	2128	+207
37	2513	2339	+174
38	2686	2544	+142
39	2851	2734	+117
40	3004	2903	+101

Table 17-8	In utero fetal weight standards for normal twin pregnancies				
Gestational age (wks)	**Percentiles of Fetal Weight (g)**				
	5th	**25th**	**50th**	**75th**	**95th**
16	132	141	154	189	207
17	173	194	215	239	249
18	214	248	276	289	291
19	223	253	300	333	412
20	232	259	324	378	534
21	275	355	432	482	705
22	319	452	540	586	876
23	347	497	598	684	880
24	376	543	656	783	885
25	549	677	793	916	1118
26	722	812	931	1049	1352
27	755	978	1087	1193	1563
28	789	1145	1244	1337	1774
29	900	1266	1395	1509	1883
30	1011	1387	1546	1682	1992
31	1198	1532	1693	1875	2392
32	1385	1677	1840	2068	2793
33	1491	1771	2032	2334	3000
34	1597	1866	2224	2601	3208
35	1703	2093	2427	2716	3336
36	1809	2321	2631	2832	3465
37	2239	2540	2824	3035	3679
38	2669	2760	3017	3239	3894

From Yarkoni S, Reece EA, Holford T, et al: Estimated fetal weight in the evaluation of growth in twin gestations: a prospective longitudinal study. Obstet Gynecol 1987;69:636-639. Weights calculated from formula in Shepard MJ, Richards VA, Berkowitz RL, et al: An evaluation of two equations for predicting fetal weight by ultrasound. Am J Obstet Gynecol 1982;142:47-54.

Table 17-7 compares the 10th percentile weights of Hadlock et al[12] with Doubilet et al.[13] The data derived by Hadlock et al[12] is consistently larger than that by Doubilet et al.[13] The maximum difference of 284 g at 32 weeks equates to a 21% increase over the weight obtained by Doubilet et al.[12] These marked differences highlight the importance of each institution comparing their data with published reports. Ideally, each institution should derive its own weight percentile table by gestational age. At our institution the data of Hadlock et al[12] results in a significant increase in normal fetuses being considered small for gestational age. Most fetal weight standards are for singleton pregnancies. Yarkoni et al's[14] data for twin pregnancies is outlined in Table 17-8.

References

1. Hadlock FP, Deter RL, Harrist RB, Park SK: Computer assisted analysis of fetal age in the third trimester using multiple fetal growth parameters. J Clin Ultrasound 1983;11:313-316.
2. Hadlock FP, Harrist RB, Martinez-Poyer J: How accurate is second trimester fetal dating? J Ultrasound Med 1991;10:557-561.
3. Chervenak FA, Skupski DW, Romero R, et al: How accurate is fetal biometry in the assessment of fetal age? Am J Obstet Gynecol 1998;178:678-687.
4. Hadlock FP, Deter RL, Harrist RB, et al: Estimating fetal age: computer-assisted analysis of multiple fetal growth parameters. Radiology 1984;152:497-501.
5. Hadlock FP, Deter RL, Carpenter RJ, et al: Estimating fetal age: effect of head shape on BPD. Am J Roentgenol 1981;137:83-85.
6. Hohler CW, Quetel TA: Comparison of ultrasound femur length and biparietal diameter in late pregnancy. Am J Obstet Gynecol 1981;141:759.

7. Hadlock, FP, Deter RI, Harrist RD, et al: A date-independent predictor of intrauterine growth retardation: femur length/abdominal circumference ratio. Am J Roentgenol 1987;1141:979-984.

8. Snijders RJ, Nicolaides KH: Fetal biometry at 14-40 weeks' gestation. Ultrasound Obstet Gynecol 1994;4:34-48.

9. Hadlock FP: Sonographic estimation of fetal age and weight. Radiol Clin North Am 1990;28:39-50.

10. Hill LM, Guzick D, Hixson J, et al: Composite assessment of gestational age: a comparison of institutionally derived and published regression equations. Am J Obstet Gynecol 1992;166:551-555.

11. Lubchenco LO, Hansman C, Dressler M, Boyd E: Intrauterine growth as estimated from liveborn birthweight data at 24 to 42 weeks of gestation. Pediatrics 1963;32: 793-800.

12. Hadlock FP, Harrist RB, Martinez-Poyer J: In utero analysis of fetal growth: a sonographic weight standard. Radiology 1991;181: 129-133.

13. Doubilet PM, Benson CB, Nadel AS, Ringer SA: Improved birth weight table for neonates developed from gestations dated by early ultrasonography. J Ultrasound Med 1997;16:241-249.

14. Yarkoni S, Reece EA, Holford T, et al: Estimated fetal weight in the evaluation of growth in twin gestations: a prospective longitudinal study. Obstet Gynecol 1987;69: 636-639.

CHAPTER 18

Lyndon Hill

Fetal Bowel

Introduction

The sonographic diagnosis of markedly dilated fetal bowel is not difficult. However, the detection of the early stages of bowel dilatation requires a knowledge of the normal increase in the diameter of small bowel and colon as menstrual age advances.

Materials/Methods

The colon can be identified by its location around the periphery of the abdominal cavity. The small bowel is centrally located. The maximal internal diameter of the bowel loops are measured.

DISCUSSION

There is a linear correlation (r = 0.82[1] to 0.859[2]) between colon diameter and menstrual age. The diameter of the colon increases from 4 to 6 mm at 22 weeks' menstrual age to 10 to 18 mm at term (Fig. 18-1).[1] There is a gradual increase in meconium content as gestation advances. As a result, the colonic contents gradually become more echodense (Fig. 18-2). The sigmoid colon is significantly larger than the ascending colon; the difference between the other parts of the colon is not significant.[2] In order to diagnose dilated bowel, the confidence intervals about the mean diameter are required. Table 18-1 provides the mean and 95% confidence intervals

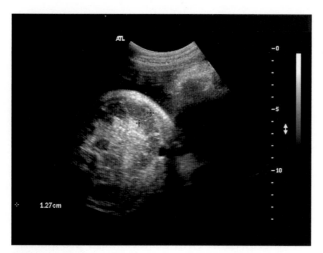

Figure 18-1
Large bowel diameter (calipers) at 37 weeks'
menstrual age.

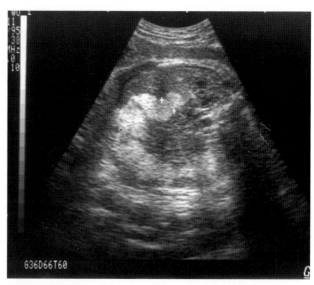

Figure 18-2
Meconium-filled large bowel (calipers) at 40 weeks'
menstrual age.

Table 18-1	Descending colon and rectal diameters according to gestational age				
		Descending colon diameter (mm)		Rectal diameter (mm)	
Week of gestation	Number	Mean	95% CI	Mean	95% CI
19-20	10	3.52	0.79-6.26	3.64	1.45-5.82
21	16	3.59	0.86-6.32	3.79	1.61-5.97
22	28	3.69	0.96-6.41	3.95	1.78-6.13
23	29	3.82	1.09-6.54	4.14	1.97-6.31
24	29	3.98	1.26-6.7	4.34	2.17-6.52
25	29	4.18	1.46-6.9	4.57	2.40-6.74
26	13	4.43	1.70-7.15	4.82	2.64-6.99
27	7	4.71	1.99-7.43	5.08	2.91-7.26
28	7	5.04	2.32-7.76	5.38	3.20-7.55
29	7	5.42	2.69-8.14	5.69	3.52-7.87
30	8	5.84	3.12-8.57	6.04	3.86-8.21
31	10	6.32	3.60-9.05	6.41	4.23-8.58
32	11	6.86	4.13-9.58	6.80	4.63-8.98
33	17	7.45	4.72-10.17	7.23	5.05-9.40
34	14	8.10	5.37-10.82	7.68	5.51-9.85
35	29	8.81	6.09-11.53	8.17	5.99-10.34
36	32	9.59	6.87-12.31	8.68	6.51-10.85
37	18	10.44	7.71-13.16	9.23	7.06-11.40
38	26	11.35	8.63-14.08	9.81	7.64-11.98
39	17	12.34	9.61-15.07	10.43	8.25-12.61
40	22	13.40	10.66-16.15	11.08	8.89-13.26

From Zalel Y, Perlitz Y, Gamzu R, et al: In-utero development of the fetal colon and rectum: sonographic evaluation. Ultrasound Obstet Gynecol 2003;21:161-164.

Table 18-2 Descending colon diameter (mm) at various menstrual ages

Menstrual Age (wks)	Descending Colon (mm)		
	Malas[5]	Zalel[3]	Goldstein[6]
21	3.22	3.59	—
22	4.08	3.69	—
23	4.44	3.82	—
24	4.80	3.98	—
25	5.00	4.18	—
26	6.00	4.43	5
27	6.11	4.71	5
28	6.55	5.04	6
29	7.10	5.42	7
30	7.33	5.84	8
31	8.11	6.32	8
32	8.66	6.86	9
33	8.70	7.45	10
34	8.86	8.10	11
35	9.00	8.81	11
36	9.20	9.59	12
37	10.23	10.44	13
38	10.30	11.35	14
39	10.66	12.34	15
40	11.33	13.40	16
N	131	379	289
Study	Autopsy	Sonographic	Sonographic
Country	Turkey	Israel	USA
Measurement	Outer-to-outer diameter	Internal diameter	Outer-to-outer diameter

for the maximum internal diameter of the descending colon. Malas et al[2] measured the ascending, transverse, descending, and sigmoid colon diameters from the outermost edges in 131 autopsied fetuses who did not have external pathology or anomalies. The descending colon diameter was consistent with the sonographically obtained inner diameter measurement reported by Zalel et al (Table 18-2).[3] The maximum colon diameter reported by Zalel et al[3] of 18 mm is in accordance with the findings of Nyberg et al.[1] The data in Table 18-3 do not provide the confidence intervals for the menstrual age groups evaluated. The largest diameter obtained of 28 mm may, therefore, be an outlier.

The small bowel diameter increases from 1 mm at 13 weeks' menstrual age to 4.4 mm in post-term fetuses[4]; the diameter of the jejunum is greater than the diameter of the ileum during the fetal period (p < 0.05).[5] The maximum diameter of fetal small bowel has been reported as between 6[1] and 8[3] mm (Figs. 18-3 and 18-4; see Table 18-3). The only sonographic data on small bowel diameter throughout gestation is in Table 18-3. Unfortunately, this study is methodologically flawed because it does not provide either the standard deviation or confidence intervals for each 5-week interval. A recent autopsy study obtained the outer-to-outer small bowel diameters in Table 18-4. The postmortem measurement of a flaccid loop of bowel may be significantly different from the diameter of a dynamic loop of bowel in a normal fetus. However, the different diameters of small bowel obtained in the autopsy and sonographic studies after the first trimester are in marked contrast to the comparable large bowel diameters throughout gestation (see Table 18-2). Because the same authors measured the small and large bowel in the autopsy series, the limited sonographic data on small bowel diameter may be inaccurate.

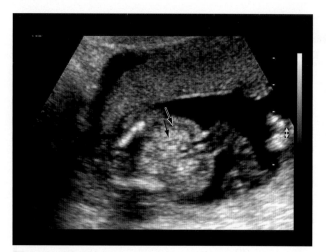

Figure 18-3
Normal small bowel diameter (*arrows*).

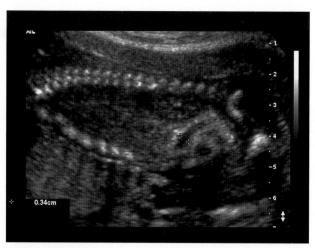

Figure 18-4
Dilated loop of small bowel (0.34 cm) at 22 weeks' menstrual age.

Table 18-3	Lumen diameters (mm) of small bowel and colon at various menstrual ages				
		Small bowel lumen size (mm)		Colon lumen size (mm)	
Menstrual Age (wks)	*N*	Average	Largest	Average	Largest
>40	9	4.4	6	18.7	28
35-40	44	3.7	8	16.8	26
30-35	36	2.9	6	11.4	16
25-30	44	1.8	3	8.0	13
20-25	44	1.4	2	4.4	6
15-20	34	1.2	2	3.6	5
10-15	32	1.0	1	1.5	2

From Parulekar SG: Sonography of normal fetal bowel. J Ultrasound Med 1991;10:211-220.

Table 18-4	Small bowel diameter (mm) at various menstrual ages		
		Small bowel diameter (mm)	
Menstrual Age (wks)	*N*	Jejunum	Ileum
10-12	10	1.431 ± 0.317	1.000 ± 0.311
13-25	63	2.997 ± 0.996	2.392 ± 0.832
26-37	43	5.472 ± 1.808	4.883 ± 1.803
38-40	15	7.379 ± 2.301	6.356 ± 1.743

From Malas MA, Aslankoç R, Üngör B, et al: The development of jejunum and ileum during the fetal period. Early Hum Dev 2003;74: 109-124.

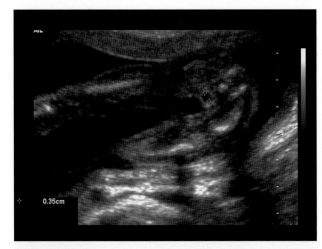

Figure 18-5
Rectal diameter at 20 weeks' menstrual age.

The internal diameter of the fetal rectum (Fig. 18-5) has been measured in a transverse plane by Zalel et al[3] at the level of the fetal bladder (see Table 18-1).

References

1. Nyberg DA, Mack LA, Patten RM, et al: Fetal bowel. Normal sonographic findings. J Ultrasound Med 1987;6:3-6.
2. Malas MA, Aslankoç R, Üngör B, et al: The development of large intestine during the fetal period. Early Hum Dev 2004;78:1-13.
3. Zalel Y, Perlitz Y, Gamzu R, et al: In-utero development of the fetal colon and rectum: sonographic evaluation. Ultrasound Obstet Gynecol 2003;21:161-164.
4. Parulekar SG: Sonography of normal fetal bowel. J Ultrasound Med 1991;10:211-220.
5. Malas MA, Aslankoç R, Üngör B, et al: The development of jejunum and ileum during the fetal period. Early Hum Dev 2003;74:109-124.
6. Goldstein I, Lockwood C, Hobbins JC: Ultrasound assessment of fetal intestinal development in the evaluation of gestational age. Obstet Gynecol 1987;70:682-686.

CHAPTER 19

Lyndon Hill

Fetal Foot Length

Introduction

Because the foot was usually available in fetal autopsy specimens, it was chosen as a means of assessing menstrual age.

Materials/Methods

The foot is measured from heel to the big toe[1,2] or to the first or second toe, whichever is longer,[3,4] in either the plantar (Fig. 19-1) or longitudinal (Fig. 19-2) planes.[5]

DISCUSSION

The results of several ultrasound studies are consistent with Streeter's original data of pathologic specimens[2] (Table 19-1). Hern,[6] in a more recent autopsy study, found a curvilinear correlation between foot length and menstrual age from 10 to 26 weeks. As with most autopsy

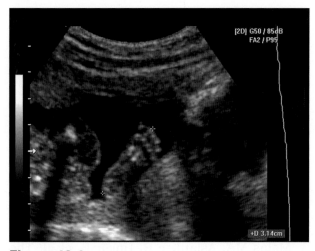

Figure 19-1
Plantar measurement of fetal foot length.

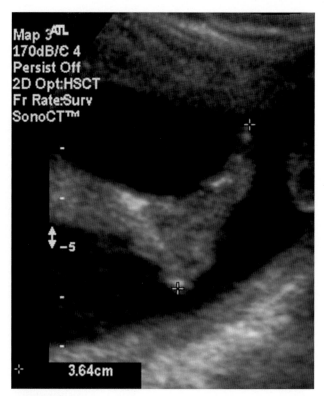

Figure 19-2
Longitudinal measurement of foot length.

Table 19-1	Comparison of fetal foot length for menstrual age between autopsy and sonographic studies						
	Mean Foot Length (cm)						
Menstrual Age (wks)	**Autopsy Streeter**[2]	**Hern**[6]	**Mercer**[2]	**Platt**[4]	***Ultrasound* Goldstein**[1]	**Meriowitz**[3]	**Chitty**[7]
14	1.4	1.4	1.6	1.5	1.8	—	1.5
16	2.0	2.1	2.1	2.1	2.3	2.1	2.1
18	2.7	2.5	2.7	2.7	2.6	2.7	2.7
20	3.3	3.3	3.3	3.3	3.3	3.2	3.3
22	4.0	3.9	3.8	3.9	3.5	3.9	3.9
24	4.5	4.5	4.4	4.6	4.6	4.5	4.4
26	5.0	5.1	5.1	5.2	4.7	5.1	5.0
28	5.5	—	5.8	5.8	5.3	5.6	5.5
30	5.9	—	6.1	—	6.1	6.1	6.0
32	6.3	—	6.3	—	5.6	6.5	6.5
34	6.8	—	6.8	—	6.5	7.0	6.9
36	7.4	—	7.4	—	—	7.5	7.3
38	7.9	—	7.8	—	—	—	7.7
40	8.3	—	8.2	—	—	—	8.0
N	—	1800	160	120	223	5372	450
Year	1920	1984	1987	1988	1988	2000	2002

Table 19-2 Fetal foot length percentiles by menstrual age*

Menstrual Age (wks)	N	CV (%)	Fetal Foot Length Percentiles (Smoothed)				
			5th	10th	50th	90th	95th
15	18	12.7	1.4	1.5	1.8	2.2	2.3
16	146	10.4	1.6	1.7	2.1	2.5	2.6
17	375	9.7	1.9	2.0	2.4	2.8	2.9
18	613	9.8	2.2	2.3	2.7	3.1	3.2
19	1160	8.9	2.5	2.6	3.0	3.3	3.4
20	929	9.3	2.8	2.9	3.2	3.6	3.7
21	552	8.5	3.1	3.2	3.5	3.9	4.0
22	360	8.9	3.4	3.5	3.9	4.2	4.3
23	222	8.1	3.7	3.8	4.2	4.6	4.7
24	177	7.0	4.0	4.1	4.5	4.9	5.0
25	125	7.1	4.3	4.4	4.8	5.1	5.2
26	123	7.0	4.6	4.7	5.1	5.4	5.5
27	108	6.3	4.8	4.9	5.3	5.7	5.8
28	74	5.4	5.1	5.2	5.6	5.9	6.0
29	66	6.2	5.3	5.4	5.8	6.2	6.3
30	65	5.2	5.6	5.7	6.1	6.4	6.5
31	62	5.7	5.8	5.9	6.3	6.7	6.8
32	65	5.3	6.0	6.1	6.5	6.9	7.0
33	39	4.4	6.3	6.4	6.8	7.1	7.2
34	37	6.8	6.5	6.6	7.0	7.4	7.5
35	24	6.2	6.8	6.9	7.3	7.6	7.7
36	15	5.5	7.0	7.1	7.5	7.9	8.0
37	17	5.3	7.3	7.4	7.7	8.1	8.2

*Values for percentiles are in centimeters.
CV, coefficient of variation; N, Number of fetuses.
From Meirowitz NB, Ananth CV, Smulian JC, et al: Foot length in fetuses with abnormal growth. J Ultrasound Med 2000;19:201-205.

studies of the time, a scattergram of the data had a wide variation in foot length values at a given menstrual age because of inaccurately reported menstrual dates. In order to compensate for this potential error, Hern[6] restricted his foot length data to those measurements falling within two standard deviations of the median. The data from the two autopsy studies in Table 19-1 are strikingly similar. Subsequent ultrasound studies have attempted to more rigorously define menstrual age.

The percentile values for fetal foot length at specific menstrual ages are outlined in Table 19-2. As with other fetal parameters, the standard deviation of fetal foot length increases with gestational age.[7]

Meirowitz et al[3] have reported that 29.4% of foot lengths from large-for-gestational age fetuses are above the 90th percentile, and 60.6% of foot lengths in small-for-gestational age fetuses are less than the 10th percentile. Hence foot length cannot be used to accurately assess menstrual age in fetuses with growth abnormalities. Acromelia refers to shortening of the hands and feet. However, most of the skeletal dysplasias do not affect the foot. The fetal foot length is approximately equal to the femur length throughout gestation. As a result, a femur length/foot ratio of less than 0.84 has been used to detect skeletal dysplasias.[8]

References

1. Goldstein I, Reece A, Hobbins JC: Sonographic appearance of the fetal heel ossification centers and foot length measurements provide independent markers for gestational age estimation. Am J Obstet Gynecol 1988;159:923-926.

2. Mercer BM, Sklar S, Shariatmadar A, et al: Fetal foot length as a predictor of

gestational age. Am J Obstet Gynecol 1987; 156:350-355.

3. Meirowitz NB, Ananth CV, Smulian JC, et al: Foot length in fetuses with abnormal growth. J Ultrasound Med 2000;19:201-205.

4. Platt LD, Medearis AL, DeVore GR, et al: Fetal foot length: relationship to menstrual age and fetal measurements in the second trimester, Obstet Gynecol 1988;71:526-531.

5. Shalev E, Weiner E, Zuckerman H, et al: Reliability of sonographic measurement of the fetal foot. J Ultrasound Med 1989;8: 259-262.

6. Hern WM: Correlation of fetal age and measurements between 10 and 26 weeks of gestation. Obstet Gynecol 1984;63:26-32.

7. Chitty LS, Altman DG: Charts of fetal size: limb bones. Br J Obstet Gynaecol, 2002;109: 919-929.

8. Brons JTJ, Van der Harten JJ, Van Geijn HP, et al: Ratios between growth parameters for the prenatal ultrasonographic diagnosis of skeletal dysplasias. Eur J Obstet Gynecol Reprod Biol 1990;34:37-46.

CHAPTER 20

Lyndon Hill

Fetal Head Circumference

Introduction

Head circumference (HC) is incorporated into menstrual age assessment in the second and third trimester. The head circumference is an especially important parameter to use when there has been an alteration in the shape of the head that could result in a large error in menstrual age assessment from the biparietal diameter.

Materials/Methods

The landmarks for obtaining the HC are the same as for the biparietal diameter and include midline thalami and the third ventricle. In order to ensure the proper alignment with the skull base, the cavum septum pellucidum should be visualized anteriorly and the tentorium posteriorly. The circumference measurement should be taken around the calvarium, not around the scalp. Currently, the HC can be measured in two ways: by directly tracing around the calvarium or by a formula that utilizes the two long axes of the HC image. The former is consistently 1% larger than the latter.[1,2] The ellipse mode in ultrasound equipment (Fig. 20-1) uses a derived formula from the two maximum diameters of the ellipse.[1] The measurement technique employed should be consistent with the HC chart adopted for gestational age assessment.

DISCUSSION

Several authors have evaluated the relationship of HC to menstrual age (Tables 20-1 and 20-2).

The percentile values for head circumference derived from Hadlock[2] are in Table 20-3. There is a widening of the 5th and 95th percentiles

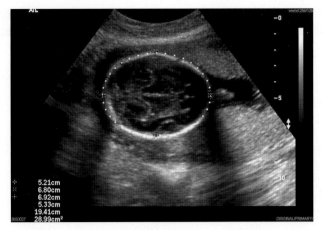

Figure 20-1

Head circumference at 22 weeks' menstrual age utilizing the ellipse function. The head circumference (19.41 cm) is calculated from the two maximum diameters.

Table 20-1	Predicted menstrual age in weeks for head circumference measurements (8.5-36.0 cm)		
Head Circumference (cm)	**Menstrual Age (wks)**	**Head Circumference (cm)**	**Menstrual Age (wks)**
8.5	13.7	22.5	24.4
9.0	14.0	23.0	24.9
9.5	14.3	23.5	25.4
10.0	14.6	24.0	25.9
10.5	15.0	24.5	26.4
11.0	15.3	25.0	26.9
11.5	15.6	25.5	27.5
12.0	15.9	26.0	28.0
12.5	16.3	26.5	28.6
13.0	16.6	27.0	29.2
13.5	17.0	27.5	29.8
14.0	17.3	28.0	30.3
14.5	17.7	28.5	31.0
15.0	18.1	29.0	31.6
15.5	18.4	29.5	32.2
16.0	18.8	30.0	32.8
16.5	19.2	30.5	33.5
17.0	19.6	31.0	34.2
17.5	20.0	31.5	34.9
18.0	20.4	32.0	35.5
18.5	20.8	32.5	36.3
19.0	21.2	33.0	37.0
19.5	21.6	33.5	37.7
20.0	22.1	34.0	38.5
20.5	22.5	34.5	39.2
21.0	23.0	35.0	40.0
21.5	23.4	35.5	40.8
22.0	23.9	36.0	41.6

From Callen PW (ed): Ultrasonography in Obstetrics and Gynecology, 3rd ed. Philadelphia, WB Saunders, 1994. Modified from Hadlock FP, Deter RL, Harrist RB, Park SK: Fetal head circumference: relation to menstrual age. AJR Am J Roentgenol 1982;138:649-653.

Table 20-2 Predicted head circumference (mm) for menstrual age in weeks

Menstrual Age (wks)	Chitty[1] A	Chitty[1] B	Kurmanavicius[5]	Hadlock[6]	Deter[7]
12	68.1	69.6	72.1	—	—
14	96.0	97.7	99.9	—	106
16	123.1	125.1	126.8	122	125
18	149.3	151.6	152.7	148	154
20	174.5	177.0	177.5	177	176
22	198.5	201.3	201.0	193	201
24	221.2	224.3	223.1	221	230
26	242.6	246.0	243.7	241	249
28	262.5	266.2	262.7	271	269
30	280.7	284.8	280.0	276	285
32	297.3	301.6	295.3	292	311
34	312.0	316.7	308.7	308	326
36	324.8	329.8	319.9	322	332
38	335.5	340.8	328.8	336	352
40	344	349.7	335.4	345	362
42	350.3	356.3	339.4	—	—
N	594	594	5462	402	252
Measurement	Derived	Measured	Derived	Measured	Measured technique
Country	UK	UK	UK	USA	USA

Table 20-3 Percentile values for fetal head circumference, from the 3rd through the 97th percentile for menstrual age in weeks

Menstrual Week	Head Circumference (cm) 3rd	10th	50th	90th	97th	Menstrual Week	Head Circumference (cm) 3rd	10th	50th	90th	97th
14	8.8	9.1	9.7	10.3	10.6	28	24.2	25.1	26.6	28.1	29.0
15	10.0	10.4	11.0	11.6	12.0	29	25.0	25.9	27.5	29.1	30.0
16	11.3	11.7	12.4	13.1	13.5	30	25.8	26.8	28.4	30.0	31.0
17	12.6	13.0	13.8	14.6	15.0	31	26.7	27.6	29.3	31.0	31.9
18	13.7	14.2	15.1	16.0	16.5	32	27.4	28.4	30.1	31.8	32.8
19	14.9	15.5	16.4	17.4	17.9	33	28.0	29.0	30.8	32.6	33.6
20	16.1	16.7	17.7	18.7	19.3	34	28.7	29.7	31.5	33.3	34.3
21	17.2	17.8	18.9	20.0	20.6	35	29.3	30.4	32.2	34.1	35.1
22	18.3	18.9	20.1	21.3	21.9	36	29.9	30.9	32.8	34.7	35.8
23	19.4	20.1	21.3	22.5	23.2	37	30.3	31.4	33.3	35.2	36.3
24	20.4	21.1	22.4	23.7	24.3	38	30.8	31.9	33.8	35.8	36.8
25	21.4	22.2	23.5	24.9	25.6	39	31.1	32.2	34.2	36.2	37.3
26	22.4	23.2	24.6	26.0	26.8	40	31.5	32.6	34.6	36.6	37.7
27	23.3	24.1	25.6	27.1	27.9						

From Callen PW (ed): Ultrasonography in Obstetrics and Gynecology, 3rd ed. Philadelphia, WB Saunders, 1994. Modified from Hadlock FP, Deter RL, Harrist RB, Park SK: Estimating fetal age: computer-assisted analysis of multiple fetal growth parameters. Radiology 1984;152:497-501.

Table 20-4	Variability (±2 SD) (wks) in head circumference assessment of menstrual age	
Menstrual Age (wks)	**Hadlock[6]**	**Benson[8]**
14-20	1.4	1.2
20-26	1.6	1.9
26-32	3.0	3.4
30-36	3.0	—
32-42	—	3.8
36-42	2.5	—

Table 20-5	Evaluation of race as a factor in head circumference assessment of menstrual age				
Author	**Ref**	**N**	**Study Design**	**Race**	**Significant Difference**
Jacquemyn	9	524	Cross-sectional; populations compared in study	Belgian Moroccan Turkish	Yes
Arenson	10	126	Longitudinal; compared with published charts	Oriental	No
Westerway	11	300	Cross-sectional; compared with published charts	Australian—no Aborigines	Yes

toward term because of the increasing variability associated with estimating menstrual age as pregnancy advances (Table 20-4).

The head circumference, in contrast to the biparietal diameter (BPD), is independent of head shape. Chervenak et al[4] found that the HC was the best predictor of menstrual age between 14 and 22 weeks' gestation with a random error of 3.35 days.

Two of three studies on Table 20-5 found a racial difference in head circumference measurements for menstrual age. The one investigation that did not find a difference compared the study group to published charts. Because the study group is compared with a standard instead of with a control group, this type of comparison may obscure small differences among populations.

References

1. Chitty LS, Altman DG, Henderson A, et al: Charts of fetal size: 2. Head measurements. Br J Obstet Gynaecol 1994;101: 35-43.

2. Hadlock FP, Kent WR, Loyd JL, et al: An evaluation of two methods for measuring head and body circumferences. J Ultrasound Med 1982;1:359-360.

3. Callen PW: Ultrasonography in Obstetrics and Gynecology, 3rd ed. Philadelphia, WB Saunders, 1994.

4. Chervenak FA, Skupski DW, Romero R, et al: How accurate is fetal biometry in the assessment of fetal age? Am J Obstet Gynecol 1998;178:678-687.

5. Kurmanavicius J, Wright EM, Royston P, et al: Fetal ultrasound biometry: 1. Head reference values. Br J Obstet Gynaecol 1999;106:126-135.

6. Hadlock FP, Deter RL, Harrist RB, et al: Fetal head circumference: Relation to menstrual age. Am J Roentgenol 1982;138: 649-653.

7. Deter RL, Harrist RB, Hadlock FP, et al: Fetal head and abdominal circumferences: II. A critical re-evaluation of the relationship to menstrual age. J Clin Ultrasound 1982;10:365-372.

8. Benson CB, Doubilet PM: Sonographic prediction of gestational age: accuracy of

second- and third-trimester fetal measurements. Am J Roentgenol 1991;157:1275-1277.

9. Jacquemyn Y, Sys SU, Verdonk P: Fetal biometry in different ethnic groups. Early Hum Develop 2000;57:1-13.

10. Arenson AM, Chan P-L, Withers C, et al: Value of standardized gestational age charts for fetuses of first generation Oriental immigrants to Canada. Can Assoc Radiol J 1995; 46:111-113.

11. Westerway SC, Davison A, Cowell S: Ultrasonic fetal measurements: new Australian standards for the new millennium. Aust NZ J Obstet Gynaecol 2000;40:297-302.

CHAPTER 21

Lyndon Hill

Fetal Liver Length

Introduction

The hepatic diverticulum grows rapidly to fill most of the abdominal cavity by 8 weeks' gestation. Initially, the left and right lobes are the same size, but gradually, as gestation advances, the right lobe becomes larger.[1] Intrauterine growth restriction (IUGR) is associated with a decrease in liver size. Fetuses affected by severe Rh disease may have enlarged livers because of extramedullary hematopoesis,[2] while fetuses of diabetic women have an increased liver size because of hyperinsulinemia.[3] Hepatomegaly may also occur with intrauterine infections.[2] Consequently, several authors have evaluated liver length throughout gestation in an attempt to better delineate the aforementioned conditions.

Materials/Methods

Since the right lobe of the liver is much larger than the left, investigators have concentrated on using a linear measurement of the right lobe as indicative of overall liver size. In order to appropriately measure the right lobe of the liver, the aorta is first imaged in a longitudinal plane. The transducer is then moved parallel to this plane until the tip of the right lobe and right hemidiaphragm are imaged. Occasionally, the transducer has to be tipped in order to visualize both the diaphragm and the right lobe of the liver. This is a coronal image of the fetal abdomen. The length of the fetal liver is measured from where the right margin of the heart is in contact with the hemidiaphragm to the tip of the right lobe (Fig. 21-1). The right lobe of the liver cannot be measured if the left side of the fetus is closest to the transducer (Fig. 21-2).

DISCUSSION

Table 21-1 provides the mean liver length (±2 SD) for 20 to 41 weeks' menstrual age. The number of measurements prior to 23 weeks and after 38 weeks are so few that the data are not reliable. Because the purpose of obtaining liver length is to confirm that it is the proper size for menstrual age, a table of liver length predicted by menstrual age is appropriate. Table 21-2 compares liver length values at different menstrual ages by four authors. The data of Senoh et al[4] and Murao et al[5,6] from a Japanese population are similar to the liver lengths of

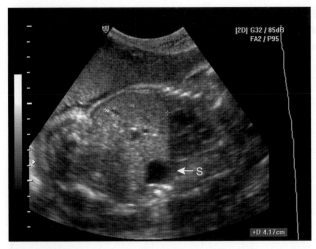

Figure 21-1
The right lobe of the fetal liver at 29 weeks'
menstrual age (between the graticules)
(S = stomach).

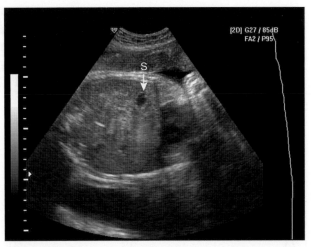

Figure 21-2
With the left side of the fetus up, the right lobe of
the liver cannot be measured (S = stomach).

Table 21-1	Ultrasound measurement of the fetal liver from 20 weeks' menstrual age to term		
Menstrual Age (wks)	**No. of measurements**	**Arithmetic mean (mm)**	**±2SD* (mm)**
20	8	27.3	6.4
21	2	28.0	1.5
22	4	30.6	6.7
23	13	30.9	4.5
24	10	32.9	6.7
25	14	33.6	5.3
26	10	35.7	6.3
27	20	36.6	3.3
28	14	38.4	4.0
29	13	39.1	5.0
30	10	38.7	5.0
31	13	39.6	5.7
32	11	42.7	7.5
33	14	43.8	6.6
34	11	44.8	7.1
35	14	47.8	9.1
36	10	49.0	8.4
37	10	52.0	6.8
38	12	52.9	4.2
39	5	55.4	6.7
40	1	59.0	—
41	2	49.3	2.4

*Standard deviation.
From Vintzileos AM, Neckles S, Campbell WA, et al: Fetal liver ultrasound measurements during normal pregnancy. Obstet Gynecol
1985;66:477-480.

Table 21-2   Liver length values (mm) obtained by different authors for menstrual age

Menstrual Age (wks)	Liver Length (mm)				
	Vintzileos et al[10] (mean)	Murao et al[5] (P)+	Murao et al[6] (P)	Senoh et al[4] (P)	Roberts[2] (G)
15	—	—	—	17	16
16	—	—	—	19	17
17	—	—	—	20	19
18	—	20	24	22	20
19	—	22	26	24	22
20	27	24	27	27	24
21	28	25	29	28	26
22	31	27	30	30	28
23	31	29	32	32	29
24	33	31	33	34	31
25	34	32	35	36	33
26	36	34	37	38	35
27	37	36	38	40	37
28	38	37	40	42	39
29	39	39	41	44	40
30	39	41	43	46	42
31	40	42	45	48	43
32	43	44	46	50	45
33	44	46	48	51	46
34	45	47	49	53	47
35	48	49	51	54	48
36	49	51	52	56	49
37	52	52	54	57	50
38	53	54	56	59	50
39	55	56	57	60	51
40	59	57	59	61	51
R^2 of mathematical function (%)	86	86.5	88.4	91.9	88
N	221	378	573	162	350

P, predicted value; G, graphic data; +, provided by Senoh et al[4]; R^2, coefficient of determination.
Adapted from Senoh D, Hata T, Kitao M: Fetal liver length measurement does not provide a superior means for prediction of a small for gestational age fetus. Am J Perinatol 1994;11:344-347.

Vintzileos et al[7] who studied a mixed racial group, except Orientals.

The right lobe of the liver is thought to be more severely affected than the left lobe in intrauterine growth restriction.[8] However, liver length is not a sufficiently sensitive marker for the detection of IUGR.[4,9]

Serial liver measurements have been found to be a useful adjunct to the evaluation of isoimmunized pregnancies. In one series, eight of eight fetuses with severe isoimmunization had an elongated liver length, while the abdominal circumference was only increased in three fetuses.[10] In another study, 21 of 21 isoimmunized pregnancies with a hemoglobin less than 100 g/L had a liver length greater than the 90th percentile.[2] In a larger study between 1986 and 1999, Roberts et al[11] measured liver length in 200 fetuses at risk for anemia; 45 also had the peak systolic velocity (PSV) measured in the middle cerebral artery. Liver length was greater than the 95th percentile in 93% of the 69 anemic fetuses. The PSV in the middle cerebral artery was greater than the 95th percentile in 15 of 19 fetuses (79%); the remaining 4 fetuses had a peak systolic velocity consistent with mild anemia.

Recently, an evaluation of fetal liver volume has replaced linear measurements. Three-dimensional ultrasound has documented a 14-fold increase in liver volume over the second half of pregnancy.[12] Kuno et al[13] have reported that three-dimensional liver volume was below the normal range in 10 of 10 small-for-gestational-age fetuses; two-dimensional liver length was normal in 7 of 10 fetuses. Boito et al[14], in a study of 24 growth-restricted fetuses and 85 controls, found that hepatic volume was significantly reduced in fetuses with growth restriction. In this latter study, hepatic volume was not a better discriminator of growth restriction than the abdominal circumference.

References

1. Hata T, Fujiwaki R, Senoh D, et al: Intrauterine sonographic assessment of embryonal liver length. Human Reprod 1996; 11:2758-2761.
2. Roberts AB, Mitchell JM, Pattison NS: Fetal liver length in normal and isoimmunized pregnancies. Am J Obstet Gynecol 1989;161: 42-46.
3. Roberts AB, Mitchell JM, Murphy C, et al: Fetal liver length in diabetic pregnancies. Am J Obstet Gynecol 1994;170:1308-1312.
4. Senoh D, Hata T, Kitao M: Fetal liver length measurement does not provide a superior means for prediction of a small for gestational age fetus. Am J Perinatol 1994;11: 344-347.
5. Murao F, Takamori H, Hata K, et al: Fetal liver measurements by ultrasonography. Int J Gynaecol Obstet 1987;25:381-385.
6. Murao F, Senoh D, Takamiya O, et al: Ultrasonic evaluation of liver development in the fetus in utero. Gynecol Obstet Invest 1989; 28:198-201.
7. Vintzileos AM, Neckles S, Campbell WA, et al: Fetal liver ultrasound measurements during normal pregnancy. Obstet Gynecol 1985;66:477-480.
8. Gruenwald P: Degenerative changes in the right half of the liver resulting from intrauterine anoxia. Am J Clin Pathol 1949;19: 801-813.
9. Roberts AB, Mitchell JM, McCowan LM, et al: Ultrasonographic measurement of liver length in the small-for-gestational-age fetus. Am J Obstet Gynecol 1999;180:634-638.
10. Vintzileos AM, Campbell WA, Storlazzi E, et al: Fetal liver ultrasound measurements in isoimmunized pregnancies. Obstet Gynecol 1986;68:162-167.
11. Roberts AB, Mitchel JM, Lake Y, et al: Ultrasonographic surveillance in red blood cell alloimmunication. Am J Obstet Gynecol 2001;184:1251-1255.
12. Laudy JAM, Janssen MMM, Struijk PC, et al: Fetal liver volume measurement by three-dimensional ultrasonography: a preliminary study. Ultrasound Obstet Gynecol 1998;12:93-96.
13. Kuno A, Hayashi Y, Akiyama M, et al: Three-dimensional sonographic measurement of liver volume in the small-for-gestational-age fetus. J Ultrasound Med 2002;21:361-366.
14. Boito SME, Laudy JAM, Struijk PC, et al: Three-dimensional US assessment of hepatic volume, head circumference, and abdominal circumference in healthy and growth-restricted fetuses. Radiology 2002; 223:661-665.

Lyndon Hill

CHAPTER 22

Fetal Long Bones

Introduction

The femur was the original long bone that was measured to help determine menstrual age.

Materials/Methods

The femur length is the primary long bone that is utilized to assess menstrual age. The femoral diaphysis should be measured with the transducer aligned perpendicular to the long axis of the bone (Fig. 22-1). A femur measured in the axial plane (parallel to the ultrasound beam) (Fig. 22-2) between 18 and 35 weeks' gestation is significantly shorter than one measured perpendicular to the shaft.[1] When the femur length is measured axially, the difference in the measurement equates to a reduction in the estimation of menstrual age by up to 2 weeks.[2] All the studies on fetal femoral length are based on perpendicular measurements.

DISCUSSION

Table 22-1 provides the predicted menstrual age from femur length. Table 22-2 compares menstrual age in weeks derived from femur lengths in three different studies.[3-5] The variability in predicting menstrual age from femur length by various authors is outlined in Table 22-3. As with other fetal measurements, most authors have found that the variability in predicting menstrual age from the femur length increases with advancing gestation.[6] Jeanty et al[4] used the Bartlett test to assess significance and did not find an increase in variation with advancing menstrual age. Warda[7] noted that Jeanty et al[4] had a small sample size. Hence the Bartlett test was not appropriate and their results may not have been reliable.

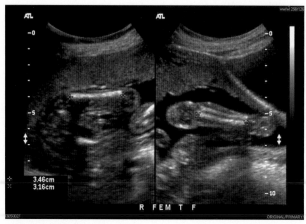

Figure 22-1
20 weeks' menstrual age. Femur length (left) and tibial length (right).

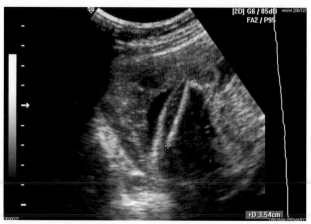

Figure 22-2
A femur length incorrectly measured in the axial plane.

Table 22-1 Predicted menstrual age in weeks for specific femur lengths (1.0 to 7.9 cm)

Femur Length (cm)	Menstrual Age (wks)	Femur Length (cm)	Menstrual Age (wks)
1.0	12.8	4.5	24.5
1.1	13.1	4.6	24.9
1.2	13.4	4.7	25.3
1.3	13.6	4.8	25.7
1.4	13.9	4.9	26.1
1.5	14.2	5.0	26.5
1.6	14.5	5.1	27.0
1.7	14.8	5.2	27.4
1.8	15.1	5.3	27.8
1.9	15.4	5.4	28.2
2.0	15.7	5.5	28.7
2.1	16.0	5.6	29.1
2.2	16.3	5.7	29.6
2.3	16.6	5.8	30.0
2.4	16.9	5.9	30.5
2.5	17.2	6.0	30.9
2.6	17.6	6.1	31.4
2.7	17.9	6.2	31.9
2.8	18.2	6.3	32.3
2.9	18.6	6.4	32.8
3.0	18.9	6.5	33.3
3.1	19.2	6.6	33.8
3.2	19.6	6.7	34.2
3.3	19.9	6.8	34.7
3.4	20.3	6.9	35.2
3.5	20.7	7.0	35.7
3.6	21.0	7.1	36.2
3.7	21.4	7.2	36.7
3.8	21.8	7.3	37.2
3.9	22.1	7.4	37.7
4.0	22.5	7.5	38.3
4.1	22.9	7.6	38.8
4.2	23.3	7.7	39.3
4.3	23.7	7.8	39.8
4.4	24.1	7.9	40.4

From Callen PW (ed): Ultrasonography in Obstetrics and Gynecology, 3rd ed. Philadelphia, WB Saunders, 1994. Modified from Hadlock FP, Harrist RB, Deter RL, Park SK: Fetal femur length as a predictor of menstrual age: sonographically measured. AJR Am J Roentgenol 1982;138:875-878.

Percentiles of femur length between 12 and 42 weeks are provided in Table 22-4.

The femur length has a linear relationship to the biparietal diameter. After 22 weeks' gestation, the femur length/biparietal diameter ratio is 79% ± 6% (90% confidence interval).[8] This ratio can, therefore, be used as an internal verification of the measurements that have been obtained. The femur/abdominal circumference ratio after 21 weeks' gestation is also independent of menstrual age [22% ± 2% (mean ± SD)].[9]

There is controversy over the generalizability of data from racially mixed populations to fetuses of a specific race.[10-14] Some studies compared individual values with a previously published chart. This type of comparison could obscure small differences between populations because groups are compared with a standard instead of with each other. Table

Table 22-2	Menstrual age (wks) derived from femur lengths by three different authors		
	Gestational Age (wks)		
Femur Length (mm)	**Hadlock**[3]	**Jeanty**[4]	**Hohler**[5]
10	12.8	12.6	13.3
12	13.4	13.3	13.6
14	13.6	13.9	14.0
16	14.5	14.6	14.4
18	15.1	15.2	14.8
20	15.7	15.9	15.3
22	16.3	16.6	15.8
24	16.9	17.3	16.3
26	17.6	18.0	16.9
28	18.2	18.7	17.4
30	18.9	19.4	18.1
32	19.6	20.1	18.7
34	20.3	20.9	19.4
36	21.0	21.6	20.1
38	21.8	22.4	20.8
40	22.5	23.1	21.5
42	23.3	23.9	22.3
44	24.1	24.7	23.1
46	24.9	25.4	24.0
48	25.7	26.2	24.9
50	26.5	27.0	25.8
52	27.4	27.8	26.7
54	28.2	28.6	27.6
56	29.1	29.5	28.6
58	30.0	30.3	29.7
60	30.9	31.1	30.7
62	31.9	32.0	31.8
64	32.8	32.9	32.9
66	33.8	33.7	34.0
68	34.7	34.6	35.2
70	35.7	35.5	36.4
72	36.7	36.4	37.6
74	37.7	37.3	38.8
76	38.8	38.2	40.1
78	38.8	38.2	40.1
80	40.4	40.0	42.8
N	338	—	310

22-5 outlines the results from six studies that looked at race as a factor in the assessment of gestational age by femur length. Three of the six studies compared their data with previously published charts—none of these studies found that race was a significant factor in assessing gestational age from femur length. The study of Ruvolo et al[15] only examined fetuses between 19 and 32 completed weeks' gestation. The two largest studies that compared subpopulations within their study found a significant difference between races in gestational age assessment from femur length. Ethnic differences seem to be absent prior to 20 weeks' gestation.[13] The difference in femur lengths between races is less than the variability estimates for menstrual

Table 22-3	Variability (±SD) (wks) in predicting menstrual age from femur length		
Gestational Age (wks)	Jeanty[4]	Hadlock[3]	Benson[22]
12-18	2.8	±1.0	1.4
18-24	2.8	±1.8	2.5
24-30	2.8	±2.0	—
30-36	2.8	±2.4	3.1
36-42	2.8	±3.2	3.5

Table 22-4	Percentile values of fetal femur length from the 3rd through 97th percentile for given menstrual ages (wks)				
Menstrual Week	Femur Length (cm)				
	3rd	10th	50th	90th	97th
14	1.2	1.3	1.4	2.5	1.6
15	1.5	1.6	1.7	1.9	1.9
16	1.7	1.8	2.0	2.2	2.3
17	2.1	2.2	2.4	2.6	2.7
18	2.3	2.5	2.7	2.9	3.1
19	2.6	2.7	3.0	3.3	3.4
20	2.8	3.0	3.3	3.6	3.8
21	3.0	3.2	3.5	3.8	4.0
22	3.3	3.5	3.8	4.1	4.3
23	3.5	3.7	4.1	4.5	4.7
24	3.8	4.0	4.4	4.8	5.0
25	4.0	4.2	4.6	5.0	5.2
26	4.2	4.5	4.9	5.3	5.6
27	4.4	4.6	5.1	5.6	5.8
28	4.6	4.9	5.4	5.9	6.2
29	4.8	5.1	5.6	6.1	6.4
30	5.0	5.3	5.8	6.3	6.6
31	5.2	5.5	6.0	6.5	6.8
32	5.3	5.6	6.2	6.8	7.1
33	5.5	5.8	6.4	7.0	7.3
34	5.7	6.0	6.6	7.2	7.5
35	5.9	6.2	6.8	7.4	7.8
36	6.0	6.4	7.0	7.6	8.0
37	6.2	6.6	7.2	7.9	8.2
38	6.4	6.7	7.4	8.1	8.4
39	6.5	6.8	7.5	8.2	8.6
40	6.6	7.0	7.7	8.4	8.8

From Callen PW (ed): Ultrasonography in Obstetrics and Gynecology, 3rd ed. Philadelphia, W.B. Saunders, 1994. Adapted from Hadlock FP, Deter RL, Harrist RB, Park SK: Estimating fetal age: computer-assisted analysis of multiple fetal growth parameters. Radiology 1984;152:497-501.

age. However, the difference may be significant enough to consider incorporating race into the assessment of gestational age by femur length in the third trimester.[16]

Other Long Bones

INTRODUCTION

Any of the long bones can be used to assess fetal age. The percentile values for menstrual age have also been established. These data are helpful in the evaluation of fetuses with a suspected skeletal dysplasia.

MATERIALS/METHODS

The long bone diaphysis should be measured with the transducer aligned perpendicular to the long axis of the bone. This method is identical to that used to measure the femoral length (see Fig. 22-1).

DISCUSSION

The determination of menstrual age from the humerus, ulna, and tibia is provided in Tables 22-6, 22-7, and 22-8.[4,16-18] Table 22-9 compares three cross-sectional studies that estimated menstrual age from the length of the humerus, radius, and ulna (Fig. 22-3).[4,17,18] Despite the different populations studied and advances in ultrasound technology over the 18 years that spanned the three investigations, the 50th percentile values are strikingly similar.

Zelop et al[19] compared humeral length at different menstrual ages in 4202 African-American, 2269 Hispanic, 639 Asian, and 4168 white fetuses. Race and ethnicity did not affect the humeral length between 15 and 22 weeks' gestation. Chervenak et al[20] have previously shown that most formulas are accurate across populations in the second trimester.

The 50th percentile for the radius length (see Fig. 22-3) by three different authors is outlined

Table 22-5 | Evaluation of race as a factor in femur length assessment of menstrual age

Author	Ref	N	Study Design	Significant Difference
Davis	14	2831	1743—1 exam; 1088—≥2 exams; populations compared in study	Yes
Jacquemyn	13	524	Cross-sectional; populations compared in study	Yes
Humphrey	12	192	Longitudinal; populations compared in study	No
Arenson	11	126	Longitudinal; compared with published charts	No
Westerway	10	3135	Cross-sectional; compared with published charts	No
Ruvolo	15	314	Cross-sectional; compared with published charts	No

Table 22-6 | The 5th through 95th percentiles for given menstrual ages (wks) for humeral length (mm)

Bone Length (mm)	Humerus Percentile			Bone Length (mm)	Humerus Percentile		
	5th	50th	95th		5th	50th	95th
10	9 + 6	12 + 4	15 + 2	40	21 + 4	24 + 2	27 + 1
11	10 + 1	12 + 6	15 + 4	41	22	24 + 6	27 + 4
12	10 + 3	13 + 1	15 + 6	42	22 + 4	25 + 2	28
13	10 + 6	13 + 4	16 + 1	43	23	25 + 5	28 + 4
14	11 + 1	13 + 6	16 + 4	44	23 + 4	26 + 1	29
15	11 + 3	14 + 1	16 + 6	45	24	26 + 5	29 + 4
16	11 + 6	14 + 4	17 + 2	46	24 + 4	27 + 1	30
17	12 + 1	14 + 6	17 + 4	47	25	27 + 5	30 + 4
18	12 + 4	15 + 1	18	48	25 + 4	28 + 1	31
19	12 + 6	15 + 4	18 + 2	49	26	28 + 6	31 + 4
20	13 + 1	15 + 6	18 + 5	50	26 + 4	29 + 2	32
21	13 + 4	16 + 2	19 + 1	51	27 + 1	29 + 6	32 + 4
22	13 + 6	16 + 5	19 + 3	52	27 + 4	30 + 2	33 + 1
23	14 + 2	17 + 1	19 + 6	53	28 + 1	30 + 6	33 + 4
24	14 + 5	17 + 3	20 + 1	54	28 + 5	31 + 3	34 + 1
25	15 + 1	17 + 6	20 + 4	55	29 + 1	32	34 + 5
26	15 + 4	18 + 1	21	56	29 + 6	32 + 4	35 + 2
27	15 + 6	18 + 4	21 + 3	57	30 + 2	33 + 1	35 + 6
28	16 + 2	19	21 + 6	58	30 + 6	33 + 4	36 + 3
29	16 + 5	19 + 3	22 + 1	59	31 + 3	34 + 1	36 + 6
30	17 + 1	19 + 6	22 + 4	60	32	34 + 6	37 + 4
31	17 + 4	20 + 2	23	61	32 + 4	35 + 2	38 + 1
32	18	20 + 5	23 + 4	62	33 + 1	35 + 6	38 + 5
33	18 + 3	21 + 1	23 + 6	63	33 + 6	36 + 4	39 + 2
34	18 + 6	21 + 4	24 + 2	64	34 + 3	37 + 1	39 + 6
35	19 + 2	22	24 + 6	65	35	37 + 5	40 + 4
36	19 + 5	22 + 4	25 + 1	66	35 + 4	38 + 2	41 + 1
37	20 + 1	22 + 6	25 + 5	67	36 + 1	38 + 6	41 + 5
38	20 + 4	23 + 3	26 + 1	68	36 + 6	39 + 4	42 + 2
39	21 + 1	23 + 6	26 + 4	69	37 + 3	40 + 1	42 + 6

From Jeanty P, Rodesch F, Delbeke D, Dumont JE: Estimation of gestational age from measurements of fetal long bones. J Ultrasound Med 1984;3:75-79.

| Table 22-7 | The 5th through 95th percentiles for given menstrual ages (wks + days) for ulna length (mm) |

Bone Length (mm)	Ulna Percentile			Bone Length (mm)	Ulna Percentile		
	5th	50th	95th		5th	50th	95th
10	10 + 1	13 + 1	16 + 1	38	22 + 1	25 + 1	28 + 1
11	10 + 4	13 + 4	16 + 4	39	22 + 4	25 + 4	28 + 5
12	10 + 6	13 + 6	16 + 6	40	23 + 1	26 + 1	29 + 1
13	11 + 1	14 + 1	17 + 2	41	23 + 4	26 + 5	29 + 5
14	11 + 4	14 + 4	17 + 5	42	24 + 1	27 + 1	30 + 2
15	11 + 6	15	18	43	24 + 5	27 + 5	30 + 6
16	12 + 2	15 + 3	18 + 3	44	25 + 1	28 + 2	31 + 2
17	12 + 5	15 + 5	18 + 6	45	25 + 6	28 + 6	31 + 6
18	13 + 1	16 + 1	19 + 1	46	26 + 2	29 + 3	32 + 3
19	13 + 4	16 + 4	19 + 4	47	26 + 6	29 + 6	33
20	13 + 6	16 + 6	20	48	27 + 3	30 + 4	33 + 4
21	14 + 2	17 + 2	20 + 3	49	28	31 + 1	34 + 1
22	14 + 5	17 + 5	20 + 6	50	28 + 4	31 + 4	34 + 5
23	15 + 1	18 + 1	21 + 1	51	29 + 1	32 + 1	35 + 2
24	15 + 4	18 + 4	21 + 4	52	29 + 5	32 + 6	35 + 6
25	16	19	22 + 1	53	30 + 2	33 + 3	36 + 3
26	16 + 3	19 + 3	22 + 4	54	30 + 6	34	37
27	16 + 6	19 + 6	22 + 6	55	31 + 4	34 + 4	37 + 5
28	17 + 2	20 + 2	23 + 3	56	32 + 1	35 + 1	38 + 2
29	17 + 5	20 + 6	23 + 6	57	32 + 6	35 + 6	38 + 6
30	18 + 1	21 + 1	24 + 2	58	33 + 3	36 + 3	39 + 4
31	18 + 4	21 + 5	24 + 6	59	34	37 + 1	40 + 1
32	19 + 1	22 + 1	25 + 1	60	34 + 4	37 + 5	40 + 6
33	19 + 4	22 + 5	25 + 5	61	35 + 2	38 + 2	41 + 3
34	20 + 1	23 + 1	26 + 1	62	35 + 6	39	42
35	20 + 4	23 + 4	26 + 5	63	36 + 4	39 + 4	42 + 5
36	21 + 1	24 + 1	27 + 1	64	37 + 1	40 + 2	43 + 2
37	21 + 4	24 + 4	27 + 5				

From Jeanty P, Rodesch F, Delbeke D, Dumont JE: Estimation of gestational age from measurements of fetal long bones. J Ultrasound Med 1984;3:75-79.

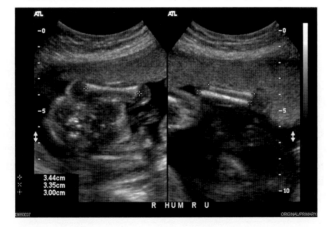

Figure 22-3
20 weeks' menstrual age. Humeral length (left) (+ . . . . +) Radius length (right) (+ . . . . +) Ulnar length (right) (x . . . . . x).

Table 22-8	The 5th through 95th percentiles for given menstrual ages (wks + days) for tibial length (mm)							

Bone Length (mm)	Tibia Percentile			Bone Length (mm)	Tibia Percentile		
	5th	50th	95th		5th	50th	95th
10	10 + 4	13 + 3	16 + 2	40	22 + 3	25 + 2	28 + 1
11	10 + 6	13 + 5	16 + 4	41	22 + 6	25 + 5	28 + 4
12	11 + 1	14 + 1	17	42	23 + 2	26 + 1	29 + 1
13	11 + 4	14 + 3	17 + 2	43	23 + 5	26 + 4	29 + 4
14	11 + 6	14 + 6	17 + 5	44	24 + 1	27 + 1	30
15	12 + 1	15 + 1	18	45	24 + 4	27 + 4	30 + 4
16	12 + 4	15 + 4	18 + 3	46	25 + 1	28	30 + 6
17	13	15 + 6	18 + 6	47	25 + 4	28 + 4	31 + 3
18	13 + 2	16 + 1	19 + 1	48	26 + 1	29	31 + 6
19	13 + 5	16 + 4	19 + 4	49	26 + 4	29 + 3	32 + 2
20	14 + 1	17	19 + 6	50	27	29 + 6	32 + 6
21	14 + 4	17 + 3	20 + 2	51	27 + 4	30 + 3	33 + 2
22	14 + 6	17 + 6	20 + 5	52	28	30 + 6	33 + 6
23	15 + 1	18 + 1	21 + 1	53	28 + 4	31 + 3	34 + 2
24	15 + 4	18 + 4	21 + 3	54	29	31 + 6	34 + 6
25	16	18 + 6	21 + 6	55	29 + 4	32 + 3	35 + 2
26	16 + 3	19 + 2	22 + 1	56	30	32 + 6	35 + 6
27	16 + 6	19 + 5	22 + 4	57	30 + 4	33 + 3	36 + 2
28	17 + 1	20 + 1	23	58	31	33 + 6	36 + 6
29	17 + 4	20 + 4	23 + 4	59	31 + 4	34 + 3	37 + 2
30	18 + 1	21	23 + 6	60	32	34 + 6	37 + 6
31	18 + 4	21 + 3	24 + 2	61	32 + 4	35 + 3	38 + 2
32	18 + 6	21 + 6	24 + 5	62	33	35 + 6	38 + 6
33	19 + 2	22 + 1	25 + 1	63	33 + 4	36 + 4	39 + 3
34	19 + 5	22 + 4	25 + 4	64	34 + 1	37	39 + 6
35	20 + 1	23 + 1	26	65	34 + 4	37 + 4	40 + 3
36	20 + 4	23 + 4	26 + 3	66	35 + 1	38	41
37	21	23 + 6	26 + 6	67	35 + 5	38 + 4	41 + 4
38	21 + 4	24 + 3	27 + 2	68	36 + 1	39 + 1	42
39	21 + 6	24 + 6	27 + 5	69	36 + 6	39 + 5	42 + 4

From Jeanty P, Rodesch F, Delbeke D, Dumont JE: Estimation of gestational age from measurements of fetal long bones. J Ultrasound Med 1984;3:75-79.

in Table 22-10. All three studies were cross-sectional. All of the radius lengths for menstrual age are within 3 mm. Hill et al[16] reported that the slopes for Caucasian and African-American study groups were distinctly different—a 10-day difference in gestational age assessment was noted in the third trimester (Table 22-11). Although this difference lies below the variability of radius length for gestational age, it was felt by the authors to be significant enough to warrant incorporating race into the assessment of menstrual age by radius length. Long bone measurement in percentiles versus gestational age in weeks is presented in Table 22-12.

Table 22-9	Different authors' measurement of the 50th percentile (mm) for a given menstrual age (in wks)								
	50th Percentile (mm)								
Menstrual Age (wks)	**Humerus**			**Ulna**			**Tibia**		
	Jeanty[4]	Chitty[17]	Merz[18]	Jeanty[4]	Chitty[17]	Merz[18]	Jeanty[4]	Chitty[17]	Merz[18]
12	—	7.1	—	—	7.3	—	—	7.6	—
14	15	14.1	12	13	12.4	10	12	11.4	10
16	21	20.4	17	18	18.2	16	18	16.9	16
18	26	26.2	23	23	24.0	22	23	22.8	22
20	31	31.5	29	27	29.4	27	28	28.5	27
22	35	36.3	33	32	34.4	31	33	33.8	32
24	40	40.7	38	35	38.8	36	37	38.8	37
26	44	44.8	43	40	42.8	40	42	43.2	42
28	48	48.5	47	44	46.5	44	46	47.3	45
30	52	51.9	50	47	49.8	47	50	51.0	48
32	55	55.0	54	51	52.7	50	54	54.4	52
34	59	57.8	58	54	55.4	54	58	57.5	57
36	62	60.3	60	57	57.9	55	62	60.3	60
38	66	62.6	64	60	60.2	58	66	62.9	62
40	69	64.7	66	64	62.2	60	69	65.2	65
N	—	663	530	—	663	530	—	663	530

Table 22-10	50th percentile for radius length (mm) by different authors for a given menstrual age (in weeks)		
Menstrual Age (wks)	**Hill[16]**	**Chitty[17]**	**Merz[18]**
12	—	5.5	—
14	10.0	11.0	8.0
16	16.0	16.7	14.0
18	21.0	21.9	19.0
20	25.5	26.7	24.0
22	30.0	30.9	28.0
24	33.5	34.7	33.0
26	37.0	38.1	36.0
28	40.0	41.2	39.0
30	43.5	43.9	41.0
32	46.0	46.4	44.0
34	49.0	48.6	47.0
36	51.5	50.6	49.0
38	53.5	52.5	51.0
40	56.0	54.2	53.0
N	353	663	530

Table 22-11	Menstrual age for 5th, 50th, and 95th percentile prediction intervals for radius length in a Caucasian population (values for African-Americans in parentheses)		
Radius (cm)	**5th Percentile**	**50th Percentile**	**95th Percentile**
0.6	11.7 (12.3)	12.9 (12.9)	14.3 (13.6)
0.7	11.9 (12.6)	13.2 (13.2)	14.6 (13.9)
0.8	12.2 (12.9)	13.5 (13.5)	15.0 (14.2)
0.9	12.5 (13.1)	13.8 (13.8)	15.4 (14.5)
1.0	12.7 (13.4)	14.2 (14.1)	15.7 (14.8)
1.1	13.0 (13.7)	14.5 (14.4)	16.1 (15.1)
1.2	13.3 (14.0)	14.8 (14.7)	16.4 (15.5)
1.3	13.6 (14.3)	15.1 (15.1)	16.8 (15.8)
1.4	13.9 (14.7)	15.5 (15.4)	17.2 (16.2)
1.5	14.3 (15.0)	15.8 (15.7)	17.6 (16.5)
1.6	14.6 (15.3)	16.2 (16.1)	18.0 (16.9)
1.7	14.9 (15.7)	16.6 (16.4)	18.4 (17.2)
1.8	15.3 (16.0)	17.0 (16.8)	18.8 (17.6)
1.9	15.6 (16.4)	17.3 (17.2)	19.3 (18.0)
2.0	16.0 (16.7)	17.7 (17.5)	19.7 (18.4)
2.1	16.3 (17.1)	18.1 (17.9)	20.1 (18.8)
2.2	16.7 (17.5)	18.6 (18.3)	20.6 (19.3)
2.3	17.1 (17.8)	19.0 (18.7)	21.0 (19.7)
2.4	17.5 (18.2)	19.4 (19.2)	21.5 (20.1)
2.5	17.9 (18.6)	19.9 (19.6)	22.0 (20.6)
2.6	18.3 (19.1)	20.3 (20.0)	22.5 (21.0)
2.7	18.7 (19.5)	20.8 (20.5)	23.1 (21.5)
2.8	19.1 (19.6)	21.2 (20.9)	23.5 (22.0)
2.9	19.6 (20.3)	21.7 (21.4)	24.1 (22.4)
3.0	20.0 (20.8)	22.2 (21.9)	24.7 (22.9)
3.1	20.5 (21.3)	22.7 (22.3)	25.2 (23.4)
3.2	20.9 (21.7)	23.2 (22.8)	25.8 (24.0)
3.3	21.4 (22.2)	23.8 (23.3)	26.4 (24.5)
3.4	21.9 (22.7)	24.3 (23.8)	27.0 (25.0)
3.5	22.4 (23.2)	24.9 (24.4)	27.6 (25.6)
3.6	22.9 (23.7)	25.5 (24.9)	28.3 (26.2)
3.7	23.5 (24.2)	26.0 (25.5)	28.9 (26.7)
3.8	24.0 (24.8)	26.6 (26.0)	29.6 (27.3)
3.9	24.5 (25.3)	27.2 (26.6)	30.2 (27.9)
4.0	25.1 (25.9)	27.9 (27.2)	30.9 (28.6)
4.1	25.7 (26.5)	28.5 (27.8)	31.6 (29.2)
4.2	26.3 (27.0)	29.1 (28.4)	32.4 (29.8)
4.3	26.9 (27.6)	29.8 (29.0)	33.1 (30.5)
4.4	27.5 (28.2)	30.5 (29.7)	33.9 (31.2)
4.5	28.1 (28.9)	31.2 (30.3)	34.6 (31.9)
4.6	28.7 (29.5)	31.9 (31.0)	35.4 (32.6)
4.7	29.4 (30.2)	32.6 (31.7)	36.2 (33.3)
4.8	30.1 (30.8)	33.4 (32.4)	37.1 (34.0)
4.9	30.7 (31.5)	34.1 (33.1)	37.9 (34.8)
5.0	31.4 (32.2)	34.9 (33.8)	38.8 (35.5)
5.1	32.2 (32.9)	35.7 (34.6)	39.7 (36.3)
5.2	32.9 (33.6)	36.5 (35.3)	40.5 (37.1)
5.3	33.6 (34.4)	37.4 (36.1)	41.5 (38.0)
5.4	34.4 (35.1)	38.2 (36.9)	42.5 (38.8)
5.5	35.2 (35.9)	39.1 (37.7)	43.4 (39.7)
5.6	36.0 (36.7)	40.0 (38.6)	44.4 (40.5)
5.7	36.8 (37.5)	40.9 (39.4)	45.4 (41.4)
5.8	— (38.3)	— (40.3)	— (42.2)

From Hill LM, Guzick D, Thomas ML, Fries JK: Fetal radius length: a critical evaluation of race as a factor in gestational age assessment. Am J Obstet Gynecol 1989;161:193-199.

Table 22-12	Reference values of major long bones								
	Femur (mm)[a]			**Tibia (mm)**[b]			**Fibuia (mm)**[c]		
	Percentiles			**Percentiles**			**Percentiles**		
GA (wk)	**5th**	**50th**	**95th**	**5th**	**50th**	**95th**	**5th**	**50th**	**95th**
12	3.9	8.1	12.3	3.3	7.2	11.2	1.7	5.7	9.6
13	6.8	11.0	15.2	5.6	9.6	13.6	4.7	8.7	12.7
14	9.7	13.9	18.1	8.1	12.0	16.0	7.7	11.7	15.6
15	12.6	16.8	21.0	10.6	14.6	18.6	10.6	14.6	18.6
16	15.4	19.7	23.9	13.1	17.1	21.2	13.3	17.4	21.4
17	18.3	22.5	26.8	15.6	19.7	23.8	16.1	20.1	24.2
18	21.1	25.4	29.7	18.2	22.3	26.4	18.7	22.8	26.9
19	23.9	28.2	32.6	20.8	24.9	29.0	21.3	25.4	29.5
20	26.7	31.0	35.4	23.3	27.5	31.6	23.8	27.9	32.0
21	29.4	33.8	38.2	25.8	30.0	34.2	26.2	30.3	34.5
22	32.1	36.5	40.9	28.3	32.5	36.7	28.5	32.7	36.9
23	34.7	39.2	43.6	30.7	34.9	39.1	30.8	35.0	39.2
24	37.4	41.8	46.3	33.1	37.3	41.6	33.0	37.2	41.5
25	39.9	44.4	48.9	35.4	39.7	43.9	35.1	39.4	43.6
26	42.4	46.9	51.4	37.6	41.9	46.2	37.2	41.5	45.7
27	44.9	49.4	53.9	39.8	44.1	48.4	39.2	43.5	47.8
28	47.3	51.8	56.4	41.9	46.2	50.5	41.1	45.4	49.7
29	49.6	54.2	58.7	43.9	48.2	52.6	42.9	47.2	51.6
30	51.8	56.4	61.0	45.8	50.1	54.5	44.7	49.0	53.4
31	54.0	58.6	63.2	47.6	52.0	56.4	46.3	50.7	55.1
32	56.1	60.7	65.4	49.4	53.8	58.2	47.9	52.4	56.8
33	58.1	62.7	67.4	51.1	55.5	60.0	49.5	53.9	58.4
34	60.0	64.7	69.4	52.7	57.2	61.6	50.9	55.4	59.9
35	61.8	66.5	71.2	54.2	58.7	63.2	52.3	56.8	61.3
36	63.5	68.3	73.0	55.8	60.3	64.8	53.6	58.2	62.7
37	65.1	69.9	74.7	57.2	61.8	66.3	54.9	59.4	64.0
38	66.6	71.4	76.2	58.7	63.2	67.8	56.0	60.6	65.2
39	68.0	72.8	77.7	60.1	64.7	69.3	57.1	61.7	66.3
40	69.3	74.2	79.0	61.5	66.1	70.7	58.1	62.8	67.4

Table 22-12	Reference values of major long bones—cont'd								
	Humerus (mm)[d]			Radius (mm)[e]			Ulna (mm)[f]		
	Percentiles			Percentiles			Percentiles		
GA (wk)	5th	50th	95th	5th	50th	95th	5th	50th	95th
12	4.8	8.6	12.3	3.0	6.9	10.8	2.9	6.8	10.7
13	7.6	11.4	15.1	5.6	9.5	13.4	5.8	9.7	13.7
14	10.3	14.1	17.9	8.1	12.0	16.0	8.6	12.6	16.6
15	13.1	16.9	20.7	10.5	14.5	18.5	11.4	15.4	19.4
16	15.8	19.7	23.5	12.9	16.9	20.9	14.1	18.1	22.1
17	18.5	22.4	26.3	15.2	19.3	23.3	16.7	20.8	24.8
18	21.2	25.1	29.0	17.5	21.5	25.6	19.3	23.3	27.4
19	23.8	27.7	31.6	19.7	23.8	27.9	21.8	25.8	29.9
20	26.3	30.3	34.2	21.8	25.9	30.0	24.2	28.3	32.4
21	28.8	32.8	36.7	23.9	28.0	32.2	26.5	30.6	34.8
22	31.2	35.2	39.2	25.9	30.1	34.2	28.7	32.9	37.1
23	33.5	37.5	41.6	27.9	32.0	36.2	30.9	35.1	39.3
24	35.7	39.8	43.8	29.7	34.0	38.2	33.0	37.2	41.5
25	37.9	41.9	46.0	31.6	35.8	40.0	35.1	39.3	43.5
26	39.9	44.0	48.1	33.3	37.6	41.9	37.0	41.3	45.6
27	41.9	46.0	50.1	35.0	39.3	43.6	38.9	43.2	47.5
28	43.7	47.9	52.0	36.7	41.0	45.3	40.7	45.0	49.3
29	45.5	49.7	53.9	38.3	42.6	46.9	42.5	46.8	51.1
30	47.2	51.4	55.6	39.8	44.1	48.5	44.1	48.5	52.8
31	48.9	53.1	57.3	41.2	45.6	50.0	45.7	50.1	54.5
32	50.4	54.7	58.9	42.6	47.0	51.4	47.2	51.6	56.1
33	52.0	56.2	60.5	44.0	48.4	52.8	48.7	53.1	57.5
34	53.4	57.7	62.0	45.2	49.7	54.1	50.0	54.5	59.0
35	54.8	59.2	63.5	46.4	50.9	55.4	51.3	55.8	60.3
36	56.2	60.6	64.9	47.6	52.1	56.6	52.6	57.1	61.6
37	57.6	62.0	66.4	48.7	53.2	57.7	53.7	58.2	62.8
38	59.0	63.4	67.8	49.7	54.2	58.8	54.8	59.3	63.9
39	60.4	64.8	69.3	50.6	55.2	59.8	55.8	60.4	64.9
40	61.9	66.3	70.8	51.5	56.2	60.8	56.7	61.3	65.9

GA, gestational age.

*Femur (mean) = −25.252 + 2.555 × GA + 0.027566 × GA² − 0.00073286 × GA³ (Jeanty et al., 1984).

*Tibia (mean) = 5.555 − 0.915554 × GA + 0.23359 × GA² − 0.00638 × GA³ + 0.000055801 × GA⁴ (Jeanty et al., 1984).

*Fibula (mean) = −36.563 + 3.963 × GA − 0.037 × GA² (Exacoustos et al., 1991).

*Humerus (mean) = −16.24 + 0.76315 × GA + 0.1683 × GA² − 0.0056212 × GA³ + 0.000055666 × GA⁴.

*Radius (mean) = −29.09 + 3.371 × GA − 0.031 × GA² (Exacoustos et al., 1991).

*Ulna (mean) = −34.313 + 3.8685 × GA − 0.036949 × GA² (Jeanty et al., 1984).

Derived from compilation of data: Jeanty P, Cousaert E, Cantraine F, Hobbins JC, Tack B, et al. A longitudinal study of fetal limb growth. Am J Perinatol 1984;1:136–144; Merz E, Grubner A, Kern F. Mathematical modeling of fetal limb growth. J Clin Ultrasound 1989;17:179–185; and Exacoustos C, Rosati P, Rizzo G, Arduini D. Ultrasound measurements of fetal limb bones. Ultrasound Obstet Gynecol 1991;1:325–330.

From Diagnostic Imaging of Fetal Anomalies; Nyberg DA, McGahan JP, Pretorius DH, Pilu G; Lippincott Williams & Wilkins, 2003.

References

1. Abramowicz J, Jaffe R: Comparison between lateral and axial ultrasonic measurements of the fetal femur. Am J Obstet Gynecol 1988;159:921-922.
2. Lessoway VA, Schulzer M, Wittman BK: Sonographic measurement of the fetal femur: factors affecting accuracy. J Clin Ultrasound 1990;18:471-476.
3. Hadlock FP, Harrist RB, Deter RL: Fetal femur length as a predictor of menstrual age: sonographically measured. Am J Roentgenol 1982;138:875-878.
4. Jeanty P, Rodesch F, Delbeke D: Estimation of gestational age from measurements of fetal long bones. J Ultrasound Med 1984; 3:75-79.
5. Hohler CW, Quetel TA: Fetal femur length: equation for computer calculation of gestational age from ultrasound measurements. Am J Obstet Gynecol 1982;143:479-481.
6. Altman DG, Chitty LS: Chart of fetal size: 1. Methodology. Br J Obstet Gynaecol 1994;101:29-34.
7. Warda AH, Deter RL, Rossavik IK, et al: Fetal femur length: a critical re-evaluation of the relationship to menstrual age. Obstet Gynecol 1985;66:69-75.
8. Hohler CW, Quetel TA: Comparison of ultrasound femur length and biparietal diameter in late pregnancy. Am J Obstet Gynecol 1981;141:759-762.
9. Hadlock FP, Deter RL, Harrist RB, et al: A date-independent predictor of intrauterine growth retardation: femur length/abdominal circumference ratio. Am J Roentgenol 1983;141:979-984.
10. Westerway SC, Davison A, Cowell S: Ultrasonic fetal measurements: new Australian standards for the new millennium. Aust NZ J Obstet Gynaecol 2000;40:297-302.
11. Arenson AM, Chan P-L, Withers C, et al: Value of standardized gestational age charts for fetuses of first-generation Oriental immigrants to Canada. Can Assoc Radiol J 1995;46:111-113.
12. Humphrey M, Holzheimer D: Fetal growth charts for Aboriginal fetuses. Aust NZ J Obstet Gynaecol 2000;40:388-393.
13. Jacquemyn Y, Sys SU, Vendonk P: Fetal biometry in different ethnic groups. Early Human Devel 2000;57:1-13.
14. Davis RD, Cutter GR, Goldenberg RL, et al: Fetal biparietal diameter, head circumference and femur length. A comparison by race and sex. J Reprod Med 1993;38:201-206.
15. Ruvolo KA, Filly RA, Callen PW: Evaluation of fetal femur length for prediction of gestational age in a racially mixed obstetric population. J Ultrasound Med 1987;6:417-419.
16. Hill LM, Guzick D, Thomas ML, Fries JK: Fetal radius length: a critical evaluation of race as a factor in gestational age assessment. Am J Obstet Gynecol 1989;161:193-199.
17. Chitty LS, Altman DG: Chart of fetal size: limb bones. Br J Obstet Gynaecol 2002; 109:919-929.
18. Merz E, Kim-Kern M-S, Pehl S: Ultrasonic menstruation of fetal limb bones in the second and third trimesters. J Clin Ultrasound 1987;15:175-183.
19. Zelop CM, Borgida AF, Egan JFX: Variation of fetal humeral length in second-trimester fetuses according to race and ethnicity. J Ultrasound Med 2003;22:691-693.
20. Chervenak FA, Skupski DW, Romero R, et al: How accurate is fetal biometry in the assessment of fetal age? Am J Obstet Gynecol 1998;178:678-687.
21. Callen PW: Ultrasonography in Obstetrics and Gynecology, 3rd ed. Philadelphia, WB Saunders Company, 1994. Modified from Hadlock FP, Harrist RB, Deter RL: Fetal femur length as a predictor of menstrual age: sonographically measured. Am J Roentgenol 1982;138:875-878.
22. Benson CB, Doubilet PM: Sonographic prediction of gestational age: accuracy of second- and third-trimester fetal measurements. Am J Roentgenol 1991;157:1275-1277.

Fetal Mandible

Introduction

Mandibular anomalies are present in more than 100 genetic syndromes.[1] It is important to distinguish between a recessed chin (retrognathia) and a chin that is too small (micrognathia). Sixty-six percent of cases with micrognathia have been associated with chromosomal abnormalities.[2] Even in chromosomally normal fetuses, the outcome is quite poor with few survivors.[2] However, the data from which these outcome statistics are derived may have included only the most severe cases that are subjectively apparent. With the advent of the mandibular measurements outlined below, more subtle cases with better outcomes will be detected. Hence, the percent of micrognathic fetuses with chromosomal abnormalities, as well as the perinatal mortality, will decline. Polyhydramnios has been reported in 70% of cases of micrognathia after 21 to 22 weeks' gestation.[3]

Materials/Methods

A number of different sonographic measurements have been used to define micrognathia:

1. Mandibular length.
2. Anteroposterior and transverse mandibular measurement compared with menstrual age norms.
3. Jaw index: anteroposterior mandibular diameter divided by biparietal diameter (<23 = microganthia).
4. Mandibular width divided by maxillary width (<0.785 = micrognathia).

DISCUSSION

Chitty et al[4] measured the mandible in a plane that visualized one ramus of the jaw, so the ultrasound beam was at right angles to the jaw (Fig. 23-1). They developed percentiles for menstrual age (Table 23-1). Beyond 28 weeks' menstrual age, it became difficult to obtain a reliable measurement. The mandibular lengths reported by Otto and Platt[5] are nearly identical (Table 23-2).

Watson and Katz[6] measured the anteroposterior and transverse mandible measurements with the hypopharynx as a reference point (Fig. 23-2). They felt that this measurement was more reliable than attempting to accurately measure the length of the mandible.

The jaw index is calculated by dividing the anteroposterior mandibular diameter (see Fig. 23-2) by the biparietal diameter. A jaw index less than 23 in one study had a 100% sensitiv-

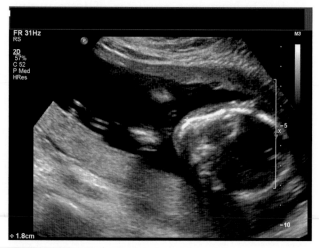

Figure 23-1
Mandibular jaw length.

Table 23-1	Mean mandibular measurements with fitted 2nd, 50th, and 97th percentiles from 12 to 28 weeks' menstrual age (exact weeks)		
	Percentile		
Gestation (wks)	**2nd (mm)**	**50th (mm)**	**97th (mm)**
12	6.3	8.0	9.7
13	8.2	10.2	12.3
14	10.0	12.4	14.7
15	11.7	14.4	17.2
16	13.4	16.4	19.5
17	15.0	18.4	21.8
18	16.5	20.2	24.0
19	18.0	22.1	26.2
20	19.4	23.9	28.3
21	20.8	25.6	30.4
22	22.2	27.3	32.4
23	23.5	28.9	34.4
24	24.8	30.6	36.4
25	26.0	32.2	38.3
26	27.3	33.7	40.2
27	28.4	35.2	42.1
28	29.6	36.7	43.9

From Chitty LS, Campbell S, Altman DG: Measurement of the fetal mandible—feasibility and construction of a percentile chart. Prenat Diagn 1993;13:749-756.

Table 23-2	Mean mandibular length (mm) based on menstrual age	
Menstrual Age (wks)	**Otto[5]**	**Chitty[4]**
14	12	12
15	14	14
16	16	16
17	19	18
18	21	20
19	23	22
20	25	24
21	26	26
22	28	27
23	30	29
24	32	31
25	33	32
26	35	34
27	37	35
28	38	37

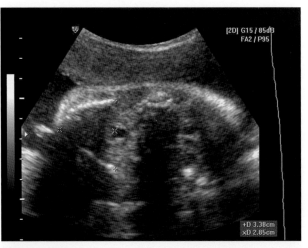

Figure 23-2
Anteroposterior (x . . . x) and transverse (+ . . . .+) mandibular measurements with the hypopharynx as a reference point.

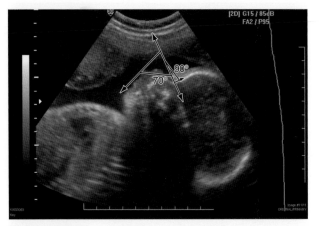

Figure 23-3
Sagittal view of the fetal face showing an inferior facial angle of 70 degrees.

ity and a 68.7% positive predictive value for the diagnosis of micrognathia.[7]

Rotten et al[8] proposed using an inferior facial angle (Fig. 23-3) of less than 50° between 18 and 28 weeks' menstrual age to define retrognathia. These authors defined micrognathia as a mandibular width/maxillary width ratio during the same menstrual age interval of less than 0.785. The inferior facial angle (IFA) was obtained on a sagittal view by the crossing of (1) a line orthogonal to the vertical part of the forehead drawn at the synostosis of the nasal bone and (2) a line joining the tip of the mentum and the anterior border of the most protrusive lip (Fig. 23-4). Because two defined points are not available for the line orthogonal to the forehead, this angle is consistently difficult to reproduce. By using a

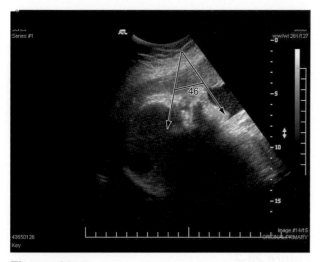

Figure 23-4
Sagittal view of a fetal face with micrognathia
(inferior facial angle: 46 degrees).

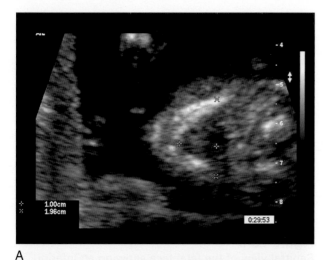

A

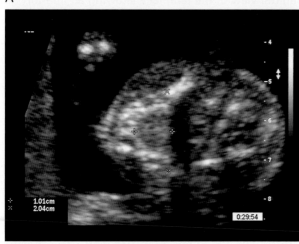

B

Figure 23-5
Axial view of the fetal jaw. **A,** Measuring the
mandibular width. **B,** Measuring the maxilla width.
The width of the mandible and maxilla are nearly
equal, indicating that micrognathia is not present.

line perpendicular to the forehead at the level of the synostosis of the nasal bone, the variation in drawing the IFA is reduced.

The mandibular (MD) (Fig. 23-5A) and maxillary (MX) (Fig. 23-5B) widths are measured on an axial plane. A line orthogonal to the sagittal axis is drawn 1 cm posteriorly to the anterior osseus border. The measurement is then made from one external bone table to the other. The MD/MX ratio is derived from these two measurements.

In an evaluation of 12 fetuses with mandible anomalies, the IFA had a specificity of 100% and a positive predictive value of 75%. The advantage of the technique proposed by Rotten et al[8] is the differentiation of retro- from micrognathia. The utilization of three-dimensional (3D) reconstructed views will reduce the amount of time required in obtaining the three images for a more detailed assessment of the fetal jaw. Additional studies will be required to confirm and extend the findings of Rotten et al.[8]

References

1. Jones KL: Smith's Recognizable Patterns of Human Malformation, 5th ed. London, WB Saunders, 1997.
2. Nicolaides KH, Salvesen DR, Snijders RJB, et al: Micrognathia fetal facial defects: associated malformations and chromosomal abnormalities. Fetal Diagn Ther 1993;8:1-9.
3. Bromley B, Benacerraf BR: Fetal micrognathia: associated anomalies and outcome. J Ultrasound Med 1994;13:529-533.
4. Chitty LS, Campbell S, Altman DG: Measurement of the fetal mandible-feasibility and construction of a centile chart. Prenat Diagn 1993;13:749-756.
5. Otto C, Platt LD: The fetal mandible measurement: an objective determination of fetal jaw size. Ultrasound Obstet Gynecol 1991;1: 12-17.
6. Watson WJ, Katz VL: Sonographic measurement of the fetal mandible: standards for normal pregnancy. Am J Perinatol 1993;10: 226-228.
7. Paladini D, Morra T, Teodoro A, et al: Objective diagnosis of micrognathia in the fetus. The jaw index. Obstet Gynecol 1999;93:382-386.
8. Rotten D, Levaillant JM, Martinez H, et al: The fetal mandible: a 2D and 3D sonographic approach to the diagnosis of retrognathia and micrognathia. Ultrasound Obstet Gynecol 2002;19:122-130.

Lyndon Hill

CHAPTER 24

Fetal Nasal Bone

Introduction

A number of "soft" markers have been used in an attempt to prenatally diagnose Down's syndrome. Flattening of the nasal profile is one acknowledged feature of Down's syndrome.

Several prenatal studies have therefore been undertaken to compare the nasal bone in Down's syndrome fetuses and controls.

Materials/Methods

A midsagittal profile must be obtained in order to measure the nasal bone. An off-axis fetal profile will produce an erroneous measurement. The nasal bone is measured from its base to its

tip (Figs. 24-1 and 24-2). Several studies have been performed to measure the fetal nose and are reproduced in Tables 24-1 and 24-2.

DISCUSSION

A flattening of the facial profile is an acknowledged feature of Down's syndrome. Keeling et al[1] evaluated radiographs of fetuses between 12 and 24 weeks' gestation and found that 19 of 31 (61%) fetuses with Down's syndrome had an absent or shortened nasal bone. Cicero et al[2] have reported that an absence of the nasal bone at 11 to 14 weeks' gestation has a sensitivity of 73% and a false positive rate of 0.5% for the detection of Down's syndrome (see Fig. 24-1).

The FASTER (First and Second Trimester Evaluation of Risk) Trial, a multi-institutional study in the United States, did not find the first trimester presence or absence of the nasal bone to be a useful tool for Down syndrome screening.[3] Additional first trimester studies using a standard protocol are therefore required.

The value of an absent or hypoplastic nasal bone in the second trimester detection of Down's syndrome has also been evaluated. Bromley

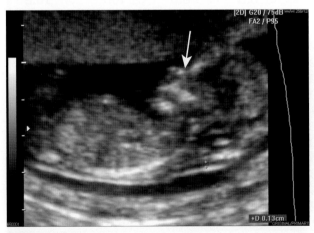

Figure 24-1
Fetal profile (13 weeks) with the nasal bone present (*arrow*).

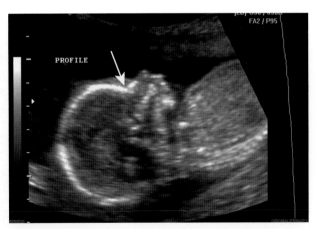

Figure 24-2
Fetal nasal bone at 19 weeks' menstrual age (*arrow*).

Table 24-1 Mean nasal bone length (mm), for a specific menstrual age (wks)

Author Country *N* Menstrual Age (wks)	Sonek[6] USA 3537	Chen[8] China 198	Guis[10] France 376	Bunduki[11] Brazil 1923
14	3.8	—	4.2	—
16	4.7	4.1	5.2	5.9
18	5.7	5.0	6.3	6.5
20	6.7	5.8	7.6	7.0
22	7.5	6.7	8.2	7.6
24	8.3	—	9.4	8.0
26	8.9	—	9.7	—
28	9.8	—	10.7	—
30	10.0	—	11.3	—
32	10.5	—	11.6	—
34	10.9	—	12.3	—

Table 24-2 Normal percentile ranges for nasal bone lengths (mm) (*n* = 3537) for a specific menstrual age (wks)

Gestational Age (wks)	Subjects (*n*)	Percentile				
		2.5th	5th	50th	95th	97.5th
11	16	1.3	1.4	2.3	3.3	3.4
12	54	1.7	1.8	2.8	4.2	4.3
13	59	2.2	2.3	3.1	4.6	4.8
14	82	2.2	2.5	3.8	5.3	5.7
15	103	2.8	3.0	4.3	5.7	6.0
16	134	3.2	3.4	4.7	6.2	6.2
17	203	3.7	4.0	5.3	6.6	6.9
18	252	4.0	4.3	5.7	7.0	7.3
19	388	4.6	5.0	6.3	7.9	8.2
20	440	5.0	5.2	6.7	8.3	8.6
21	322	5.1	5.6	7.1	9.0	9.3
22	208	5.6	5.8	7.5	9.3	10.2
23	157	6.0	6.4	7.9	9.6	9.9
24	121	6.6	6.8	9.3	10.0	10.3
25	123	6.3	6.5	8.5	10.7	10.8
26	96	6.8	7.4	8.9	10.9	11.3
27	80	7.0	7.5	9.2	11.3	11.6
28	103	7.2	7.6	9.8	12.1	13.4
29	95	7.2	7.7	9.8	11.8	12.3
30	104	7.3	7.9	10.0	12.6	13.2
31	92	7.9	8.2	10.4	12.6	13.2
32	66	8.1	8.6	10.5	13.6	13.7
33	54	8.6	8.7	10.8	12.8	13.0
34	41	9.0	9.1	10.9	12.8	13.5
35	37	7.5	8.5	11.0	14.1	15.0
36	40	7.3	7.8	10.8	12.8	13.6
37	36	8.4	8.7	11.4	14.5	15.0
38	13	9.2	9.3	11.7	15.7	16.6
39	12	9.1	9.2	10.9	14.0	14.8
40	6	10.3	10.4	12.1	14.5	14.7

From Sonek JD, McKenna D, Webb D, et al: Nasal bone length throughout gestation: normal ranges based on 3537 fetal ultrasound measurements. Ultrasound Obstet Gynecol 2003;21:152-155.

et al[4] found complete absence of the nasal bone in 6 of 16 (37%) second trimester Down's syndrome fetuses. There was an absent nasal bone in only 1 of 223 (0.5%) euploid fetuses. The likelihood ratio for Down's syndrome when the nasal bone was absent on a second trimester ultrasound examination was 83. The mean nasal bone length in second trimester fetuses with Down's syndrome who had a nasal bone was smaller than for euploid fetuses. A biparietal diameter/nasal bone length ratio of 10 or greater detected 81% of fetuses with Down's syndrome and 11% of euploid fetuses. In the first trimester, Cicero et al[5] did not find a difference in nasal bone length between chromosomally normal and abnormal fetuses (see Fig. 24-2).

Sonek et al[6] did not find a difference in nasal bone length between Caucasians and Afro-Caribbean subgroups of their study population. Of note, they did find a higher incidence of absent nasal bone (8.8% vs. 5%) in the Afro-Caribbean population. This finding was confirmed by Prefumo et al.[7] Chen et al[8] have demonstrated that the nasal bone length is shorter in a Chinese population. Ethnic differences will have to be further evaluated before nasal bone length can be utilized as a second trimester marker for Down syndrome.

Lee et al[9] have voiced concern about the reproducibility of second trimester nasal bone detection. They utilized three-dimensional ultrasound in order to ensure that an appropriate sagittal view of the face is obtained. If a two-dimensional image of the face is slightly parasagittal, the frontal process of the maxilla can be mistaken for the nasal bone.

References

1. Keeling JW, Hansen BF, Kjaer I: Pattern of malformations in the axial skeleton in human trisomy 21 fetuses. Am J Med Genet 1997;68:466-471.

2. Cicero S, Curcio P, Papageorghiou A, et al: Absence of nasal bone in fetuses with trisomy 21 at 11-14 weeks' gestation: an observational study. Lancet 2001;358:1665-1667.

3. Malone FD, Ball RH, Nyberg DA, et al: First-trimester nasal bone evaluation for aneuploidy in the general population. Obstet Gynecol 2004;104:1222-1228.

4. Bromley B, Lieberman E, Shipp TD, et al: Fetal nasal bone length. A marker for Down syndrome in the second trimester. J Ultrasound Med 2002;21:1387-1394.

5. Cicero S, Binhdra R, Rembouskos G, et al: Fetal nasal bone length in chromosomally normal and abnormal fetuses at 11-14 weeks of gestation. J Mat Fet Neonat Med 2002;11:400-402.

6. Sonek JD, McKenna D, Webb D, et al: Nasal bone length throughout gestation: normal ranges based on 3537 fetal ultrasound measurements. Ultrasound Obstet Gynecol 2003;21:152-155.

7. Prefumo F, Sairam S, Bhide A, et al: Maternal ethnic origin and fetal nasal bones at 11-14 weeks of gestation. Br J Obstet Gynaecol 2004;111:109-112.

8. Chen M, Lee CP, Leung KY, et al: Pilot study on the mid-second trimester examination of fetal nasal bone in the Chinese population. Prenat Diagn 2004;24:87-91.

9. Lee W, DeVore GR, Comstock CH, et al: Nasal bone evaluation in fetuses with Down syndrome during the second and third trimesters of pregnancy. J Ultrasound Med 2003;22:55-60.

10. Guis F, Ville Y, Vincent Y, et al: Ultrasound evaluation of the length of the fetal nasal bones throughout gestation. Ultrasound Obstet Gynecol 1995;5:304-307.

11. Bunduki V, Ruano R, Miguelez J, et al: Fetal nasal bone length: reference ranges and clinical application in ultrasound screening for trisomy 21. Ultrasound Obstet Gynecol 2003;21:156-160.

Fetal Nuchal Translucency

Introduction

Various measurements have been used in an attempt to prenatally diagnose Down's syndrome. In the first trimester the most commonly used measurement is the nuchal translucency.

Materials/Methods

The nuchal translucency (NT) refers to the space between the back of the neck and the overlying skin. The measurement of the fetal nuchal translucency is highly operator dependent. Sonographers/sonologists must undergo both theoretical and practical training and then should be subject to continuous external quality control.[1] Specific criteria have been established to maximize quality and reduce the variability in nuchal translucency measurement (Fig. 25-1)[1]:

1. The crown-rump length measurement should be between 41 and 79 mm (10 weeks, 6 days and 13 weeks, 4 days).
2. A transabdominal measurement is preferred. In specific instances the transvaginal approach may be used.
3. The fetus should be in a midsagittal plane.
4. The fetal neck should be in a neutral position.
5. The image of the fetus should fill 75% of the screen.
6. The amnion must be distinguished from the fetal skin.
7. The calipers are placed perpendicular to the long axis of the fetus.
8. The calipers are placed on the inner borders of the nuchal fold.
9. Three measurements are obtained; the largest is used for risk calculation.

The nuchal translucency is 0.62 mm *greater* when the neck is extended and is 0.40 mm *less* when the neck is flexed than the mean nuchal translucency when the neck is in a neutral position.[2] Increasing magnification (60%, 100%, 200%) significantly decreases the mean NT.[3]

DISCUSSION

The association between the thickness of nuchal translucency and chromosomal abnormalities was initially reported in high-risk populations (i.e., advanced maternal age, abnormal multiple marker screen).[4] Most of the initial studies used a single cut-off across gestational age of between 2.5[5] and 3 mm (Fig. 25-2).[6]

The performance of fetal nuchal translucency measurement as a screening test for Down's syndrome depends on the prevalence of disease. Hence, the results from studies in high-risk women cannot be extrapolated to a low-risk population. Pandya et al[7] published the first study of nuchal translucency screening in a low-risk population. Snijders et al[8] reported their findings in 96,127 first trimester nuchal translucency examinations from 22 centers. The latter studies reported an 82% detection rate of trisomy 21 with an 8% false-positive rate or a 77% detection rate with a 5% false-positive rate. Snijders et al[8] calculated that there would have been 266 liveborn Down's syndrome infants at term without screening. However, 40% of Down's syndrome fetuses alive at 10 to 14 weeks' gestation will not survive until term. The latter statistic implies that at least 443 fetuses with Down's syndrome would have been alive at 10 to 14 weeks' gestation. The detection rate of 82% (266/326) would therefore have been 60% (268/443).[9]

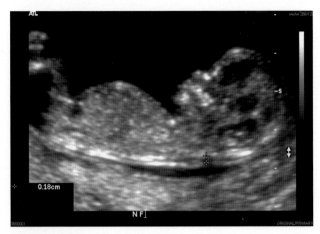

Figure 25-1
Normal nuchal translucency of 0.18 cm (between the graticules) at 13.4 weeks' gestation.

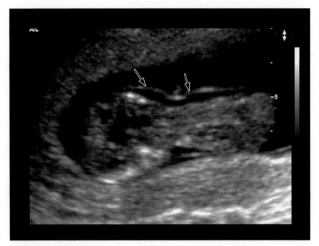

Figure 25-2
Abnormally thickened nuchal translucency (*arrows*) at 13 weeks' gestation.

Table 25-1	Sensitivity and false-positive rate for nuchal translucency aneuploidy screening at 10-14 weeks' gestation			
		Sensitivity		
Author	**Screened Patients**	**Trisomy 21**	**All Aneuploidy**	**False Positive (%)**
Thilaganathan[16]	2,920	71.0	78.0	5.0
Zoppi[17]	5,210	74.4	80.8	9.1
Snijders[8]	96,127	82.0	80.0	8.3
Schwarzler[18]	4,523	83.3	78.3	4.7

Modified from Souter VL, Nyberg DA: Sonographic screening for fetal aneuploidy: first trimester. J Ultrasound Med 2001;20:775-790.

Table 25-2	Combined first trimester nuchal translucency and serum screening for trisomy 21		
Author	**Screened Patients**	**Sensitivity (%)**	**False Positive (%)**
Wald[19]	39,983	80.0	3.4
Crossley[20]	17,229	62.0	5.0
Bindra[21]	14,383	92.0	7.1
Krantz[22]	5,809	91.0	5.0
Schuchter[23]	4,939	86.0	5.0

Modified from Malone FD, D'Alton ME; Society for Maternal-Fetal Medicine: first-trimester sonographic screening for Down's syndrome. Obstet Gynecol 2003;102(5 Pt 1):1066-1079.

Because the nuchal translucency increases significantly with menstrual age, Snijders et al[10] converted each NT measurement for a given crown-rump length to the logarithm of the multiple of the median (MoM). This has become the accepted way to interpret the thickness of the nuchal translucency, rather than utilizing a fixed cut-off (Table 25-1).

Mol et al[11] have raised the issue of ascertainment or verification bias in nuchal translucency-based screening. Verification bias occurs when selection for verification of the diagnosis is based on the results of the test that is being studied. In fetal nuchal translucency studies karyotyping is restricted to women with an increased nuchal thickness. Mol et al[11] divided nuchal translucency studies into those with and without verification bias. The difference in sensitivity for the detection of Down's syndrome was 77% for studies with verification bias, in contrast to 55% for those studies without bias.

In chromosomally normal fetuses with an NT greater than or equal to 3.5 mm there is also an increased risk of miscarriage, intrauterine demise, cardiac and other structural defects, and developmental delay.[12–15]

The addition of biochemical markers (pregnancy-associated plasma protein A and free β-human chorionic gonadotropin) to nuchal translucency measurement improves the efficacy of first trimester screening (Table 25-2). Hence as a first trimester genetic screen, a combination of an NT measurement and biochemical markers is recommended.

References

1. Wapner R, Thom E, Simpson JL, et al: First-trimester screening for trisomies 21 and 18. N Engl J Med 2003;349:1405-1413.
2. Whitlow BJ, Chatzippos IK, Economides DL: The effect of fetal neck position on nuchal translucency measurement. Br J Obstet Gynaecol 1998;105:872-876.
3. Edwards A, Mulvey S, Wallace EM: The effect of image size on nuchal translucency measurement. Prenat Diagn 2003;23:284-286.
4. Nicolaides KH, Brizot ML, Snijders RJM: Fetal nuchal translucency: ultrasound screening for fetal trisomy in the first trimester of pregnancy. Br J Obstet Gynaecol 1994;101:782-786.
5. Hafner E, Schuchter K, Liebhart E, et al: Results of routine fetal nuchal translucency measurement at weeks 10-13 in 4223 unselected pregnant women. Prenat Diagn 1998;18:29-34.
6. Pandya PP, Brizot ML, Kuhn P, et al: First-trimester fetal nuchal translucency thickness and risk for trisomies. Obstet Gynecol 1994;84:420-423.
7. Pandya P, Goldberg H, Walton B, et al: The implementation of first-trimester scanning at 10 to 13 weeks' gestation and the measurement of fetal nuchal translucency thickness in two maternity units. Ultrasound Obstet Gynecol 1995;5:20-25.
8. Snijders RJM, Noble P, Sebire N, et al: UK multicentre project on assessment of risk of trisomy 21 by maternal age and fetal nuchal-translucency thickness at 10-14 weeks of gestation. Lancet 1998;352:343-346.
9. Haddow JE: Antenatal screening for Down's syndrome: where are we and where next. Lancet 1998;352:336-337.
10. Snijders RJM, Thom EA, Zachary JM, et al: First-trimester trisomy screening: nuchal translucency measurement training and quality assurance to correct and unify technique. Ultrasound Obstet Gynecol 2002;19:353-359.
11. Mol BW, Lijmer JG, Van der Meulen J, et al: Effect of study design on the association between nuchal translucency measurement and Down's syndrome. Obstet Gynecol 1999;94:864-869.
12. Makrydimos G, Sotiriadis A, Ioannidis JP: Screening performance of first-trimester nuchal translucency for major cardiac defects: a meta-analysis. Am J Obstet Gynecol 2003;189:1330-1335.
13. Souka AP, Krampl E, Bakalis S et al: Outcome of pregnancy in chromosomally normal fetuses with increased nuchal translucency in the first trimester. Ultrasound Obstet Gynecol 2001;18:9-17.
14. Senat MV, De Keersmaeker B, Audibert F, et al: Pregnancy outcomes in fetuses with increased nuchal translucency and normal karyotype. Prenat Diagn 2002;22:345-349.
15. Mavrides E, Cobian-Sanchez F, Tekay A, et al: Limitations of using first trimester nuchal translucency measurements in routine screening for major congenital heart defects. Ultrasound Obstet Gynecol 2001;17:106-110.
16. Thilaganathan B, Slack A, Wathen NC: Effect of first-trimester nuchal translucency on second-trimester maternal serum biochemical screening for Down's syndrome. Ultrasound Obstet Gynecol 1997;10:261-264.
17. Zoppi MA, Ibba RM, Putzolu M, et al: Assessment of risk for chromosomal abnormalities at 10-14 weeks of gestation by nuchal translucency and maternal age in 5,210 fetuses at a single center. Fetal Diagn Ther 2000;15:170-173.
18. Schwarzler P, Carvalho JS, Senat MV, et al: Screening for fetal aneuploidy and fetal cardiac abnormalities by nuchal translucency thickness measurement at 10-14

weeks' gestation as part of routine antenatal care in an unselected population. Br J Obstet Gynaecol 1999;106:1029-1034.

19. Wald NJ, Rodeck C, Hackshaw AK, et al: First and second trimester antenatal screening for Down's syndrome: the results of the Serum Urine and Ultrasound Screening Study (SURUSS). J Med Screen 2003; 10:56-104.

20. Crossley JA, Aitken DA, Cameron AD, et al: Combined ultrasound and biochemical screening for Down's syndrome in the first trimester: a Scottish multicentre study. Br J Obstet Gynaecol, 2002;109:667-676.

21. Bindra R, Health V, Liao A, et al: One-stop clinic for assessment of risk for trisomy 21 at 11-14 weeks: a prospective study of 15,030 pregnancies. Ultrasound Obstet Gynecol 2002;20:219-225.

22. Krantz DA, Hallahan TW, Orlandi F, et al: First-trimester Down's syndrome screening using dried blood biochemistry and nuchal translucency. Obstet Gynecol 2000;96:207-213.

23. Schuchter K, Hafner E, Stangl G, et al: The first trimester "combined test" for the detection of Down's syndrome pregnancies in 4939 unselected pregnancies. Prenat Diagn 2002;22:211-215.

CHAPTER 26

Fetal Ocular Biometry

Lyndon Hill

Introduction

Fetal ocular biometry has been used to diagnose hypo- and hypertelorism in utero. Hypotelorism is frequently present with holo-prosencephaly. Hypertelorism may occur with median cleft syndromes and frontal cephaloceles.[1]

Materials/Methods

Fetal orbital measurements are most commonly made by taking an axial scan through the fetal face. This scan includes the bony orbits and bridge of the nose. Measurements may include the inner orbital diameter, with measurements from one medial wall of the orbit to the medial wall of the other orbit (Fig. 26-1). The outer orbital diameter (binocular distance) is made from the outer bony orbit to the other outer bony orbit (Fig. 26-2). The orbital diameter is from the medial to lateral bony orbital wall (Fig. 26-3).

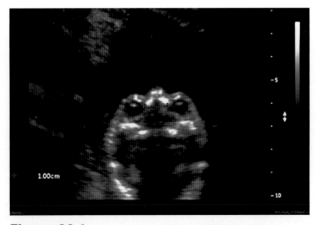

Figure 26-1
Second trimester inner orbital diameter (calipers).

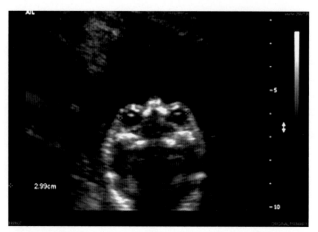

Figure 26-2
Second trimester outer orbital diameter (calipers).

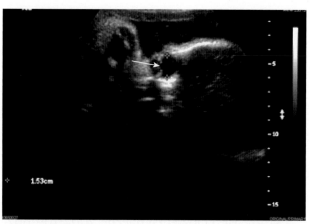

Figure 26-3
34 weeks' gestation orbital diameter (calipers). Lens of the eye (*arrow*).

Table 26-1	Mean fetal binocular distance with standard deviation, 5th, 50th, and 95th percentile for gestational age (GA)					
GA (Wks)	No of Exam *(n)*	Mean (cm)	SD (cm)	5th percentile	50th percentile	95th percentile
14	19	1.91	0.25	1.60	1.90	2.30
15	20	2.15	0.25	1.70	2.10	2.35
16	20	2.24	0.24	1.71	2.31	2.69
17	20	2.55	0.21	2.10	2.51	2.80
18	22	2.78	0.27	2.30	2.81	3.24
19	20	2.97	0.25	2.56	3.00	3.53
20	21	3.07	0.21	2.70	3.10	3.54
21	22	3.29	0.23	2.85	3.25	3.74
22	20	3.46	0.19	3.02	3.50	3.80
23	20	3.67	0.22	3.21	3.66	4.01
24	21	3.77	0.27	3.48	3.75	4.27
25	22	4.03	0.23	3.60	4.06	4.40
26	19	4.16	0.21	3.82	4.15	4.58
27	20	4.33	0.24	3.95	4.31	4.75
28	20	4.49	0.22	4.10	4.52	5.03
29	22	4.67	0.24	4.30	4.61	5.19
30	21	4.76	0.21	4.41	4.79	5.23
31	21	4.98	0.26	4.50	5.04	5.40
32	22	5.05	0.20	4.71	5.12	5.40
33	20	5.17	0.23	4.73	5.20	5.63
34	21	5.39	0.26	4.85	5.41	5.82
35	22	5.46	0.23	4.95	5.60	6.05
36	19	5.56	0.24	5.02	5.62	5.95
37	20	5.65	0.27	5.09	5.70	6.10
38	20	5.81	0.28	5.31	5.80	6.24
39	20	5.82	0.27	5.32	5.90	6.29
40	21	5.95	0.27	5.40	6.00	6.40

From Tongsong T, Wanapirak C, Jesadapornchai S, Tathayathikom E: Fetal binocular distance as a predictor of menstrual age. Int J Gynaecol Obstet 1992;38:87-91.

DISCUSSION

The 5th, 50th, and 95th percentile binocular distance for menstrual age are in Table 26-1. The predicted menstrual age for binocular distance are provided in Table 26-2. The binocular distances for specific menstrual ages, as derived from four different studies, are outlined in Table 26-3 —the values are consistent with one another.

The inner orbital diameter may be a more accurate measurement than the binocular distance to detect hypertelorism.[1] The inner orbital diameter from two studies are compared in Table 26-4 and, as with binocular distance, are quite consistent.

The mean and percentile values for orbital diameter are presented in Table 26-5. The orbital diameter from two studies are compared in Table 26-6. Orbital diameter could be used to predict micro-opthalmia. A study evaluating the efficacy of this measurement has not yet been published.

Table 26-2 Predicted menstrual age for binocular distances

BN (cm)	GA (wks)	BN (cm)	GA (wks)	BN (cm)	GA (wks)
1.6	12.8	3.2	20.80	4.8	30.29
1.7	13.3	3.3	21.34	4.9	30.94
1.8	13.78	3.4	21.90	5.0	31.59
1.9	14.24	3.5	22.46	5.1	32.25
2.0	14.71	3.6	23.02	5.2	32.91
2.1	15.18	3.7	23.59	5.3	33.58
2.2	15.66	3.8	24.17	5.4	34.26
2.3	16.15	3.9	24.76	5.5	34.94
2.4	16.64	4.0	25.35	5.6	35.63
2.5	17.14	4.1	25.94	5.7	36.33
2.6	17.64	4.2	26.54	5.8	37.03
2.7	18.15	4.3	27.15	5.9	37.74
2.8	18.67	4.4	27.77	6.0	38.45
2.9	19.19	4.5	28.39	6.1	39.17
3.0	19.72	4.6	29.02	6.2	39.90
3.1	20.25	4.7	29.65	6.3	40.63

From Tongsong T, Wanapirak C, Jesadapornchai S, Tathayathikom E: Fetal binocular distance as a predictor of menstrual age. Int J Gynaecol Obstet 1992;38:87-91.
BN, binocular distance; GA, gestational age.

Table 26-3 Binocular distance (mm) (50th percentile)

Menstrual Age (wks)	Trout[1]	Jeanty[3]	Mayden[4]	Tongsong[5]
14	18	21	—	1.9
16	23	24	—	2.3
18	27	28	—	2.8
20	32	31	34	3.1
22	36	35	37	3.5
24	39	38	41	3.8
26	43	41	44	4.2
28	46	45	47	4.5
30	49	48	50	4.8
32	51	51	52	5.1
34	53	55	54	5.4
N	442	188	180	555
Country	USA	USA	USA	Thailand

Table 26-4	Inner orbital diameter (mm) (50th percentile)	
Menstrual Age (wks)	Trout[1]	Mayden[4]
14	8	—
16	9	—
18	11	—
20	12	13
22	13	14
24	14	15
26	16	17
28	17	17
30	18	18
32	19	18
34	20	19
N	442	180

Table 26-6	Fetal orbital diameter (mm) at various menstrual ages	
Menstrual Age (wks)	Orbital Diameter (mm)	
	Goldstein[6]	Dilmen[7]
15	6.1	5.3
16	6.6	6.4
17	—	7.7
18	—	8.7
19	—	8.8
20	—	9.6
21	10.5	9.8
22	10.4	11.1
23	10.7	11.4
24	11.6	11.6
25	11.2	13.1
26	12.7	13.1
27	13.0	13.3
28	13.0	13.7
29	13.9	14.1
N	349	335
Country	Israel	Turkey

Table 26-5	The fetal orbital diameter (mm)							
				Percentiles				
Menstrual Age (wks)	N	Mean	95% CI	10th	25th	50th	75th	90th
14	10	5.2	4.8-5.7	4.5	5.0	5.3	5.7	5.7
15	26	6.1	5.9-6.3	5.4	5.5	6.2	6.5	6.7
16	25	6.6	6.3-6.9	5.8	6.2	6.5	7.0	7.6
17-18	19	7.3	6.7-7.8	6.2	6.5	6.7	9.0	9.0
19-20	23	9.8	9.3-10.2	8.6	9.0	10.0	10.1	11.3
21	19	10.5	10.0-10.9	9.4	9.9	10.0	11.0	12.0
22	26	10.4	10.0-10.7	9.5	9.6	10.5	11.0	11.3
23	21	10.7	10.4-11.1	9.6	10.0	10.5	11.4	11.5
24	10	11.6	11.3-11.8	10.7	11.0	11.5	12.0	12.5
25	13	11.2	11.4-12.4	10.3	11.0	12.2	12.5	12.8
26	16	12.7	12.0-13.4	11.0	11.0	12.7	13.8	14.5
27	14	13.0	12.4-13.5	11.9	12.0	12.9	13.4	14.8
28	21	13.0	12.7-13.3	12.1	12.0	13.1	13.3	14.1
29	23	13.9	13.4-14.4	12.6	13.0	13.7	14.6	15.7
30-31	24	14.2	13.8-14.5	13.3	13.0	13.9	14.7	15.4
32-33	24	14.4	13.7-15.1	12.2	13.0	14.1	14.8	17.5
34-36	26	15.8	15.4-16.2	14.6	15.0	15.7	16.5	16.9

From Goldstein I, Tamir A, Zimmer EZ, Itskovitz-Eldor J: Growth of the fetal orbit and lens in normal pregnancies. Ultrasound Obstet Gynecol 1998;12:175-179.

Transvaginal sonography has been used to obtain orbital dimensions between 10 and 16 weeks' menstrual age.[2]

References

1. Trout T, Budorick NE, Pretorius DH, et al: Significance of orbital measurements in the fetus. J Ultrasound Med 1994;13:937-943.
2. Guariglia L, Rosati P: Early transvaginal biometry of fetal orbits: a cross-sectional study. Fetal Diagn Ther 2002;17:42-47.
3. Jeanty P, Cantraine F, Cousaert F, et al: The binocular distance: a new way to estimate fetal age. J Ultrasound Med 1984;3:241-243.
4. Mayden KL, Tortora M, Berkowitz RL, et al: Orbital diameters: a new parameter prenatal diagnosis and dating. Am J Obstet Gynecol 1982;144:289-297.
5. Tongsong T, Wanapirak C, Jesadapornchai S, et al: Fetal binocular distance as a predictor of menstrual age. Int J Gynecol Obstet 1992;38:87-91.
6. Goldstein I, Tamir A, Zimmer EZ, et al: Growth of the fetal orbit and lens in normal pregnancies. Ultrasound Obstet Gynecol 1998;12:175-179.
7. Dilmen G, Köktener A, Turban NÖ, et al: Growth of the fetal lens and orbit. Int J Gynecol Obstet 2002;76:267-271.

CHAPTER 27

Fetal Renal Length

Lyndon Hill

Introduction

Normal fetal renal length for menstrual age has been evaluated by a number of authors.[1-4] These data can be used to identify abnormalities in the size of kidneys (e.g., hypoplasia, nephromegaly). The functional effect of a unilateral renal malformation can be assessed by determining if there is contralateral renal compensatory growth.[5]

Materials/Methods

Exclusion criteria for obtaining a normal fetal renal length include a failure to identify the renal borders, abnormal renal morphology, or significant pyelocaliectasis. In the past, the last fetal rib would sometime make visualization of the upper end of the kidney difficult. The better resolution of more recent equipment has considerably reduced the technical difficulties associated with the measurement of an accurate renal length.

DISCUSSION

Sagi et al[1] have reported that renal length increases linearly with menstrual age. In a more recent publication, Gloor et al[2] found that the best model of renal length to menstrual age was a quadratic function. Cohen et al[3] provided confidence intervals and the number of patients per week for their tabulation of renal length by menstrual week. As a result, their data are reproduced in Table 27-1. The two most recent studies[2,3] reported similar renal lengths from 22 weeks' menstrual age until term. The smaller renal lengths reported by Sagi et al[1] and Bertagnoli et al[4] may be because of population and/or methodologic differences (Table 27-2).

Table 27-1	Mean renal lengths for various gestational ages			
Menstrual Age (wks)	**Mean Length (cm)**	**SD**	**95% CI**	**N**
18	2.2	0.3	1.6-2.8	14
19	2.3	0.4	1.5-3.1	23
20	2.6	0.4	1.8-3.4	22
21	2.7	0.3	2.1-3.2	20
22	2.7	0.3	2.0-3.4	18
23	3.0	0.4	2.2-3.7	13
24	3.1	0.6	1.9-4.4	13
25	3.3	0.4	2.5-4.2	9
26	3.4	0.4	2.4-4.4	9
27	3.5	0.4	2.7-4.4	15
28	3.4	0.4	2.6-4.2	19
29	3.6	0.7	2.3-4.8	12
30	3.8	0.4	2.9-4.6	24
31	3.7	0.5	2.8-4.6	23
32	4.1	0.5	3.1-5.1	23
33	4.0	0.3	3.3-4.7	28
34	4.2	0.4	3.3-5.0	36
35	4.2	0.5	3.2-5.2	17
36	4.2	0.4	3.3-5.0	36
37	4.2	0.4	3.3-5.1	40
38	4.4	0.6	3.2-5.6	32
39	4.2	0.3	3.5-4.8	17
40	4.3	0.5	3.2-5.3	10
41	4.5	0.3	3.9-5.1	4

From Cohen HL, Cooper J, Eisenberg P, et al: Normal length of fetal kidneys: sonographic study in 397 obstetric patients. AJR Am J Roentgenol 1991;157:545-548.

Table 27-2	Renal length from 20 to 38 weeks' menstrual age by different authors			
	Renal Length (mm)			
Menstrual Age (wks)	**Sagi[1]***	**Gloor[2]**	**Cohen[3]**	**Bertagnoli[4]**
20	15.9	21	26	—
22	19.1	25	27	—
24	22.4	29	31	24.5
26	25.1	32	34	25.8
28	27.8	35	34	27.2
30	30.5	38	38	28.8
32	33.3	40	41	30.4
34	36.0	41	42	32.2
36	38.2	42	42	34.0
38	40.3	43	44	36.0
N	660	100	397	280
Country	Israel; South Africa	USA	USA	Italy
Year	1987	1997	1991	1983

*Calculated.

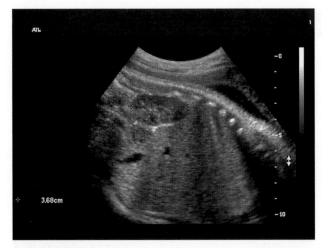

Figure 27-1
Renal length at 35 weeks' menstrual age.

In the study by Cohen et al,[3] renal length did not change significantly from 35 weeks' menstrual age until term. This finding is not consistent with the continued growth noted in other fetal organs. Autopsy studies[6,7] from 27 weeks' menstrual age until term consistently indicate continued growth of renal length. This would suggest that technical factors may have made the accurate sonographic measurement of renal length in the third trimester difficult. Additional ultrasound studies of fetal renal length in the third trimester would be helpful to validate or modify the findings of Cohen et al.[3]

Figure 27-1 shows measurement of renal length at 35 weeks' menstrual age.

References

1. Sagi J, Vagman I, David MP, et al: Fetal kidney size related to gestational age. Gynecol Obstet Invest 1987;23:1-4.
2. Gloor JM, Breckle RJ, Gehrking WC, et al: Fetal renal growth evaluated by prenatal ultrasound examination. Mayo Clin Proc 1997;72:124-129.
3. Cohen HL, Cooper J, Eisenberg P, et al: Normal length of fetal kidneys: sonographic study in 397 obstetric patients. AJR Am J Roentgenol 1991;157:545-548.
4. Bertagnoli L, Lalatta L, Gallicchio R, et al: Quantitative characterization of the growth of the fetal kidney. J Clin Ultrasound 1983;11:349-356.
5. Hill LM, Nowak A, Hartle R, et al: Fetal compensatory renal hypertrophy with a unilateral functioning kidney. Ultrasound Obstet Gynecol 2000;15:191-193.
6. Gonzales J, Gonzales M, Mary JY: Size and weight study of human kidney growth velocity during the last three months of pregnancy. Eur Urol 1980;6:37-44.
7. Chiara A, Chirico G, Barbarini M, et al: Ultrasonic evaluation of kidney length in term and preterm infants. Eur J Pediatr 1989;149:94-95.

CHAPTER 28

Lyndon Hill

Fetal Rib Length

Introduction

The fetal ribs are oriented horizontally. As a result, individual ribs can be imaged on a standard transverse view of the fetal chest.

Table 28-1	Gestational age predicted by rib length (mean ± 2SE)						
	Gestational Age (wks)				**Gestational Age (wks)**		
Rib length (cm)	**+2SE**	**Mean**	**+2SE**	**Rib length (cm)**	**+2SE**	**Mean**	**+2SE**
1.50	7.2	11.8	16.5	4.75	21.7	26.3	30.9
1.75	8.4	13.1	17.7	5.00	22.6	27.2	31.8
2.00	9.7	14.4	19.0	5.25	23.6	28.3	32.9
2.25	10.6	15.2	19.9	5.50	24.8	29.4	34.0
2.50	11.7	16.3	21.0	5.75	25.9	30.6	35.2
2.75	12.8	17.4	22.0	6.00	26.9	31.6	36.2
3.00	13.8	18.5	23.1	6.25	28.1	32.7	37.3
3.25	14.9	19.5	24.2	6.50	29.2	33.8	38.5
3.50	16.0	20.7	25.3	6.75	30.3	34.9	39.6
3.75	17.2	21.8	26.4	7.00	31.2	35.8	40.5
4.00	18.2	22.9	27.5	7.25	32.5	37.1	41.7
4.25	19.3	23.9	28.6	7.50	33.4	38.0	42.6
4.50	20.4	25.1	29.7	8.00	35.5	40.2	44.8

From Abuhamad AZ, Sedule-Murphy SJ, Kolm P, et al: Prenatal ultrasonographic fetal rib length measurement: correlation with gestational age. Ultrasound Obstet Gynecol 1996;7:193-196.

Materials/Methods

The fetal rib at the level of the four-chamber view of the heart is measured. The calipers trace the anterior rib to the lateral edge of the vertebra (Fig. 28-1).

DISCUSSION

Rib length correlates with menstrual age in a linear fashion (R = 0.94). Gestational age predicted by rib length is outlined in Table 28-1. The wide standard error indicates that rib length should not be added to the standard biometric data of biparietal diameter, head circumference, abdominal circumference, and femur length.

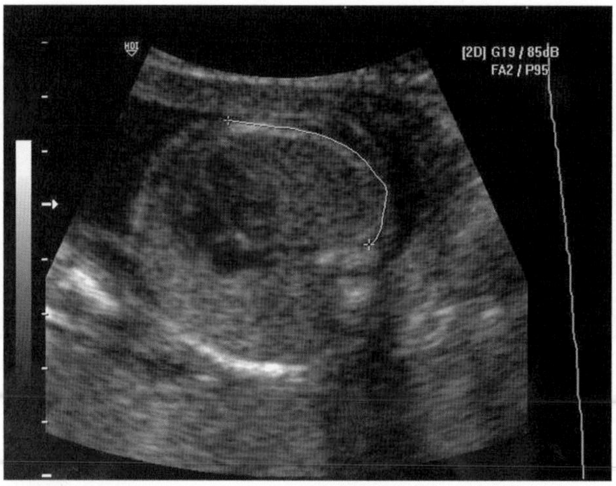

Abuhamad et al[1] have proposed that rib length may be helpful in the evaluation of a fetus for skeletal dysplasia. However, the authors did not investigate this possibility. It remains to be determined if rib length is a better predictor of severe skeletal dysplasia than chest circumference.

Reference

1. Abuhamad AZ, Sedule-Murphy SJ, Kolm P, et al: Prenatal ultrasonographic fetal rib length measurement: correlation with gestational age. Ultrasound Obstet Gynecol 1996; 7:193-196.

Figure 28-1
Anterior rib length at 20 weeks' menstrual age.

CHAPTER 29

Lyndon Hill

Fetal Scapular Length

Introduction

Scapular length has been evaluated by a few authors[1-3] as an additional measurement to assess menstrual age.

Materials/Methods

Scapular length is measured between the acromion and inferior angle (Figs. 29-1 and 29-2).

DISCUSSION

Table 29-1 provides menstrual age as predicted by scapular length. The mean scapular length for menstrual age from two studies is incorporated in Table 29-2. The study performed in the United States[2] consistently reported shorter scapular lengths for menstrual age. The disparity in scapular lengths between the two studies equates to a 2- to 5-week difference in menstrual age assessment after 18 weeks' gestation. This difference suggests a difference in the measurement technique between the two studies. Dilmen et al[3] measured with hand-held calipers rather than by means of a measurement package within the ultrasound unit. As a result, the menstrual age predicted by scapular length from Sherer et al[2] is provided (see Table 29-1).

The correlation coefficient between scapular length and menstrual age has been reported as 0.93,[1] 0.94,[2] and 0.94[3] in three separate investigations. Dilmen et al[3] divided their study group into two subgroups, 16 to 28 weeks and 29 to

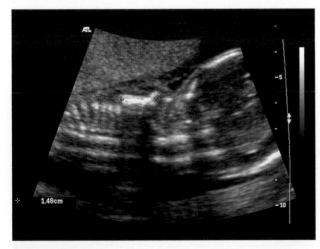

Figure 29-1
Scapular length (calipers) at 18 weeks' menstrual age.

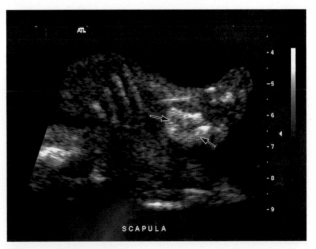

Figure 29-2
Parasagittal view of the fetal scapula (*arrows*) at 19 weeks' menstrual age.

Table 29-1 Menstrual age predicted by scapular length (mean ± 2SD calculated on basis of regression equation)

Scapular Length (cm)	Menstrual Age (wks + days)			Scapular Length (cm)	Menstrual Age (wks + days)		
	−2SD	Mean	+2SD		−2SD	Mean	+2SD
0.7	7 + 3	11 + 5	15~6	2.3	23 + 2	27 + 3	31 + 5
0.8	8 + 3	12 + 5	16 + 6	2.4	24 + 2	28 + 3	32 + 5
0.9	9 + 3	13 + 5	17 + 6	2.5	25 + 2	29 + 3	33 + 4
1.0	10 + 3	14 + 4	18 + 6	2.6	26 + 1	30 + 3	34 + 4
1.1	11 + 3	15 + 4	19 + 6	2.7	27 + 1	31 + 3	35~4
1.2	12 + 3	16 + 4	20 + 6	2.8	28 + 1	32 + 3	36 + 4
1.3	13 + 3	17 + 4	21 + 6	2.9	29 + 1	33 + 3	37 + 4
1.4	14 + 3	18 + 4	22 + 6	3.0	30 + 1	34 + 2	38 + 4
1.5	15 + 2	19 + 4	23 + 5	3.1	31 + 1	35 + 2	39 + 4
1.6	16 + 2	20 + 4	24 + 5	3.2	32 + 1	36 + 2	40 + 4
1.7	17 + 2	21 + 4	25 + 5	3.3	33 + 1	37 + 2	41 + 4
1.8	18 + 2	22 + 4	26 + 5	3.4	34 + 1	38 + 2	42 + 4
1.9	19 + 2	23 + 4	27 + 5	3.5	35 + 0	39 + 2	43 + 3
2.0	20 + 2	24 + 3	28 + 5	3.6	36 + 0	40 + 2	44 + 3
2.1	21 + 2	25 + 3	29 + 5	3.7	37 + 0	41 + 2	45 + 3
2.2	22 + 2	26 + 3	30 + 5	3.8	38 + 0	42 + 2	46 + 3

From Sherer DM, Plessinger MA, Allen TA: Fetal scapular length in the ultrasonographic assessment of gestational age. J Ultrasound Med 1994;13:523-528.

Table 29-2 Scapular length by menstrual age

Menstrual Age (wks)	Scapular Length (cm)		
	Sherer[2]	Dilmen[3]	Difference Sherer-Dilmen
16	1.2	1.26	−0.06
17	1.3	1.40	−0.1
18	1.4	1.62	−0.22
19	1.5	1.82	−0.32
20	1.6	1.86	−0.26
21	1.7	2.04	−0.34
22	1.8	2.20	−0.40
23	1.9	2.27	−0.37
24	2.0	2.40	−0.40
25	2.1	2.52	−0.42
26	2.2	2.56	−0.36
27	2.3	2.73	−0.43
28	2.4	2.83	−0.43
29	2.4	2.92	−0.52
30	2.5	2.95	−0.45
31	2.6	3.12	−0.52
32	2.7	3.21	−0.51
33	2.8	3.25	−0.55
34	2.9	3.36	−0.46
35	3.0	3.40	−0.40
36	3.1	3.50	−0.40
37	3.2	3.68	−0.48
38	3.3	3.67	−0.37
39	3.4	3.86	−0.46
40	3.5	3.88	−0.38
41	3.6	3.92	−0.32
N	515	343	
Country	USA	Turkey	

41 weeks; the correlation coefficients were 0.92 and 0.74, respectively.

In terms of menstrual age assessment, the standard deviation (SD), or more precisely the confidence intervals, of a specific measurement are as important as the correlation coefficient. In Table 29-1 the two SD range around a predicted menstrual age is constant throughout gestation. Fetal measurements have increasing variation with increasing menstrual age.[4] Therefore it seems that the model selected by the authors did not allow the standard deviation to change with advancing gestation. As a result, the plus or minus two SD values are too far apart early in pregnancy and too close together in the third trimester. Because of these methodological problems, as well as the reported variation in menstrual age assessment by scapular length, this measurement should not be added to standard fetal biometry.

References

1. Murao F, Shibukawa T, Takamiya O, et al: Antenatal measurement of scapular length using ultrasound. Gynecol Obstet Invest 1989;28:195-197.
2. Sherer DM, Plessinger MA, Allen TA: Fetal scapular length in the ultrasonographic assessment of gestational age. J Ultrasound Med 1994;13:523-528.
3. Dilmen G, Turhan N, Toppare M, et al: Scapular length measurement for assessment of fetal growth and development. Ultrasound in Med Biol 1995;21:139-142.
4. Altman DG, Chitty LS: Charts of fetal size: 1 methodology. Br J Obstet Gynaecol 1994; 101:29-34.

CHAPTER 30

Fetal Splenic Circumference

Lyndon Hill

Introduction

The fetal spleen is hematopoietically active from 12 to 24 menstrual weeks. After 24 weeks the bone marrow begins to function. As a result, red cell production by the liver and spleen decreases.[1]

Fetal splenomegaly may occur secondary to anemia, intrauterine infection, or inborn errors of metabolism (i.e., Gaucher's or Niemann-Pick's disease).[1]

Materials/Methods

On a transverse view of the fetal abdomen, the spleen is posterior to the fetal stomach (Fig. 30-1). The left adrenal is occasionally imaged between the spine medially and the spleen laterally.

DISCUSSION

Splenic length and circumference (length + transverse dimension × 1.57) have been correlated to menstrual age. Splenic circumference was more closely correlated to menstrual age ($R^2 = 0.935$) than was splenic volume ($R^2 = 0.829$), calculated from three measurements (longitudinal, transverse, and coronal).[1]

Table 30-1 compares the splenic length and circumference obtained by different authors. The splenic length provided by Hata et al[2] and Aoki et al[3] are quite similar. However, this is not surprising because the two studies are performed by the same group. The data from Japan[2,3] are consistently smaller than the values obtained from a population in the United States.[1]

Table 30-2 provides the mean, 5th, and 95th percentile of splenic circumference by menstrual age. The parametric method was used in the authors' data analysis (i.e., the 5th and 95th percentiles were calculated as mean plus or minus 1.65 multiplied by the standard deviation [SD]). However, there are only two to six patients per week (total: 79). As a result, the width of the 95% confidence interval for the 5th and 95th percentiles will be quite large. In addi-

Table 30-1	Splenic length and circumference by menstrual age					
	Length (cm)			Circumference (cm)		
Menstrual Age (wks)	Schmidt[1] (m*)	Hata[2] (p†)	Aoki[3] (p†)	Schmidt[1] (m*)	Aoki[3] (p†)	Bahado-Singh[4] (p†)
20	1.8	1.4	1.5	4.5	4.2	3.7
24	2.5	2.0	2.2	6.1	6.1	5.0
28	3.1	2.5	2.9	7.4	7.9	6.3
32	3.8	3.1	3.5	8.9	9.5	7.6
36	4.8	3.6	4.0	10.9	11.0	8.9
40	6.2	4.2	4.3	13.8	12.3	—
N	79	49	229	79	229	121
Country	USA	Japan	Japan	USA	Japan	USA

*Mean
†Predicted

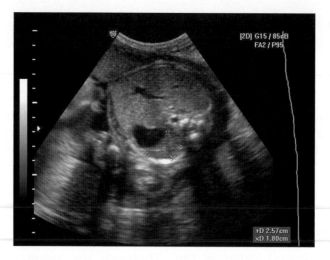

Figure 30-1

Transverse scan of the fetal abdomen at 29 weeks' menstrual age. The calipers demarcate the length (+ . . . +) and transverse (× . . . ×) diameters.

Menstrual Age (wks)	Circumference (mm) 5th	Mean	95th
18	2.3	3.5	4.7
19	2.7	3.9	5.1
20	3.3	4.5	5.7
21	3.5	4.7	5.9
22	4.1	5.3	6.5
23	4.5	5.7	6.9
24	4.9	6.1	7.2
25	5.3	6.4	7.7
26	5.5	6.7	7.9
27	5.9	7.1	8.3
28	6.2	7.4	8.6
29	6.5	7.7	8.9
30	6.9	8.1	9.3
31	7.3	8.5	9.7
32	7.7	8.9	10.1
33	8.1	9.3	10.5
34	8.6	9.8	11.0
35	9.1	10.3	11.5
36	9.7	10.9	12.1
37	10.4	11.6	12.8
38	11.1	12.3	13.4
39	11.8	13.0	14.2
40	12.7	13.8	15.1

Table 30-2 Splenic circumference (mm)

From Schmidt W, Yarkoni S, Jeanty P, et al: Sonographic measurements of the fetal spleen: clinical implications. J Ultrasound Med 1985;4:667-672.

There is a significant correlation between splenic circumference and severe fetal anemia.[4,5] Sonographically detected splenomegaly has between a 72.7% and 83% sensitivity with a 14% false-positive rate for the detection of severe fetal anemia before the first intrauterine transfusion.[4,5]

Measurement of the peak systolic velocity of the middle cerebral artery has replaced other, more indirect biometry measurements in the detection of fetal anemia prior to the onset of spleno- or hepatomegaly.[6]

tion, the authors utilized the same standard deviation throughout gestation. Because there is increasing variation in all fetal measurements as menstrual age advances, the SD upon which the percentile calculation is based should also vary. The 5th and 95th percentile values in the third trimester should therefore be greater than those recorded on the table.

References

1. Schmidt W, Yarkoni S, Jeanty P, et al: Sonographic measurement of the fetal spleen: clinical implications. J Ultrasound Med 1985;4:667-672.
2. Hata T, Aoki S, Takamori H, et al: Ultrasonographic in utero identification and measurement of the normal fetal spleen. Gynecol Obstet Invest 1987;23:124-128.
3. Aoki S, Hata T, Kitao M: Ultrasonographic assessment of fetal and neonatal spleen. Am J Perinatol 1992;9:361-367.
4. Bahado-Singh R, Oz U, Mari G, et al: Fetal splenic size in anemia due to Rh-alloimmunization. Obstet Gynecol 1998;92:828-832.
5. Oepkes D, Meerman RH, Vandenbusche FPHA, et al: Ultrasonographic fetal spleen measurements in red blood cell alloimmunized pregnancies. Am J Obstet Gynecol 1993;109:121-128.
6. Mari G, Deter RL, Carpenter RL, et al: Noninvasive diagnosis by Doppler ultrasonography of fetal anemia due to maternal red-cell alloimmunization. Collaborative Group for Doppler Assessment of the Blood Velocity in Anemic Fetuses. N Engl J Med 2000;342:9-14.

CHAPTER 31

Fetal Transverse Cerebellar Diameter

Lyndon Hill

Introduction

One of the fetal measurements that has been used to estimate menstrual age is the cerebellar transverse diameter.

Materials/Methods

The cerebellum is visualized by angling the transducer posteriorly from the level of the biparietal diameter (Fig. 31-1). The vermis should be equidistant between the cerebellar hemispheres.

DISCUSSION

Nomograms have been established for transverse cerebellar diameter and menstrual age throughout pregnancy.[1,2] Between 14 and 20 weeks' menstrual age, the transverse cerebellar diameter in millimeters is equivalent to the menstrual age in weeks. The predicted menstrual ages for transverse cerebellar diameters from 14 to 56 mm are outlined in Table 31-1. The transverse cerebellar diameter for menstrual age derived by Hill et al[1] and Goldstein et al[2] are compared in Table 31-2. The divergence of the data after 32 weeks may be because of the limited number of patients in both studies after this menstrual age. The variability associated with predicting gestational age from the transverse cerebellar diameter is outlined in Table 31-3.

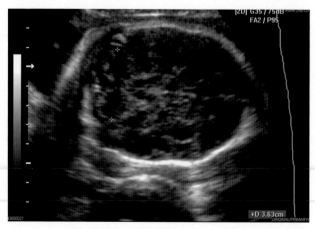

Figure 31-1
A transverse cerebellar diameter measurement (between the graticules) at 30 weeks' menstrual age.

Table 31-1 Predicted menstrual ages for transverse cerebellar diameters of 14 to 56 mm

Cerebellum (mm)	Gestational Age (wks)	Cerebellum (mm)	Gestational Age (wks)
14	15.2	35	29.4
15	15.8	36	30.0
16	16.5	37	30.6
17	17.2	38	31.2
18	17.9	39	31.8
19	18.6	40	32.3
20	19.3	41	32.8
21	20.0	42	33.4
22	20.7	43	33.9
23	21.4	44	34.4
24	22.1	45	34.8
25	22.8	46	35.3
26	23.5	47	35.7
27	24.2	48	36.1
28	24.9	49	36.5
29	25.5	50	36.8
30	26.2	51	37.2
31	26.9	52	37.5
32	27.5	54	38.0
33	28.1	55	38.3
34	28.8	56	38.5

From Hill LM, Guzick D, Fries J, et al: The transverse cerebellar diameter in estimating gestational age in the large for gestational age fetus. Obstet Gynecol 1990;75:981-985.

Table 31-2 Transverse cerebellar diameter (mm)

Menstrual Age (wks)	Hill[1]	Goldstein[2]
16	15	16
18	18	18
20	21	20
22	24	23
24	27	25
26	30	29
28	33	31
30	36	35
32	39	38
34	43	40
36	48	43
38	54	48.5
40	—	—

Table 31-3 Variability in determining menstrual age from the transverse cerebellar diameter

Menstrual Age (wks)	Variability Weeks (±2SD)
12-17	±1.0
18-23	±1.8
24-29	±2.0
30-35	±2.4
≥36	±3.2

From Hill LM, Guzick D, Fries J, et al: The transverse cerebellar diameter in estimating gestational age in the large for gestational age fetus. Obstet Gynecol 1990;75:981-985.

References

1. Hill LM, Guzick D, Fries J, et al: The transverse cerebellar diameter in estimating gestational age in the large for gestational age fetus. Obstet Gynecol 1990;75:981-988.

2. Goldstein I, Reece A, Pilu G, et al: Cerebellar measurements with ultrasonography in the evaluation of fetal growth and development. Am J Obstet Gynecol 1987;156:1065-1069.

CHAPTER 32

Lyndon Hill

Twins: Second and Third Trimester Biometric Data, Excluding Fetal Weight

Introduction

Twinning occurs spontaneously approximately once in every 80 pregnancies. The growth rate of twins, as well as higher multiples, has been evaluated by a number of different authors.

Because they are far more common, second trimester biometric measurements are more readily available for twins.

Materials/Methods

Retrospective cross-sectional studies,[1] as well as prospective longitudinal studies,[2] have been conducted to compare fetal biometry of singleton and twins by menstrual age. Smaller, more focused studies have evaluated biometry in twins versus triplets,[3] as well as fetal biometry of mono- and dichorionic twins.[4]

DISCUSSION

Tables 32-1 through 32-3 compare twin biparietal diameters (BPD), femur lengths (FL), and abdominal circumferences (AC) with singleton controls—the BPD and AC of twins are significantly smaller than singletons at 32 weeks' menstrual age and beyond; femur length is the same for singletons and twins throughout gestation.[1,5-8] Although the BPD is significantly less in twins compared with singletons, the head circumference is unaffected.[2,5] The difference in the BPD is, therefore, because of the effect of fetal crowding on head shape.[9]

Tables 32-4 and 32-5 compare twin values obtained by three different authors. The data of Kuno et al[2] are consistently less than the mean values from the other two studies. The difference between the means at 26 weeks' menstrual age for Ong et al[1] and Kuno et al[2] was calculated and found to be significant ($P < 0.01$). The smaller ACs reported by Kuno et al[2] may

Table 32-1	Mean twin and singleton fetal biparietal diameter (BPD) for 27 to 37 weeks' menstrual age				
		Mean Twin			
Menstrual Age (wks)	**N**	**BPD (cm)**	**SD (cm)**	**Singleton BPD (cm)**	**P Value***
27	20	6.9	0.4	6.9	0.999
28	20	7.4	0.4	7.2	0.057
29	22	7.4	0.4	7.4	0.919
30	26	7.4	0.5	7.6	0.028
31	18	7.8	0.5	7.9	0.466
32	20	7.9	0.4	8.1	0.028
33	24	8.1	0.4	8.3	0.047
34	16	8.2	0.3	8.5	0.002
35	18	8.4	0.4	8.7	0.006
36	14	8.5	0.3	8.9	0.005
37	6	8.5	0.3	9.1	0.003

* Student's t test.
From Grumbach K, Coleman BG, Arger PH, et al: Twin and singleton growth patterns compared using US. Radiology 1986;158:237-241.

Table 32-2	Mean twin and singleton fetal femur length (FFL) for 27 to 37 menstrual weeks				
		Mean Twin			
Menstrual Age (wks)	**N**	**FFL (cm)**	**SD (cm)**	**Mean Singleton FFL (cm)**	**P Value***
27	10	5.1	0.3	5.1	0.99
28	8	5.7	0.2	5.4	0.60
29	4	5.2	0.3	5.6	0.60
30	16	5.9	0.4	5.8	0.12
31	8	5.9	0.6	6.0	0.44
32	10	6.3	0.5	6.3	0.99
33	10	6.4	0.5	6.5	0.68
34	10	6.6	0.3	6.7	0.62
35	8	6.9	0.3	6.9	0.22
36	8	6.9	0.3	7.1	0.24
37	4	7.2	0.3	7.3	0.62

* Student's t test.
From Grumbach K, Coleman BG, Arger PH, et al: Twin and singleton growth patterns compared using US. Radiology 1986;158:237-241.

be because of ethnic differences of the two populations.

Weissman et al[10] evaluated fetal biometry in triplets. They found that all four biometric parameters (BPD, HC, AC, FL) differed from singleton controls. The mean BPD, HC, and AC for triplets approaches the 10th percentile for singletons at 34, 34, and 28 weeks' menstrual age, respectively. The femur length of triplets parallels the 5th percentile for singletons throughout gestation.

Shussan et al[3] compared BPD and FL in twins and triplets. They found a significant difference in both measurements between 25 and 37 weeks' menstrual age.

Third trimester fetuses of multiple gestations tend to be smaller than singletons at the same gestational age. This indicates that using sin-

Table 32-3 Mean twin and singleton abdominal circumference (AC) for 27 to 37 menstrual weeks

Menstrual Age (wks)	N	Mean Twin AC (cm)	SD (cm)	Mean Singleton AC (cm)	P Value*
27	12	23.6	1.7	22.7	0.07
28	19	23.9	2.7	23.8	0.68
29	12	24.9	2.5	24.9	0.56
30	18	25.3	1.9	26.0	0.11
31	12	26.9	1.9	27.1	0.68
32	18	27.2	1.8	28.2	0.035
33	14	27.1	2.1	29.3	0.002
34	14	28.9	1.9	30.4	0.012
35	14	29.6	1.7	31.5	0.001
36	10	29.8	1.6	32.6	0.001
37	8	29.2	2.6	33.7	0.009

* Student's t test.
From Grumbach K, Coleman BG, Arger PH, et al: Twin and singleton growth patterns compared using US. Radiology 1986;158:237-241.

Table 32-4 Mean values for abdominal circumference in twins (mm)

Menstrual Age (wks)	Ong[1]	Kuno[2]	Grumbach[6]
24	197.9	183	—
26	224.7	202	—
28	237.7	219	239
30	259.1	235	253
32	280.7	250	272
34	295.8	264	289
36	311.0	277	298
N	884	52	103
Study	Cross-sectional	Longitudinal	Longitudinal
Country	Scotland	Japan	USA

Table 32-5 Mean values for femur length in twins (mm)

Menstrual Age (wks)	Ong[1]	Kuno[2]	Grumbach[6]
24	197.9	183	—
24	43.1	40	—
26	48.1	45	—
28	51.8	49	57
30	57.1	53	59
32	60.7	56	63
34	65.6	59	66
36	68.2	62	69
38	70.6	64	—
N	884	52	103
Study	Cross-sectional	Longitudinal	Longitudinal
Country	Scotland	Japan	USA

gleton charts to determine gestational age from the abdominal circumference in third trimester multiple gestations will have a larger standard deviation. Because femur length and head circumference are not affected in twins, they should be used to determine third trimester gestational age in multiple pregnancies. If twin data are used to determine menstrual age, each institution should determine which chart is most appropriate for its indigenous population.

References

1. Ong S, Lim M-N, Fitzmaurice A, et al: The creation of twin centile curves for size. Br J Obstet Gynaecol 2002;109:753-758.
2. Kuno A, Akiyama M, Yanagihara T, et al: Comparison of fetal growth in singleton, twin, and triplet pregnancies. Hum Reprod 1999;14:1352-1360.
3. Shushan A, Mordel N, Zajicek G, et al: A comparison of sonographic growth curves of triplet and twin fetuses. Am J Perinatol 1993;10:388-391.
4. Snijder MJ, Wladimiroff JW: Fetal biometry and outcome in monochorionic vs. dichorionic twin pregnancies: a retrospective cross-sectional matched-control study. Ultrasound in Med Biol 1998;24:197-201.
5. Socol ML, Tamura RK, Sabbagha RE, et al: Diminished biparietal diameter and abdominal circumference growth in twins. Obstet Gynecol 1984;64:235-238.
6. Grumbach K, Coleman B, Aryer P, et al: Twins and singleton growth patterns compared using ultrasound. Radiology 1986;158:237-241.
7. Reece EA, Yarkoni S, Abdulla M, et al: A prospective longitudinal study of growth in twin gestations compared with growth in singleton pregnancies. II: the fetal limbs. J Ultrasound Med 1991;10:445-450.
8. Haines CJ, Langlois S, Jones WR: Ultrasonic measurement of fetal femoral length in singleton and twin pregnancies. Am J Obstet Gynecol 1986;155:838-841.
9. Reece EA, Yarkoni S, Abdulla M, et al: A prospective longitudinal study of growth in twin gestations compared with growth in singleton pregnancies. I: the fetal head. J Ultrasound Med 1991;10:439-443.
10. Weissman A, Jakobi P, Yoffe N, et al: Sonographic growth measurements in triplet pregnancies. Obstet Gynecol 1990;75:324-328.

Obstetrical Doppler

Two-Dimensional and Pulsed Doppler Examination of the Fetal Ductus Arteriosus

Introduction

The ductus arteriosus is a unique vessel that is normally only present during fetal life. It courses between the main pulmonary artery and the thoracic aorta and can best be visualized using the transverse view of the chest, just above the three-vessel view (Figs. 33-1 and 33-2).[1] This vessel is responsible for directing more than 50% of the cardiac output to the lower body and placenta. Spontaneous constriction of the ductus arteriosus has been reported to be associated with fetal hydrops, right ventricular hypertrophy, right ventricular dysfunction, tricuspid regurgitation, and abnormal flow patterns of the ductus venosus. In addition to spontaneous premature closure, specific drugs, especially indomethacin, have been associated with premature closure of the ductus arteriosus and the associated increase in peak systolic and diastolic Doppler velocities, as well as a decrease in the pulsatility index.[1,2] Low-dose aspirin, often used in the treatment of patients at risk for adverse pregnancy outcome, has not been shown to constrict the ductus arteriosus if given up through 40 weeks of gestation.[3] Reverse flow through the ductus arteriosus has been reported with atrial flutter, as well as a number of complex heart defects, the most common being the hypoplastic left heart syndrome.[4] Given these findings, an argument could be made to examine the ductus arteriosus

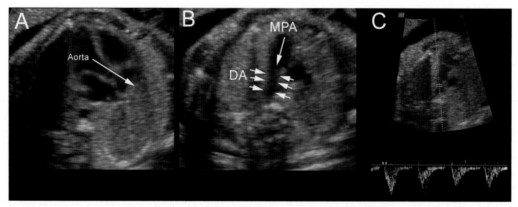

Figure 33-1
B-mode imaging of the ductus arteriosus obtained from the transverse plane of the chest. **A,** Orientation of the five-chamber view with the apex at 12 o'clock. **B,** Orientation of the main pulmonary artery (*MPA*) and ductus arteriosus (*DA*). **C,** The pulsed Doppler waveform of the ductus arteriosus. Although this is the ideal position for recording the pulsed Doppler waveform, the measurement of the diameter of the ductus arteriosus is less reliable because the vessel is parallel to the ultrasound beam. For accurate measurement of the ductus arteriosus diameter, it is best to image the vessel tangential or perpendicular to the ultrasound beam (see Fig. 33-2).[4]

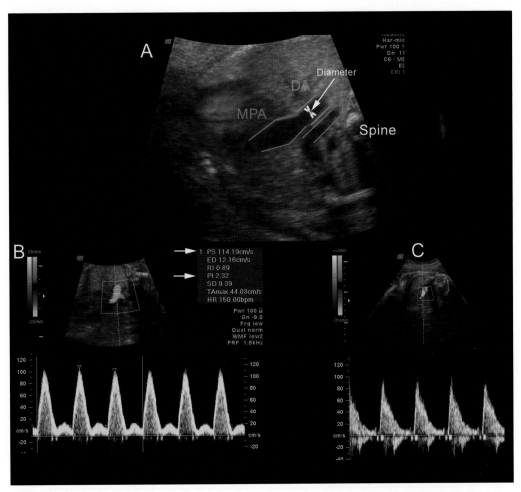

Figure 33-2
A, This image is obtained cephalad to the three-vessel view and contains the main pulmonary artery (*MPA*), ductus arteriosus (*DA*), and transverse arch of the aorta (*TA*). In this orientation, the boundary of the vessel walls are readily identified and measurement of the diameters of the ductus arteriosus and main pulmonary artery can be performed. **B,** The pulsed Doppler waveform of the ductus arteriosus is recorded and the peak velocity (PS) measured, as well as the pulsatility index (PI). **C,** Pulsed Doppler of the main pulmonary artery.

with Doppler ultrasound to look for evidence of ductal constriction and/or reverse flow.

B-Mode Evaluation of the Ductus Arteriosus

Tan et al[5] reported measurements of the ductal arch in 1992. (Fig. 33-3; Table 33-1). More recently, Mielke and Benda[6] reported results of their studies in which they measured the ductus arteriosus at three different levels, as well as its length (Fig. 33-4; Table 33-2).[6] Both sets of investigators found that the ductus arteriosus increased in size as a function of gestational age.

Pulsed Doppler Examination of the Ductus Arteriosus

During the 1990s a number of investigators reported an increase in the peak velocity of the ductus arteriosus between 12 and 40 weeks of gestation.[7] In 2000, Mielke and Benda[8] reported their results from examining fetuses between 13 and 40 weeks of gestation. They compared the peak velocity of the ductus arteriosus and the main pulmonary artery and found the peak systolic velocity increased between 13 and 40 weeks of gestation and was not influenced by a decreasing heart rate (Fig. 33-5; Table 33-3). The pulsatility index did not decrease with

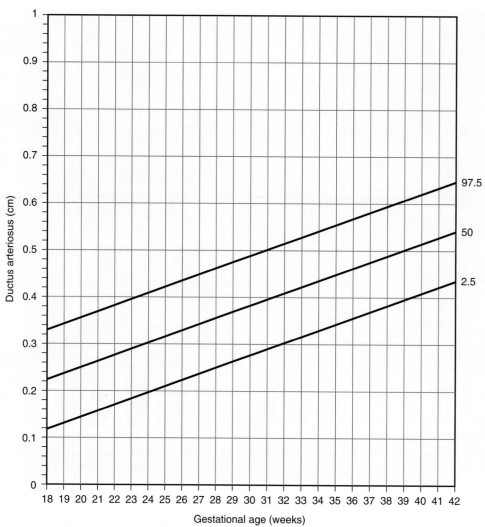

Figure 33-3
B-Mode measurement of the ductus arteriosus.[5]

Table 33-1	Measurements from the ductal arch[5]						
	Diameter of the Ductus Arteriosus (cm)				**Diameter of the Ductus Arteriosus (cm)**		
Gestation (wks)	**2.5th Percentile**	**50th Percentile**	**95th Percentile**	**Weeks Gestation**	**2.5th Percentile**	**50th Percentile**	**95th Percentile**
18	0.12	0.22	0.33	31	0.29	0.40	0.50
19	0.13	0.24	0.34	32	0.30	0.41	0.51
20	0.15	0.25	0.35	33	0.32	0.42	0.53
21	0.16	0.26	0.37	34	0.33	0.44	0.54
22	0.17	0.28	0.38	35	0.34	0.45	0.55
23	0.19	0.29	0.39	36	0.36	0.46	0.57
24	0.20	0.30	0.41	37	0.37	0.47	0.58
25	0.21	0.32	0.42	38	0.38	0.49	0.59
26	0.23	0.33	0.43	39	0.40	0.50	0.61
27	0.24	0.34	0.45	40	0.41	0.51	0.62
28	0.25	0.36	0.46	41	0.42	0.53	0.63
29	0.26	0.37	0.47	42	0.44	0.54	0.65
30	0.28	0.38	0.49				

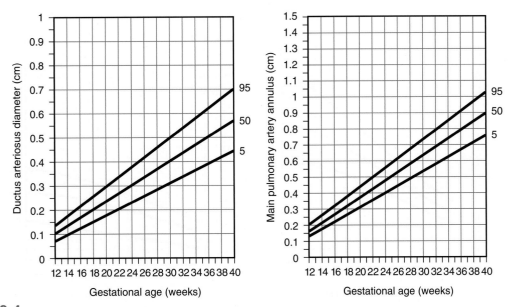

Figure 33-4
Diameter of the ductus arteriosus and main pulmonary artery annulus.[6]

Table 33-2	Diameter of the ductus arteriosus and main pulmonary artery[6]					
	Diameter of the Ductus Arteriosus (cm)			**Diameter of the Main Pulmonary Artery Annulus (cm)**		
Gestation (wks)	**5th Percentile**	**50th Percentile**	**95th Percentile**	**5th Percentile**	**50th Percentile**	**95th Percentile**
12	0.07	0.10	0.14	0.12	0.16	0.20
13	0.08	0.12	0.16	0.14	0.19	0.23
14	0.10	0.13	0.18	0.17	0.21	0.26
15	0.11	0.15	0.20	0.19	0.24	0.29
16	0.12	0.17	0.22	0.21	0.26	0.32
17	0.14	0.18	0.24	0.24	0.29	0.35
18	0.15	0.20	0.26	0.26	0.32	0.38
19	0.16	0.22	0.28	0.28	0.34	0.41
20	0.18	0.24	0.30	0.30	0.37	0.43
21	0.19	0.25	0.32	0.33	0.40	0.46
22	0.20	0.27	0.34	0.35	0.42	0.49
23	0.22	0.29	0.36	0.37	0.45	0.52
24	0.23	0.30	0.38	0.40	0.47	0.55
25	0.24	0.32	0.40	0.42	0.50	0.58
26	0.26	0.34	0.42	0.44	0.53	0.61
27	0.27	0.35	0.44	0.46	0.55	0.64
28	0.28	0.37	0.46	0.49	0.58	0.67
29	0.30	0.39	0.48	0.51	0.60	0.70
30	0.31	0.40	0.50	0.53	0.63	0.73
31	0.32	0.42	0.52	0.56	0.66	0.76
32	0.34	0.44	0.54	0.58	0.68	0.79
33	0.35	0.45	0.56	0.60	0.71	0.82
34	0.36	0.47	0.58	0.62	0.73	0.84
35	0.38	0.49	0.60	0.65	0.76	0.87
36	0.39	0.50	0.62	0.67	0.79	0.90
37	0.41	0.52	0.64	0.69	0.81	0.93
38	0.42	0.54	0.66	0.72	0.84	0.96
39	0.43	0.55	0.68	0.74	0.87	0.99
40	0.45	0.57	0.70	0.76	0.89	1.02

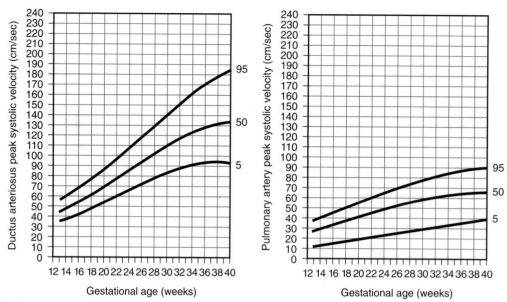

Figure 33-5
Peak systolic velocity of the ductus arteriosus and main pulmonary artery.[8]

Table 33-3	Peak systolic velocity of the ductus arteriosus and main pulmonary artery[8]					
	Peak Systolic Velocity of the Ductus Arteriosus (cm/sec)			Peak Velocity of the Main Pulmonary Artery (cm/sec)		
Gestation (wks)	5th Percentile	50th Percentile	95th Percentile	5th Percentile	50th Percentile	95th Percentile
13	34	43	56	28	38	47
14	36	47	59	30	40	50
15	39	50	63	32	43	53
16	42	54	67	34	45	56
17	45	58	71	36	48	59
18	48	61	76	38	50	62
19	51	65	81	40	53	65
20	54	70	86	42	55	68
21	57	74	91	43	57	71
22	60	78	96	45	60	74
23	63	82	102	47	62	77
24	67	86	107	49	65	80
25	70	90	113	51	67	82
26	73	94	118	53	69	85
27	75	98	124	54	72	87
28	78	102	130	56	74	90
29	81	106	135	57	76	92
30	83	109	141	59	78	94
31	86	113	146	60	80	96
32	88	116	151	62	82	98
33	89	119	156	63	83	100
34	91	122	161	64	85	102
35	92	124	165	65	86	103
36	93	127	170	66	87	105
37	94	129	174	66	88	106
38	94	130	178	67	89	107
39	94	132	181	67	90	108
40	93	133	184	67	91	108

gestational age (2.45 [SD 0.30]) but was affected by changes in heart rate.

References

1. Yoo SJ, Lee YH, Cho KS, Kim DY: Sequential segmental approach to fetal congenital heart disease. Cardiol Young 1999;9:430-444.
2. Levy R, Matitiau A, Ben Arie A, et al: Indomethacin and corticosteroids: an additive constrictive effect on the fetal ductus arteriosus. Am J Perinatol 1999;16:379-383.
3. Grab D, Paulus WE, Erdmann M, et al: Effects of low-dose aspirin on uterine and fetal blood flow during pregnancy: results of a randomized, placebo-controlled, double-blind trial. Ultrasound Obstet Gynecol 2000;15:19-27.
4. Berning RA, Silverman NH, Villegas M, et al: Reversed shunting across the ductus arteriosus or atrial septum in utero heralds severe congenital heart disease. J Am Coll Cardiol 1996;27:481-486.
5. Tan J, Silverman NH, Hoffman JI, et al: Cardiac dimensions determined by cross-sectional echocardiography in the normal human fetus from 18 weeks to term. Am J Cardiol 1992;70:1459-1467.
6. Mielke G, Benda N: Reference ranges for two-dimensional echocardiographic examination of the fetal ductus arteriosus. Ultrasound Obstet Gynecol 2000;15:219-225.
7. van der MK, Barendregt LG, Wladimiroff JW: Flow velocity wave forms in the human fetal ductus arteriosus during the normal second half of pregnancy. Pediatr Res 1991;30:487-490.
8. Mielke G, Benda N: Blood flow velocity waveforms of the fetal pulmonary artery and the ductus arteriosus: reference ranges from 13 weeks to term. Ultrasound Obstet Gynecol 2000;15:213-218.

CHAPTER 34

Greggory R. DeVore

M-Mode Measurement of the Fetal Heart

Introduction

In the late 1970s and early 1980s, M-mode ultrasound was used to elucidate fetal arrhythmias and to measure ventricular chamber size, ventricular wall thickness, ventricular contractility, atrioventricular valve size, and the dimensions of the aortic and pulmonary outflow tracts.[1-7] M-mode is still a useful adjunct to the fetal cardiovascular examination because it enables the physician or sonographer to obtain exact measurements of these structures. This section describes how to obtain the M-mode recording and an approach to making the necessary measurements.

Placement of the M-Mode Cursor

Unlike the postnatal examination in which an electrocardiogram can be obtained to identify systole and diastole, an electrocardiogram of the fetus cannot be obtained for this purpose. Therefore it is important to place the M-mode cursor through the heart so that the mechanical equivalent of ventricular systole and diastole can be identified. To accomplish this, the M-mode cursor is placed perpendicular to the interventricular septum at the level of the mitral and tricuspid valves and the M-mode recorded

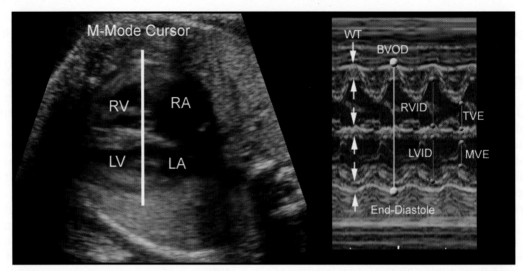

Figure 34-1

Recording of the M-mode from the four-chamber view. Measurements are made from the M-mode tracing at end-diastole. This is defined as the point where the tricuspid and mitral valves close. BVOD, biventricular outer dimension; LA, left atrium; LV, left ventricle; LVID, left ventricular internal dimension; MVE, mitral valve excursion; RA, right atrium; RV, right ventricle; RVID, right ventricular internal dimension; TVE, tricuspid valve excursion; WT, wall thickness.

(Fig. 34-1). This allows the examiner to identify end-systole (maximal inward excursion of the ventricular walls) and end-diastole (closure of the atrioventricular valves). Once end-systole and end-diastole are identified, a number of measurements can be made (Fig. 34-2).

Adjusting for Gestational Age

Several studies have been published in which the M-mode measurements have been compared with gestational age that was determined from ultrasound measurements of noncardiovascular structures.[6,7] From these data, confidence intervals were constructed. The problem with this approach is that gestational age is a derived value from regression analysis of measurements of the fetal head, abdomen, and femur that introduces an additional error. In the postnatal period, cardiac measurements are compared with the size of the individual and not his or her age. For these reasons, it is preferable to compare M-mode measurements with the fetal biparietal diameter, femur length, or abdominal circumference.[2-5] This allows for the comparison of heart size with the size of the fetus, independent of its age.

Measurements of Ventricular Chamber Size

Three measurements are used to determine ventricular size, all of which are obtained at end-diastole. Biventricular outer dimension is measured from the epicardium of the left ventricle to the epicardium of the right ventricle. This measurement includes the thickness of the right and left ventricular walls and interventricular septum, as well as the dimensions of the ventricular chambers (Figs. 34-1 to 34-4; Tables 34-1 and 34-2). The right ventricular inner dimension is measured from the endocardium of the right ventricular wall to the endocardium of the right side of the interventricular septum. This is the widest dimension of the right ventricle (see Figs. 34-1 to 34-4; see Tables 34-1 and 34-2). The left ventricular inner dimension is measured from the endocardium of the left ventricular wall to the endocardium of the left side of the ventricular septum. This is the widest dimension of the left ventricle (see Figs. 34-1 to 34-4; see Tables 34-1 and 34-2). The ratio of the end-diastolic right ventricular inner dimension to the end-diastolic left ventricular inner dimension can also be computed

Text continued on p. 124

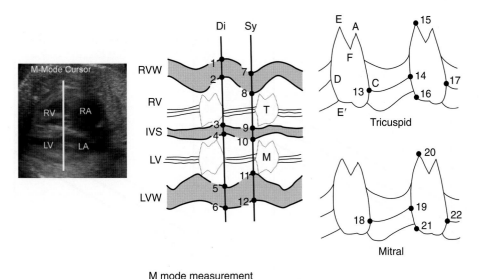

M mode measurement

	Point	Point
Right ventricle		
(A) Internal dimension – diastole	2	3
(B) Internal dimension – systole	8	9
(C) Wall thickness – diastole	1	2
Left ventricle		
(D) Internal dimension – diastole	4	5
(E) Internal dimension – systole	10	11
(F) Wall thickness – diastole	5	6
Interventricular septum		
(G) Wall thickness – diastole	3	4
(H) Wall thickness – systole	9	10
Biventricular dimensions		
(I) Inner dimension – diastole	2	5
(J) Inner dimension – systole	8	11
(K) Outer dimension – diastole	1	6
(L) Outer dimension – systole	7	12
Tricuspid valve		
(M) Opening excursion (E–E′)	16	16
(N) Systolic time	13	14
(O) Diastolic time	14	17
(P) Duration of cardiac cycle	13	17
Mitral valve		
(Q) Opening excursion (E–E′)	20	21
(R) Systolic time	18	19
(S) Diastolic time	19	22
(T) Duration of cardiac cycle	18	22

Figure 34-2
M-Mode measurements obtained from the four-chamber view. The reference points define the measurements from the M-mode recording.[5]

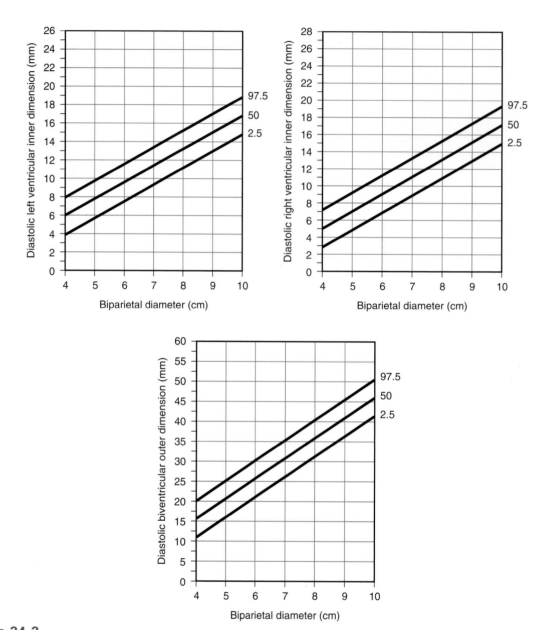

Figure 34-3
M-mode measurements of the ventricular chambers at end-diastole using the biparietal diameter as the reference.[5]

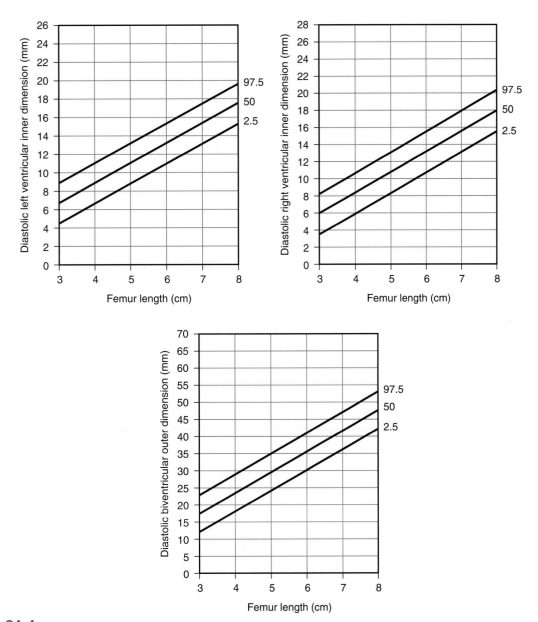

Figure 34-4
M-mode measurements of the ventricular chambers at end-diastole using the femur length as the reference.[4]

Table 34-1   End-diastolic M-mode measurements of the ventricular chambers using the biparietal diameter (BPD) as the reference[5]

BPD (cm)	Left Ventricular Inner Dimension (mm)			Right Ventricular Inner Dimension (mm)			Biventricular Outer Dimension (mm)		
	2.5th Percentile	50th Percentile	97.5th Percentile	2.5th Percentile	50th Percentile	97.5th Percentile	2.5th Percentile	50th Percentile	97.5th Percentile
4.0	3.9	5.9	7.9	3.0	5.1	7.3	10.6	15.3	20.0
4.1	4.0	6.1	8.1	3.2	5.3	7.5	11.2	15.8	20.5
4.2	4.2	6.3	8.3	3.4	5.5	7.7	11.7	16.3	21.0
4.3	4.4	6.4	8.5	3.6	5.7	7.9	12.2	16.9	21.5
4.4	4.6	6.6	8.6	3.8	5.9	8.1	12.7	17.4	22.0
4.5	4.8	6.8	8.8	4.0	6.1	8.3	13.2	17.9	22.6
4.6	4.9	7.0	9.0	4.2	6.3	8.5	13.7	18.4	23.1
4.7	5.1	7.2	9.2	4.4	6.5	8.7	14.2	18.9	23.6
4.8	5.3	7.3	9.4	4.6	6.7	8.9	14.7	19.4	24.1
4.9	5.5	7.5	9.5	4.8	6.9	9.1	15.2	19.9	24.6
5.0	5.7	7.7	9.7	5.0	7.1	9.3	15.7	20.4	25.1
5.1	5.9	7.9	9.9	5.2	7.3	9.5	16.2	20.9	25.6
5.2	6.0	8.1	10.1	5.4	7.5	9.7	16.8	21.4	26.1
5.3	6.2	8.2	10.3	5.6	7.7	9.9	17.3	21.9	26.6
5.4	6.4	8.4	10.4	5.8	7.9	10.1	17.8	22.5	27.1
5.5	6.6	8.6	10.6	6.0	8.1	10.3	18.3	23.0	27.6
5.6	6.8	8.8	10.8	6.2	8.3	10.5	18.8	23.5	28.2
5.7	6.9	9.0	11.0	6.4	8.5	10.7	19.3	24.0	28.7
5.8	7.1	9.1	11.2	6.6	8.7	10.9	19.8	24.5	29.2
5.9	7.3	9.3	11.4	6.8	8.9	11.1	20.3	25.0	29.7
6.0	7.5	9.5	11.5	7.0	9.1	11.3	20.8	25.5	30.2
6.1	7.7	9.7	11.7	7.2	9.3	11.5	21.3	26.0	30.7
6.2	7.8	9.9	11.9	7.4	9.5	11.7	21.8	26.5	31.2
6.3	8.0	10.1	12.1	7.6	9.7	11.9	22.4	27.0	31.7
6.4	8.2	10.2	12.3	7.8	9.9	12.1	22.9	27.5	32.2
6.5	8.4	10.4	12.4	8.0	10.2	12.3	23.4	28.1	32.7
6.6	8.6	10.6	12.6	8.2	10.4	12.5	23.9	28.6	33.2
6.7	8.7	10.8	12.8	8.4	10.6	12.7	24.4	29.1	33.8
6.8	8.9	11.0	13.0	8.6	10.8	12.9	24.9	29.6	34.3
6.9	9.1	11.1	13.2	8.8	11.0	13.1	25.4	30.1	34.8
7.0	9.3	11.3	13.3	9.0	11.2	13.3	25.9	30.6	35.3
7.1	9.5	11.5	13.5	9.2	11.4	13.5	26.4	31.1	35.8
7.2	9.7	11.7	13.7	9.4	11.6	13.7	26.9	31.6	36.3
7.3	9.8	11.9	13.9	9.6	11.8	13.9	27.4	32.1	36.8
7.4	10.0	12.0	14.1	9.8	12.0	14.1	28.0	32.6	37.3
7.5	10.2	12.2	14.2	10.0	12.2	14.3	28.5	33.1	37.8
7.6	10.4	12.4	14.4	10.2	12.4	14.5	29.0	33.7	38.3
7.7	10.6	12.6	14.6	10.4	12.6	14.7	29.5	34.2	38.8
7.8	10.7	12.8	14.8	10.6	12.8	14.9	30.0	34.7	39.4
7.9	10.9	12.9	15.0	10.8	13.0	15.1	30.5	35.2	39.9
8.0	11.1	13.1	15.2	11.0	13.2	15.3	31.0	35.7	40.4
8.1	11.3	13.3	15.3	11.2	13.4	15.5	31.5	36.2	40.9
8.2	11.5	13.5	15.5	11.4	13.6	15.7	32.0	36.7	41.4
8.3	11.6	13.7	15.7	11.6	13.8	15.9	32.5	37.2	41.9
8.4	11.8	13.9	15.9	11.8	14.0	16.1	33.0	37.7	42.4
8.5	12.0	14.0	16.1	12.0	14.2	16.3	33.6	38.2	42.9
8.6	12.2	14.2	16.2	12.2	14.4	16.5	34.1	38.7	43.4
8.7	12.4	14.4	16.4	12.4	14.6	16.7	34.6	39.3	43.9
8.8	12.5	14.6	16.6	12.6	14.8	16.9	35.1	39.8	44.4
8.9	12.7	14.8	16.8	12.8	15.0	17.1	35.6	40.3	45.0
9.0	12.9	14.9	17.0	13.0	15.2	17.3	36.1	40.8	45.5
9.1	13.1	15.1	17.1	13.2	15.4	17.5	36.6	41.3	46.0
9.2	13.3	15.3	17.3	13.4	15.6	17.7	37.1	41.8	46.5
9.3	13.5	15.5	17.5	13.6	15.8	17.9	37.6	42.3	47.0
9.4	13.6	15.7	17.7	13.8	16.0	18.1	38.1	42.8	47.5
9.5	13.8	15.8	17.9	14.0	16.2	18.3	38.6	43.3	48.0
9.6	14.0	16.0	18.1	14.2	16.4	18.5	39.2	43.8	48.5
9.7	14.2	16.2	18.2	14.4	16.6	18.7	39.7	44.3	49.0
9.8	14.4	16.4	18.4	14.7	16.8	18.9	40.2	44.9	49.5
9.9	14.5	16.6	18.6	14.9	17.0	19.1	40.7	45.4	50.0
10.0	14.7	16.7	18.8	15.1	17.2	19.3	41.2	45.9	50.6

Table 34-2 End-diastolic M-mode measurements of the ventricular chambers using the femur length (FL) as the reference[4]

FL (cm)	Left Ventricular Inner Dimension (mm)			Right Ventricular Inner Dimension (mm)			Biventricular Outer Dimension (mm)		
	2.5th Percentile	50th Percentile	97.5th Percentile	2.5th Percentile	50th Percentile	97.5th Percentile	2.5th Percentile	50th Percentile	97.5th Percentile
3.0	4.5	6.7	8.8	3.6	6.0	8.3	12.0	17.5	23.0
3.1	4.7	6.9	9.0	3.9	6.2	8.6	12.7	18.1	23.6
3.2	4.9	7.1	9.2	4.1	6.5	8.8	13.3	18.8	24.2
3.3	5.1	7.3	9.5	4.4	6.7	9.1	13.9	19.4	24.8
3.4	5.4	7.5	9.7	4.6	6.9	9.3	14.5	20.0	25.5
3.5	5.6	7.7	9.9	4.8	7.2	9.5	15.1	20.6	26.1
3.6	5.8	8.0	10.1	5.1	7.4	9.8	15.7	21.2	26.7
3.7	6.0	8.2	10.3	5.3	7.7	10.0	16.3	21.8	27.3
3.8	6.2	8.4	10.6	5.6	7.9	10.3	16.9	22.4	27.9
3.9	6.5	8.6	10.8	5.8	8.2	10.5	17.5	23.0	28.5
4.0	6.7	8.8	11.0	6.0	8.4	10.8	18.1	23.6	29.1
4.1	6.9	9.1	11.2	6.3	8.6	11.0	18.8	24.2	29.7
4.2	7.1	9.3	11.4	6.5	8.9	11.2	19.4	24.9	30.3
4.3	7.3	9.5	11.6	6.8	9.1	11.5	20.0	25.5	31.0
4.4	7.6	9.7	11.9	7.0	9.4	11.7	20.6	26.1	31.6
4.5	7.8	9.9	12.1	7.3	9.6	12.0	21.2	26.7	32.2
4.6	8.0	10.1	12.3	7.5	9.9	12.2	21.8	27.3	32.8
4.7	8.2	10.4	12.5	7.7	10.1	12.4	22.4	27.9	33.4
4.8	8.4	10.6	12.7	8.0	10.3	12.7	23.0	28.5	34.0
4.9	8.6	10.8	13.0	8.2	10.6	12.9	23.6	29.1	34.6
5.0	8.9	11.0	13.2	8.5	10.8	13.2	24.3	29.7	35.2
5.1	9.1	11.2	13.4	8.7	11.1	13.4	24.9	30.4	35.8
5.2	9.3	11.5	13.6	8.9	11.3	13.7	25.5	31.0	36.5
5.3	9.5	11.7	13.8	9.2	11.5	13.9	26.1	31.6	37.1
5.4	9.7	11.9	14.0	9.4	11.8	14.1	26.7	32.2	37.7
5.5	10.0	12.1	14.3	9.7	12.0	14.4	27.3	32.8	38.3
5.6	10.2	12.3	14.5	9.9	12.3	14.6	27.9	33.4	38.9
5.7	10.4	12.5	14.7	10.2	12.5	14.9	28.5	34.0	39.5
5.8	10.6	12.8	14.9	10.4	12.8	15.1	29.1	34.6	40.1
5.9	10.8	13.0	15.1	10.6	13.0	15.3	29.8	35.2	40.7
6.0	11.0	13.2	15.4	10.9	13.2	15.6	30.4	35.9	41.3
6.1	11.3	13.4	15.6	11.1	13.5	15.8	31.0	36.5	42.0
6.2	11.5	13.6	15.8	11.4	13.7	16.1	31.6	37.1	42.6
6.3	11.7	13.9	16.0	11.6	14.0	16.3	32.2	37.7	43.2
6.4	11.9	14.1	16.2	11.9	14.2	16.6	32.8	38.3	43.8
6.5	12.1	14.3	16.4	12.1	14.4	16.8	33.4	38.9	44.4
6.6	12.4	14.5	16.7	12.3	14.7	17.0	34.0	39.5	45.0
6.7	12.6	14.7	16.9	12.6	14.9	17.3	34.6	40.1	45.6
6.8	12.8	14.9	17.1	12.8	15.2	17.5	35.3	40.7	46.2
6.9	13.0	15.2	17.3	13.1	15.4	17.8	35.9	41.4	46.8
7.0	13.2	15.4	17.5	13.3	15.7	18.0	36.5	42.0	47.5
7.1	13.4	15.6	17.8	13.5	15.9	18.2	37.1	42.6	48.1
7.2	13.7	15.8	18.0	13.8	16.1	18.5	37.7	43.2	48.7
7.3	13.9	16.0	18.2	14.0	16.4	18.7	38.3	43.8	49.3
7.4	14.1	16.3	18.4	14.3	16.6	19.0	38.9	44.4	49.9
7.5	14.3	16.5	18.6	14.5	16.9	19.2	39.5	45.0	50.5
7.6	14.5	16.7	18.8	14.8	17.1	19.5	40.1	45.6	51.1
7.7	14.8	16.9	19.1	15.0	17.3	19.7	40.8	46.2	51.7
7.8	15.0	17.1	19.3	15.2	17.6	19.9	41.4	46.9	52.3
7.9	15.2	17.3	19.5	15.5	17.8	20.2	42.0	47.5	53.0
8.0	15.4	17.6	19.7	15.7	18.1	20.4	42.6	48.1	53.6

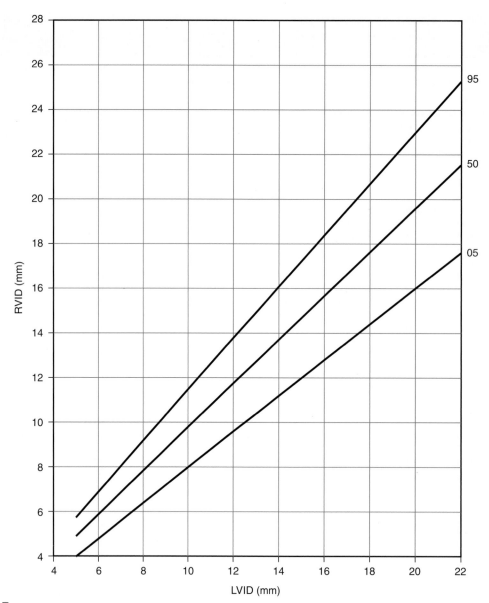

Figure 34-5
Ratio of the right ventricular internal dimension (RVID) with the left ventricular inner dimension (LVID) measured at end-diastole.[5]

to evaluate chamber disproportion (Fig. 34-5; Table 34-3).

Measurements of Ventricular Wall Thickness

There are two methods to evaluate the thickness of ventricular walls and interventricular septum. The first method is to evaluate the total wall thickness, which includes the right and left ventricular walls and the interventricular septum. This is computed by measuring the end-diastolic biventricular outer dimension and subtracting the right and left end-diastolic inner dimensions (Figs. 34-2 and 34-6; Table 34-4). The second method is to measure the end-diastolic right and left ventricular walls and the interventricular septum separately (Figs. 34-2, 34-7, and 34-8; Tables 34-5 and 34-6). For screening purposes, the first method has been found to be the easiest to use.

Text continued on p. 131

Table 34-3 Ratio of the end-diastolic right ventricular inner dimension (RVID) to the end-diastolic left ventricular inner dimension (LVID)[5]

LVID (mm)	RVID 5th Percentile (mm)	RVID 50th Percentile (mm)	RVID 95th Percentile (mm)	LVID (mm)	RVID 5th Percentile (mm)	RVID 50th Percentile (mm)	RVID 95th Percentile (mm)
1.0	0.8	1.0	1.2	14.0	11.2	13.7	16.1
2.0	1.6	2.0	2.3	15.0	12.0	14.7	17.3
3.0	2.4	2.9	3.5	16.0	12.8	15.7	18.4
4.0	3.2	3.9	4.6	17.0	13.6	16.7	19.6
5.0	4.0	4.9	5.8	18.0	14.4	17.6	20.7
6.0	4.8	5.9	6.9	19.0	15.2	18.6	21.9
7.0	5.6	6.9	8.1	20.0	16.0	19.6	23.0
8.0	6.4	7.8	9.2	21.0	16.8	20.6	24.2
9.0	7.2	8.8	10.4	22.0	17.6	21.6	25.3
10.0	8.0	9.8	11.5	23.0	18.4	22.5	26.5
11.0	8.8	10.8	12.7	24.0	19.2	23.5	27.6
12.0	9.6	11.8	13.8	25.0	20.0	24.5	28.8
13.0	10.4	12.7	15.0				

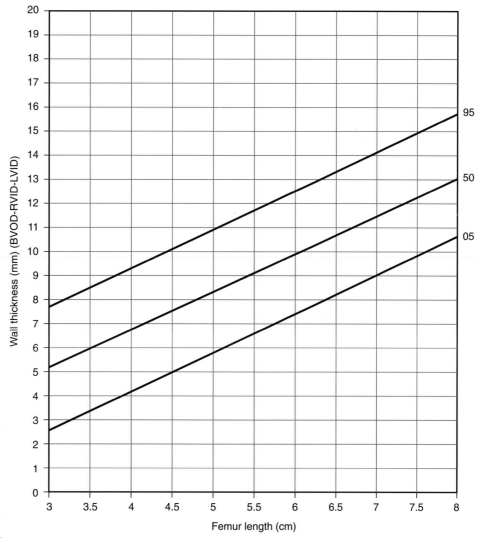

Figure 34-6
Combined thickness of the right and left ventricular walls and the interventricular septum is determined by measuring the end-diastolic biventricular outer dimension (BVOD) and subtracting the end-diastolic right (RVID) and left ventricular (LVID) inner chamber dimensions. Following this computation, the total thickness of the walls can be determined.

Table 34-4	Combined wall thickness of the ventricles measured at end-diastole using the femur length (FL) as the reference		

| FL (cm) | Combined Wall Thickness (BVOD-RVID-LVID) (mm) | | |
	5th Percentile	50th Percentile	95th Percentile
3.0	2.6	5.2	7.7
3.1	2.8	5.3	7.9
3.2	2.9	5.5	8.0
3.3	3.1	5.6	8.2
3.4	3.2	5.8	8.3
3.5	3.4	5.9	8.5
3.6	3.6	6.1	8.7
3.7	3.7	6.3	8.8
3.8	3.9	6.4	9.0
3.9	4.0	6.6	9.1
4.0	4.2	6.7	9.3
4.1	4.4	6.9	9.5
4.2	4.5	7.0	9.6
4.3	4.7	7.2	9.8
4.4	4.8	7.4	9.9
4.5	5.0	7.5	10.1
4.6	5.2	7.7	10.3
4.7	5.3	7.8	10.4
4.8	5.5	8.0	10.6
4.9	5.6	8.1	10.7
5.0	5.8	8.3	10.9
5.1	6.0	8.4	11.1
5.2	6.1	8.6	11.2
5.3	6.3	8.8	11.4
5.4	6.4	8.9	11.5
5.5	6.6	9.1	11.7
5.6	6.8	9.2	11.9
5.7	6.9	9.4	12.0
5.8	7.1	9.5	12.2
5.9	7.2	9.7	12.3
6.0	7.4	9.9	12.5
6.1	7.6	10.0	12.7
6.2	7.7	10.2	12.8
6.3	7.9	10.3	13.0
6.4	8.0	10.5	13.1
6.5	8.2	10.6	13.3
6.6	8.4	10.8	13.5
6.7	8.5	10.9	13.6
6.8	8.7	11.1	13.8
6.9	8.8	11.3	13.9
7.0	9.0	11.4	14.1
7.1	9.2	11.6	14.3
7.2	9.3	11.7	14.4
7.3	9.5	11.9	14.6
7.4	9.6	12.0	14.7
7.5	9.8	12.2	14.9
7.6	10.0	12.4	15.1
7.7	10.1	12.5	15.2
7.8	10.3	12.7	15.4
7.9	10.4	12.8	15.5
8.0	10.6	13.0	15.7

BVOD, Biventricular outer dimension; LVID, left ventricular inner dimension; RVID, right ventricular inner dimension.

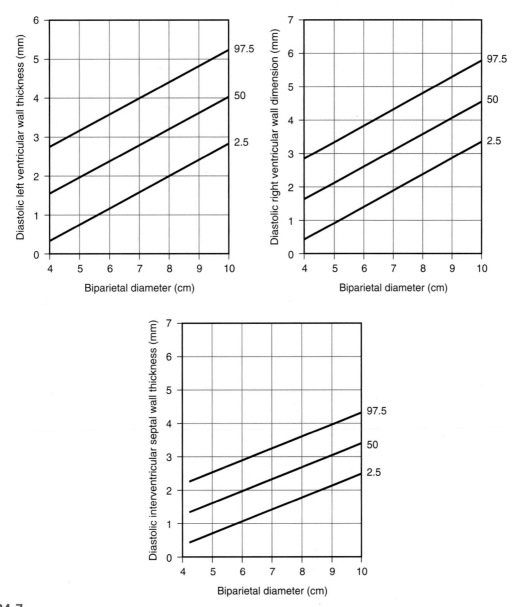

Figure 34-7

End-diastolic thickness of the ventricular walls and the interventricular septum using the biparietal diameter as the reference.[5]

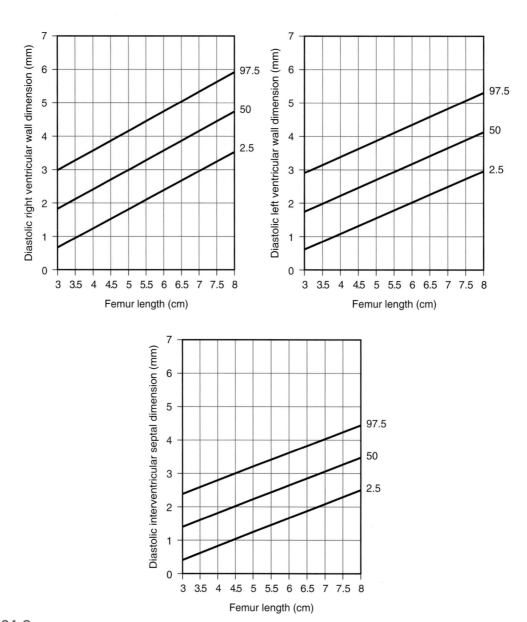

Figure 34-8
End-diastolic thickness of the ventricular walls and the interventricular septum using the femur length as the reference.[4]

| Table 34-5 | End-diastolic measurements of the ventricular wall thickness using the biparietal diameter (BPD) as the reference[5] | | | | | | | | |

BPD (cm)	Left Ventricular Wall Thickness (mm)			Right Ventricular Wall Thickness (mm)			Interventricular Septall Wall Thickness (mm)		
	2.5th Percentile	50th Percentile	97.5th Percentile	2.5th Percentile	50th Percentile	97.5th Percentile	2.5th Percentile	50th Percentile	97.5th Percentile
4.0	0.3	1.6	2.8	0.4	1.6	2.8	0.3	1.2	2.2
4.1	0.4	1.6	2.8	0.4	1.6	2.9	0.4	1.3	2.2
4.2	0.4	1.6	2.8	0.5	1.7	2.9	0.4	1.3	2.2
4.3	0.5	1.7	2.9	0.5	1.7	3.0	0.4	1.3	2.3
4.4	0.5	1.7	2.9	0.6	1.8	3.0	0.5	1.4	2.3
4.5	0.6	1.8	3.0	0.6	1.8	3.1	0.5	1.4	2.3
4.6	0.6	1.8	3.0	0.7	1.9	3.1	0.5	1.4	2.4
4.7	0.6	1.8	3.0	0.7	1.9	3.2	0.6	1.5	2.4
4.8	0.7	1.9	3.1	0.8	2.0	3.2	0.6	1.5	2.4
4.9	0.7	1.9	3.1	0.8	2.0	3.3	0.6	1.6	2.5
5.0	0.8	2.0	3.2	0.9	2.1	3.3	0.7	1.6	2.5
5.1	0.8	2.0	3.2	0.9	2.1	3.4	0.7	1.6	2.5
5.2	0.8	2.0	3.3	1.0	2.2	3.4	0.7	1.7	2.6
5.3	0.9	2.1	3.3	1.0	2.2	3.5	0.8	1.7	2.6
5.4	0.9	2.1	3.3	1.1	2.3	3.5	0.8	1.7	2.7
5.5	1.0	2.2	3.4	1.1	2.3	3.6	0.8	1.8	2.7
5.6	1.0	2.2	3.4	1.2	2.4	3.6	0.9	1.8	2.7
5.7	1.0	2.3	3.5	1.2	2.4	3.6	0.9	1.8	2.8
5.8	1.1	2.3	3.5	1.3	2.5	3.7	1.0	1.9	2.8
5.9	1.1	2.3	3.5	1.3	2.5	3.7	1.0	1.9	2.8
6.0	1.2	2.4	3.6	1.3	2.6	3.8	1.0	1.9	2.9
6.1	1.2	2.4	3.6	1.4	2.6	3.8	1.1	2.0	2.9
6.2	1.2	2.5	3.7	1.4	2.7	3.9	1.1	2.0	2.9
6.3	1.3	2.5	3.7	1.5	2.7	3.9	1.1	2.1	3.0
6.4	1.3	2.5	3.7	1.5	2.8	4.0	1.2	2.1	3.0
6.5	1.4	2.6	3.8	1.6	2.8	4.0	1.2	2.1	3.0
6.6	1.4	2.6	3.8	1.6	2.9	4.1	1.2	2.2	3.1
6.7	1.5	2.7	3.9	1.7	2.9	4.1	1.3	2.2	3.1
6.8	1.5	2.7	3.9	1.7	3.0	4.2	1.3	2.2	3.1
6.9	1.5	2.7	3.9	1.8	3.0	4.2	1.3	2.3	3.2
7.0	1.6	2.8	4.0	1.8	3.1	4.3	1.4	2.3	3.2
7.1	1.6	2.8	4.0	1.9	3.1	4.3	1.4	2.3	3.3
7.2	1.7	2.9	4.1	1.9	3.2	4.4	1.5	2.4	3.3
7.3	1.7	2.9	4.1	2.0	3.2	4.4	1.5	2.4	3.3
7.4	1.7	2.9	4.2	2.0	3.3	4.5	1.5	2.4	3.4
7.5	1.8	3.0	4.2	2.1	3.3	4.5	1.6	2.5	3.4
7.6	1.8	3.0	4.2	2.1	3.4	4.6	1.6	2.5	3.4
7.7	1.9	3.1	4.3	2.2	3.4	4.6	1.6	2.5	3.5
7.8	1.9	3.1	4.3	2.2	3.5	4.7	1.7	2.6	3.5
7.9	1.9	3.2	4.4	2.3	3.5	4.7	1.7	2.6	3.5
8.0	2.0	3.2	4.4	2.3	3.6	4.8	1.7	2.7	3.6
8.1	2.0	3.2	4.4	2.4	3.6	4.8	1.8	2.7	3.6
8.2	2.1	3.3	4.5	2.4	3.6	4.9	1.8	2.7	3.6
8.3	2.1	3.3	4.5	2.5	3.7	4.9	1.8	2.8	3.7
8.4	2.1	3.4	4.6	2.5	3.7	5.0	1.9	2.8	3.7
8.5	2.2	3.4	4.6	2.6	3.8	5.0	1.9	2.8	3.7
8.6	2.2	3.4	4.6	2.6	3.8	5.1	1.9	2.9	3.8
8.7	2.3	3.5	4.7	2.7	3.9	5.1	2.0	2.9	3.8
8.8	2.3	3.5	4.7	2.7	3.9	5.2	2.0	2.9	3.9
8.9	2.4	3.6	4.8	2.8	4.0	5.2	2.1	3.0	3.9
9.0	2.4	3.6	4.8	2.8	4.0	5.3	2.1	3.0	3.9
9.1	2.4	3.6	4.8	2.9	4.1	5.3	2.1	3.0	4.0
9.2	2.5	3.7	4.9	2.9	4.1	5.4	2.2	3.1	4.0
9.3	2.5	3.7	4.9	3.0	4.2	5.4	2.2	3.1	4.0
9.4	2.6	3.8	5.0	3.0	4.2	5.5	2.2	3.1	4.1
9.5	2.6	3.8	5.0	3.1	4.3	5.5	2.3	3.2	4.1
9.6	2.6	3.8	5.1	3.1	4.3	5.6	2.3	3.2	4.1
9.7	2.7	3.9	5.1	3.2	4.4	5.6	2.3	3.3	4.2
9.8	2.7	3.9	5.1	3.2	4.4	5.7	2.4	3.3	4.2
9.9	2.8	4.0	5.2	3.3	4.5	5.7	2.4	3.3	4.2
10.0	2.8	4.0	5.2	3.3	4.5	5.8	2.4	3.4	4.3

Table 34-6 End-diastolic measurements of the ventricular wall thickness using the femur length (FL) as the reference[4]

FL (cm)	Left Ventricular Wall Thickness (mm)			Right Ventricular Wall Thickness (mm)			Interventricular Septal Wall Thickness (mm)		
	2.5th Percentile	50th Percentile	97.5th Percentile	2.5th Percentile	50th Percentile	97.5th Percentile	2.5th Percentile	50th Percentile	97.5th Percentile
3.0	0.6	1.8	2.9	0.6	1.8	3.0	0.4	1.4	2.4
3.1	0.6	1.8	3.0	0.7	1.9	3.0	0.5	1.4	2.4
3.2	0.7	1.9	3.0	0.8	1.9	3.1	0.5	1.5	2.5
3.3	0.7	1.9	3.1	0.8	2.0	3.2	0.5	1.5	2.5
3.4	0.8	1.9	3.1	0.9	2.0	3.2	0.6	1.6	2.5
3.5	0.8	2.0	3.2	0.9	2.1	3.3	0.6	1.6	2.6
3.6	0.9	2.0	3.2	1.0	2.2	3.3	0.7	1.7	2.6
3.7	0.9	2.1	3.3	1.0	2.2	3.4	0.7	1.7	2.7
3.8	1.0	2.1	3.3	1.1	2.3	3.5	0.8	1.7	2.7
3.9	1.0	2.2	3.4	1.2	2.3	3.5	0.8	1.8	2.8
4.0	1.1	2.2	3.4	1.2	2.4	3.6	0.8	1.8	2.8
4.1	1.1	2.3	3.5	1.3	2.5	3.6	0.9	1.9	2.8
4.2	1.2	2.3	3.5	1.3	2.5	3.7	0.9	1.9	2.9
4.3	1.2	2.4	3.6	1.4	2.6	3.7	1.0	1.9	2.9
4.4	1.3	2.4	3.6	1.5	2.6	3.8	1.0	2.0	3.0
4.5	1.3	2.5	3.7	1.5	2.7	3.9	1.1	2.0	3.0
4.6	1.3	2.5	3.7	1.6	2.7	3.9	1.1	2.1	3.1
4.7	1.4	2.6	3.7	1.6	2.8	4.0	1.1	2.1	3.1
4.8	1.4	2.6	3.8	1.7	2.9	4.0	1.2	2.2	3.1
4.9	1.5	2.7	3.8	1.7	2.9	4.1	1.2	2.2	3.2
5.0	1.5	2.7	3.9	1.8	3.0	4.2	1.3	2.2	3.2
5.1	1.6	2.8	3.9	1.9	3.0	4.2	1.3	2.3	3.3
5.2	1.6	2.8	4.0	1.9	3.1	4.3	1.3	2.3	3.3
5.3	1.7	2.9	4.0	2.0	3.2	4.3	1.4	2.4	3.3
5.4	1.7	2.9	4.1	2.0	3.2	4.4	1.4	2.4	3.4
5.5	1.8	3.0	4.1	2.1	3.3	4.4	1.5	2.5	3.4
5.6	1.8	3.0	4.2	2.2	3.3	4.5	1.5	2.5	3.5
5.7	1.9	3.1	4.2	2.2	3.4	4.6	1.6	2.5	3.5
5.8	1.9	3.1	4.3	2.3	3.4	4.6	1.6	2.6	3.6
5.9	2.0	3.1	4.3	2.3	3.5	4.7	1.6	2.6	3.6
6.0	2.0	3.2	4.4	2.4	3.6	4.7	1.7	2.7	3.6
6.1	2.1	3.2	4.4	2.4	3.6	4.8	1.7	2.7	3.7
6.2	2.1	3.3	4.5	2.5	3.7	4.9	1.8	2.7	3.7
6.3	2.2	3.3	4.5	2.6	3.7	4.9	1.8	2.8	3.8
6.4	2.2	3.4	4.6	2.6	3.8	5.0	1.9	2.8	3.8
6.5	2.3	3.4	4.6	2.7	3.9	5.0	1.9	2.9	3.9
6.6	2.3	3.5	4.7	2.7	3.9	5.1	1.9	2.9	3.9
6.7	2.4	3.5	4.7	2.8	4.0	5.1	2.0	3.0	3.9
6.8	2.4	3.6	4.8	2.9	4.0	5.2	2.0	3.0	4.0
6.9	2.5	3.6	4.8	2.9	4.1	5.3	2.1	3.0	4.0
7.0	2.5	3.7	4.9	3.0	4.1	5.3	2.1	3.1	4.1
7.1	2.5	3.7	4.9	3.0	4.2	5.4	2.1	3.1	4.1
7.2	2.6	3.8	4.9	3.1	4.3	5.4	2.2	3.2	4.1
7.3	2.6	3.8	5.0	3.1	4.3	5.5	2.2	3.2	4.2
7.4	2.7	3.9	5.0	3.2	4.4	5.6	2.3	3.3	4.2
7.5	2.7	3.9	5.1	3.3	4.4	5.6	2.3	3.3	4.3
7.6	2.8	4.0	5.1	3.3	4.5	5.7	2.4	3.3	4.3
7.7	2.8	4.0	5.2	3.4	4.6	5.7	2.4	3.4	4.4
7.8	2.9	4.1	5.2	3.4	4.6	5.8	2.4	3.4	4.4
7.9	2.9	4.1	5.3	3.5	4.7	5.9	2.5	3.5	4.4
8.0	3.0	4.2	5.3	3.6	4.7	5.9	2.5	3.5	4.5

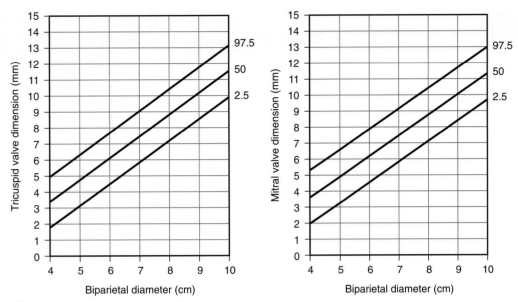

Figure 34-9
Mitral and tricuspid valve opening excursion using the biparietal diameter as the reference.[5]

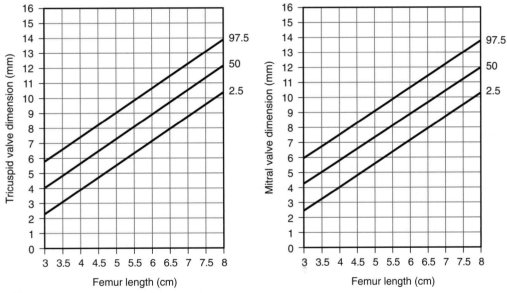

Figure 34-10
Mitral and tricuspid valve opening excursion using the femur length as the reference.[4]

Measurements of Mitral and Tricuspid Valve Excursion

By placing the M-mode cursor through the mitral and tricuspid leaflets, the examiner can determine their maximal excursion. This is done by measuring the leaflet dimension after the leaflets open (E wave) during the rapid filling phase of the diastolic cycle (Figs. 34-2, 34-9, and 34-10; Tables 34-7 and 34-8).

Measurements of the Aortic Valve

In 1985 DeVore et al[2] published results regarding the measurement of the aortic root and valve using M-mode echocardiography and comparing these measurements with the biparietal diameter, head circumference, abdominal circumference, femur length, biventricular inner dimension, left ventricular inner dimension, and mitral valve excursion (Figs. 34-11 and

Table 34-7	Mitral and tricuspid valve opening excursion using the biparietal diameter (BPD) as the reference[5]					
	Mitral Valve Opening Excursion (mm)			**Tricuspid Valve Opening Excursion (mm)**		
BPD (cm)	**2.5th Percentile**	**50th Percentile**	**97.5th Percentile**	**2.5th Percentile**	**50th Percentile**	**97.5th Percentile**
4.0	2.0	3.6	5.3	1.8	3.4	5.0
4.1	2.1	3.7	5.4	1.9	3.5	5.1
4.2	2.2	3.9	5.5	2.0	3.6	5.3
4.3	2.3	4.0	5.7	2.2	3.8	5.4
4.4	2.5	4.1	5.8	2.3	3.9	5.5
4.5	2.6	4.3	5.9	2.4	4.0	5.7
4.6	2.7	4.4	6.1	2.6	4.2	5.8
4.7	2.9	4.5	6.2	2.7	4.3	5.9
4.8	3.0	4.6	6.3	2.8	4.5	6.1
4.9	3.1	4.8	6.4	3.0	4.6	6.2
5.0	3.2	4.9	6.6	3.1	4.7	6.3
5.1	3.4	5.0	6.7	3.3	4.9	6.5
5.2	3.5	5.2	6.8	3.4	5.0	6.6
5.3	3.6	5.3	7.0	3.5	5.1	6.8
5.4	3.8	5.4	7.1	3.7	5.3	6.9
5.5	3.9	5.6	7.2	3.8	5.4	7.0
5.6	4.0	5.7	7.3	3.9	5.5	7.2
5.7	4.1	5.8	7.5	4.1	5.7	7.3
5.8	4.3	5.9	7.6	4.2	5.8	7.4
5.9	4.4	6.1	7.7	4.3	6.0	7.6
6.0	4.5	6.2	7.9	4.5	6.1	7.7
6.1	4.7	6.3	8.0	4.6	6.2	7.8
6.2	4.8	6.5	8.1	4.7	6.4	8.0
6.3	4.9	6.6	8.2	4.9	6.5	8.1
6.4	5.1	6.7	8.4	5.0	6.6	8.3
6.5	5.2	6.8	8.5	5.2	6.8	8.4
6.6	5.3	7.0	8.6	5.3	6.9	8.5
6.7	5.4	7.1	8.8	5.4	7.0	8.7
6.8	5.6	7.2	8.9	5.6	7.2	8.8
6.9	5.7	7.4	9.0	5.7	7.3	8.9
7.0	5.8	7.5	9.2	5.8	7.5	9.1
7.1	6.0	7.6	9.3	6.0	7.6	9.2
7.2	6.1	7.7	9.4	6.1	7.7	9.3
7.3	6.2	7.9	9.5	6.2	7.9	9.5
7.4	6.3	8.0	9.7	6.4	8.0	9.6
7.5	6.5	8.1	9.8	6.5	8.1	9.7
7.6	6.6	8.3	9.9	6.7	8.3	9.9
7.7	6.7	8.4	10.1	6.8	8.4	10.0
7.8	6.9	8.5	10.2	6.9	8.5	10.2
7.9	7.0	8.7	10.3	7.1	8.7	10.3
8.0	7.1	8.8	10.4	7.2	8.8	10.4
8.1	7.2	8.9	10.6	7.3	8.9	10.6
8.2	7.4	9.0	10.7	7.5	9.1	10.7
8.3	7.5	9.2	10.8	7.6	9.2	10.8
8.4	7.6	9.3	11.0	7.7	9.4	11.0
8.5	7.8	9.4	11.1	7.9	9.5	11.1
8.6	7.9	9.6	11.2	8.0	9.6	11.2
8.7	8.0	9.7	11.3	8.2	9.8	11.4

Table 34-7	Mitral and tricuspid valve opening excursion using the biparietal diameter (BPD) as the reference[5]—cont'd					
	Mitral Valve Opening Excursion (mm)			**Tricuspid Valve Opening Excursion (mm)**		
BPD (cm)	**2.5th Percentile**	**50th Percentile**	**97.5th Percentile**	**2.5th Percentile**	**50th Percentile**	**97.5th Percentile**
8.8	8.2	9.8	11.5	8.3	9.9	11.5
8.9	8.3	9.9	11.6	8.4	10.0	11.7
9.0	8.4	10.1	11.7	8.6	10.2	11.8
9.1	8.5	10.2	11.9	8.7	10.3	11.9
9.2	8.7	10.3	12.0	8.8	10.4	12.1
9.3	8.8	10.5	12.1	9.0	10.6	12.2
9.4	8.9	10.6	12.3	9.1	10.7	12.3
9.5	9.1	10.7	12.4	9.2	10.9	12.5
9.6	9.2	10.8	12.5	9.4	11.0	12.6
9.7	9.3	11.0	12.6	9.5	11.1	12.7
9.8	9.4	11.1	12.8	9.6	11.3	12.9
9.9	9.6	11.2	12.9	9.8	11.4	13.0
10.0	9.7	11.4	13.0	9.9	11.5	13.2

Table 34-8	Mitral and tricuspid valve opening excursion using the femur length (FL) as the reference[4]					
	Mitral Valve Opening Excursion (mm)			**Tricuspid Valve Opening Excursion (mm)**		
FL (cm)	**2.5th Percentile**	**50th Percentile**	**97.5th Percentile**	**2.5th Percentile**	**50th Percentile**	**97.5th Percentile**
3.0	2.4	4.1	5.9	2.2	3.9	5.7
3.1	2.5	4.3	6.1	2.3	4.1	5.9
3.2	2.7	4.5	6.2	2.5	4.3	6.0
3.3	2.8	4.6	6.4	2.7	4.4	6.2
3.4	3.0	4.8	6.5	2.8	4.6	6.4
3.5	3.2	4.9	6.7	3.0	4.8	6.5
3.6	3.3	5.1	6.8	3.2	4.9	6.7
3.7	3.5	5.2	7.0	3.3	5.1	6.8
3.8	3.6	5.4	7.2	3.5	5.2	7.0
3.9	3.8	5.5	7.3	3.6	5.4	7.2
4.0	3.9	5.7	7.5	3.8	5.6	7.3
4.1	4.1	5.9	7.6	4.0	5.7	7.5
4.2	4.3	6.0	7.8	4.1	5.9	7.7
4.3	4.4	6.2	7.9	4.3	6.1	7.8
4.4	4.6	6.3	8.1	4.5	6.2	8.0
4.5	4.7	6.5	8.3	4.6	6.4	8.2
4.6	4.9	6.6	8.4	4.8	6.6	8.3
4.7	5.0	6.8	8.6	5.0	6.7	8.5
4.8	5.2	7.0	8.7	5.1	6.9	8.7
4.9	5.4	7.1	8.9	5.3	7.1	8.8
5.0	5.5	7.3	9.0	5.5	7.2	9.0
5.1	5.7	7.4	9.2	5.6	7.4	9.2
5.2	5.8	7.6	9.4	5.8	7.6	9.3
5.3	6.0	7.7	9.5	6.0	7.7	9.5

Table 34-8	Mitral and tricuspid valve opening excursion using the femur length (FL) as the reference[4]—cont'd					
	Mitral Valve Opening Excursion (mm)			Tricuspid Valve Opening Excursion (mm)		
FL (cm)	2.5th Percentile	50th Percentile	97.5th Percentile	2.5th Percentile	50th Percentile	97.5th Percentile
5.4	6.1	7.9	9.7	6.1	7.9	9.6
5.5	6.3	8.1	9.8	6.3	8.0	9.8
5.6	6.5	8.2	10.0	6.4	8.2	10.0
5.7	6.6	8.4	10.1	6.6	8.4	10.1
5.8	6.8	8.5	10.3	6.8	8.5	10.3
5.9	6.9	8.7	10.5	6.9	8.7	10.5
6.0	7.1	8.8	10.6	7.1	8.9	10.6
6.1	7.2	9.0	10.8	7.3	9.0	10.8
6.2	7.4	9.2	10.9	7.4	9.2	11.0
6.3	7.6	9.3	11.1	7.6	9.4	11.1
6.4	7.7	9.5	11.2	7.8	9.5	11.3
6.5	7.9	9.6	11.4	7.9	9.7	11.5
6.6	8.0	9.8	11.5	8.1	9.9	11.6
6.7	8.2	9.9	11.7	8.3	10.0	11.8
6.8	8.3	10.1	11.9	8.4	10.2	12.0
6.9	8.5	10.3	12.0	8.6	10.4	12.1
7.0	8.6	10.4	12.2	8.8	10.5	12.3
7.1	8.8	10.6	12.3	8.9	10.7	12.4
7.2	9.0	10.7	12.5	9.1	10.8	12.6
7.3	9.1	10.9	12.6	9.2	11.0	12.8
7.4	9.3	11.0	12.8	9.4	11.2	12.9
7.5	9.4	11.2	13.0	9.6	11.3	13.1
7.6	9.6	11.4	13.1	9.7	11.5	13.3
7.7	9.7	11.5	13.3	9.9	11.7	13.4
7.8	9.9	11.7	13.4	10.1	11.8	13.6
7.9	10.1	11.8	13.6	10.2	12.0	13.8
8.0	10.2	12.0	13.7	10.4	12.2	13.9

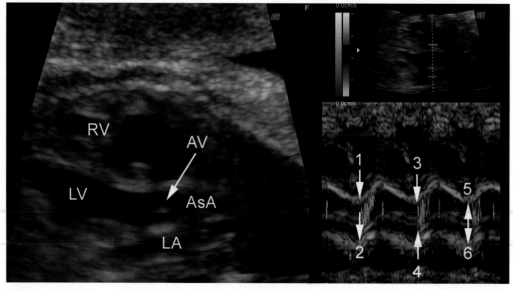

Figure 34-11
M-Mode recording of the aortic valve, demonstrating measurements of the vessel diameter (1 to 2 outer to inner; 5 to 6 inner to inner) and the valve excursion (3 to 4).[2]

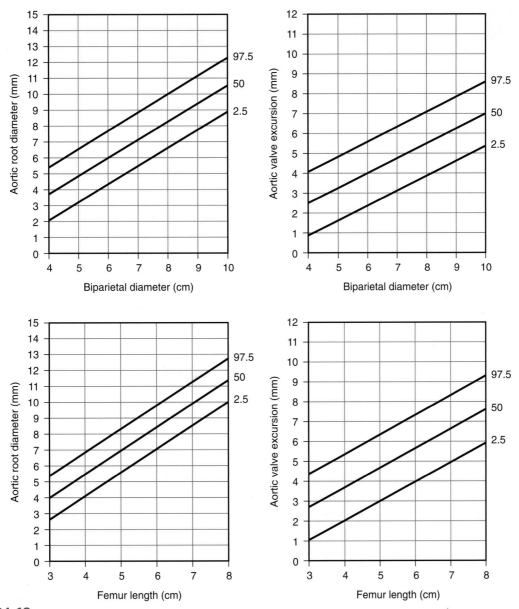

Figure 34-12
Aortic root diameter and aortic valve excursion using the biparietal diameter and the femur length as references.[2]

34-12; Tables 34-9 and 34-10). In 1988 DeVore et al[1] published their findings using this technique to identify fetuses at risk for tetralogy of Fallot. The aortic root and valve, as well as the main pulmonary artery and valve, have been measured by other investigators (Figs. 34-13 and 34-14; Table 34-11).[8,9]

Text continued on p. 140

Table 34-9	Aortic root diameter and valve excursion using the biparietal diameter (BPD) as the reference[2]					
	Aortic Valve Diameter (mm)			Aortic Valve Excursion (mm)		
BPD (cm)	2.5th Percentile	50th Percentile	97.5th Percentile	2.5th Percentile	50th Percentile	97.5th Percentile
4.0	2.0	3.7	5.4	1.9	3.5	5.1
4.1	2.1	3.8	5.5	2.0	3.6	5.2
4.2	2.2	3.9	5.6	2.1	3.7	5.3
4.3	2.3	4.0	5.7	2.2	3.8	5.4
4.4	2.4	4.1	5.8	2.2	3.9	5.5
4.5	2.5	4.2	5.9	2.3	4.0	5.6
4.6	2.6	4.4	6.1	2.4	4.0	5.7
4.7	2.8	4.5	6.2	2.5	4.1	5.8
4.8	2.9	4.6	6.3	2.6	4.2	5.8
4.9	3.0	4.7	6.4	2.7	4.3	5.9
5.0	3.1	4.8	6.5	2.8	4.4	6.0
5.1	3.2	4.9	6.6	2.8	4.5	6.1
5.2	3.3	5.0	6.7	2.9	4.6	6.2
5.3	3.4	5.2	6.9	3.0	4.6	6.3
5.4	3.6	5.3	7.0	3.1	4.7	6.4
5.5	3.7	5.4	7.1	3.2	4.8	6.4
5.6	3.8	5.5	7.2	3.3	4.9	6.5
5.7	3.9	5.6	7.3	3.4	5.0	6.6
5.8	4.0	5.7	7.4	3.5	5.1	6.7
5.9	4.1	5.8	7.5	3.5	5.2	6.8
6.0	4.2	6.0	7.7	3.6	5.3	6.9
6.1	4.4	6.1	7.8	3.7	5.3	7.0
6.2	4.5	6.2	7.9	3.8	5.4	7.1
6.3	4.6	6.3	8.0	3.9	5.5	7.1
6.4	4.7	6.4	8.1	4.0	5.6	7.2
6.5	4.8	6.5	8.2	4.1	5.7	7.3
6.6	4.9	6.6	8.3	4.1	5.8	7.4
6.7	5.1	6.8	8.5	4.2	5.9	7.5
6.8	5.2	6.9	8.6	4.3	5.9	7.6
6.9	5.3	7.0	8.7	4.4	6.0	7.7
7.0	5.4	7.1	8.8	4.5	6.1	7.7
7.1	5.5	7.2	8.9	4.6	6.2	7.8
7.2	5.6	7.3	9.0	4.7	6.3	7.9
7.3	5.7	7.4	9.1	4.8	6.4	8.0
7.4	5.9	7.6	9.3	4.8	6.5	8.1
7.5	6.0	7.7	9.4	4.9	6.6	8.2
7.6	6.1	7.8	9.5	5.0	6.6	8.3
7.7	6.2	7.9	9.6	5.1	6.7	8.4
7.8	6.3	8.0	9.7	5.2	6.8	8.4
7.9	6.4	8.1	9.8	5.3	6.9	8.5
8.0	6.5	8.2	9.9	5.4	7.0	8.6
8.1	6.7	8.4	10.1	5.4	7.1	8.7
8.2	6.8	8.5	10.2	5.5	7.2	8.8
8.3	6.9	8.6	10.3	5.6	7.2	8.9
8.4	7.0	8.7	10.4	5.7	7.3	9.0
8.5	7.1	8.8	10.5	5.8	7.4	9.0
8.6	7.2	8.9	10.6	5.9	7.5	9.1
8.7	7.3	9.0	10.8	6.0	7.6	9.2

Table 34-9	Aortic root diameter and valve excursion using the biparietal diameter (BPD) as the reference[2]—cont'd					
	Aortic Valve Diameter (mm)			**Aortic Valve Excursion (mm)**		
BPD (cm)	**2.5th Percentile**	**50th Percentile**	**97.5th Percentile**	**2.5th Percentile**	**50th Percentile**	**97.5th Percentile**
8.8	7.5	9.2	10.9	6.1	7.7	9.3
8.9	7.6	9.3	11.0	6.1	7.8	9.4
9.0	7.7	9.4	11.1	6.2	7.9	9.5
9.1	7.8	9.5	11.2	6.3	7.9	9.6
9.2	7.9	9.6	11.3	6.4	8.0	9.7
9.3	8.0	9.7	11.4	6.5	8.1	9.7
9.4	8.1	9.8	11.6	6.6	8.2	9.8
9.5	8.3	10.0	11.7	6.7	8.3	9.9
9.6	8.4	10.1	11.8	6.7	8.4	10.0
9.7	8.5	10.2	11.9	6.8	8.5	10.1
9.8	8.6	10.3	12.0	6.9	8.5	10.2
9.9	8.7	10.4	12.1	7.0	8.6	10.3
10.0	8.8	10.5	12.2	7.1	8.7	10.3

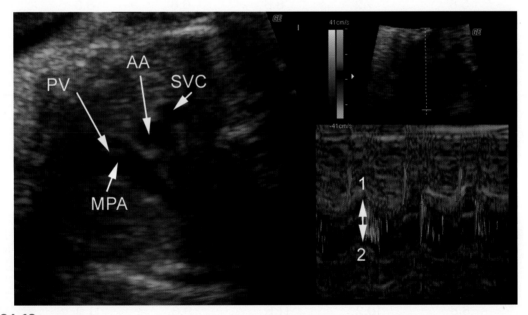

Figure 34-13
M-Mode recording of the pulmonary valve, demonstrating measurements of the vessel dimension (1 to 2 inner to inner).[2]

Table 34-10	Aortic root diameter and valve excursion using the femur length (FL) as the reference[2]					
	Aortic Valve Diameter (mm)			**Aortic Valve Excursion (mm)**		
FL (cm)	**2.5th Percentile**	**50th Percentile**	**97.5th Percentile**	**2.5th Percentile**	**50th Percentile**	**97.5th Percentile**
3.0	2.6	3.9	5.3	3.3	5.0	6.7
3.1	2.7	4.1	5.5	3.4	5.1	6.8
3.2	2.9	4.2	5.6	3.6	5.3	7.0
3.3	3.0	4.4	5.8	3.7	5.4	7.1
3.4	3.2	4.5	5.9	3.9	5.6	7.3
3.5	3.3	4.7	6.1	4.0	5.7	7.4
3.6	3.5	4.8	6.2	4.2	5.9	7.6
3.7	3.6	5.0	6.4	4.3	6.0	7.7
3.8	3.8	5.1	6.5	4.5	6.2	7.9
3.9	3.9	5.3	6.7	4.6	6.3	8.0
4.0	4.1	5.4	6.8	4.8	6.5	8.2
4.1	4.2	5.6	7.0	4.9	6.6	8.3
4.2	4.4	5.7	7.1	5.1	6.8	8.5
4.3	4.5	5.9	7.3	5.2	6.9	8.6
4.4	4.7	6.0	7.4	5.4	7.1	8.8
4.5	4.8	6.2	7.6	5.5	7.2	8.9
4.6	5.0	6.3	7.7	5.7	7.4	9.1
4.7	5.1	6.5	7.9	5.8	7.5	9.2
4.8	5.2	6.6	8.0	6.0	7.7	9.4
4.9	5.4	6.8	8.2	6.1	7.8	9.5
5.0	5.5	6.9	8.3	6.3	8.0	9.7
5.1	5.7	7.1	8.5	6.4	8.1	9.8
5.2	5.8	7.2	8.6	6.6	8.3	9.9
5.3	6.0	7.4	8.8	6.7	8.4	10.1
5.4	6.1	7.5	8.9	6.9	8.6	10.2
5.5	6.3	7.7	9.1	7.0	8.7	10.4
5.6	6.4	7.8	9.2	7.2	8.9	10.5
5.7	6.6	8.0	9.4	7.3	9.0	10.7
5.8	6.7	8.1	9.5	7.5	9.2	10.8
5.9	6.9	8.3	9.7	7.6	9.3	11.0
6.0	7.0	8.4	9.8	7.8	9.5	11.1
6.1	7.2	8.6	10.0	7.9	9.6	11.3
6.2	7.3	8.7	10.1	8.1	9.8	11.4
6.3	7.5	8.9	10.3	8.2	9.9	11.6
6.4	7.6	9.0	10.4	8.4	10.1	11.7
6.5	7.8	9.2	10.6	8.5	10.2	11.9
6.6	7.9	9.3	10.7	8.7	10.4	12.0
6.7	8.1	9.5	10.9	8.8	10.5	12.2
6.8	8.2	9.6	11.0	9.0	10.6	12.3
6.9	8.4	9.8	11.2	9.1	10.8	12.5
7.0	8.5	9.9	11.3	9.3	10.9	12.6
7.1	8.7	10.1	11.5	9.4	11.1	12.8
7.2	8.8	10.2	11.6	9.6	11.2	12.9
7.3	9.0	10.4	11.8	9.7	11.4	13.1
7.4	9.1	10.5	11.9	9.9	11.5	13.2
7.5	9.3	10.7	12.1	10.0	11.7	13.4
7.6	9.4	10.8	12.2	10.2	11.8	13.5
7.7	9.6	11.0	12.4	10.3	12.0	13.7
7.8	9.7	11.1	12.5	10.5	12.1	13.8
7.9	9.9	11.3	12.7	10.6	12.3	14.0
8.0	10.0	11.4	12.8	10.8	12.4	14.1

Table 34-11	Diameter of the main pulmonary artery and aortic root using the biparietal diameter (BPD) as the reference[8]					
	Pulmonary Valve Diameter (mm)			**Aortic Valve Diameter (mm)**		
BPD (cm)	**2.5th Percentile**	**50th Percentile**	**97.5th Percentile**	**2.5th Percentile**	**50th Percentile**	**97.5th Percentile**
40	0.4	2.4	4.4	1.0	2.6	4.2
41	0.5	2.5	4.5	1.1	2.7	4.3
42	0.7	2.7	4.7	1.2	2.8	4.4
43	0.8	2.8	4.8	1.4	3.0	4.6
44	0.9	2.9	4.9	1.5	3.1	4.7
45	1.1	3.1	5.1	1.6	3.2	4.8
46	1.2	3.2	5.2	1.7	3.3	4.9
47	1.3	3.3	5.3	1.8	3.4	5.0
48	1.5	3.5	5.5	1.9	3.5	5.1
49	1.6	3.6	5.6	2.0	3.6	5.2
50	1.7	3.7	5.7	2.2	3.8	5.4
51	1.9	3.9	5.9	2.3	3.9	5.5
52	2.0	4.0	6.0	2.4	4.0	5.6
53	2.1	4.1	6.1	2.5	4.1	5.7
54	2.3	4.3	6.3	2.6	4.2	5.8
55	2.4	4.4	6.4	2.7	4.3	5.9
56	2.6	4.6	6.6	2.9	4.5	6.1
57	2.7	4.7	6.7	3.0	4.6	6.2
58	2.8	4.8	6.8	3.1	4.7	6.3
59	3.0	5.0	7.0	3.2	4.8	6.4
60	3.1	5.1	7.1	3.3	4.9	6.5
61	3.2	5.2	7.2	3.4	5.0	6.6
62	3.4	5.4	7.4	3.6	5.2	6.8
63	3.5	5.5	7.5	3.7	5.3	6.9
64	3.6	5.6	7.6	3.8	5.4	7.0
65	3.8	5.8	7.8	3.9	5.5	7.1
66	3.9	5.9	7.9	4.0	5.6	7.2
67	4.0	6.0	8.0	4.1	5.7	7.3
68	4.2	6.2	8.2	4.3	5.9	7.5
69	4.3	6.3	8.3	4.4	6.0	7.6
70	4.4	6.4	8.4	4.5	6.1	7.7
71	4.6	6.6	8.6	4.6	6.2	7.8
72	4.7	6.7	8.7	4.7	6.3	7.9
73	4.8	6.8	8.8	4.8	6.4	8.0
74	5.0	7.0	9.0	5.0	6.6	8.2
75	5.1	7.1	9.1	5.1	6.7	8.3
76	5.2	7.2	9.2	5.2	6.8	8.4
77	5.4	7.4	9.4	5.3	6.9	8.5
78	5.5	7.5	9.5	5.4	7.0	8.6
79	5.6	7.6	9.6	5.5	7.1	8.7
80	5.8	7.8	9.8	5.7	7.3	8.9
81	5.9	7.9	9.9	5.8	7.4	9.0
82	6.0	8.0	10.1	5.9	7.5	9.1
83	6.2	8.2	10.2	6.0	7.6	9.2
84	6.3	8.3	10.3	6.1	7.7	9.3
85	6.5	8.5	10.5	6.2	7.8	9.4
86	6.6	8.6	10.6	6.4	8.0	9.6
87	6.7	8.7	10.7	6.5	8.1	9.7

Table 34-11	Diameter of the main pulmonary artery and aortic root using the biparietal diameter (BPD) as the reference[8]—cont'd					
	Pulmonary Valve Diameter (mm)			**Aortic Valve Diameter (mm)**		
BPD (cm)	**2.5th Percentile**	**50th Percentile**	**97.5th Percentile**	**2.5th Percentile**	**50th Percentile**	**97.5th Percentile**
88	6.9	8.9	10.9	6.6	8.2	9.8
89	7.0	9.0	11.0	6.7	8.3	9.9
90	7.1	9.1	11.1	6.8	8.4	10.0
91	7.3	9.3	11.3	6.9	8.5	10.1
92	7.4	9.4	11.4	7.1	8.7	10.3
93	7.5	9.5	11.5	7.2	8.8	10.4
94	7.7	9.7	11.7	7.3	8.9	10.5
95	7.8	9.8	11.8	7.4	9.0	10.6

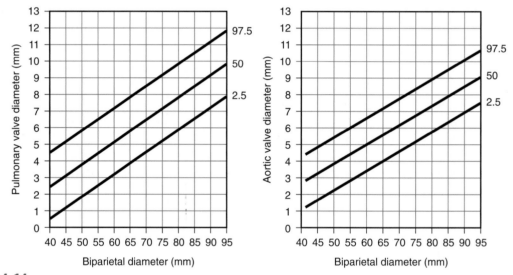

Figure 34-14
M-Mode measurements of the aortic and pulmonic valve diameters measured from inner to inner (see Figs. 34-11 and 34-13).[8]

References

1. DeVore GR, Siassi B, Platt LD: Fetal echocardiography. VIII. Aortic root dilatation—a marker for tetralogy of Fallot. Am J Obstet Gynecol 1988;159:129-136.
2. DeVore GR, Siassi B, Platt LD: Fetal echocardiography. V. M-mode measurements of the aortic root and aortic valve in second- and third-trimester normal human fetuses. Am J Obstet Gynecol 1985;152:543-550.
3. DeVore GR, Siassi B, Platt LD: The use of the abdominal circumference as a means of assessing M-mode ventricular dimensions during the second and third trimesters of pregnancy in the normal human fetus. J Ultrasound Med 1985;4:175-182.
4. De Vore GR, Siassi B, Platt LD: Use of femur length as a means of assessing M-mode ventricular dimensions during second and third trimesters of pregnancy in normal fetus. J Clin Ultrasound 1985;13:619-625.
5. DeVore GR, Siassi B, Platt LD: Fetal echocardiography. IV. M-mode assessment of ventricular size and contractility during the second and third trimesters of pregnancy in the normal fetus. Am J Obstet Gynecol 1984;150:981-988.

6. John Sutton MG, Gewitz MH, Shah B, et al: Quantitative assessment of growth and function of the cardiac chambers in the normal human fetus: a prospective longitudinal echocardiographic study. Circulation 1984;69: 645-654.

7. Allan LD, Joseph MC, Boyd EG, et al: M-mode echocardiography in the developing human fetus. Br Heart J 1982;47:573-583.

8. Deng J, Cheng PX, Gao SY, Wen LZ: Echocardiographic evaluation of the valves and roots of the pulmonary artery and aorta in the developing fetus. J Clin Ultrasound 1992;20: 3-9.

9. Cartier MS, Davidoff A, Warneke LA, et al: The normal diameter of the fetal aorta and pulmonary artery: echocardiographic evaluation in utero. Am J Roentgenol 1987;149:1003-1007.

CHAPTER 35

Greggory R. DeVore

B-Mode Measurement of the Fetal Heart

Introduction

In the early 1980s ultrasound technology did not allow the examiner to obtain end-diastolic or end-systolic real-time B-mode images of the heart from which to make adequate cardiac measurements. Therefore investigators used real-time-directed M-mode ultrasound to measure dimensions of the ventricular chambers, ventricular and septal wall thickness, and dimensions of the aorta and main pulmonary artery.[1-6] However, as the frequency of the transducers increased and the ability to record and evaluate computer-digitized B-mode images with the cine loop function evolved, accurate measurements could be made. In 1992 two groups of investigators, Sharland and Allan[7] and Tan et al,[8] reported measuring cardiac structures in normal fetuses. In 1998 Shapiro et al[9] included younger fetuses (14 weeks) in their analysis. In 2001 Firpo et al[10] expanded the original study of Tan et al.[8] After reviewing the literature, several studies have been selected for reference values for this communication.

Sharland and Allan, 1992

In this study the authors measured ventricular chamber dimensions and outflow tract dimensions.[7] In preparation of this manuscript, the graphic display of the mean plus 95% confidence intervals was reviewed and errors were found in which the graphic display did not correspond to the regression equations provided by the authors. Therefore data from this paper are not included.

Tan et al, 1992 and Firpo et al, 2001

In the study by Firpo et al[10] the investigators expanded the previous study reported by Tan et al.[8] During the creation of graphs and tables, several errors were identified in the recent report by Firpo et al[10] in which the graphic analysis did not match the corresponding equations.

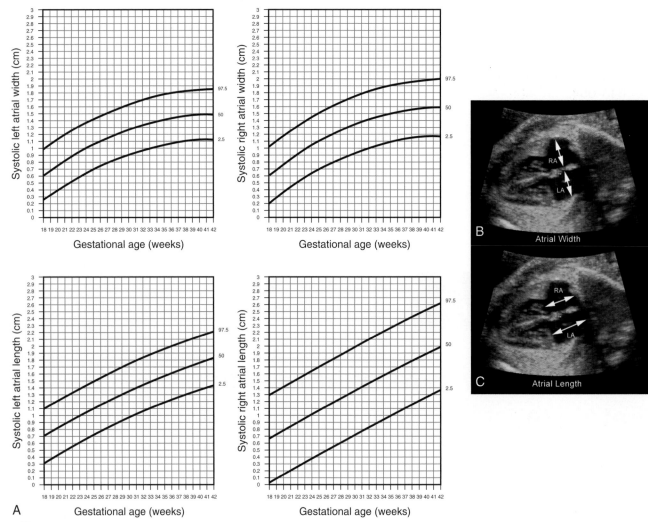

Figure 35-1
Atrial width and length measured from the four-chamber view.[8] **A,** Measurements of atrial width at end-ventricular systole. The atrial width is measured from the lateral wall to the line between two portions of the foramen ovale. **B,** Measurements of atrial length at end-ventricular systole. The atrial length is measured from the coapted atrioventricular valve leaflet to the posterior wall of the atrial chamber. *LA,* left atrium; *RA,* Right atrium.

Therefore the original data from Tan et al[8] have been used and the following measurements have been selected for reporting:

1. Width and length of the atrial chambers (Fig. 35-1, Table 35-1).
2. Width and length of the ventricular chambers (Fig. 35-2, Table 35-2)
3. Width of the right and left ventricular walls and the interventricular septum (Fig. 35-3, Table 35-3).
4. Measurements from the aortic arch (Fig. 35-4, Table 35-4).
5. Measurements from the ductal arch (Fig. 35-5, Table 35-5).

6. Measurements from the aorta and main pulmonary artery (Fig. 35-6, Table 35-6).

An observation from this study is that the confidence intervals are the same, irrespective of gestational age. One would expect that the confidence intervals for a specific cardiac measurement early in gestation would be less than when it is obtained later in gestation.

Shapiro et al, 1998

This study measured fewer cardiac structures than the study by Tan et al.[8] However, the

Text continued on p. 151

Table 35-1   Atrial width and length measured from the four-chamber view and the corresponding percentiles[8]

Gestation (wks)	Left Atrial Width (cm)			Right Atrial Width (cm)			Left Atrial Length (cm)			Right Atrial Length (cm)		
	2.5th Percentile	50th Percentile	95th Percentile	2.5th Percentile	50th Percentile	95th Percentile	2.5th Percentile	50th Percentile	95th Percentile	2.5th Percentile	50th Percentile	95th Percentile
18	0.24	0.60	0.96	0.19	0.59	1.00	0.31	0.70	1.09	0.04	0.67	1.30
19	0.31	0.67	1.03	0.27	0.67	1.08	0.37	0.77	1.16	0.10	0.73	1.36
20	0.38	0.74	1.10	0.34	0.75	1.16	0.43	0.83	1.22	0.16	0.79	1.42
21	0.44	0.81	1.17	0.42	0.82	1.23	0.49	0.89	1.28	0.22	0.85	1.48
22	0.51	0.87	1.23	0.49	0.89	1.30	0.55	0.94	1.34	0.28	0.91	1.54
23	0.57	0.93	1.29	0.55	0.96	1.36	0.61	1.00	1.39	0.34	0.97	1.60
24	0.62	0.99	1.35	0.61	1.02	1.43	0.66	1.06	1.45	0.40	1.03	1.66
25	0.68	1.04	1.40	0.67	1.08	1.48	0.72	1.11	1.50	0.45	1.09	1.72
26	0.73	1.09	1.45	0.73	1.13	1.54	0.77	1.16	1.56	0.51	1.14	1.78
27	0.78	1.14	1.50	0.78	1.19	1.59	0.82	1.22	1.61	0.57	1.20	1.83
28	0.82	1.18	1.55	0.83	1.24	1.64	0.87	1.27	1.66	0.63	1.26	1.89
29	0.86	1.22	1.59	0.88	1.28	1.69	0.92	1.31	1.71	0.68	1.31	1.95
30	0.90	1.26	1.62	0.92	1.32	1.73	0.97	1.36	1.75	0.74	1.37	2.00
31	0.94	1.30	1.66	0.96	1.36	1.77	1.02	1.41	1.80	0.79	1.43	2.06
32	0.97	1.33	1.69	0.99	1.40	1.80	1.06	1.45	1.85	0.85	1.48	2.11
33	1.00	1.36	1.72	1.03	1.43	1.84	1.10	1.50	1.89	0.90	1.54	2.17
34	1.02	1.38	1.75	1.05	1.46	1.87	1.15	1.54	1.93	0.96	1.59	2.22
35	1.05	1.41	1.77	1.08	1.49	1.89	1.19	1.58	1.97	1.01	1.64	2.28
36	1.06	1.43	1.79	1.10	1.51	1.91	1.23	1.62	2.01	1.07	1.70	2.33
37	1.08	1.44	1.81	1.12	1.53	1.93	1.27	1.66	2.05	1.12	1.75	2.38
38	1.09	1.46	1.82	1.14	1.54	1.95	1.30	1.69	2.09	1.17	1.80	2.44
39	1.10	1.47	1.83	1.15	1.56	1.96	1.34	1.73	2.12	1.22	1.86	2.49
40	1.11	1.47	1.84	1.16	1.56	1.97	1.37	1.76	2.16	1.28	1.91	2.54
41	1.12	1.48	1.84	1.16	1.57	1.98	1.40	1.80	2.19	1.33	1.96	2.59
42	1.12	1.48	1.84	1.17	1.57	1.98	1.44	1.83	2.22	1.38	2.01	2.64

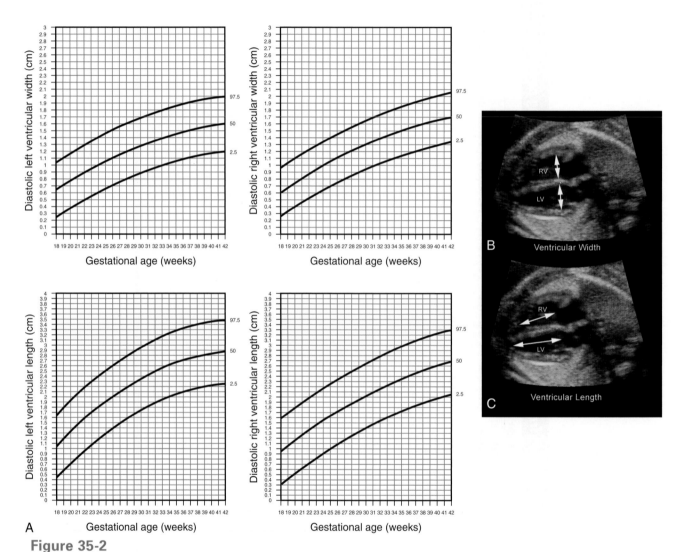

Figure 35-2

Ventricular width and length.[8] **A,** Measurements of ventricular width at end-ventricular diastole. This is measured below the coapted atrioventricular valve, from the septum to the wall of each ventricular chamber. **B,** Measurements of ventricular length at end-ventricular diastole from the coapted atrioventricular valve to the apex of the ventricle. *LV,* left ventricle; *RV,* Right ventricle.

Table 35-2 Ventricular width and length measured from the four-chamber view and the corresponding percentiles[8]

Gestation (wks)	Left Ventricular Width (cm)			Right Ventricular Width (cm)			Left Ventricular Length (cm)			Right Ventricular Length (cm)		
	2.5th Percentile	50th Percentile	95th Percentile	2.5th Percentile	50th Percentile	95th Percentile	2.5th Percentile	50th Percentile	95th Percentile	2.5th Percentile	50th Percentile	95th Percentile
18	0.24	0.64	1.04	0.25	0.61	0.97	0.45	1.06	1.67	0.31	0.94	1.57
19	0.31	0.71	1.11	0.32	0.68	1.04	0.58	1.19	1.80	0.42	1.05	1.68
20	0.37	0.77	1.17	0.39	0.75	1.11	0.72	1.33	1.94	0.52	1.15	1.79
21	0.43	0.83	1.23	0.46	0.81	1.17	0.84	1.45	2.06	0.62	1.26	1.89
22	0.49	0.89	1.29	0.52	0.88	1.23	0.96	1.57	2.18	0.72	1.35	1.99
23	0.55	0.95	1.35	0.58	0.94	1.30	1.08	1.69	2.30	0.82	1.45	2.08
24	0.60	1.00	1.40	0.64	1.00	1.35	1.19	1.80	2.41	0.91	1.54	2.17
25	0.66	1.06	1.46	0.70	1.05	1.41	1.29	1.90	2.51	1.00	1.63	2.26
26	0.71	1.11	1.51	0.75	1.11	1.47	1.39	2.00	2.61	1.08	1.72	2.35
27	0.75	1.15	1.55	0.80	1.16	1.52	1.49	2.10	2.71	1.17	1.80	2.43
28	0.80	1.20	1.60	0.85	1.21	1.57	1.58	2.19	2.80	1.25	1.88	2.51
29	0.84	1.24	1.64	0.90	1.26	1.62	1.66	2.27	2.88	1.33	1.96	2.59
30	0.88	1.28	1.68	0.95	1.31	1.66	1.74	2.35	2.96	1.40	2.03	2.66
31	0.92	1.32	1.72	0.99	1.35	1.71	1.81	2.42	3.03	1.47	2.10	2.73
32	0.96	1.36	1.76	1.03	1.39	1.75	1.88	2.49	3.10	1.54	2.17	2.80
33	0.99	1.39	1.79	1.07	1.43	1.79	1.94	2.55	3.16	1.60	2.24	2.87
34	1.03	1.43	1.83	1.11	1.47	1.83	2.00	2.61	3.22	1.67	2.30	2.93
35	1.05	1.45	1.85	1.15	1.51	1.86	2.05	2.66	3.27	1.72	2.36	2.99
36	1.08	1.48	1.88	1.18	1.54	1.90	2.09	2.70	3.31	1.78	2.41	3.04
37	1.11	1.51	1.91	1.21	1.57	1.93	2.13	2.74	3.35	1.83	2.46	3.10
38	1.13	1.53	1.93	1.24	1.60	1.96	2.17	2.78	3.39	1.88	2.51	3.15
39	1.15	1.55	1.95	1.27	1.63	1.99	2.20	2.81	3.42	1.93	2.56	3.19
40	1.17	1.57	1.97	1.30	1.66	2.01	2.22	2.83	3.44	1.97	2.61	3.24
41	1.18	1.58	1.98	1.32	1.68	2.04	2.24	2.85	3.46	2.01	2.65	3.28
42	1.20	1.60	2.00	1.34	1.70	2.06	2.26	2.87	3.48	2.05	2.68	3.32

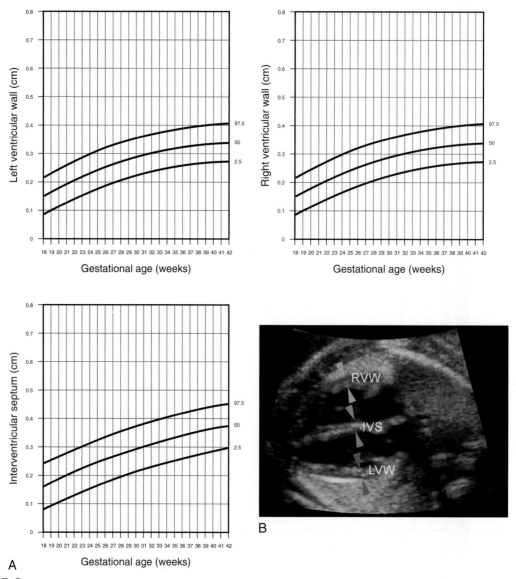

Figure 35-3
Measurement of the width of the right and left ventricular walls and the interventricular septum and end-diastole.[8] *IVS*, interventricular septum; *LVW*, left ventricular wall; *RVW*, Right ventricular wall.

Table 35-3 Width of the ventricular walls and the interventricular septum measured from the four-chamber view and the corresponding percentiles[8]

Gestation (wks)	Left Ventricular Wall Width (cm)			Interventricular Septal Wall Width (cm)			Right Ventricular Wall Width (cm)		
	2.5th Percentile	50th Percentile	95th Percentile	2.5th Percentile	50th Percentile	95th Percentile	2.5th Percentile	50th Percentile	95th Percentile
18	0.08	0.15	0.22	0.08	0.16	0.24	0.08	0.15	0.22
19	0.10	0.17	0.23	0.09	0.17	0.25	0.10	0.16	0.23
20	0.11	0.18	0.25	0.11	0.19	0.27	0.11	0.18	0.25
21	0.13	0.19	0.26	0.12	0.20	0.28	0.12	0.19	0.26
22	0.14	0.21	0.27	0.13	0.21	0.29	0.14	0.20	0.27
23	0.15	0.22	0.28	0.14	0.22	0.30	0.15	0.22	0.29
24	0.16	0.23	0.30	0.15	0.23	0.31	0.16	0.23	0.30
25	0.17	0.24	0.31	0.16	0.24	0.32	0.17	0.24	0.31
26	0.19	0.25	0.32	0.17	0.25	0.33	0.18	0.25	0.32
27	0.19	0.26	0.33	0.18	0.26	0.34	0.19	0.26	0.33
28	0.20	0.27	0.34	0.19	0.27	0.35	0.20	0.27	0.34
29	0.21	0.28	0.34	0.20	0.28	0.36	0.21	0.28	0.35
30	0.22	0.29	0.35	0.21	0.29	0.37	0.22	0.29	0.36
31	0.23	0.29	0.36	0.22	0.30	0.38	0.23	0.30	0.36
32	0.24	0.30	0.37	0.23	0.31	0.39	0.23	0.30	0.37
33	0.24	0.31	0.37	0.24	0.32	0.40	0.24	0.31	0.38
34	0.25	0.31	0.38	0.25	0.33	0.41	0.25	0.31	0.38
35	0.25	0.32	0.38	0.25	0.33	0.41	0.25	0.32	0.39
36	0.26	0.32	0.39	0.26	0.34	0.42	0.26	0.32	0.39
37	0.26	0.33	0.39	0.27	0.35	0.43	0.26	0.33	0.39
38	0.26	0.33	0.40	0.27	0.35	0.43	0.26	0.33	0.40
39	0.27	0.33	0.40	0.28	0.36	0.44	0.26	0.33	0.40
40	0.27	0.34	0.40	0.28	0.36	0.44	0.27	0.33	0.40
41	0.27	0.34	0.40	0.29	0.37	0.45	0.27	0.34	0.40
42	0.27	0.34	0.40	0.29	0.37	0.45	0.27	0.34	0.40

Table 35-4 Measurements from the aortic arch and the corresponding percentiles[8]

Gestation (wks)	Annulus of the Aortic Arch (cm)			Ascending Aorta (cm)			Descending Aorta (cm)		
	2.5th Percentile	50th Percentile	95th Percentile	2.5th Percentile	50th Percentile	95th Percentile	2.5th Percentile	50th Percentile	95th Percentile
18	0.14	0.32	0.50	0.15	0.31	0.47	0.13	0.29	0.45
19	0.17	0.35	0.52	0.17	0.33	0.49	0.15	0.31	0.47
20	0.19	0.37	0.55	0.19	0.35	0.51	0.17	0.33	0.49
21	0.22	0.40	0.57	0.21	0.37	0.53	0.18	0.34	0.50
22	0.24	0.42	0.60	0.23	0.39	0.55	0.20	0.36	0.52
23	0.27	0.45	0.62	0.25	0.41	0.57	0.22	0.38	0.54
24	0.29	0.47	0.65	0.27	0.43	0.59	0.24	0.40	0.56
25	0.32	0.50	0.67	0.29	0.45	0.61	0.25	0.41	0.57
26	0.34	0.52	0.70	0.31	0.47	0.63	0.27	0.43	0.59
27	0.37	0.55	0.72	0.33	0.49	0.65	0.29	0.45	0.61
28	0.39	0.57	0.75	0.35	0.51	0.67	0.31	0.47	0.63
29	0.42	0.60	0.77	0.37	0.53	0.69	0.32	0.48	0.64
30	0.44	0.62	0.80	0.39	0.55	0.71	0.34	0.50	0.66
31	0.47	0.65	0.82	0.41	0.57	0.73	0.36	0.52	0.68
32	0.49	0.67	0.85	0.43	0.59	0.75	0.37	0.54	0.70
33	0.52	0.70	0.87	0.45	0.61	0.77	0.39	0.55	0.71
34	0.54	0.72	0.90	0.47	0.63	0.79	0.41	0.57	0.73
35	0.57	0.75	0.92	0.49	0.65	0.81	0.43	0.59	0.75
36	0.59	0.77	0.95	0.51	0.67	0.83	0.44	0.60	0.76
37	0.62	0.80	0.97	0.53	0.69	0.85	0.46	0.62	0.78
38	0.64	0.82	1.00	0.55	0.71	0.87	0.48	0.64	0.80
39	0.67	0.85	1.02	0.57	0.73	0.89	0.50	0.66	0.82
40	0.69	0.87	1.05	0.59	0.75	0.91	0.51	0.67	0.83
41	0.72	0.90	1.07	0.61	0.77	0.93	0.53	0.69	0.85
42	0.74	0.92	1.10	0.63	0.79	0.95	0.55	0.71	0.87

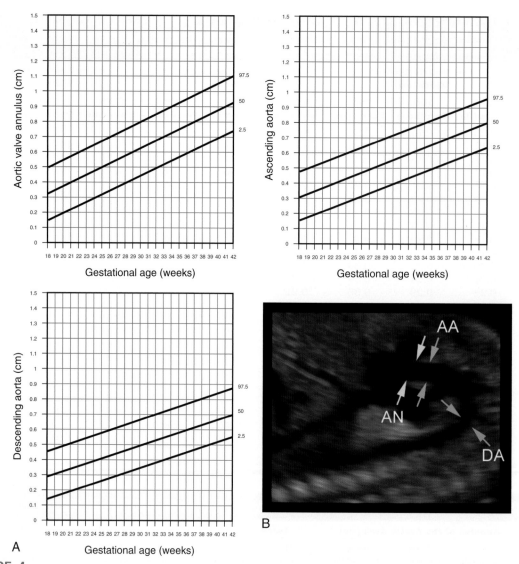

Figure 35-4
Measurements from the aortic arch. The aortic annulus (AN) is measured at the level of the aortic valve. The ascending aorta (AA) is measured above the aortic valve. The descending aorta (DA) is measured above the entrance of the ductus arteriosus.[8]

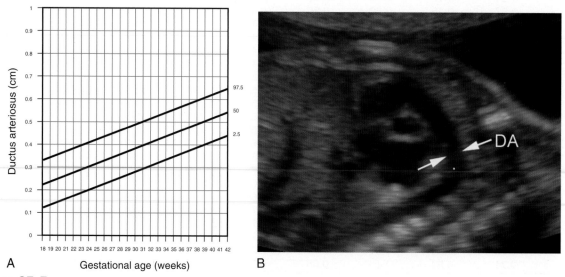

Figure 35-5
Measurements from the middle of the ductal arch obtained in the short-axis view. *DA*, Ductus arteriosus.[8]

Table 35-5 Measurements from the ductal arch and the corresponding percentiles[8]

Gestation (wks)	Ductal Arch (cm)			Weeks Gestation	Ductal Arch (cm)		
	2.5th Percentile	50th Percentile	95th Percentile		2.5th Percentile	50th Percentile	95th Percentile
18	0.12	0.22	0.33	31	0.29	0.40	0.50
19	0.13	0.24	0.34	32	0.30	0.41	0.51
20	0.15	0.25	0.35	33	0.32	0.42	0.53
21	0.16	0.26	0.37	34	0.33	0.44	0.54
22	0.17	0.28	0.38	35	0.34	0.45	0.55
23	0.19	0.29	0.39	36	0.36	0.46	0.57
24	0.20	0.30	0.41	37	0.37	0.47	0.58
25	0.21	0.32	0.42	38	0.38	0.49	0.59
26	0.23	0.33	0.43	39	0.40	0.50	0.61
27	0.24	0.34	0.45	40	0.41	0.51	0.62
28	0.25	0.36	0.46	41	0.42	0.53	0.63
29	0.26	0.37	0.47	42	0.44	0.54	0.65
30	0.28	0.38	0.49				

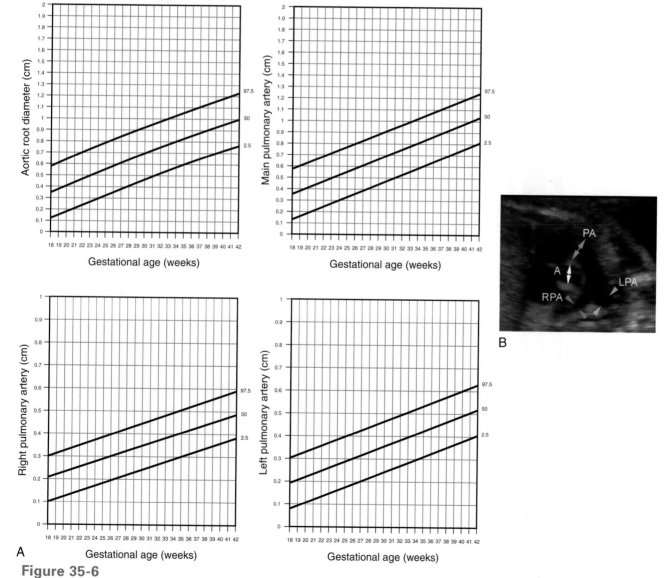

Figure 35-6

Measurements of the aorta, main pulmonary artery, and the right and left pulmonary arteries from the short-axis view.[8] *A*, aorta; *LPA*, left pulmonary artery; *PA*, Main pulmonary artery; *RPA*, right pulmonary artery.

Table 35-6   Measurements of the aorta, main pulmonary artery, and the right and left pulmonary arteries from the short-axis view and the corresponding percentiles[8]

Gestation (wks)	Aortic Root Diameter (cm)			Main Pulmonary Artery Diameter (cm)			Left Pulmonary Artery Diameter (cm)			Right Pulmonary Artery Diameter (cm)		
	2.5th Percentile	50th Percentile	95th Percentile	2.5th Percentile	50th Percentile	95th Percentile	2.5th Percentile	50th Percentile	95th Percentile	2.5th Percentile	50th Percentile	95th Percentile
18	0.11	0.34	0.57	0.13	0.35	0.57	0.08	0.19	0.30	0.10	0.20	0.30
19	0.14	0.37	0.60	0.16	0.38	0.60	0.09	0.20	0.32	0.12	0.22	0.32
20	0.18	0.41	0.64	0.19	0.41	0.63	0.10	0.22	0.33	0.13	0.23	0.33
21	0.21	0.44	0.67	0.21	0.43	0.65	0.12	0.23	0.34	0.14	0.24	0.34
22	0.24	0.47	0.70	0.24	0.46	0.68	0.13	0.24	0.36	0.15	0.25	0.35
23	0.27	0.50	0.73	0.27	0.49	0.71	0.15	0.26	0.37	0.16	0.26	0.36
24	0.29	0.52	0.75	0.30	0.52	0.74	0.16	0.27	0.38	0.18	0.28	0.38
25	0.32	0.55	0.78	0.33	0.55	0.77	0.17	0.28	0.40	0.19	0.29	0.39
26	0.35	0.58	0.81	0.35	0.57	0.79	0.19	0.30	0.41	0.20	0.30	0.40
27	0.38	0.61	0.84	0.38	0.60	0.82	0.20	0.31	0.42	0.21	0.31	0.41
28	0.41	0.64	0.87	0.41	0.63	0.85	0.21	0.33	0.44	0.22	0.32	0.42
29	0.44	0.67	0.90	0.44	0.66	0.88	0.23	0.34	0.45	0.23	0.33	0.43
30	0.46	0.69	0.92	0.47	0.69	0.91	0.24	0.35	0.46	0.25	0.35	0.45
31	0.49	0.72	0.95	0.49	0.71	0.93	0.25	0.37	0.48	0.26	0.36	0.46
32	0.52	0.75	0.98	0.52	0.74	0.96	0.27	0.38	0.49	0.27	0.37	0.47
33	0.54	0.77	1.00	0.55	0.77	0.99	0.28	0.39	0.51	0.28	0.38	0.48
34	0.57	0.80	1.03	0.58	0.80	1.02	0.30	0.41	0.52	0.29	0.39	0.49
35	0.60	0.83	1.06	0.60	0.82	1.04	0.31	0.42	0.53	0.30	0.40	0.50
36	0.62	0.85	1.08	0.63	0.85	1.07	0.32	0.43	0.55	0.32	0.42	0.52
37	0.65	0.88	1.11	0.66	0.88	1.10	0.34	0.45	0.56	0.33	0.43	0.53
38	0.67	0.90	1.13	0.69	0.91	1.13	0.35	0.46	0.57	0.34	0.44	0.54
39	0.69	0.92	1.15	0.72	0.94	1.16	0.36	0.48	0.59	0.35	0.45	0.55
40	0.72	0.95	1.18	0.74	0.96	1.18	0.38	0.49	0.60	0.36	0.46	0.56
41	0.74	0.97	1.20	0.77	0.99	1.21	0.39	0.50	0.61	0.37	0.47	0.57
42	0.76	0.99	1.22	0.80	1.02	1.24	0.40	0.52	0.63	0.39	0.49	0.59

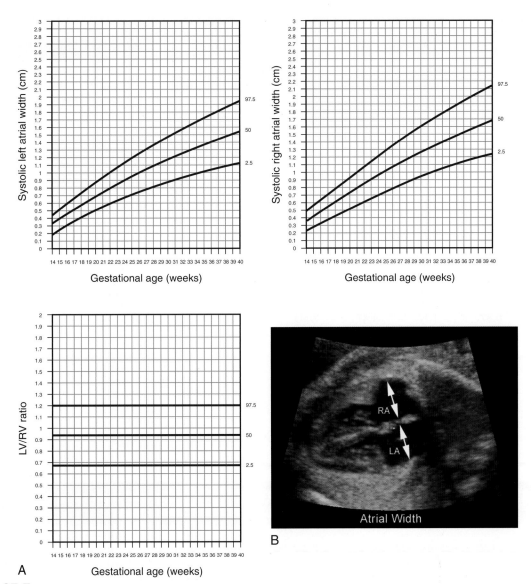

Figure 35-7
Measurements of the right and left atrial chamber width and their ratio. Measurements are obtained at end-ventricular systole. Atrial width is measured below the coapted atrioventricular valve, from the septum to the lateral wall of each ventricular chamber.[9]

confidence intervals are smaller earlier in gestation than later in gestation, and they provided ratios between the measured structures. From this study the following measurements have been selected for reporting:

1. Width of the atrial chambers and their ratio (Fig. 35-7, Table 35-7).
2. Width of the ventricular chambers and their ratio (Fig. 35-8, Table 35-8).
3. Dimension of the aorta and main pulmonary artery and their ratio (Fig. 35-9, Table 35-9).

Given the smaller range for the confidence intervals early in gestation when compared with the paper by Tan et al,[8] it would be important for the reader to compare the graphical display of normal measurements with known cases of pathology to determine which analysis best meets the user's needs. Fig. 35-10 illustrates the comparison of the mean and 95% confidence intervals for atrial and ventricular width and the dimensions of the aorta and ductus arteriosus between the studies of Tan et al[8] and Shapiro et al.[9]

Table 35-7   Measurements of the right and left atrial width and their ratio obtained at end-ventricular systole and the corresponding percentiles[9]

Gestation (wks)	Left Atrial Width (cm)			Right Atrial Width (cm)			Left Atrial/Right Atrial Ratio		
	2.5th Percentile	50th Percentile	95th Percentile	2.5th Percentile	50th Percentile	95th Percentile	2.5th Percentile	50th Percentile	95th Percentile
14	0.18	0.32	0.44	0.22	0.35	0.49	0.67	0.94	1.21
15	0.25	0.38	0.51	0.28	0.42	0.57	0.67	0.94	1.20
16	0.30	0.44	0.59	0.33	0.48	0.64	0.67	0.94	1.20
17	0.35	0.50	0.66	0.38	0.55	0.72	0.67	0.94	1.20
18	0.40	0.56	0.73	0.43	0.61	0.79	0.67	0.94	1.20
19	0.45	0.62	0.80	0.48	0.67	0.86	0.67	0.94	1.20
20	0.49	0.68	0.87	0.52	0.73	0.94	0.67	0.94	1.20
21	0.54	0.73	0.93	0.57	0.79	1.01	0.67	0.94	1.20
22	0.58	0.79	1.00	0.61	0.85	1.08	0.67	0.94	1.20
23	0.62	0.84	1.06	0.66	0.90	1.15	0.67	0.93	1.20
24	0.66	0.89	1.12	0.70	0.96	1.21	0.67	0.93	1.20
25	0.70	0.94	1.19	0.74	1.01	1.28	0.67	0.93	1.20
26	0.74	0.99	1.25	0.78	1.06	1.34	0.67	0.93	1.20
27	0.77	1.04	1.30	0.82	1.11	1.41	0.67	0.93	1.20
28	0.81	1.08	1.36	0.86	1.16	1.47	0.67	0.93	1.20
29	0.84	1.13	1.42	0.90	1.21	1.53	0.67	0.93	1.20
30	0.87	1.17	1.47	0.93	1.26	1.59	0.67	0.93	1.20
31	0.90	1.21	1.52	0.96	1.31	1.65	0.67	0.93	1.20
32	0.93	1.25	1.58	1.00	1.35	1.71	0.67	0.93	1.20
33	0.96	1.29	1.63	1.03	1.40	1.77	0.67	0.93	1.19
34	0.99	1.33	1.67	1.06	1.44	1.82	0.67	0.93	1.19
35	1.01	1.37	1.72	1.09	1.48	1.88	0.67	0.93	1.19
36	1.04	1.40	1.77	1.12	1.52	1.93	0.67	0.93	1.19
37	1.06	1.43	1.81	1.15	1.56	1.98	0.67	0.93	1.19
38	1.08	1.47	1.85	1.17	1.60	2.03	0.67	0.93	1.19
39	1.10	1.50	1.90	1.20	1.64	2.08	0.67	0.93	1.19
40	1.12	1.53	1.94	1.22	1.67	2.13	0.67	0.93	1.19

Table 35-8   Measurements of the right and left ventricular width and their ratio obtained at end-ventricular diastole and the corresponding percentiles[9]

Gestation (wks)	Left Ventricular Width (cm)			Right Ventricular Width (cm)			Left Ventricular/Right Ventricular Ratio		
	2.5th Percentile	50th Percentile	95th Percentile	2.5th Percentile	50th Percentile	95th Percentile	2.5th Percentile	50th Percentile	95th Percentile
14	0.10	0.23	0.37	0.12	0.25	0.37	0.75	0.99	1.23
15	0.16	0.30	0.45	0.17	0.31	0.45	0.74	0.99	1.23
16	0.21	0.37	0.53	0.23	0.38	0.53	0.74	0.99	1.23
17	0.26	0.43	0.61	0.28	0.44	0.61	0.74	0.99	1.24
18	0.31	0.50	0.68	0.32	0.51	0.69	0.73	0.99	1.24
19	0.36	0.56	0.75	0.37	0.57	0.76	0.73	0.98	1.24
20	0.40	0.61	0.82	0.42	0.63	0.84	0.72	0.98	1.24
21	0.45	0.67	0.89	0.46	0.69	0.91	0.72	0.98	1.24
22	0.49	0.72	0.96	0.51	0.74	0.98	0.71	0.97	1.24
23	0.53	0.77	1.02	0.55	0.80	1.05	0.71	0.97	1.23
24	0.56	0.82	1.08	0.59	0.85	1.12	0.70	0.97	1.23
25	0.59	0.87	1.14	0.63	0.91	1.19	0.69	0.96	1.23
26	0.62	0.91	1.20	0.66	0.96	1.25	0.69	0.96	1.23
27	0.65	0.95	1.25	0.70	1.01	1.32	0.68	0.95	1.22
28	0.68	0.99	1.30	0.74	1.06	1.38	0.67	0.95	1.22
29	0.70	1.03	1.35	0.77	1.10	1.44	0.66	0.94	1.22
30	0.73	1.06	1.40	0.80	1.15	1.50	0.65	0.93	1.21
31	0.74	1.09	1.44	0.83	1.20	1.56	0.64	0.93	1.21
32	0.76	1.12	1.49	0.86	1.24	1.62	0.63	0.92	1.20
33	0.78	1.15	1.53	0.89	1.28	1.67	0.62	0.91	1.20
34	0.79	1.18	1.56	0.92	1.32	1.73	0.61	0.90	1.19
35	0.80	1.20	1.60	0.94	1.36	1.78	0.60	0.89	1.18
36	0.81	1.22	1.63	0.97	1.40	1.83	0.59	0.88	1.18
37	0.81	1.24	1.66	0.99	1.44	1.88	0.58	0.87	1.17
38	0.82	1.25	1.69	1.01	1.47	1.93	0.56	0.86	1.16
39	0.82	1.27	1.72	1.03	1.51	1.98	0.55	0.85	1.15
40	0.82	1.28	1.74	1.05	1.54	2.03	0.54	0.84	1.15

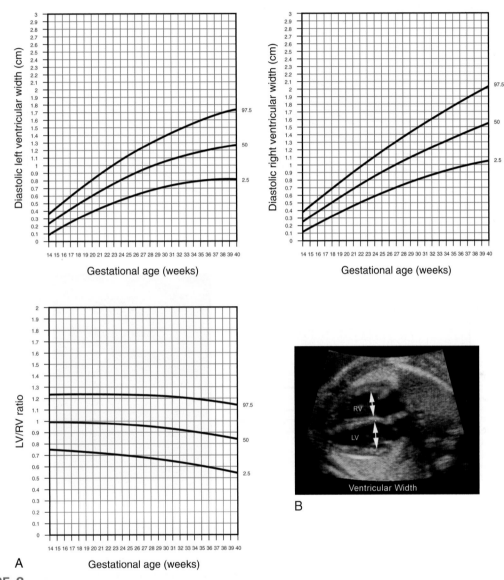

Figure 35-8

Measurements of the right and left ventricular chamber width and their ratio. Measurements are obtained at end-ventricular diastole. Ventricular width is measured below the coapted atrioventricular valve, from the septum to the lateral wall of each ventricular chamber.[9]

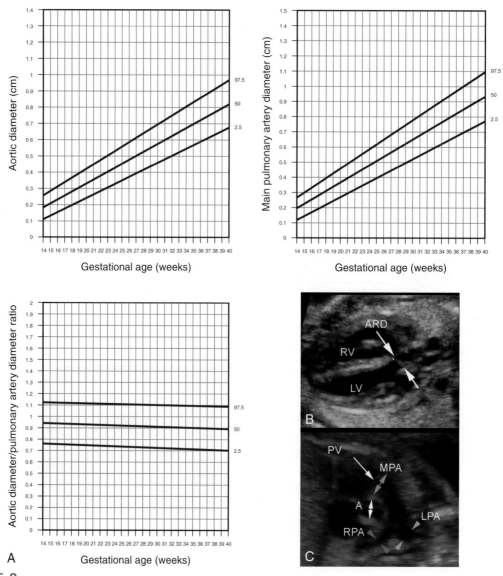

Figure 35-9

Measurements of the width of the aorta and main pulmonary artery and their ratio.[9] **A,** The long-axis view of the left ventricle from which the aortic root dimension was measured at the level of the aortic valve. **B,** The short-axis view of the outflow tracts from which the dimension of the main pulmonary artery is measured at the level of the pulmonary valve. *A,* aorta; *ARD,* aortic root dimension at the level of the aortic valve; *LPA,* left pulmonary artery; *LV,* left ventricle; *MPA,* main pulmonary artery; *PV,* pulmonary valve; *RA,* right atrium; *RPA,* right pulmonary artery; *RV,* Right ventricle.

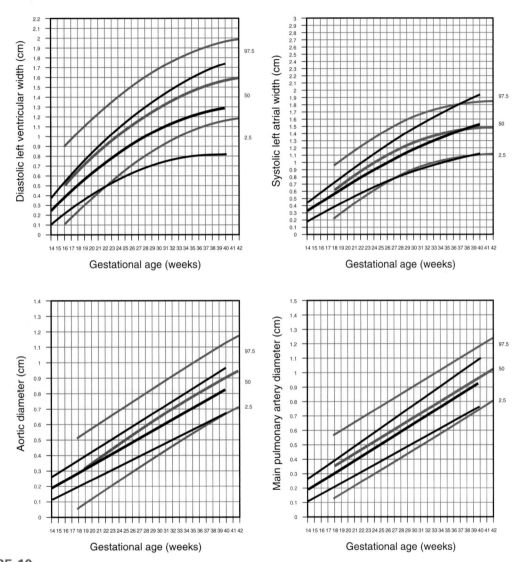

Figure 35-10
Mean and 95% confidence intervals of atrial and ventricular width, aortic diameter, and main pulmonary artery diameter between Tan et al[8] (red lines) and Shapiro et al[9] (black lines).

Table 35-9 Measurements of the aorta and main pulmonary artery and their ratio and the corresponding percentiles[9]

Gestation (wks)	Aorta Diameter (cm)			Main Pulmonary Artery (cm)			Aorta/Main Pulmonary Artery Ratio		
	2.5th Percentile	50th Percentile	95th Percentile	2.5th Percentile	50th Percentile	95th Percentile	2.5th Percentile	50th Percentile	95th Percentile
14	0.11	0.18	0.25	0.12	0.19	0.26	0.75	0.93	1.12
15	0.13	0.21	0.28	0.15	0.22	0.30	0.75	0.93	1.11
16	0.15	0.23	0.31	0.17	0.25	0.33	0.75	0.93	1.11
17	0.18	0.26	0.34	0.19	0.28	0.36	0.75	0.93	1.11
18	0.20	0.28	0.36	0.22	0.30	0.39	0.74	0.93	1.11
19	0.22	0.31	0.39	0.24	0.33	0.42	0.74	0.93	1.11
20	0.24	0.33	0.42	0.27	0.36	0.45	0.74	0.92	1.11
21	0.26	0.35	0.45	0.29	0.39	0.49	0.74	0.92	1.11
22	0.29	0.38	0.47	0.32	0.42	0.52	0.74	0.92	1.11
23	0.31	0.40	0.50	0.34	0.45	0.55	0.73	0.92	1.10
24	0.33	0.43	0.53	0.37	0.47	0.58	0.73	0.92	1.10
25	0.35	0.45	0.56	0.39	0.50	0.61	0.73	0.92	1.10
26	0.37	0.48	0.58	0.42	0.53	0.65	0.73	0.91	1.10
27	0.39	0.50	0.61	0.44	0.56	0.68	0.72	0.91	1.10
28	0.42	0.53	0.64	0.47	0.59	0.71	0.72	0.91	1.10
29	0.44	0.55	0.67	0.49	0.62	0.74	0.72	0.91	1.10
30	0.46	0.58	0.69	0.52	0.64	0.77	0.72	0.91	1.10
31	0.48	0.60	0.72	0.54	0.67	0.80	0.72	0.91	1.09
32	0.50	0.63	0.75	0.57	0.70	0.84	0.71	0.90	1.09
33	0.53	0.65	0.78	0.59	0.73	0.87	0.71	0.90	1.09
34	0.55	0.68	0.80	0.62	0.76	0.90	0.71	0.90	1.09
35	0.57	0.70	0.83	0.64	0.79	0.93	0.71	0.90	1.09
36	0.59	0.73	0.86	0.67	0.81	0.96	0.71	0.90	1.09
37	0.61	0.75	0.89	0.69	0.84	1.00	0.70	0.90	1.09
38	0.63	0.77	0.91	0.71	0.87	1.03	0.70	0.89	1.08
39	0.66	0.80	0.94	0.74	0.90	1.06	0.70	0.89	1.08
40	0.68	0.82	0.97	0.76	0.93	1.09	0.70	0.89	1.08

References

1. Allan LD, Joseph MC, Boyd EG, et al: M-mode echocardiography in the developing human fetus. Br Heart J 1982;47:573-583.
2. De Vore GR, Siassi B, Platt LD: Use of femur length as a means of assessing M-mode ventricular dimensions during second and third trimesters of pregnancy in normal fetus. J Clin Ultrasound 1985;13:619-625.
3. DeVore GR, Siassi B, Platt LD: Fetal echocardiography. IV. M-mode assessment of ventricular size and contractility during the second and third trimesters of pregnancy in the normal fetus. Am J Obstet Gynecol 1984;150:981-988.
4. DeVore GR, Siassi B, Platt LD: The use of the abdominal circumference as a means of assessing M-mode ventricular dimensions during the second and third trimesters of pregnancy in the normal human fetus. J Ultrasound Med 1985;4:175-182.
5. DeVore GR, Siassi B, Platt LD: Fetal echocardiography. V. M-mode measurements of the aortic root and aortic valve in second- and third-trimester normal human fetuses. Am J Obstet Gynecol 1985;152:543-550.
6. John Sutton MG, Gewitz MH, Shah B, et al: Quantitative assessment of growth and function of the cardiac chambers in the normal human fetus: a prospective longitudinal echocardiographic study. Circulation 1984;69:645-654.
7. Sharland GK, Allan LD: Normal fetal cardiac measurements derived by cross-sectional echocardiography. Ultrasound Obstet Gynecol 1992;2:175-181.

8. Tan J, Silverman NH, Hoffman JI, Villegas M, Schmidt KG: Cardiac dimensions determined by cross-sectional echocardiography in the normal human fetus from 18 weeks to term. Am J Cardiol 1992;70: 1459-1467.

9. Shapiro I, Degani S, Leibovitz Z, et al: Fetal cardiac measurements derived by trans-vaginal and transabdominal cross-sectional echocardiography from 14 weeks of gestation to term. Ultrasound Obstet Gynecol 1998;12:404-418.

10. Firpo C, Hoffman JI, Silverman NH: Evaluation of fetal heart dimensions from 12 weeks to term. Am J Cardiol 2001;87: 594-600.

CHAPTER 36

Greggory R. DeVore

Pulsed Doppler Examination of the Fetal Heart

Introduction

Pulsed Doppler examination provides important information and demonstrates the direction and the characteristics of blood flow within the heart. Pulsed Doppler devices use one crystal that transmits and receives the ultrasound signal. This is performed by placing a small box that is a sample volume on the cursor that can be steered through any sector line or depth of the image (Fig. 36-1). Doppler signals that are received from moving red blood cells are then displayed either above or below the baseline (see Fig. 36-1). They are displayed above the baseline if the red blood cells are traveling toward the transducer and displayed below the baseline if the red blood cells are flowing away from the transducer. It is ideal to obtain the Doppler signal parallel to the main direction of blood flow, as the more perpendicular the Doppler sample volume recording is to the flowing blood, the less is the frequency shift of the displayed Doppler waveform (Fig. 36-2). The Doppler frequency, which returns to the transducer, is the frequency shift that can be displayed as a signal on the output of the ultrasound monitor. Older ultrasound equipment measured and displayed the frequency shift, whereas most current equipment, using state-of-the-art pulsed-wave Doppler technology, automatically uses fast Fourier analysis to convert the frequency shift into a velocity display (Table 36-1). Velocity display is obtained from the formula in which

$$V = (f_d \times c)/(2f_0 \times \cos \emptyset)$$

Using this formula, the velocity (V) is recorded in meters per second and recorded on the video output of the ultrasound monitor. C is the velocity of sound in water, which is a constant at 1560 m/sec, and f_0 is the transmitted frequency (i.e., the frequency used within the transducer, such as 3 MHz). f_d is the frequency shift in hertz, which is the returning frequency that is recorded by the ultrasound equipment. $\cos \emptyset$ is the angle of insonation of the ultrasound beam (f_0) as it interrogates the red blood cells. Thus if the ultrasound beam is parallel to the flow of red blood cells, the angle is zero and $\cos \emptyset$ is 1. If the ultrasound beam is perpendicular to the flow of red blood cells, the angle is 90 degrees and the $\cos \emptyset$ is 0. The angle $\emptyset$ should always be less than 60 degrees and ideally less than 30 degrees for most accurate measurements. Thus using this formula, velocity is recorded in meters per second.

Velocities can be measured using continuous-wave instrumentation. With continuous-wave

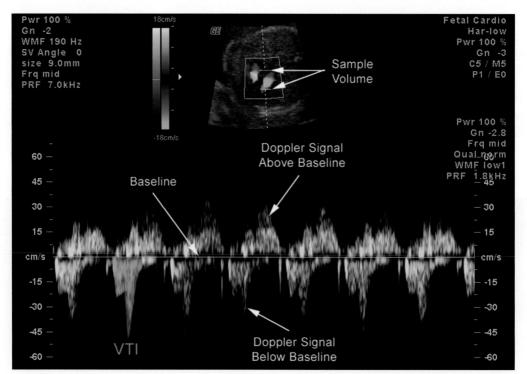

Figure 36-1

Doppler waveform and sample volume. The sample volume is placed over the left ventricle, and the pulsed Doppler waveform recorded. The pulsed Doppler waveform is recorded demonstrating a waveform above and below the baseline. The velocity time integral (VTI) is the area under the curve of the Doppler waveform, which represents one cardiac cycle.

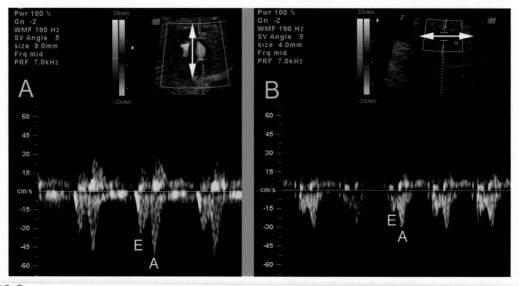

Figure 36-2

Comparing the Doppler waveforms obtained parallel and perpendicular to flow. **A,** The pulsed Doppler waveform obtained when the sample volume was placed parallel (*white double arrow*) to blood flow identified with the color Doppler. **B,** The four-chamber view is perpendicular (*white double arrow*), and the Doppler waveform recorded. Because the angle is 90 degrees, the pulsed Doppler waveform is decreased in size for the same Doppler scale used in **A.**

Table 36-1	Doppler measurements	
Measurement[a]	**Method**	**Units**
Peak or maximal velocity	Zero line to peak of the waveform	cm/sec or m/sec
Mean velocity	Time velocity integral/time of cardiac cycle	cm/sec or m/sec
Volume flow	Mean velocity × area[b] × 60	mL/min or L/min
Time-to-peak velocity or acceleration time	Time from onset to the peak of the waveform	msec
Deceleration time	Time from peak to zero line along slope of descent	msec
Velocity time integral	Area under the curve of the Doppler waveform	

[a] Velocities should be measured within 30 degrees of estimated direction of flow or be angle-corrected.
[b] Area obtained from diameters measured with two-dimensional ultrasound.

instrumentation, two transducers are used—one to transmit and the other to receive the Doppler signal. Use of continuous-wave Doppler is nonselective in that all signals along the ultrasound beam are recorded. Therefore most individuals use pulsed-wave Doppler for examining the fetal heart.

Doppler ultrasound also exposes the fetus to higher levels of ultrasound energy than real-time imaging or M-mode ultrasound. As such, the amount of time one uses in performing pulsed Doppler ultrasound of the fetus should be limited. For this reason most clinicians will use color Doppler to identify the structure of interest and then place the sample volume for pulsed Doppler recording. This shortens the time required to obtain the pulsed Doppler waveform. It is known that the Doppler ultrasound energy should be kept below 100 mW/cm^2 spatial peak-temporal average.

Measurement of blood volume (Q) requires measurement of the cross-sectional area (A) through which blood is flowing, which is then multiplied by an average velocity.

$$Q = V \times A$$

Let us examine how the above equation can be used to compute blood volume. The average velocity (V) can be computed by multiplying the velocity time integral (VTI) by the heart rate. The VTI is the area under the curve of the Doppler waveform (see Fig. 36-1). Multiplying the VTI by the heart rate (beats/minute) provides an estimate of the average velocity of blood flow during 1 minute. The second component of

the equation to compute blood volume is to measure the area of the orifice through which blood is flowing. Because all structures in the fetal heart (mitral, tricuspid, aortic, and pulmonary valve) are circular, measurements of their diameter can be obtained and the area computed ([diameter/2]^2 × 3.14). Once these values are measured, then the volume of blood flow can be determined as follows:

$$Q = 3.14 \times (D/2)^2 \times VTI \times HR$$

Intracardiac Doppler

Intracardiac Doppler examination can be performed for either the tricuspid or mitral valve. In most instances it is best to have the pulsed Doppler cursor placed as parallel to the moving red blood cells as possible. As such, it is best to image the four-chamber view of the heart so that the interventricular septum is parallel to the ultrasound beam (see Fig. 36-2A). Velocities can be angle-corrected, but small errors in estimation of the angle may result in an unacceptably large error of velocity measurements (see Fig. 36-2). Ideally, angle measurement between the ultrasound beam and the direction of the flowing blood should be less than 30 degrees and must always be less than 60 degrees.

When examining either the tricuspid or mitral valve, the Doppler sample volume is placed immediately distal to the valve leaflets in the right or left ventricle, respectively (Fig. 36-3). When velocity flow is detected across the tricuspid or mitral valve with the cursor placed within

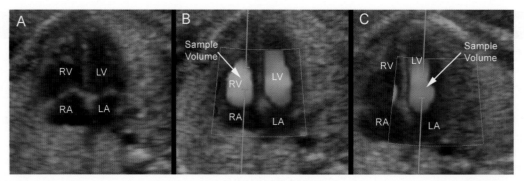

Figure 36-3
Placement of the Doppler sample volume. **A,** The four-chamber view when the mitral and tricuspid valves are closed during ventricular systole. **B,** The four-chamber view when the mitral and tricuspid valves are open, as identified by color Doppler ultrasound. The sample volume is placed within the right ventricular chamber and increased in size to record as much of the blood flow entering the chamber as possible. **C,** The sample volume is placed within the left ventricular chamber and increased in size to record as much of the blood flow entering the chamber as possible. *LA,* left atrium; *LV,* left ventricle; *RA,* right atrium; *RV,* Right ventricle.

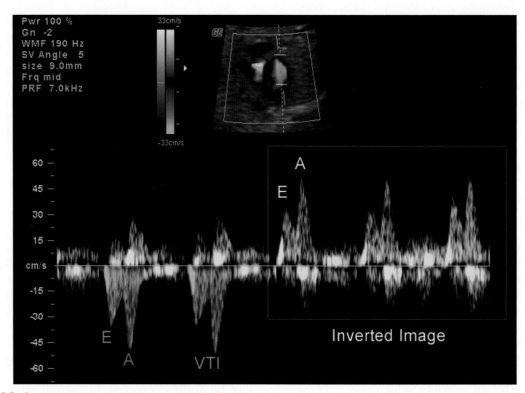

Figure 36-4
The sample volume is placed within the left ventricular chamber. Because the spine is at 1 o'clock, the flow into the ventricular chambers is away from the baseline. The colored portions of the waveform represent the E and A waves and the velocity time integral (VTI). The inverted image illustrates the waveforms if the blood flow were above the baseline.

either of their respective ventricles, there is usually a biphasic Doppler signal (Fig. 36-4). The flow velocity waveform across the valve is characterized by an E component, followed by a higher A component. The E component is a result of the rapid filling phase of diastole and is entirely passive. The A component is the result of atrial contraction (see Fig. 36-4). Several studies have examined the velocities of the E and A wave as a function of gestational age and reported an increase in the E wave, with little or no change in the A wave (Table

Table 36-2	Diastolic function of the right and left ventricles in normal fetuses[2]			
	All Subjects	**17-24 weeks**	**25-31 weeks**	**32-39 weeks**
Gestational age (wks)	27 ± 7	21 ± 2	27 ± 2	35 ± 2
Heart rate (beats/min)	142 ± 10	146 ± 9	140 ± 10	138 ± 11
Left Ventricle				
Mitral valve studies	307	130	91	86
E wave peak velocity (cm/sec)	31 ± 7	26 ± 4	31 ± 5	38 ± 6
A wave peak velocity (cm/sec)	44 ± 11	41 ± 6	45 ± 7	47 ± 6
E/A Ratio	0.7 ± 0.11	0.63 ± 0.07	0.70 ± 0.09	0.80 ± 0.10
Right Ventricle				
Tricuspid valve studies	258	118	71	69
E wave peak velocity (cm/sec)	33 ± 7	29 ± 5	35 ± 6	39 ± 6
A wave peak velocity (cm/sec)	48 ± 7	45 ± 6	49 ± 8	51 ± 8
E/A Ratio	0.70 ± 0.09	0.64 ± 0.07	0.70 ± 0.08	0.77 ± 0.09

Values are mean ± 1 SD

Table 36-3	Mitral and tricuspid valve E/A ratios					
	Mitral Valve E/A Ratio			**Tricuspid Valve E/A Ratio**		
Gestation (wks)	**2.5th Percentile**	**50th Percentile**	**97.5th Percentile**	**2.5th Percentile**	**50th Percentile**	**97.5th Percentile**
20	0.40	0.59	0.77	0.47	0.65	0.83
21	0.42	0.60	0.79	0.49	0.66	0.84
22	0.43	0.62	0.80	0.50	0.68	0.85
23	0.45	0.63	0.82	0.52	0.69	0.86
24	0.46	0.65	0.83	0.53	0.70	0.87
25	0.48	0.66	0.84	0.54	0.71	0.88
26	0.49	0.68	0.86	0.55	0.72	0.89
27	0.50	0.69	0.87	0.56	0.73	0.90
28	0.52	0.70	0.88	0.57	0.74	0.90
29	0.53	0.71	0.89	0.58	0.74	0.91
30	0.54	0.73	0.90	0.58	0.75	0.91
31	0.55	0.74	0.91	0.59	0.75	0.92
32	0.56	0.75	0.92	0.59	0.76	0.92
33	0.57	0.76	0.93	0.60	0.76	0.92
34	0.58	0.76	0.93	0.60	0.76	0.92
35	0.59	0.77	0.94	0.60	0.76	0.92
36	0.59	0.78	0.95	0.60	0.76	0.92
37	0.60	0.79	0.95	0.60	0.76	0.92
38	0.61	0.79	0.96	0.60	0.76	0.92

36-2).[1,2] The E/A wave ratio increases with gestational age as a function of the increase in the E-wave velocity (Tables 36-2 and 36-3) (Fig. 36-5).[1,3] Increased velocities through the valve may indicate valvular stenosis. If valvular insufficiency is suspected, the Doppler sample may be placed through the mitral or tricuspid valve into their respective atrium for detection of valvular insufficiency (Fig. 36-6). Studies have shown changes in the E/A ratio as the result of intrauterine growth retardation, fetal inflammatory response syndrome, and maternal diabetes.[3,4]

Investigators have also attempted to measure cardiac output from the mitral and tricuspid

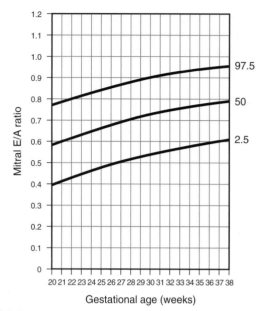

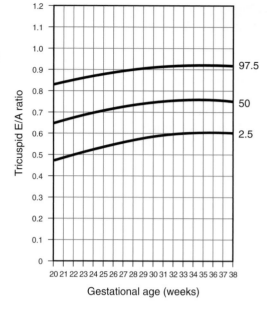

Figure 36-5
E/A ratios as a function of gestational age.[1,3]

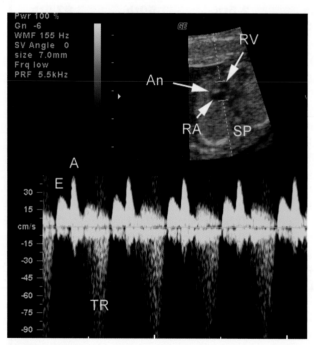

Figure 36-6
The sample volume has been placed in the right ventricle and atrium. The pulsed Doppler waveform records the inflow of blood into the right ventricle during diastole, as manifest by the E and A waveforms. During ventricular systole, there is holosystolic regurgitation of blood back into the right atrium (TR). *An,* annulus; *RA,* right atrium; *RV,* Right ventricle; *SP,* spine.

valve Doppler waveforms by measuring the VTI (see Fig. 36-4) and using the following equation to compute flow:

$$Q = 3.14 \times (D/2)^2 \times VTI \times HR$$

(Tables 36-4 and 36-5) (Figs. 36-7 and 36-8).[5]

The difficulty, however, is the determination of the area of the mitral and tricuspid valves.

Aortic and Pulmonary Outflow Tract Doppler Examination

Aortic or pulmonary arterial Doppler waveforms may be obtained from either the aorta or the pulmonary artery as they exit their respective ventricles. The aortic blood flow velocities can be obtained using the long axis of the five-chamber view of the heart (Fig. 36-9), whereas pulmonary Doppler flow velocities are best obtained from a short-axis view of the heart or through a transverse plane above the five-chamber view in the chest (Fig. 36-10). Using these approaches, the pulmonary artery and aorta are parallel to the ultrasound beam so that accurate Doppler recordings of their respective waveforms can occur. For the pulmonary artery and aorta there is usually only one peak noted on the Doppler waveform, rather than the two peaks as noted for either the tricuspid or

Table 36-4 Left and Right ventricular cardiac outputs measured from the mitral and tricuspid inflow Doppler waveforms[5]

Gestation (wks)	Left Ventricle Cardiac Output (LCO) (ml/min)			Right Ventricle Cardiac Output (RCO) (ml/min)			RCO/LCO Ratio		
	2.5th Percentile	50th Percentile	97.5th Percentile	2.5th Percentile	50th Percentile	97.5th Percentile	2.5th Percentile	50th Percentile	97.5th Percentile
18	37	57	81	40	70	97	1.01	1.33	1.65
19	36	56	80	42	72	97	1.00	1.32	1.64
20	39	61	85	47	78	103	1.00	1.32	1.64
21	44	69	96	55	89	116	1.00	1.32	1.64
22	53	83	112	67	105	135	0.99	1.31	1.63
23	66	100	135	82	126	162	0.99	1.31	1.63
24	82	123	164	101	152	194	0.99	1.30	1.63
25	101	150	199	123	183	233	0.98	1.30	1.62
26	123	181	240	148	219	279	0.98	1.30	1.62
27	148	217	287	177	260	332	0.98	1.29	1.62
28	177	258	340	210	306	391	0.97	1.29	1.61
29	209	303	398	245	357	456	0.97	1.28	1.61
30	245	353	463	284	412	529	0.97	1.28	1.61
31	284	407	534	327	473	607	0.96	1.28	1.60
32	326	466	611	373	538	693	0.96	1.27	1.60
33	371	530	693	422	609	785	0.95	1.27	1.59
34	420	598	782	474	684	883	0.95	1.26	1.59
35	472	670	877	531	765	988	0.95	1.26	1.59
36	527	747	977	590	850	1100	0.94	1.26	1.58
37	586	829	1084	653	940	1218	0.94	1.25	1.58
38	648	915	1196	719	1035	1343	0.94	1.25	1.58
39	713	1006	1315	789	1135	1475	0.93	1.24	1.57
40	782	1101	1440	862	1240	1613	0.93	1.24	1.57

Table 36-5 Reported values of volume flow estimations from the atrioventricular (AV) valves for left cardiac output (LCO), right cardiac output (RCO), and combined cardiac output (CCO) corrected for fetal weight[5]

Author	Site of Recording	LCO (ml/min)			RCO (ml/min)			
		19-21	29-31	36-40	19-21	29-31	36-40	CCO (ml/min/kg)
De Smedt	AV valves	84	333	820	105	372	915	553
Allan	AV valves	109	333	686	140	428	883	—
Rizzo	AV valves	91	320	693	134	435	890	546

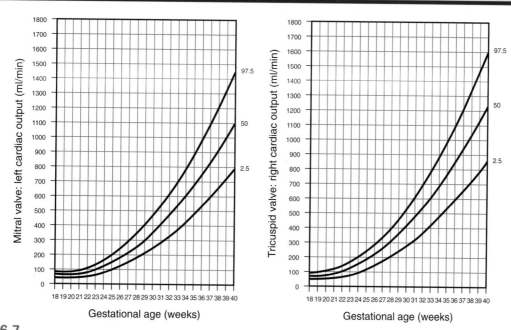

Figure 36-7

Normal values for gestation of left and right cardiac outputs obtained from the atrioventricular valves in 284 normal fetuses studied cross-sectionally.[5]

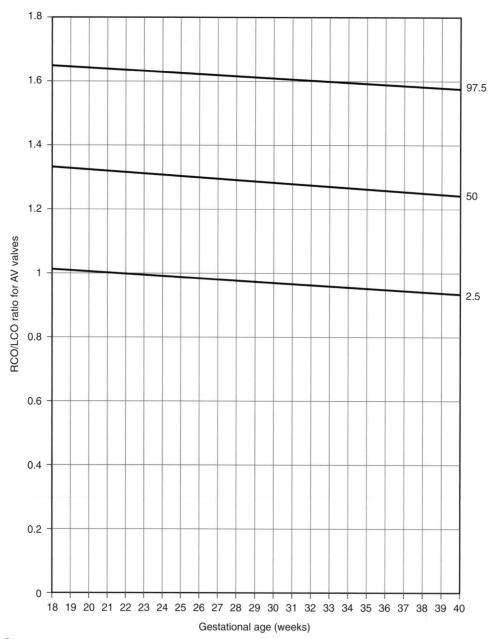

Figure 36-8
Normal values for gestation of right cardiac output (RCO) divided by left cardiac output (LCO) obtained from the atrioventricular valves in 284 normal fetuses studied cross-sectionally.[5]

mitral valve (Figs. 36-11 and 36-12). The peak or maximum velocity is obtained by measuring the highest velocity of the time velocity Doppler signal that is angle-corrected. Maximum velocities for the aorta and pulmonary artery increase as a function of gestational age (Table 36-6) (Fig. 36-13).[3] The time-to-peak velocity can be measured for each vessel and is measured from the beginning of the waveform to the point of the peak velocity (Figs. 36-11 and 36-14) (Tables 36-1 and 36-7). As gestational age increases,

the resistance in the aorta decreases as manifest by an increasing time-to-peak velocity. Conversely, the resistance in the main pulmonary artery increases as manifest by a shorter time-to-peak velocity. In addition to measuring cardiac output from the atrioventricular valves, investigators have measured cardiac output from the aorta and main pulmonary artery by using the following equation:

$$Q = 3.14 \times (D/2)^2 \times VTI \times HR$$

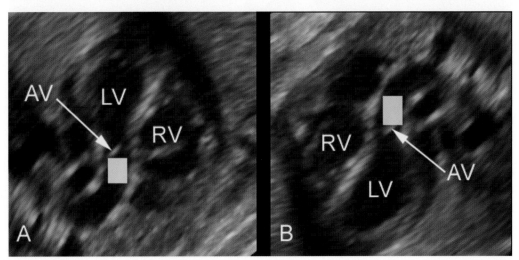

Figure 36-9
Five-chamber view of the heart demonstrating the aorta parallel to the Doppler sample volume. The sample volume is placed distal to the aortic valve and the pulsed Doppler waveform recorded. **A,** Apex of the heart at 12 o'clock; **B,** apex at 6 o'clock. *AV,* Aortic valve; *LV,* left ventricle; *RV,* right ventricle; *yellow box,* location of pulsed Doppler sample volume.

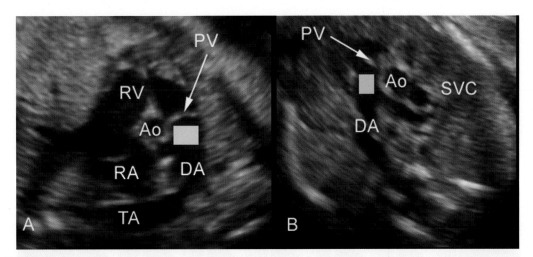

Figure 36-10
A, Short-axis view of the heart imaged in a sagittal plane demonstrating the placement of the Doppler sample volume distal to the pulmonary valve (PV). **B,** Main pulmonary artery imaged in a transverse plane of the chest, cephalad to the five-chamber view. *Ao,* aorta; *DA,* ductus arteriosus; *RA,* Right atrium; *RV* = right ventricle; *SVC,* superior vena cava; *TA,* thoracic aorta.

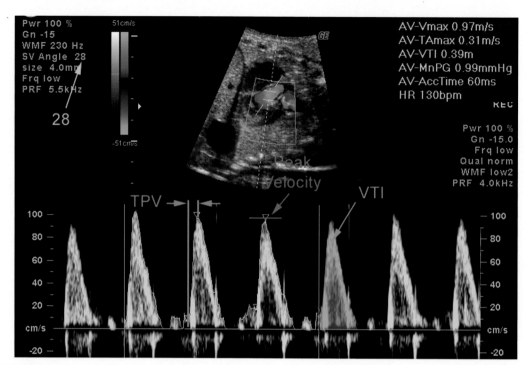

Figure 36-11
Pulsed Doppler recording from the ascending aorta with the apex of the ventricles at 6 o'clock. TPV, time-to-peak velocity or acceleration time; VTI, velocity time integral. The angle of insonation is 28 degrees. Note the computed measurements in the upper right portion of the image.

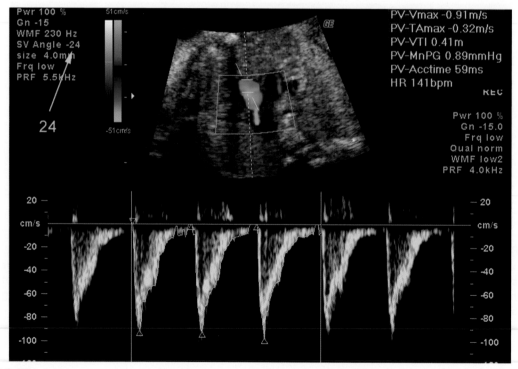

Figure 36-12
Pulsed Doppler waveform recorded distal to the pulmonary valve. The sample volume was at a 24-degree angle.

Table 36-6	Peak or maximum velocity of the aorta and main pulmonary artery					
	Aorta Peak Velocity (cm/sec)			**Pulmonary Artery Peak Velocity (cm/sec)**		
Gestation (wks)	**2.5th Percentile**	**50th Percentile**	**97.5th Percentile**	**2.5th Percentile**	**50th Percentile**	**97.5th Percentile**
20	29	62	95	23	53	80
21	30	63	96	24	54	81
22	32	65	98	25	56	82
23	33	66	99	27	57	84
24	34	67	100	28	58	85
25	36	68	101	29	59	86
26	37	70	103	30	61	87
27	38	71	104	31	62	89
28	40	72	105	32	63	90
29	41	74	107	34	64	91
30	42	75	108	35	65	92
31	44	76	109	36	67	93
32	45	77	110	37	68	95
33	46	79	112	38	69	96
34	48	80	113	39	70	97
35	49	81	114	41	72	98
36	50	82	115	42	73	100
37	52	84	117	43	74	101
38	53	85	118	44	78	102

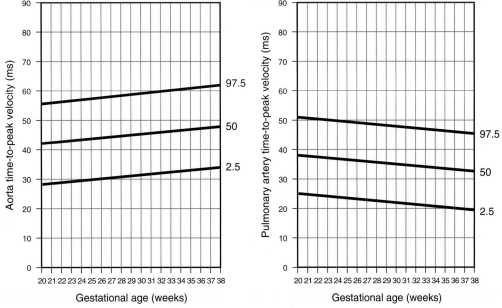

Figure 36-13
Peak velocity for the aorta and main pulmonary artery.[3]

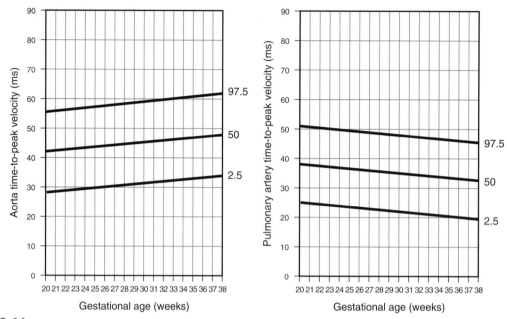

Figure 36-14
Time-to-peak velocity of the aorta and main pulmonary artery.[3] As gestational age increases, the resistance decreases in the aorta and increases in the main pulmonary artery.

Table 36-7	Aorta and pulmonary artery time-to-peak velocity					
	Aorta Time-to-Peak Velocity (msec)			**Pulmonary Artery Time-to-Peak Velocity (msec)**		
Gestation (wks)	**2.5th Percentile**	**50th Percentile**	**97.5th Percentile**	**2.5th Percentile**	**50th Percentile**	**97.5th Percentile**
20	29	43	56	25	38	51
21	29	43	56	25	38	51
22	29	43	57	24	37	50
23	29	43	57	24	37	50
24	30	44	57	24	37	50
25	30	44	58	23	36	49
26	30	44	58	23	36	49
27	31	45	58	23	36	49
28	31	45	59	22	35	48
29	31	45	59	22	35	48
30	32	46	59	22	35	48
31	32	46	60	21	34	47
32	32	46	60	21	34	47
33	32	46	60	21	34	47
34	33	47	61	20	33	46
35	33	47	61	20	33	46
36	33	47	61	20	33	46
37	34	48	62	19	32	45
38	34	48	62	19	32	45

Table 36-8 Reported values of volume flow estimations from the aorta and main pulmonary artery outflow tracts for left cardiac output (LCO), right cardiac output (RCO), and combined cardiac output (CCO) corrected for fetal weight[6]

Author	Site of Recording	LCO (ml/min)			RCO (ml/min)			CCO (ml/min/kg)
		19-21	29-31	36-40	19-21	29-31	36-40	
Kenny	Outflow Tracts	118	282	676	132	302	692	—
Allan	Outflow Tracts	70	269	647	93	361	886	450
Rizzo	Outflow Tracts	78	284	670	100	390	866	525

Table 36-9 Left and right ventricular cardiac outputs measured from the aortic and pulmonary outflow Doppler waveforms

Gestation (wks)	Left Ventricle Cardiac Output (LCO) (ml/min)			Right Ventricle Cardiac Output (RCO) (ml/min)			RCO/LCO		
	2.5th Percentile	50th Percentile	97.5th Percentile	2.5th Percentile	50th Percentile	97.5th Percentile	2.5th Percentile	50th Percentile	97.5th Percentile
18	53	83	112	38	69	92	1.65	1.32	1.00
19	50	77	104	38	66	90	1.65	1.31	1.00
20	51	77	103	42	69	94	1.65	1.31	0.99
21	55	82	109	49	76	104	1.64	1.31	0.99
22	64	94	123	59	88	119	1.64	1.31	0.99
23	76	111	145	73	105	141	1.63	1.30	0.98
24	93	134	175	89	126	169	1.63	1.30	0.98
25	113	162	212	109	153	203	1.63	1.30	0.98
26	136	197	257	131	184	243	1.62	1.30	0.97
27	164	237	309	157	220	290	1.62	1.29	0.97
28	196	282	369	186	262	342	1.61	1.29	0.97
29	231	334	437	218	308	400	1.61	1.29	0.96
30	270	391	512	253	358	464	1.60	1.29	0.96
31	313	454	596	292	414	535	1.60	1.28	0.96
32	360	523	686	333	475	611	1.60	1.28	0.95
33	411	598	785	378	540	694	1.59	1.28	0.95
34	465	678	891	425	610	782	1.59	1.28	0.95
35	524	764	1004	476	685	877	1.58	1.27	0.94
36	586	856	1126	530	765	978	1.58	1.27	0.94
37	652	953	1254	587	850	1084	1.57	1.27	0.94
38	722	1056	1391	647	940	1197	1.57	1.27	0.93

They found that the cardiac output increased as a function of gestational age (Tables 36-8 and 36-9) (Figs. 36-15 and 36-16).[3,6] Figure 36-17 compares cardiac output between that obtained from the atrioventricular valves and outflow tracts. Another indirect method to measure cardiac output is to simply measure the velocity time integral (VTI) and multiply this by the heart rate (Figs. 36-18 and 36-19) (Table 36-10). The benefit of this approach is that the examiner does not have to measure the dimension of the outflow tracts that, if an error is made, can markedly alter the computation of the cardiac output. Investigators have found that there is a decrease in cardiac output in fetuses with growth restriction and fetal anemia.[3,5,7]

The Doppler Mechanical PR Interval

Several investigators have examined the use of pulsed Doppler to identify the mechanical PR interval in utero.[8] Although the PR interval can be obtained following delivery using an electrocardiogram, this is not feasible in utero. Prolongation of the fetal mechanical PR interval has been observed with first- and second-degree heart block in fetuses at risk for complete heart block as the result of abnormal maternal

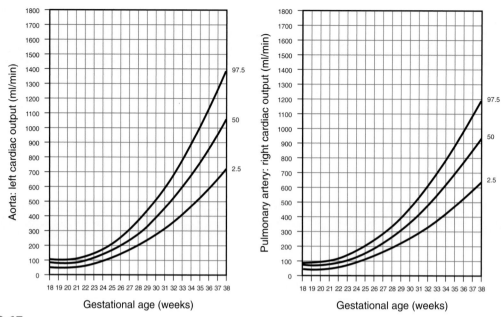

Figure 36-15
Measurement of cardiac output from the aorta and main pulmonary artery.[3]

Table 36-10	Left and right ventricular VTI × HR measured from the aortic and pulmonary outflow Doppler waveforms								
	Left Ventricle VTI × HR			**Right Ventricle VTI × HR**			**RV VTI × HR/LV VTI × HR**		
Gestation (wks)	**2.5th Percentile**	**50th Percentile**	**97.5th Percentile**	**2.5th Percentile**	**50th Percentile**	**97.5th Percentile**	**2.5th Percentile**	**50th Percentile**	**97.5th Percentile**
19	693	1147	1593	473	990	1462	0.47	0.84	1.22
20	700	1153	1600	487	1000	1473	0.47	0.85	1.23
21	708	1160	1608	500	1010	1485	0.48	0.86	1.23
22	715	1167	1615	513	1020	1497	0.49	0.87	1.24
23	723	1173	1623	527	1030	1508	0.49	0.87	1.25
24	730	1180	1630	540	1040	1520	0.50	0.88	1.26
25	738	1187	1638	553	1050	1532	0.51	0.89	1.27
26	745	1193	1645	567	1060	1543	0.51	0.90	1.28
27	753	1200	1653	580	1070	1555	0.52	0.90	1.28
28	760	1207	1660	593	1080	1567	0.53	0.91	1.29
29	768	1213	1668	607	1090	1578	0.53	0.92	1.30
30	775	1220	1675	620	1100	1590	0.54	0.93	1.31
31	783	1227	1683	633	1110	1602	0.55	0.93	1.32
32	790	1233	1690	647	1120	1613	0.55	0.94	1.33
33	798	1240	1698	660	1130	1625	0.56	0.95	1.33
34	805	1247	1705	673	1140	1637	0.57	0.96	1.34
35	813	1253	1713	687	1150	1648	0.57	0.96	1.35
36	820	1260	1720	700	1160	1660	0.58	0.97	1.36
37	828	1267	1728	713	1170	1672	0.59	0.98	1.37
38	835	1273	1735	727	1180	1683	0.59	0.99	1.38
39	843	1280	1743	740	1190	1695	0.60	0.99	1.38
40	850	1287	1750	753	1200	1707	0.61	1.00	1.39

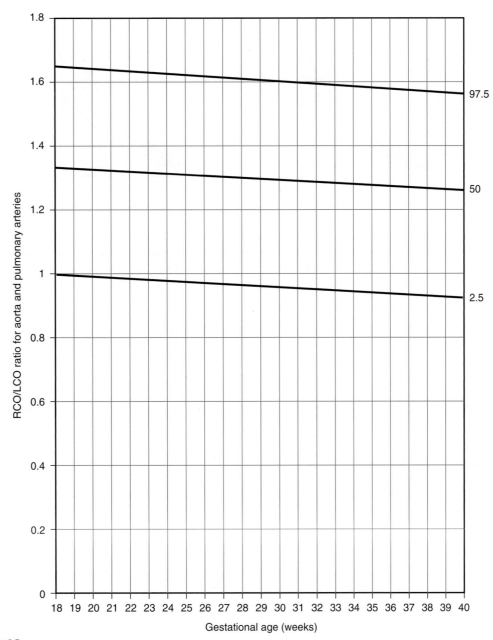

Figure 36-16
Normal values for gestation of right cardiac output (RCO) divided by left cardiac output (LCO) obtained from the pulmonary artery and aorta.[3]

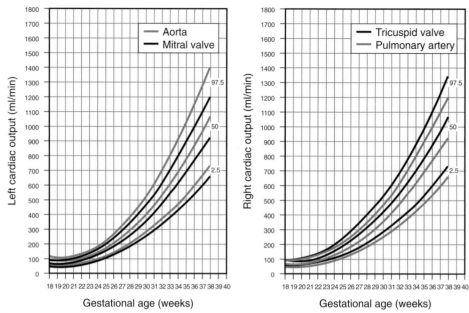

Figure 36-17
Comparison of the cardiac outputs determined by measuring either the ventricular inflow (mitral and tricuspid valves) or the outflow tracts (aorta and pulmonary artery). For the left ventricle, the range is higher for the aorta than the mitral valve. For the right ventricle the range is higher for the tricuspid valve than the pulmonary artery.[3,5]

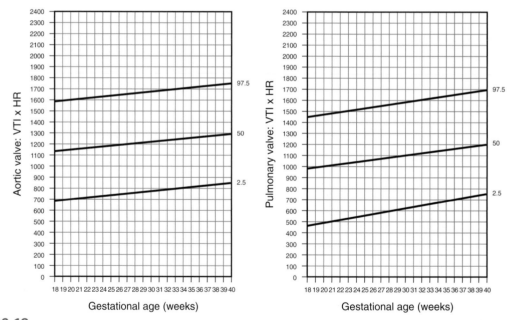

Figure 36-18
Products of time velocity integral multiplied by heart rate (TVI × HR) in aortic and pulmonary valves.[3]

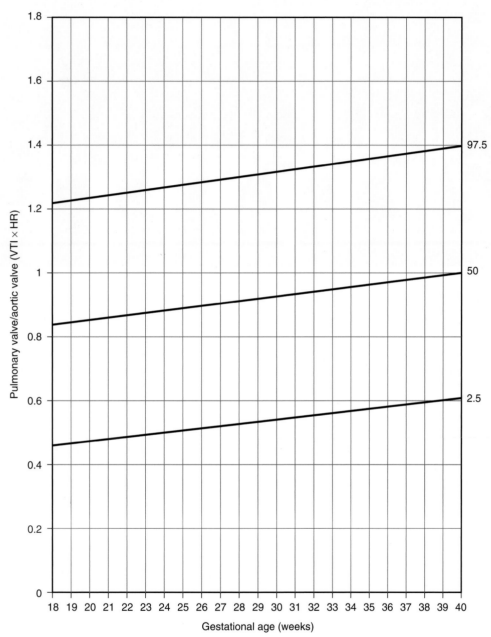

Figure 36-19
Ratio of the aortic valve (VTI × HR) to the pulmonary valve (VTI × HR).[3]

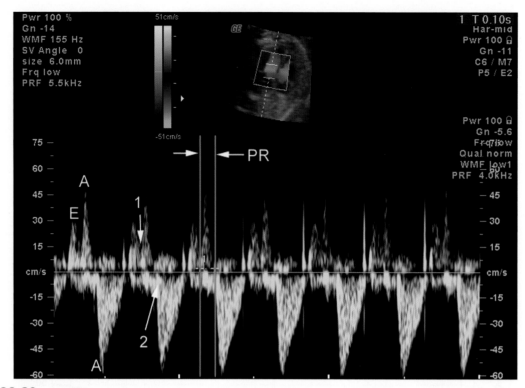

Figure 36-20
Measurement of the mechanical PR interval. This is obtained by measuring the time between the beginning of the A wave (1) to the beginning of the aortic waveform (2). In this example, the time is 10 msec.

Sjogren's antibodies, as well as other fetal conditions.[9] To obtain this waveform the sample volume is placed at the junction of the anterior mitral valve leaflet and the ascending aorta (Fig. 36-20). The Doppler mechanical PR interval is measured from the onset of the A wave of the mitral waveform to the onset of the aortic waveform. The fetal Doppler mechanical PR interval has been found to be fairly constant and is not altered by gestational age or fetal heart rate. The normal value is 120 msec (95% confidence interval 10 msec to 140 msec).

References

1. Harada K, Rice MJ, Shiota T, et al: Gestational age- and growth-related alterations in fetal right and left ventricular diastolic filling patterns. Am J Cardiol 1997;79:173-177.
2. Carceller-Blanchard AM, Fouron JC: Determinants of the Doppler Flow Velocity profile through the mitral valve of the human fetus. Br Heart J 1993;70:457-460.
3. Rizzo G, Arduini D: Fetal cardiac function in intrauterine growth retardation. Am J Obstet Gynecol 1991;165:876-882.
4. Tsyvian P, Malkin K, Artemieva O, Wladimiroff JW: Assessment of left ventricular filling in normally grown fetuses, growth-restricted fetuses and fetuses of diabetic mothers. Ultrasound Obstet Gynecol 1998;12:33-38.
5. Arduini D, Rizzo G, Romanini C: Fetal cardiac output measurements in normal and pathologic states. In Copel JA, Reed KL (eds): Doppler Ultrasound in Obstetrics and Gynecology. New York, Raven Press; 1995; pp 271-290.
6. Mielke G, Benda N: Cardiac output and central distribution of blood flow in the human fetus. Circulation 2001;103:1662-1668.
7. Severi FM, Rizzo G, Bocchi C, et al: Intrauterine growth retardation and fetal cardiac function. Fetal Diagn Ther 2000;15:8-19.
8. Glickstein J, Buyon J, Kim M, Friedman D: The fetal Doppler mechanical PR interval: a validation study. Fetal Diagn Ther 2004;19:31-34.
9. Van Bergen AH, Cuneo BF, Davis N: Prospective echocardiographic evaluation of atrioventricular conduction in fetuses with maternal Sjogren's antibodies. Am J Obstet Gynecol 2004;191:1014-1018.

CHAPTER 37

Greggory R. DeVore

Maternal Uterine Artery During Pregnancy

Introduction

The right and left uterine arteries originate from their respective internal iliac arteries, course upwards over the external iliac artery, and enter the uterus bilaterally (Fig. 37-1). The vascular bed that the uterine arteries provide blood flow to consists of the following (Fig. 37-2):

Arcuate artery. This is a vascular plexus that circumscribes the uterus and is located just below the serosa in the myometrium.

Radial arteries. Approximately 100 radial arteries originate from the arcuate plexus and enter the myometrium perpendicular to

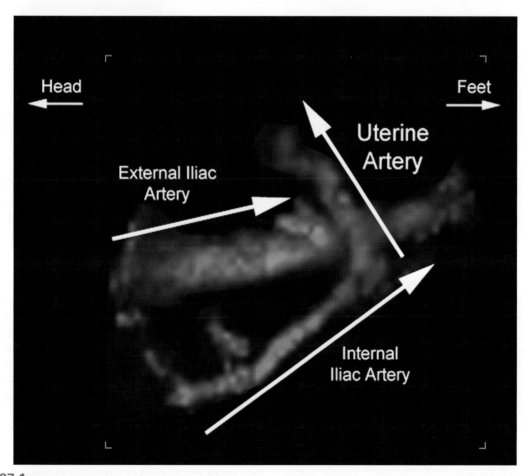

Figure 37-1
This is a B-flow image of the internal and external iliac arteries, demonstrating the uterine artery coursing over the external iliac artery.

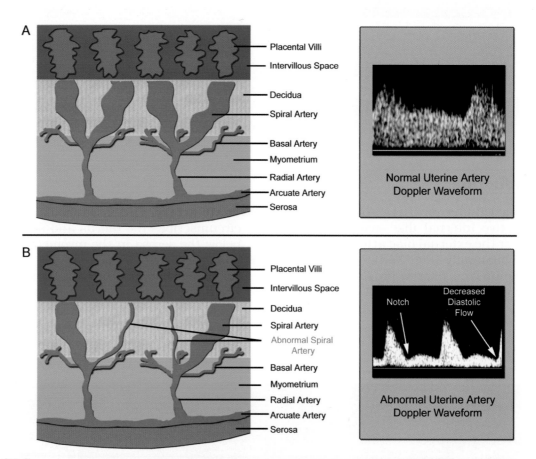

Figure 37-2
Schematic of normal and abnormal development of the spiral arteries. **A,** Normal development of the spiral arteries. **B,** Abnormal development of the spiral arteries resulting in an abnormal uterine artery Doppler waveform.

the uterine surface. They give branches to the basal artery and spiral arteries.

Basal arteries. These vessels remain in the myometrium.

Spiral arteries. The spiral arteries enter the deciduas and then branch to the intervillus space.

Cotyledons. These are supplied by the spiral arteries.

Pathological Studies

The key development of uterine blood flow during pregnancy requires changes within the spiral arteries in which they are transformed from maternal to uteroplacental vessels. This occurs in two stages during pregnancy. In the first trimester trophoblastic changes occur when these cells enter the decidual layer of spiral arteries. This results in an initial decrease in uterine artery pressure and is manifest in the uterine artery waveform. In the second trimester this process continues with trophoblastic cells entering the myometrial portion of the spiral arteries, resulting in dilation of these vessels. The diameters of the spiral arteries undergo a four- to six-fold increase in size. This results in a 10-fold increase in uterine artery blood flow (see Fig. 37-2).[1] When there is failure of the spiral arteries to undergo trophoblastic invasion, an increase in resistance to blood flow occurs, resulting in a decrease in blood flow to the placenta (see Fig. 37-2). This has been associated with adverse pregnancy outcome.[2]

Doppler Studies

In 1983 Campbell et al[3] were the first to report the association between an abnormal second and third trimester uterine artery waveform and adverse pregnancy outcome. Since the first report by Campbell et al,[3] a number of studies have identified an abnormal uterine artery Doppler waveform with adverse pregnancy outcome.[4-8]

Qualitative Evaluation of the Doppler Waveform

In the early first trimester, notching of the uterine artery may occur (Fig. 37-3). However, as the first trimester progresses the notch often disappears.[9] As the pregnancy continues, the uterine artery Doppler waveform demonstrates an increase in diastolic flow, without evidence of postsystolic notching (Fig. 37-4). If, however, notching of the uterine arteries persists, this has been associated with adverse pregnancy outcome, especially if it persists after 24 to 26 weeks of gestation (Fig. 37-5). Table 37-1

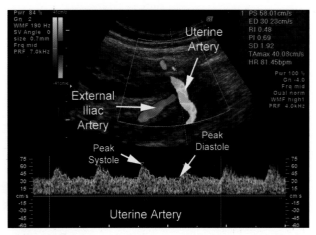

Figure 37-4
Normal uterine artery at 22 weeks of gestation.

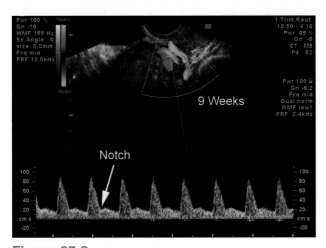

Figure 37-3
Uterine artery Doppler waveform from a 9-week pregnancy. A notch is present.

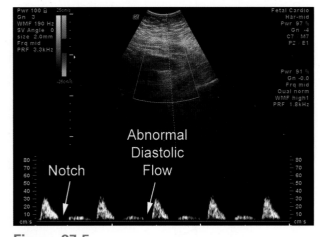

Figure 37-5
Notching of the uterine artery in a fetus with intrauterine growth restriction at 26 weeks of gestation.

Table 37-1	Incidence of unilateral and bilateral notching of the uterine artery			
Author	Gestation (wks)	Number of Patients	Unilateral Notching	Bilateral Notching
Kurmanavichius (1990)[10]	18-21	129	10.9%	3.1%
Mires (1995)[11]	18	1412	1.9%	4.2%
Harrington (1996)[4]	19-24	1326	4.7%	3.6%
Harrington (1997)[9]	12-16	652	22.8%	32.7%
Mires (1998)[12]	18-20	6579	2.9%	1.6%

lists the frequency of notching of the uterine artery.[10-12]

Quantitative Evaluation of the Doppler Waveform

Another option for evaluation of the uterine artery Doppler waveform is to measure the resistance index or the pulsatility index. Reference curves have been published for ranges that include the 90th and 95th percentiles.[13,14] Other investigators have suggested a resistance index greater than 0.58 to 0.70 as pathological (Table 37-2).[5,14-16] Recently, Merz published a reference curve for the resistance index (Table 37-3, Fig. 37-6) and the pulsatility index (Table 37-4, Fig. 37-7).[17]

Table 37-2	Incidence of an abnormal resistance index of the uterine arteries			
Author	**Gestation (wks)**	**Number of Patients**	**Resistance Index**	**Percent With Abnormal Resistance Index**
Steel (1990)[15]	24	1014	RI > 0.58	12%
Valensise (1993)[16]	22	272	RI > 0.58	9.5%
North (1994)[14]	19-24	458	RI > 90th percentile	17%
Konchak (1995)[5]	17-22	103	RI > 0.70	10.6%

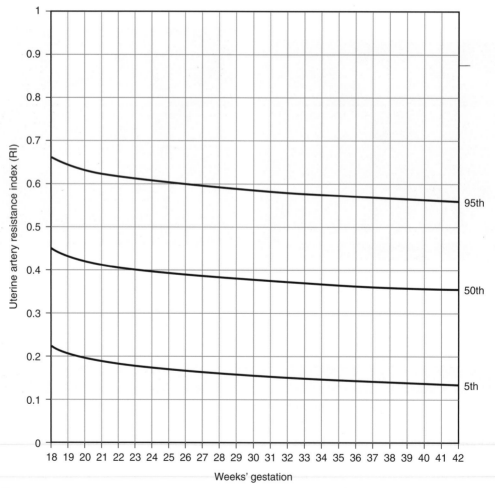

Figure 37-6

The resistance index for the uterine artery ([systolic maximal velocity-diastolic maximal velocity]/systolic maximal velocity).[17]

Table 37-3   Resistance index of the uterine artery[17]

Gestation (wks)	5th Percentile	50th Percentile	95th Percentile
18	0.222	0.447	0.659
19	0.204	0.429	0.641
20	0.194	0.419	0.630
21	0.186	0.411	0.622
22	0.180	0.405	0.615
23	0.175	0.400	0.610
24	0.171	0.395	0.605
25	0.167	0.391	0.601
26	0.163	0.387	0.597
27	0.160	0.384	0.593
28	0.157	0.380	0.590
29	0.154	0.378	0.587
30	0.152	0.375	0.584
31	0.150	0.372	0.581
32	0.147	0.370	0.578
33	0.145	0.368	0.576
34	0.144	0.366	0.574
35	0.142	0.364	0.571
36	0.140	0.362	0.569
37	0.139	0.360	0.567
38	0.137	0.358	0.566
39	0.136	0.357	0.564
40	0.135	0.355	0.562

Table 37-4   Pulsatility index of the uterine artery[17]

Gestation (wks)	5th Percentile	50th Percentile	95th Percentile
18	0.509	0.888	1.407
19	0.460	0.838	1.356
20	0.436	0.812	1.328
21	0.420	0.795	1.309
22	0.407	0.781	1.293
23	0.397	0.769	1.280
24	0.388	0.759	1.268
25	0.381	0.751	1.258
26	0.374	0.743	1.248
27	0.369	0.736	1.239
28	0.363	0.729	1.230
29	0.358	0.722	1.222
30	0.354	0.716	1.214
31	0.349	0.711	1.207
32	0.345	0.705	1.199
33	0.341	0.700	1.192
34	0.337	0.695	1.185
35	0.333	0.690	1.178
36	0.330	0.684	1.171
37	0.326	0.679	1.164
38	0.322	0.674	1.157
39	0.318	0.669	1.150
40	0.313	0.663	1.143

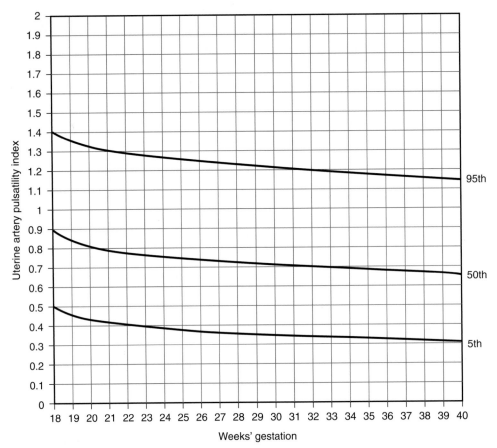

Figure 37-7
Pulsatility index for the uterine artery (systolic maximal velocity-diastolic maximal velocity/time average maximal velocity).[17]

References

1. Freese UE: The uteroplacental vascular relationship in the human. Am J Obstet Gynecol 1968;101:8-16.
2. Robertson WB, Brosens I, Dixon G: Maternal uterine vascular lesions in the hypertensive complications of pregnancy. Perspect Nephrol Hypertens 1976;5:115-127.
3. Campbell S, az-Recasens J, Griffin DR, Cohen-Overbeek TE, et al: New Doppler technique for assessing uteroplacental blood flow. Lancet 1983;1:675-677.
4. Harrington K, Cooper D, Lees C, et al: Doppler ultrasound of the uterine arteries: the importance of bilateral notching in the prediction of pre-eclampsia, placental abruption or delivery of a small-for-gestational-age baby. Ultrasound Obstet Gynecol 1996;7:182-188.
5. Konchak PS, Bernstein IM, Capeless EL: Uterine artery Doppler velocimetry in the detection of adverse obstetric outcomes in women with unexplained elevated maternal serum alpha-fetoprotein levels. Am J Obstet Gynecol 1995;173:1115-1119.
6. Madazli R, Somunkiran A, Calay Z, et al: Histomorphology of the placenta and the placental bed of growth restricted foetuses and correlation with the Doppler velocimetries of the uterine and umbilical arteries. Placenta 2003;24:510-516.
7. Martin AM, Bindra R, Curcio P, et al: Screening for pre-eclampsia and fetal growth restriction by uterine artery Doppler at 11-14 weeks of gestation. Ultrasound Obstet Gynecol 2001;18:583-586.
8. Olofsson P, Laurini RN, Marsal K: A high uterine artery pulsatility index reflects a defective development of placental bed spiral arteries in pregnancies complicated by hypertension and fetal growth retardation. Eur J Obstet Gynecol Reprod Biol 1993;49:161-168.

9. Harrington K, Goldfrad C, Carpenter RG, Campbell S: Transvaginal uterine and umbilical artery Doppler examination of 12-16 weeks and the subsequent development of pre-eclampsia and intrauterine growth retardation. Ultrasound Obstet Gynecol 1997;9:94-100.

10. Kurmanavichius J, Baumann H, Huch R, Huch A: Uteroplacental blood flow velocity waveforms as a predictor of adverse fetal outcome and pregnancy-induced hypertension. J Perinat Med 1990;18:255-260.

11. Mires GJ, Christie AD, Leslie J, et al: Are "notched" uterine arterial waveforms of prognostic value for hypertensive and growth disorders of pregnancy? Fetal Diagn Ther 1995;10:111-118.

12. Mires GJ, Williams FL, Leslie J, Howie PW: Assessment of uterine arterial notching as a screening test for adverse pregnancy outcome. Am J Obstet Gynecol 1998;179:1317-1323.

13. Bower S, Bewley S, Campbell S: Improved prediction of preeclampsia by two-stage screening of uterine arteries using the early diastolic notch and color Doppler imaging. Obstet Gynecol 1993;82:78-83.

14. North RA, Ferrier C, Long D, et al: Uterine artery Doppler flow velocity waveforms in the second trimester for the prediction of preeclampsia and fetal growth retardation. Obstet Gynecol 1994;83:378-386.

15. Steel SA, Pearce JM, McParland P, Chamberlain GV: Early Doppler ultrasound screening in prediction of hypertensive disorders of pregnancy. Lancet 1990;335:1548-1551.

16. Valensise H, Bezzeccheri V, Rizzo G, et al: Doppler velocimetry of the uterine artery as a screening test for gestational hypertension. Ultrasound Obstet Gynecol 1993;3:18-22.

17. Uteroplacental circulation, vol. 1. In Merz E (ed). Ultrasonography in Obstetrics and Gynecology. Stuttgart, New York, Thieme, 2005. pp 469-480, 613.

CHAPTER 38

Fetal Umbilical Artery

Greggory R. DeVore

Introduction

Each of two umbilical arteries originate from their respective internal iliac arteries, course around the bladder, and exit the fetus, forming two of the three components of the umbilical cord. The umbilical cord floats freely in the amniotic cavity before entering the placenta. Most examiners have elected to obtain the pulsed Doppler waveform from the umbilical artery floating within the amniotic cavity.

Identification and Recording of the Umbilical Artery

Originally the umbilical artery waveform was recorded with continuous wave Doppler. However, with the introduction of duplex pulsed-wave imaging the vessel could be identified with B-mode ultrasound and the Doppler waveform recorded.[1] The umbilical artery can be identified in one of several orientations: cross-

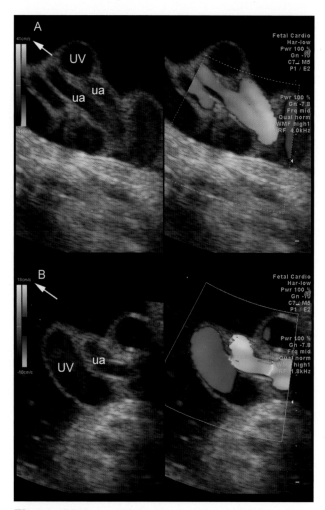

Figure 38-1
B-mode and color Doppler imaging of the umbilical cord. **A,** Identification of the umbilical artery (ua) tangential to the ultrasound beam with B-mode and color Doppler. As the result of the velocity setting of 41 cm/sec, only the umbilical artery is identified with color Doppler. **B,** The umbilical artery tangential and perpendicular to the ultrasound beam. As the result of the velocity setting of 18 cm/sec, both the umbilical vein (UV) and umbilical artery are identified with color Doppler.

sectional, longitudinal, oblique using B-mode, or in combination with color or power Doppler ultrasound (Fig. 38-1). The benefit of using a combination of modalities is that the examiner can easily identify the umbilical arteries and place the Doppler sample volume parallel to blood flow and record the waveform (Fig. 38-2). Depending on the size of the sample volume, either the arterial waveform is recorded in isolation or the umbilical venous waveform is recorded in conjunction with the arterial waveform (Fig. 38-3).

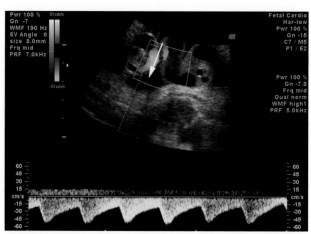

Figure 38-2
Imaging of the umbilical artery by placing the sample volume parallel to blood flow (*white arrow*).

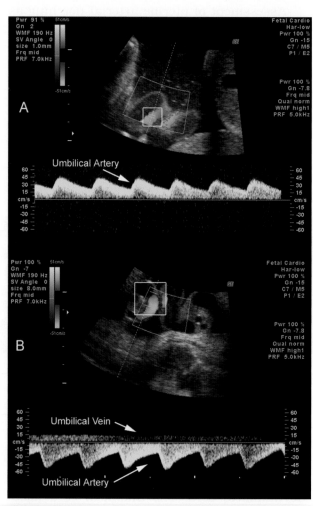

Figure 38-3
A, The sample volume is small, therefore only the umbilical artery waveform is recorded. **B,** The sample volume is increased in size, resulting in the recording of the Doppler waveform of the umbilical artery and vein.

Normal Umbilical Artery Waveform

During pregnancy the resistance to flow from the fetus to the placenta decreases, resulting in increased diastolic flow. Therefore the Doppler waveform in the first trimester of pregnancy may demonstrate absent flow (first trimester) or minimal flow during diastole. However, the presence of reverse diastolic flow may be associated with an increased risk for adverse outcome.[2] After the 14th week of gestation, diastolic flow should be present in all fetuses (see Fig. 38-3).[3]

Qualitative Evaluation of the Umbilical Artery

Investigators have used a qualitative approach in which velocity indices are not measured, but the waveform is inspected visually. An abnormal waveform demonstrates either absent or reverse flow during ventricular diastole (Fig. 38-4). As the waveform becomes progressively worse, perinatal and neonatal complications become more frequent.

Quantitative Evaluation of the Umbilical Artery

Investigators have quantified umbilical artery resistance by measuring the S/D ratio, resistance index, or pulsatility index (Fig. 38-5). In 1996 Coopens et al[3] measured the pulsatility index in fetuses between 8 and 14 weeks' gestation (Fig. 38-6, Table 38-1) and found that it significantly decreased with gestational age. DeVore et al[4] reported that the S/D ratio and resistance index did not change as a function of whether the fetus was examined at sea level or at an altitude between 4200 and 4500 feet above sea level. Clinically, most physicians measure the resistance index (Fig. 38-7, Table 38-2) or the pulsatility index (Fig. 38-8, Table 38-3).[5] Studies have shown that first trimester abnormal umbilical waveforms, coupled with abnormal uterine artery waveforms, may predict adverse outcome.

Clinical Implications of an Abnormal Umbilical Artery Doppler Waveform

The umbilical artery Doppler waveform has undergone more scrutiny than any other form of noninvasive test for fetal well-being. Meta-analysis has demonstrated that evaluation of the umbilical artery Doppler waveform, when

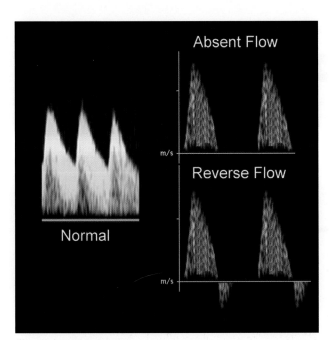

Figure 38-4
Normal and abnormal umbilical artery Doppler waveforms, illustrating absent and reverse diastolic flow.

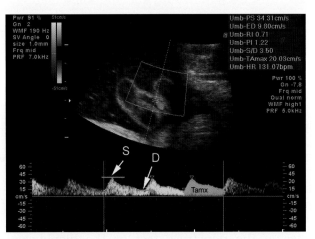

Figure 38-5
Quantification of the umbilical artery Doppler waveform. S, Peak systolic velocity; D, peak diastolic velocity; Tamx, total mean velocity. S/D ratio = peak systolic velocity/peak diastolic velocity; resistance index = (S-D)/S; pulsatility index = (S-D)/Tamx.

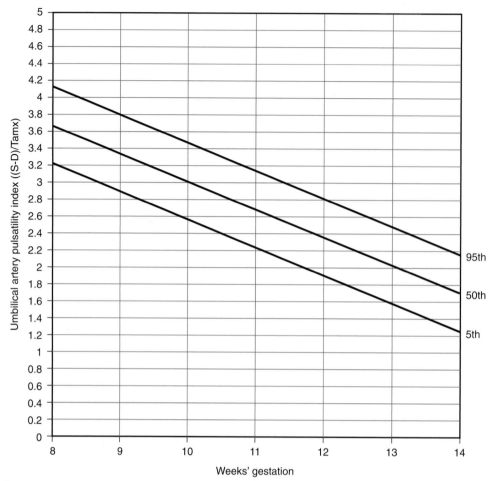

Figure 38-6
Pulsatility index between 8 and 14 weeks' gestation.

Table 38-1	Pulsatility index of the umbilical artery between 8 and 14 weeks of gestation[3]		
Weeks Gestation	**5th Percentile**	**50th Percentile**	**95th Percentile**
8	3.21	3.66	4.11
9	2.89	3.34	3.78
10	2.56	3.01	3.46
11	2.24	2.69	3.13
12	1.91	2.36	2.81
13	1.59	2.04	2.48
14	1.26	1.71	2.16

compared with the nonstress test, results in better outcome and often precedes abnormalities of the nonstress test or the biophysical profile.[6,7] However, once an abnormal umbilical artery waveform is identified, other Doppler parameters should be examined (e.g., middle cerebral artery, inferior vena cava, ductus venosus). A survey of Maternal-Fetal Medicine specialists in 1994 by DeVore[8] indicated that as the umbilical artery Doppler waveform became more severe, specialists increased the frequency of antepartum testing, increased the total number of hours of maternal bed rest, and increased the frequency of ultrasound surveillance. Recent studies have identified the relationship between abnormal umbilical artery

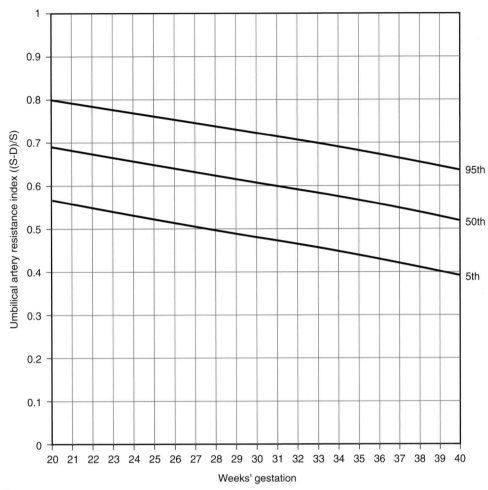

Figure 38-7
Resistance index of the umbilical artery.

Table 38-2	Resistance index of the umbilical artery between 20 and 40 weeks' gestation[5]		
Gestation (wks)	**5th Percentile**	**50th Percentile**	**95th Percentile**
20	0.567	0.690	0.802
21	0.557	0.680	0.793
22	0.548	0.671	0.784
23	0.539	0.663	0.776
24	0.530	0.655	0.768
25	0.522	0.646	0.760
26	0.514	0.639	0.752
27	0.506	0.631	0.745
28	0.498	0.623	0.737
29	0.490	0.615	0.730
30	0.482	0.608	0.723
31	0.474	0.600	0.715
32	0.465	0.592	0.707
33	0.457	0.584	0.700
34	0.449	0.576	0.692
35	0.440	0.567	0.684
36	0.431	0.559	0.675
37	0.422	0.550	0.667
38	0.412	0.540	0.657
39	0.402	0.530	0.648
40	0.390	0.519	0.637

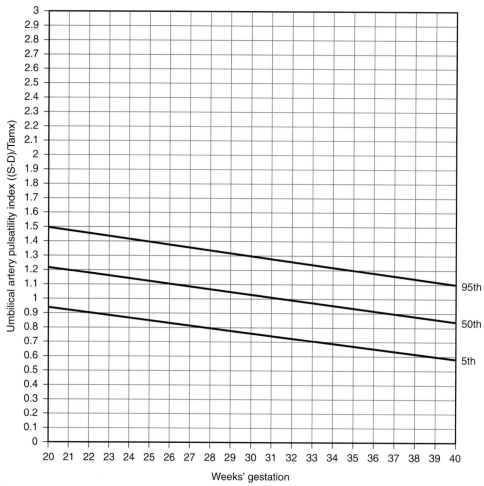

Figure 38-8
Pulsatility index of the umbilical artery.

Table 38-3	Pulsatility index of the umbilical artery between 20 and 40 weeks of gestation[5]		
Gestation (wks)	**5th Percentile**	**50th Percentile**	**95th Percentile**
20	0.940	1.216	1.505
21	0.913	1.189	1.476
22	0.890	1.165	1.450
23	0.869	1.142	1.427
24	0.849	1.122	1.405
25	0.831	1.102	1.385
26	0.813	1.084	1.365
27	0.798	1.065	1.346
28	0.780	1.048	1.327
29	0.764	1.031	1.308
30	0.748	1.014	1.290
31	0.732	0.997	1.272
32	0.716	0.980	1.254
33	0.700	0.963	1.236
34	0.684	0.946	1.218
35	0.668	0.928	1.199
36	0.651	0.910	1.180
37	0.634	0.891	1.160
38	0.615	0.872	1.139
39	0.595	0.851	1.117
40	0.573	0.828	1.093

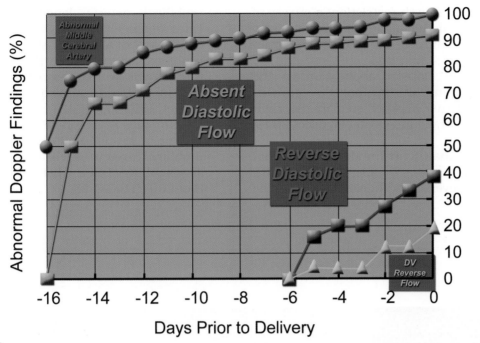

Figure 38-9
This illustrates the percent of fetuses with umbilical artery absent diastolic flow (*green*) and reverse diastolic flow (*blue*) prior to development of fetal distress at day 0. Prior to the appearance of absent diastolic flow (*green*), blood flow to the middle cerebral artery is often abnormal (*red*). After the appearance of reverse diastolic flow in the umbilical artery (*blue*), reverse flow occurs in the ductus venosus (turquoise) just prior to the development of fetal distress (day 0). (From Ferrazzi E, Bozzo M, Rigano S, et al: Temporal sequence of abnormal Doppler changes in the peripheral and central circulatory systems of the severely growth-restricted fetus. Ultrasound Obstet Gynecol 2002;19:140-146.)

Doppler waveforms and adverse fetal outcome.[9-12] Fig. 38-9 is a graphic representation of the temporal sequence of Doppler abnormalities that occur prior to an abnormal nonstress test and fetal compromise.

References

1. Brar HS, Medearis AL, DeVore GR, Platt LD: Fetal umbilical velocimetry using continuous-wave and pulsed-wave Doppler ultrasound in high-risk pregnancies: a comparison of systolic to diastolic ratios. Obstet Gynecol 1988;72:607-610.
2. Borrell A, Martinez JM, Farre MT, et al: Reversed end-diastolic flow in first-trimester umbilical artery: an ominous new sign for fetal outcome. Am J Obstet Gynecol 2001;185:204-207.
3. Coppens M, Loquet P, Kollen M, et al: Longitudinal evaluation of uteroplacental and umbilical blood flow changes in normal early pregnancy. Ultrasound Obstet Gynecol 1996;7:114-121.
4. DeVore GR, Medearis AL, Platt LD: The effect of altitude on the umbilical artery Doppler resistance. J Ultrasound Med 1992; 11:317-320.
5. Uteroplacental circulation, vol. 1 In Merz E (ed). Ultrasonography in Obstetrics and Gynecology. Stuttgart, New York, Thieme, 2005, pp 469-480, 614.
6. Harrington K, Goldfrad C, Carpenter RG, Campbell S: Transvaginal uterine and umbilical artery Doppler examination of 12-16 weeks and the subsequent development of pre-eclampsia and intrauterine growth retardation. Ultrasound Obstet Gynecol 1997;9:94-100.
7. Alfirevic Z, Neilson JP: Doppler ultrasonography in high-risk pregnancies: systematic review with meta-analysis. Am J Obstet Gynecol 1995;172:1379-1387.
8. DeVore GR: The effect of an abnormal umbilical artery Doppler on the manage-

ment of fetal growth restriction: a survey of maternal-fetal medicine specialists who perform fetal ultrasound. Ultrasound Obstet Gynecol 1994;4:294-303.

9. Baschat AA: Doppler application in the delivery timing of the preterm growth-restricted fetus: another step in the right direction. Ultrasound Obstet Gynecol 2004; 23:111-118.

10. Muller T, Nanan R, Rehn M, et al: Arterial and ductus venosus Doppler in fetuses with absent or reverse end-diastolic flow in the umbilical artery: longitudinal analysis. Fetal Diagn Ther 2003;18:163-169.

11. Seyam YS, Al Mahmeid MS, Al Tamimi HK: Umbilical artery Doppler flow velocimetry in intrauterine growth restriction and its relation to perinatal outcome. Int J Gynaecol Obstet 2002;77:131-137.

12. Valcamonico A, Accorsi P, Battaglia S, et al: Absent or reverse end-diastolic flow in the umbilical artery: intellectual development at school age. Eur J Obstet Gynecol Reprod Biol 2004;114:23-28.

CHAPTER 39

Greggory R. DeVore

Fetal Middle Cerebral Artery

Introduction

Pulsed Doppler evaluation of the middle cerebral artery was first reported in 1987 to demonstrate a decrease in the systolic/diastolic ratio in compromised fetuses.[1] In 1989 Arstrom et al[2] were the first to report the use of the ratio between the middle cerebral artery and umbilical artery. During the 1990s Doppler evaluation of the fetal middle cerebral artery was extensively investigated. Some work showed the utility of using peak systolic velocity in investigating fetal anemia. There was considerable work on association of abnormal Doppler indices of the middle cerebral artery and intrauterine growth restriction, preeclampsia, and fetal hypoxia.

Subsequent work occurring after 2000 has not only focused on detection of the growth-retarded fetus but has also established normal values of peak velocity of the middle cerebral artery in evaluation of the fetus at risk for alloisoimmunized anemia.[3] The most important studies will be reviewed in this chapter.

Imaging the Middle Cerebral Artery

The middle cerebral artery courses anteriolaterally from the circle of Willis in a circular direction (Figs. 39-1 and 39-2). Because of its location, it is easily imaged when the fetal head is in the position from which biometry (biparietal diameter, head circumference) is obtained.

Identification and Recording of the Middle Cerebral Artery

Although the examiner can identify the middle cerebral artery using B-mode ultrasound, it is easier if color Doppler is used to identify this vessel (see Fig. 39-2). To optimally image the middle cerebral artery with color Doppler, the examiner does the following:

1. Image the fetal head in the transverse plane, at the level at which biometry is measured (see Figs. 39-1 and 39-2).

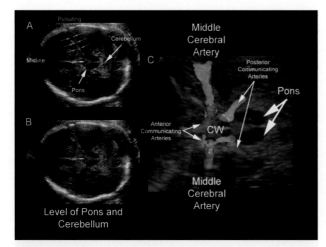

Figure 39-1
Identification of the middle cerebral artery (MCA). The fetal head is imaged in the transverse plane, at the level of the pons (A). The pulsating MCA can be observed in the B-mode image as it lies in a groove of the sphenoid bone (*green arrows*) (A). **B,** The area that is displayed in (C). The middle cerebral artery runs in a plane anterolateral to the midline, originating from the circle of Willis (CW) (C).

2. After identifying the midline, direct the ultrasound beam toward the fetal neck.
3. Identify the pons (see Figs. 39-1 and 39-2). The circle of Willis is anterior to this structure.
4. Adjust the color Doppler velocity setting to a lower setting than what may be used to image the umbilical artery.
5. Rock the transducer in a cephalad-caudal direction to visualize the middle cerebral artery (see Figs. 39-1 and 39-2).
6. Place the Doppler sample volume in the proximal mid-portion of the middle cerebral artery to record the pulsed Doppler waveform (Fig. 39-3). If the sample volume is placed in the distal portion of this vessel, there may be differences in the peak velocity, as well as quantitative indices (vida infra) (see Figs. 39-2 and 39-3).

Normal Middle Cerebral Artery Waveform

Throughout most of pregnancy there is a high resistance to blood flow in the cerebral vascular system. This is manifest by low or absent diastolic flow early in gestation. After 32 weeks of gestation the resistance decreases, resulting in an increase in diastolic flow. The change in the

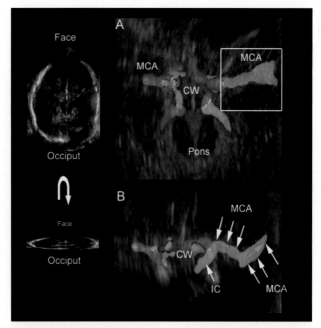

Figure 39-2
A, The middle cerebral artery (MCA) originating from the circle of Willis. The image has been rotated so that the pons is posterior, even though the image acquisition occurred when the midline was perpendicular to the ultrasound beam. **B,** The MCA after the image has been rotated 90 degrees so that the MCA is visualized from the level of the occiput, looking toward the face. This illustrates the lateral course of the MCA. Notice that this vessel angles upwards, changing its course (*blue arrow*). For this reason it is important to place the sample volume in the mid or proximal third of this vessel for accurate recording of the pulsed Doppler waveform. *CW*, Circle of Willis; *IC*, internal carotid artery.

middle cerebral blood flow is almost a mirror image of what occurs in the umbilical artery in which there is low resistance to blood flow associated with an increase in diastolic flow (Fig. 39-4).

Qualitative Evaluation of the Middle Cerebral Artery

Qualitative evaluation of the middle cerebral artery can be performed if the examiner identifies minimal or absent diastolic flow (see Fig. 39-4). The reason for this is that only when diastolic flow is increased is it indicative of increased blood flow to the brain. However, there have been several reports of reverse flow during diastole being associated with adverse outcome.[4,5]

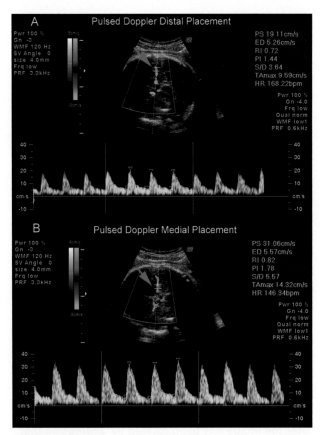

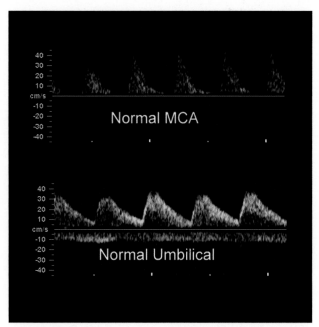

Figure 39-3
Pulsed Doppler waveforms obtained from the distal and medial portions of the middle cerebral artery (MCA). **A,** The pulsed Doppler sample volume is placed in the distal portion of the MCA. **B,** The pulsed Doppler sample volume is placed in the medial portion of the MCA. When comparing the peak velocity, resistance index (RI), pulsatilitiy index (PI), S/D ratio, and Tamx, notice that there are differences between the two sample sites.

Figure 39-4
Comparison of diastolic flow of the umbilical artery and middle cerebral arteries. Because of low resistance, the diastolic flow in the umbilical artery is increased. As the result of increased resistance, the diastolic flow in the middle cerebral artery (MCA) is decreased. When pathology occurs, the waveforms change in opposite directions. The umbilical artery demonstrates decreased diastolic flow, and the middle cerebral artery demonstrates increased diastolic flow.

Quantitative Evaluation of the Middle Cerebral Artery

INTRAUTERINE GROWTH RESTRICTION

Several indices have been measured from the middle cerebral artery waveform in the evaluation of the fetus for intrauterine growth restriction because it may reflect left ventricular afterload.[6-9] The most widely used clinically, however, are the resistance index and the pulsatility index. A number of studies have provided Doppler reference curves for the middle cerebral artery.[9-11] However, not all studies provide a reference range covering the second and third trimesters of pregnancy.[2,9-11] Mari and

Deter[9] compared a cross-sectional with a longitudinal study and found no significant differences between the two groups. Hsieh et al[12] reported a difference between the proximal third and the middle and distal third of the middle cerebral artery when the pulsatility index was measured.[12] However, there were no differences between the sites of sampling when the resistance index was measured.[12]

Resistance Index. Measurement of the resistance index has been reported in two large studies.[11,13] The study by Kurmanavicius et al[13] evaluated umbilical and middle cerebral arteries and computed the ratio between the two vessels (umbilical artery resistance index/middle cerebral artery resistance index) (Fig. 39-5, Table 39-1). Bahlmann et al[11] only computed the resistance index but found their 5th percentile to be much lower than that of Kurmanavicius et al.[13] (Figs. 39-6 and 39-7; Table 39-2).

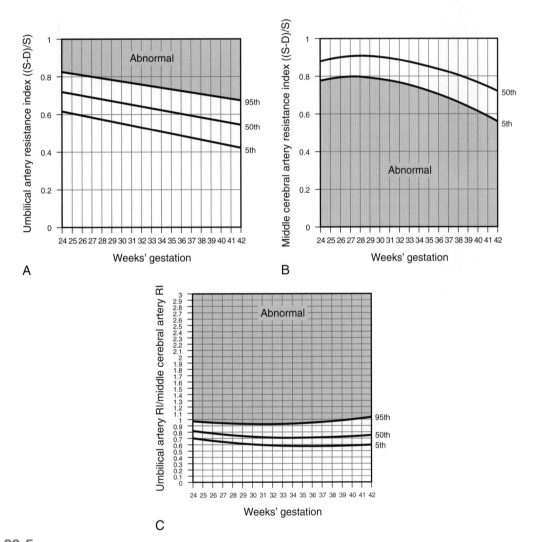

Figure 39-5
Resistance index for the **A,** umbilical artery (UA), **B,** middle cerebral artery (MCA), and **C,** UA/MCA ratio as reported by Kurmanavicius et al.[13]

| Table 39-1 | Reference values for the resistance index of umbilical and middle cerebral arteries, as well as the UA/MCA ratio from Kurmanavicius et al[13] |

Gestation (wks)	Umbilical Artery Resistance Index (UA RI)			Middle Cerebral Artery Resistance Index (MCA RI)			UA RI/MCA RI		
	5th Percentile	50th Percentile	95th Percentile	5th Percentile	50th Percentile	95th Percentile	5th Percentile	50th Percentile	95th Percentile
24	0.615	0.717	0.828	0.778	0.867	—	0.696	0.809	0.968
25	0.605	0.707	0.819	0.789	0.881	—	0.676	0.791	0.955
26	0.594	0.697	0.810	0.795	0.892	—	0.658	0.775	0.945
27	0.583	0.687	0.802	0.798	0.898	—	0.642	0.761	0.937
28	0.572	0.678	0.793	0.797	0.901	—	0.628	0.750	0.932
29	0.562	0.668	0.785	0.793	0.900	—	0.616	0.740	0.929
30	0.551	0.658	0.776	0.786	0.897	—	0.606	0.732	0.928
31	0.540	0.648	0.767	0.776	0.891	—	0.597	0.726	0.929
32	0.530	0.638	0.759	0.764	0.883	—	0.590	0.722	0.931
33	0.519	0.629	0.750	0.750	0.872	—	0.585	0.719	0.936
34	0.508	0.619	0.742	0.734	0.860	—	0.581	0.717	0.941
35	0.498	0.609	0.733	0.717	0.846	—	0.578	0.717	0.949
36	0.487	0.599	0.724	0.698	0.831	—	0.576	0.718	0.957
37	0.476	0.589	0.716	0.677	0.814	—	0.575	0.720	0.967
38	0.465	0.580	0.707	0.655	0.795	—	0.576	0.724	0.978
39	0.455	0.570	0.699	0.632	0.776	—	0.577	0.728	0.991
40	0.444	0.560	0.690	0.607	0.755	—	0.580	0.734	1.004
41	0.433	0.550	0.681	0.582	0.734	—	0.583	0.740	1.018
42	0.423	0.540	0.673	0.556	0.711	—	0.588	0.747	1.034

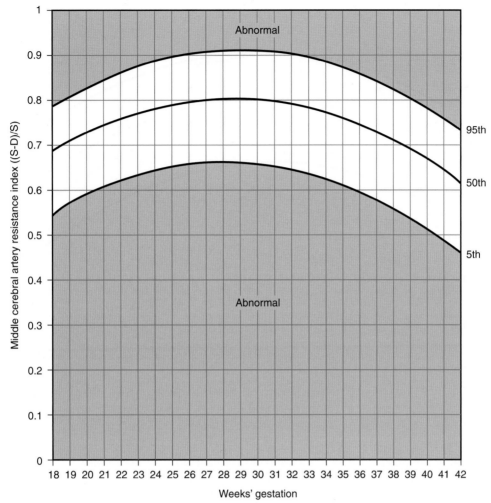

Figure 39-6
Reference values for the resistance index of the middle cerebral artery from Bahlman et al.[11] If there is brain sparing, then the RI will be below the 5th percentile. If the RI is above the 95th percentile, this could represent abnormal flow from vasoconstriction.

Table 39-2	Reference values for the resistance index of the middle cerebral artery from Bahlman et al[11]						
Gestation (wks)	5th Percentile	50th Percentile	95th Percentile	Weeks Gestation	5th Percentile	50th Percentile	95th Percentile
18	0.544	0.687	0.787	31	0.652	0.798	0.907
19	0.574	0.708	0.808	32	0.645	0.792	0.902
20	0.592	0.727	0.828	33	0.636	0.783	0.894
21	0.608	0.744	0.846	34	0.625	0.773	0.885
22	0.622	0.758	0.861	35	0.612	0.761	0.873
23	0.633	0.771	0.874	36	0.597	0.747	0.86
24	0.643	0.782	0.886	37	0.579	0.73	0.844
25	0.651	0.79	0.895	38	0.56	0.712	0.826
26	0.656	0.796	0.902	39	0.539	0.692	0.807
27	0.659	0.801	0.907	40	0.515	0.669	0.785
28	0.661	0.803	0.91	41	0.489	0.644	0.761
29	0.66	0.803	0.911	42	0.462	0.618	0.735
30	0.657	0.801	0.91				

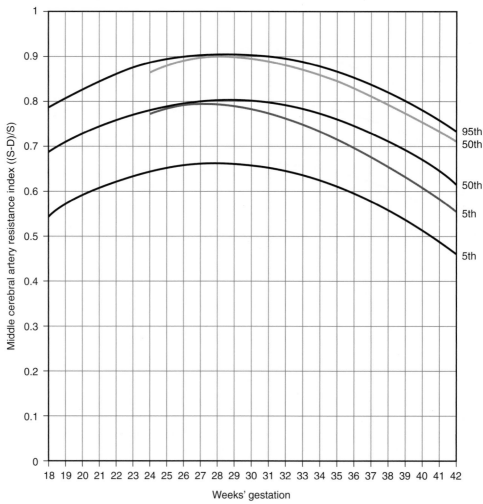

Figure 39-7
Reference values for the resistance index of the middle cerebral artery from Bahlman et al[11] (*black line*) and Kurmanavicius et al[13] (*blue lines*). The 5th percentile reference line is lower for Bahlman et al, and the 50th percentile for Kurmanavicius et al approaches the 95th reference line for Bahlman et al.

Pulsatility Index. A number of studies have evaluated the pulsatility index, but only a few have published reference ranges from 20 weeks until term.[9,11,14] Fig. 39-8 compares the pulsatility index among three studies, Mari and Deter,[9] Bascht and Gembruch,[14] and Bahlman et al[11] (Table 39-3). Although the mean and upper range of normal varies among the studies, the lower range of normal is very similar. Because the majority of fetuses with an abnormal middle cerebral blood will demonstrate pulsatility index values below the lower limits of normal (2.5th or fifth percentile), any of these three graphs can be used for analysis (Fig. 39-9). Baschat and Gembruch[14] published the only study that has evaluated the relationship between the umbilical artery pulsatility index and middle cerebral artery pulsatility index (Fig. 39-10; Table 39-4).

PREDICTION OF FETAL ANEMIA USING THE PEAK VELOCITY OF THE MIDDLE CEREBRAL ARTERY

In 2000 Mari et al[3] and Teixeira et al[15] reported the association between an increased peak velocity of the middle cerebral artery and association with fetal anemia in alloimmunized pregnancies. The data presented by Mari et al[3] allowed the examiner to easily determine the risk for anemia by plotting the maximal peak velocity against gestational age (Fig. 39-11, Table 39-5).

Table 39-3 Pulsatility index of the middle cerebral artery for three studies.[9,11,14] Although the mean and upper limits differ, the lower range of normal is very similar

	Mari and Deter (1992)[9]			Bahlmann et al (2002)[11]				Baschat and Gembruch (2003)[14]			
Gestation (wks)	2.5th Percentile	50th Percentile	97.5th Percentile	Weeks Gestation	5th Percentile	50th Percentile	95th Percentile	Weeks Gestation	2.5th Percentile	50th Percentile	97.5th Percentile
15	0.99	1.56	2.14								
16	1.08	1.70	2.33								
17	1.16	1.82	2.51								
18	1.23	1.94	2.67	18	1.01	1.51	2.02				
19	1.30	2.04	2.81	19	1.13	1.59	2.11				
20	1.35	2.13	2.93	20	1.19	1.67	2.18	20	1.22	1.65	2.09
21	1.40	2.20	3.04	21	1.26	1.73	2.25	21	1.27	1.75	2.24
22	1.44	2.27	3.13	22	1.31	1.78	2.30	22	1.30	1.83	2.38
23	1.48	2.32	3.20	23	1.35	1.83	2.35	23	1.34	1.91	2.50
24	1.51	2.36	3.25	24	1.39	1.87	2.40	24	1.36	1.97	2.61
25	1.52	2.39	3.30	25	1.41	1.90	2.43	25	1.38	2.02	2.69
26	1.54	2.40	3.32	26	1.43	1.92	2.45	26	1.40	2.06	2.76
27	1.54	2.41	3.33	27	1.44	1.93	2.47	27	1.41	2.09	2.81
28	1.54	2.40	3.32	28	1.45	1.94	2.48	28	1.41	2.10	2.85
29	1.52	2.38	3.30	29	1.44	1.94	2.48	29	1.41	2.11	2.87
30	1.50	2.35	3.26	30	1.43	1.92	2.47	30	1.40	2.10	2.87
31	1.48	2.30	3.20	31	1.40	1.90	2.45	31	1.39	2.08	2.85
32	1.44	2.24	3.12	32	1.37	1.88	2.43	32	1.37	2.05	2.82
33	1.40	2.17	3.03	33	1.33	1.84	2.39	33	1.35	2.01	2.77
34	1.35	2.09	2.92	34	1.29	1.80	2.35	34	1.32	1.95	2.70
35	1.29	2.00	2.79	35	1.23	1.74	2.30	35	1.28	1.89	2.61
36	1.22	1.89	2.65	36	1.17	1.68	2.24	36	1.24	1.81	2.51
37	1.15	1.77	2.49	37	1.09	1.61	2.17	37	1.19	1.72	2.39
38	1.07	1.64	2.32	38	1.01	1.53	2.10	38	1.14	1.62	2.26
39	0.98	1.50	2.13	39	0.92	1.45	2.02	39	1.08	1.51	2.10
40	0.89	1.34	1.92	40	0.83	1.35	1.92	40	1.02	1.39	1.93
41	0.78	1.17	1.70	41	0.72	1.25	1.82				
42	0.67	1.00	1.45	42	0.61	1.14	1.72				

Table 39-4 Umbilical artery, middle cerebral artery, and the MCA/UA ratio as reported by Baschat and Gembruch[14]

Gestation (wks)	Umbilical Artery PI			Middle Cerebral Artery PI			MCA/UA Ratio		
	5th Percentile	50th Percentile	95th Percentile	5th Percentile	50th Percentile	95th Percentile	5th Percentile	50th Percentile	95th Percentile
20	0.92	1.29	1.64	1.22	1.65	2.09	0.66	1.24	1.81
21	0.90	1.26	1.61	1.27	1.75	2.24	0.75	1.38	2.00
22	0.88	1.24	1.59	1.30	1.83	2.38	0.84	1.51	2.17
23	0.86	1.21	1.56	1.34	1.91	2.50	0.92	1.62	2.33
24	0.84	1.19	1.53	1.36	1.97	2.61	0.98	1.73	2.47
25	0.82	1.16	1.51	1.38	2.02	2.69	1.04	1.82	2.60
26	0.79	1.14	1.48	1.40	2.06	2.76	1.10	1.91	2.70
27	0.77	1.11	1.45	1.41	2.09	2.81	1.14	1.98	2.80
28	0.75	1.09	1.42	1.41	2.10	2.85	1.18	2.03	2.87
29	0.73	1.07	1.40	1.41	2.11	2.87	1.21	2.08	2.93
30	0.71	1.04	1.37	1.40	2.10	2.87	1.23	2.12	2.98
31	0.69	1.02	1.34	1.39	2.08	2.85	1.24	2.14	3.00
32	0.67	0.99	1.32	1.37	2.05	2.82	1.24	2.15	3.02
33	0.65	0.97	1.29	1.35	2.01	2.77	1.24	2.15	3.01
34	0.63	0.94	1.26	1.32	1.95	2.70	1.23	2.14	2.99
35	0.61	0.92	1.24	1.28	1.89	2.61	1.21	2.11	2.96
36	0.58	0.89	1.21	1.24	1.81	2.51	1.18	2.08	2.91
37	0.56	0.87	1.18	1.19	1.72	2.39	1.15	2.03	2.84
38	0.54	0.84	1.15	1.14	1.62	2.26	1.10	1.97	2.75
39	0.52	0.82	1.13	1.08	1.51	2.10	1.05	1.90	2.65
40	0.50	0.80	1.10	1.02	1.39	1.93	0.99	1.82	2.54

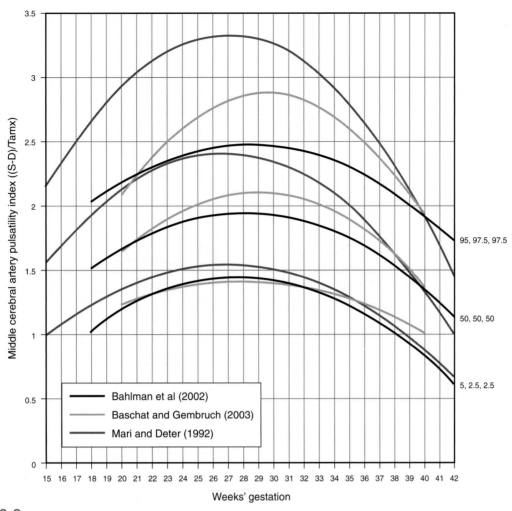

Figure 39-8
Comparison of pulsatility index among three studies. Although the mean and upper limits differ, the lower range of normal is very similar.[9,11,14]

Table 39-5	Threshold of peak velocity of systolic blood flow in the middle cerebral artery above which mild, moderate, and severe anemia occurs[3]		
	Threshold of the Peak Velocity of the Middle Cerebral Artery (cm/sec) Above Which Degree of Anemia Is Classified		
Gestation (wks)	**Mild Anemia**	**Moderate Anemia**	**Severe Anemia**
18	29.9	34.8	36.0
20	32.8	38.2	39.5
22	36.0	41.9	43.3
24	39.5	46.0	47.5
26	43.3	50.4	52.1
28	47.6	55.4	57.2
30	52.2	60.7	62.8
32	57.3	66.6	68.9
34	62.9	73.1	75.6
36	69.0	80.2	82.9
38	75.7	88.0	91.0
40	83.0	96.6	99.8

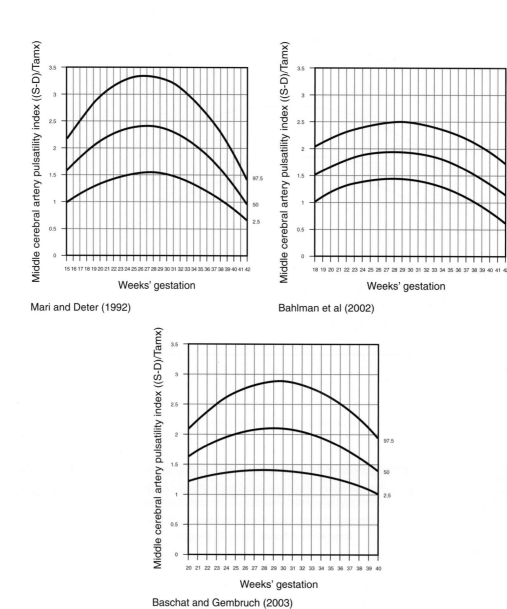

Mari and Deter (1992)

Bahlman et al (2002)

Baschat and Gembruch (2003)

Figure 39-9
Pulsatility index of the middle cerebral artery.[9,11,14]

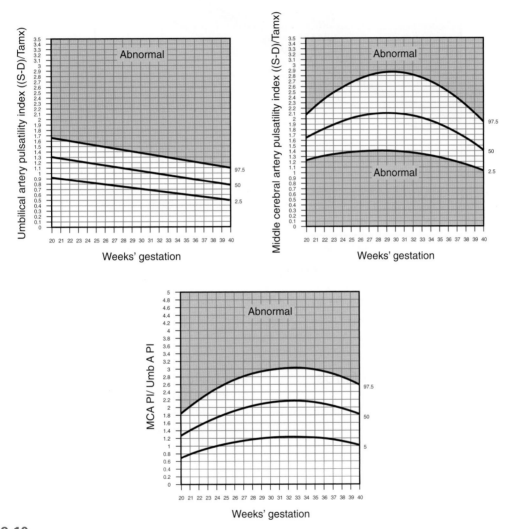

Figure 39-10
Umbilical artery, middle cerebral artery, and the MCA/UA ratio as reported by Baschat and Gembruch.[14]

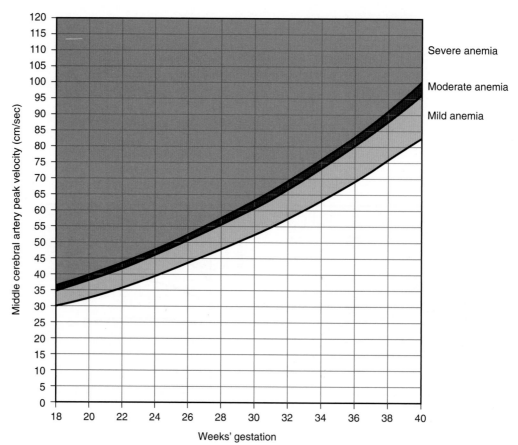

Figure 39-11
Identification of the fetus at risk for anemia by measuring the peak velocity of the middle cerebral artery.[3]

EVALUATION OF THE POST-TERM FETUS

Investigators have examined the middle cerebral artery in post-term fetuses.[16-19] Although there are several approaches, evaluating the ratio of the middle cerebral umbilical artery seems to be most promising.[17,19] Although Devine et al[17] measured the S/D ratio of the umbilical and middle cerebral arteries and found a ratio of less than 1.05 to be predictive of adverse outcome, the pulsatility index may also be used for such computations.[19] Fig. 39-12 and Table 39-6 illustrate the pulsatility index for the umbilical artery, middle cerebral artery, and the ratio of the middle cerebral/umbilical artery.[19]

Table 39-6 Normal ranges for the pulsatility index (PI) for the umbilical artery, middle cerebral artery, and the middle cerebral artery PI/umbilical artery PI in post-term pregnancies[19]

Gestation (wks)	Umbilical Artery Pulsatility Index			Middle Cerebral Pulsatility Index			Middle Cerebral PI/Umbilical Artery RI		
	5th Percentile	50th Percentile	95th Percentile	5th Percentile	50th Percentile	95th Percentile	5th Percentile	50th Percentile	95th Percentile
41 + 0	0.75	0.97	1.18	0.89	1.36	1.83	0.95	1.46	1.97
41 + 1	0.75	0.96	1.18	0.88	1.35	1.82	0.94	1.46	1.99
41 + 2	0.74	0.96	1.18	0.87	1.34	1.81	0.92	1.46	2
41 + 3	0.74	0.96	1.18	0.86	1.32	1.79	0.9	1.46	2.02
41 + 4	0.74	0.96	1.18	0.84	1.31	1.78	0.88	1.45	2.03
41 + 5	0.73	0.95	1.18	0.83	1.3	1.77	0.86	1.45	2.04
41 + 6	0.73	0.95	1.18	0.82	1.29	1.75	0.84	1.45	2.06
42 + 0	0.72	0.95	1.18	0.8	1.27	1.74	0.82	1.44	2.07
42 + 1	0.72	0.95	1.18	0.79	1.26	1.73	0.8	1.44	2.08
42 + 3	0.72	0.95	1.18	0.78	1.25	1.72	0.78	1.44	2.1
42 + 4	0.71	0.94	1.17	0.76	1.23	1.7	0.76	1.44	2.11
42 + 5	0.71	0.94	1.17	0.75	1.22	1.69	0.74	1.43	2.13
42 + 6	0.7	0.94	1.17	0.74	1.21	1.68	0.72	1.43	2.14
43 + 0	0.7	0.94	1.17	0.73	1.19	1.66	0.7	1.43	2.15

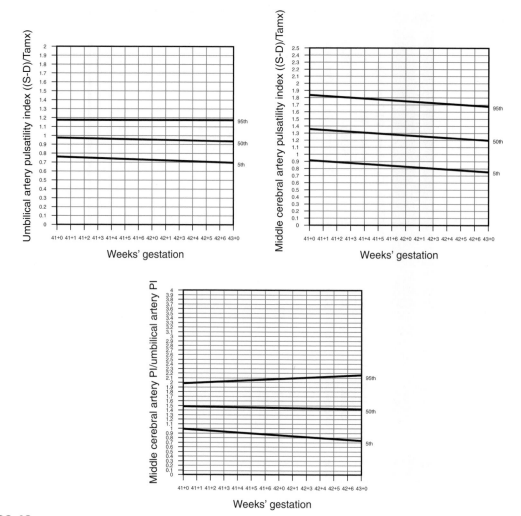

Figure 39-12
Pulsatility index for the umbilical artery, middle cerebral artery, and middle cerebral artery/umbilical artery ratio in post-term pregnancies.[19]

References

1. Woo JS, Liang ST, Lo RL, Chan FY: Middle cerebral artery Doppler flow velocity waveforms. Obstet Gynecol 1987;70:613-616.

2. Arstrom K, Eliasson A, Hareide JH, Marsal K: Fetal blood velocity waveforms in normal pregnancies. A longitudinal study. Acta Obstet Gynecol Scand 1989;68:171-178.

3. Mari G, Deter RL, Carpenter RL, et al: Non-invasive diagnosis by Doppler ultrasonography of fetal anemia due to maternal red-cell alloimmunization. Collaborative Group for Doppler Assessment of the Blood Velocity in Anemic Fetuses. N Engl J Med 2000;342:9-14.

4. Respondek M, Woch A, Kaczmarek P, Borowski D: Reversal of diastolic flow in the middle cerebral artery of the fetus during the second half of pregnancy. Ultrasound Obstet Gynecol 1997;9:324-329.

5. Sepulveda W, Shennan AH, Peek MJ: Reverse end-diastolic flow in the middle cerebral artery: an agonal pattern in the human fetus. Am J Obstet Gynecol 1996;174:1645-1647.

6. Konje JC, Bell SC, Taylor DJ: Abnormal Doppler velocimetry and blood flow volume in the middle cerebral artery in very severe intrauterine growth restriction: is the occurence of reversal of compensatory flow too late? BJOG 2001;108:973-979.

7. Baschat AA, Gembruch U, Reiss I, et al: Relationship between arterial and venous

Doppler and perinatal outcome in fetal growth restriction. Ultrasound Obstet Gynecol 2000;16:407-413.

8. Ozeren M, Dinc H, Ekmen U, et al: Umbilical and middle cerebral artery Doppler indices in patients with preeclampsia. Eur J Obstet Gynecol Reprod Biol 1999;82: 11-16.

9. Mari G, Deter RL: Middle cerebral artery flow velocity waveforms in normal and small-for-gestational-age fetuses. Am J Obstet Gynecol 1992;166:1262-1270.

10. van den Wijngaard JA, Groenenberg IA, Wladimiroff JW, Hop WC: Cerebral Doppler ultrasound of the human fetus. Br J Obstet Gynaecol 1989;96:845-849.

11. Bahlmann F, Reinhard I, Krummenauer F, et al: Blood flow velocity waveforms of the fetal middle cerebral artery in a normal population: reference values from 18 weeks to 42 weeks of gestation. J Perinat Med 2002;30:490-501.

12. Hsieh YY, Chang CC, Tsai HD, Tsai CH: Longitudinal survey of blood flow at three different locations in the middle cerebral artery in normal fetuses. Ultrasound Obstet Gynecol 2001;17:125-128.

13. Kurmanavicius J, Florio I, Wisser J, et al: Reference resistance indices of the umbilical, fetal middle cerebral and uterine arteries at 24-42 weeks of gestation. Ultrasound Obstet Gynecol 1997;10:112-120.

14. Baschat AA, Gembruch U: The cerebroplacental Doppler ratio revisited. Ultrasound Obstet Gynecol 2003;21:124-127.

15. Teixeira JM, Duncan K, Letsky E, Fisk NM: Middle cerebral artery peak systolic velocity in the prediction of fetal anemia. Ultrasound Obstet Gynecol 2000;15:205-208.

16. Anteby EY, Tadmor O, Revel A, Yagel S: Post-term pregnancies with normal cardiotocographs and amniotic fluid columns: the role of Doppler evaluation in predicting perinatal outcome. Eur J Obstet Gynecol Reprod Biol 1994;54:93-98.

17. Devine PA, Bracero LA, Lysikiewicz A, et al: Middle cerebral to umbilical artery Doppler ratio in post-date pregnancies. Obstet Gynecol 1994;84:856-860.

18. Figueras F, Lanna M, Palacio M, et al: Middle cerebral artery Doppler indices at different sites: prediction of umbilical cord gases in prolonged pregnancies. Ultrasound Obstet Gynecol 2004;24:529-533.

19. Palacio M, Figueras F, Zamora L, et al: Reference ranges for umbilical and middle cerebral artery pulsatility index and cerebroplacental ratio in prolonged pregnancies. Ultrasound Obstet Gynecol 2004;24:647-653.

CHAPTER 40

Fetal Inferior Vena Cava

Greggory R. DeVore

Introduction

The inferior vena cava drains blood from the lower extremities and abdominal cavity and returns it to the right atrium. Blood in this vessel is deoxygenated. Because blood from the inferior vena cava does not originate from the placenta, volume flow studies of this vessel are not important for fetal evaluation. The inferior vena cava waveform, however, provides information relating to compliance of the right ventricle. During ventricular systole, pressure in the right atrium is lower than the inferior vena cava, resulting in forward flow from the inferior vena cava into the right atrium. This is represented by the S wave (Fig. 40-1). At the completion of ventricular systole the tricuspid valve opens, allowing blood to flow from the right atrium into

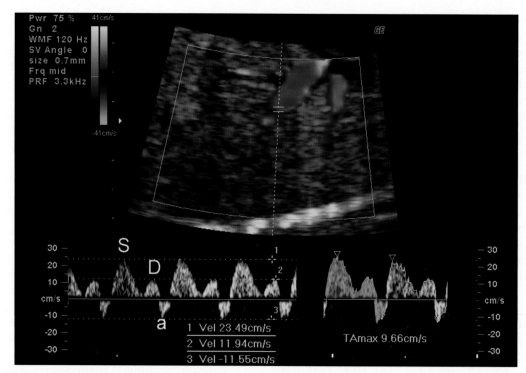

Figure 40-1
Inferior vena cava Doppler waveform. The sample volume is placed within the inferior vena cava. The Doppler waveform consists of the S (*S*), D (*D*), and A (*A*) waves. The S wave represents ventricular systole, D wave the early filling phase of atrial diastole, and A wave atrial contraction. The peak velocity for each of the waveforms is represented as follows: S = 1, D = 2, A = 3. The Tmax = Tamax and is the area under the waveform (green overlay).

the right ventricle during the early, passive filling phase. This results in forward flow from the inferior vena cava as blood continues to flow into the right atrium, which is represented by the D wave (see Fig. 40-1). At the end of the rapid filling phase of diastolic filling, the right atrium contracts against a partially filled right ventricle. Because of the stiffness of the right ventricle, there is increased resistance to blood entering the right ventricle. This may result in a negative A wave of the inferior vena cava waveform (see Fig. 40-1). Although the negative A wave may be a normal finding, an increase in ventricular stiffness results in a larger A wave than normal. Measurement of an increase in the a wave velocity, therefore, identifies fetuses with a "stiffer" right ventricle, which has been observed in fetuses with intrauterine growth restriction (IUGR) who may be compromised.[1-13]

Qualitative Assessment of the Inferior Vena Cava

Investigators have focused primarily on the relationships among the three velocity components (S, D, A) of the inferior vena cava waveform. A number of investigators have reported individual curves for inferior vena cava indices. In 1996 Rizzo et al[12] published their results after studying 209 normal fetuses and 89 with growth restriction. They measured six different indices and found that all were significantly different between control and IUGR fetuses. However, when using receiver operator curve analysis to determine which IVC index performed best, they found that the preload index (peak velocity during atrial contraction/peak velocity during ventricular systole, [a/S]) had a sensitivity of 73.8%, specificity of 72.3%, posi-

Table 40-1	Equations for the inferior vena cava[4]			
Index	**Regression Equation**	**Standard Deviation**	**R^2**	**P Value**
Preload index	$0.0001*GA + 0.1788$	0.1	0.007	0.1474
Peak velocity index	$-0.0019*GA + 1.7335$	0.41	0.0881	0.0001
Pulsatility index	$-0.0026*GA + 1.8223$	0.42	0.1487	0.0001

GA, Gestational age in weeks. To compute the 95th and 5th percentiles multiply the standard deviation by 1.66.

Table 40-2	Inferior vena cava preload index (a/S)		
	Preload Index (a/S)		
Weeks Gestation	**5th Percentile**	**50th Percentile**	**95th Percentile**
20	0.015	0.181	0.347
21	0.015	0.181	0.347
22	0.015	0.181	0.347
23	0.015	0.181	0.347
24	0.015	0.181	0.347
25	0.015	0.181	0.347
26	0.015	0.181	0.347
27	0.016	0.182	0.348
28	0.016	0.182	0.348
29	0.016	0.182	0.348
30	0.016	0.182	0.348
31	0.016	0.182	0.348
32	0.016	0.182	0.348
33	0.016	0.182	0.348
34	0.016	0.182	0.348
35	0.016	0.182	0.348
36	0.016	0.182	0.348
37	0.017	0.183	0.349
38	0.017	0.183	0.349
39	0.017	0.183	0.349
40	0.017	0.183	0.349

tive predictive value of 81.5%, and negative predictive value of 66.6%.[12] In 2003 Baschat[2] examined 237 patients and examined three indices for the inferior vena cava and found a linear relationship with gestational age (Tables 40-1 to 40-4, Figs. 40-2 to 40-4). In 2004 Baschat et al[1] used the same indices to determine if they could predict fetal acidemia at birth in high-risk fetuses by sampling the umbilical artery following delivery of a nonlaboring patient. They found that the inferior vena cava preload index (a/S) had the largest area under the receiver operator curve for predicting fetal acidemia (pH < 7.2), with a sensitivity of 74%, specificity 49%, positive predictive value 39%, and negative predictive value 82%. The pulsatility index was the next most sensitive test, while the peak velocity index was not significantly associated with the detection of an abnormal pH. Of the two indices, the preload index is the easiest to measure because it only requires a peak velocity of the S and A waves of the waveform.[1]

Fig. 40-5 is a worksheet of Doppler indices that may be useful when examining a high-risk fetus.

Table 40-3 Inferior vena cava peak velocity index (S-a)/D

Gestation (wks)	Peak Velocity Index (S-a)/D			Weeks Gestation	Peak Velocity Index (S-a)/D		
	5th Percentile	50th Percentile	95th Percentile		5th Percentile	50th Percentile	95th Percentile
20	1.015	1.696	2.376	31	0.994	1.675	2.355
21	1.013	1.694	2.374	32	0.992	1.673	2.353
22	1.011	1.692	2.372	33	0.990	1.671	2.351
23	1.009	1.690	2.370	34	0.988	1.669	2.350
24	1.007	1.688	2.369	35	0.986	1.667	2.348
25	1.005	1.686	2.367	36	0.985	1.665	2.346
26	1.004	1.684	2.365	37	0.983	1.663	2.344
27	1.002	1.682	2.363	38	0.981	1.661	2.342
28	1.000	1.680	2.361	39	0.979	1.659	2.340
29	0.998	1.678	2.359	40	0.977	1.658	2.338
30	0.996	1.677	2.357				

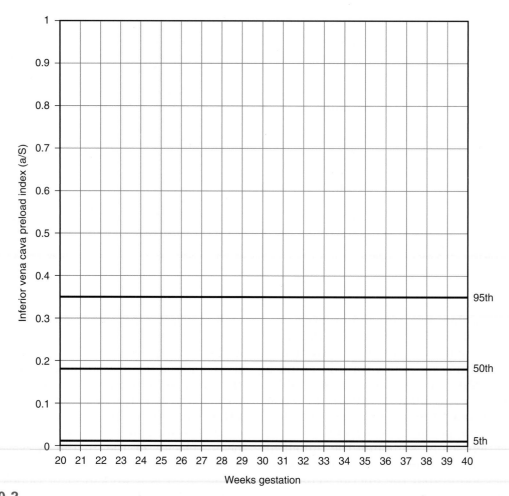

Figure 40-2

Preload index of the inferior vena cava. To compute this index, divide the A wave peak velocity by the S wave peak velocity.

Table 40-4 Inferior vena cava pulsatility index (S-a)/Tamx

Gestation (wks)	Pulsatility Index (S-a)/Tamx			Weeks Gestation	Pulsatility Index (S-a)/Tamx		
	5th Percentile	50th Percentile	95th Percentile		5th Percentile	50th Percentile	95th Percentile
20	1.073	1.770	2.468	31	1.045	1.742	2.439
21	1.071	1.768	2.465	32	1.042	1.739	2.436
22	1.068	1.765	2.462	33	1.039	1.737	2.434
23	1.065	1.763	2.460	34	1.037	1.734	2.431
24	1.063	1.760	2.457	35	1.034	1.731	2.429
25	1.060	1.757	2.455	36	1.032	1.729	2.426
26	1.058	1.755	2.452	37	1.029	1.726	2.423
27	1.055	1.752	2.449	38	1.026	1.724	2.421
28	1.052	1.750	2.447	39	1.024	1.721	2.418
29	1.050	1.747	2.444	40	1.021	1.718	2.416
30	1.047	1.744	2.442				

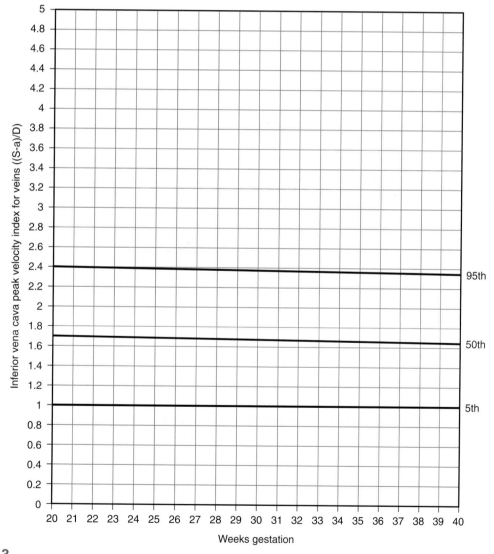

Figure 40-3
Peak velocity index of the inferior vena cava. To compute this index subtract the A wave velocity from the S wave velocity and then divide the value by the D wave velocity.

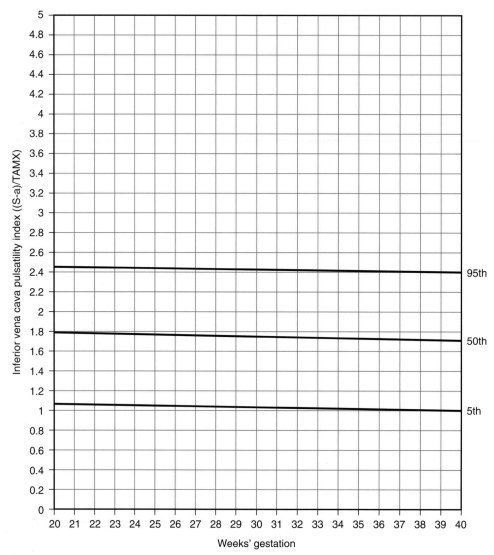

Figure 40-4
Pulsatility index of the inferior vena cava. To compute this index, subtract the A wave velocity from the S wave velocity and then divide this value by the time average mean velocity.

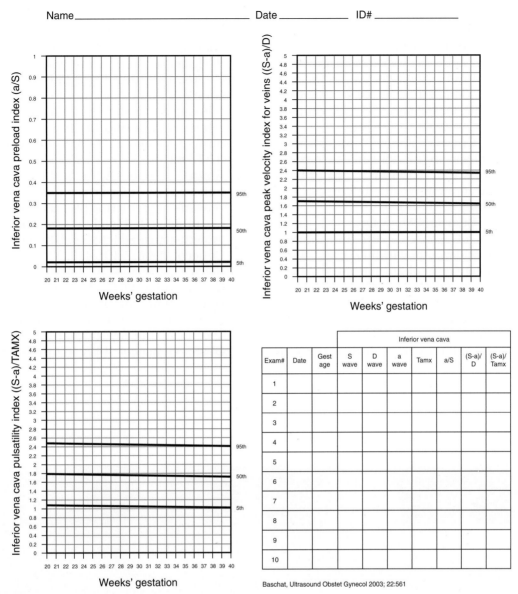

Name_____   Date_____   ID#_____

Figure 40-5
Patient flow sheet. (Redrawn from Baschat AA: Relationship between placental blood flow resistance and precordial venous Doppler indices. Ultrasound Obstet Gynecol 2003;22:561-566.)

References

1. Baschat AA, Guclu S, Kush ML, et al: Venous Doppler in the prediction of acid-base status of growth-restricted fetuses with elevated placental blood flow resistance. Am J Obstet Gynecol 2004;191:277-284.

2. Baschat AA: Relationship between placental blood flow resistance and precordial venous Doppler indices. Ultrasound Obstet Gynecol 2003;22:561-566.

3. Baschat AA, Gembruch U, Harman CR: The sequence of changes in Doppler and biophysical parameters as severe fetal growth restriction worsens. Ultrasound Obstet Gynecol 2001;18:571-577.

4. Baschat AA, Gembruch U, Reiss I, et al: Relationship between arterial and venous Doppler and perinatal outcome in fetal growth restriction. Ultrasound Obstet Gynecol 2000;16:407-413.

5. Capomolla S, Febo O, Caporotondi A, et al: Non-invasive estimation of right atrial pressure by combined Doppler echocardio-

graphic measurements of the inferior vena cava in patients with congestive heart failure. Ital Heart J 2000;1:684-690.

6. Capponi A, Rizzo G, De Angelis C, et al: Atrial natriuretic peptide levels in fetal blood in relation to inferior vena cava velocity waveforms. Obstet Gynecol 1997;89:242-247.

7. Capponi A, Rizzo G, Rinaldo D, et al: Effects of cordocentesis on inferior vena cava velocity waveforms: differences between normally grown and growth-retarded fetuses. Biol Neonate 1996;70:84-90.

8. Hecher K, Bilardo CM, Stigter RH, et al: Monitoring of fetuses with intrauterine growth restriction: a longitudinal study. Ultrasound Obstet Gynecol 2001;18:564-570.

9. Hecher K, Campbell S, Doyle P, et al: Assessment of fetal compromise by Doppler ultrasound investigation of the fetal circulation. Arterial, intracardiac, and venous blood flow velocity studies. Circulation 1995;91:129-138.

10. Makikallio K, Vuolteenaho O, Jouppila P, Rasanen J: Ultrasonographic and biochemical markers of human fetal cardiac dysfunction in placental insufficiency. Circulation 2002;105:2058-2063.

11. Okura I, Miyagi Y, Tada K, et al: The relationship between Doppler indices from inferior vena cava and hepatic veins in normal human fetuses. Acta Med Okayama 2003;57:77-82.

12. Rizzo G, Capponi A, Talone PE, et al: Doppler indices from inferior vena cava and ductus venosus in predicting pH and oxygen tension in umbilical blood at cordocentesis in growth-retarded fetuses. Ultrasound Obstet Gynecol 1996;7:401-410.

13. Rizzo G, Capponi A, Arduini D, Romanini C: The value of fetal arterial, cardiac and venous flows in predicting pH and blood gases measured in umbilical blood at cordocentesis in growth retarded fetuses. Br J Obstet Gynaecol 1995;102:963-969.

CHAPTER 41

Greggory R. DeVore

Fetal Intra-Abdominal Umbilical Vein

Introduction

Blood returns to the fetus through the umbilical vein, which enters the abdomen and becomes the intra-abdominal portion of this vessel (Fig. 41-1). The intra-abdominal umbilical vein directs oxygenated blood through the ductus venosus to the left atrium and left ventricle or to the liver (see Fig. 41-1). The umbilical vein within the abdominal cavity should be imaged so that the sample volume is placed parallel or slightly tangential to the flow of blood through the umbilical vein (see Fig. 41-1).

Qualitative Assessment of the Doppler Waveform

During the first trimester, pulsations in the umbilical vein waveform are normal but should not persist past the 13th week of gestation. From 13 weeks until term, the normal Doppler waveform of the vein demonstrates continuous, uninterrupted flow (see Fig. 41-1).[1] If, however, there is increased resistance to blood flow

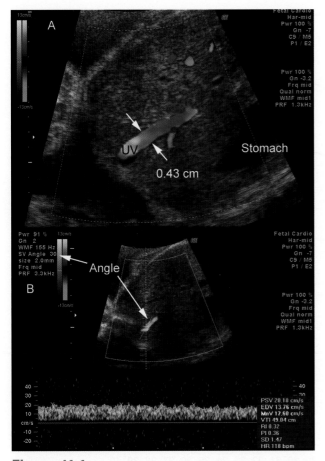

Figure 41-1

Intra-abdominal umbilical vein. **A,** The location of the umbilical vein within the abdominal cavity. The angle of the pulsed Doppler sample volume is 30 degrees. The diameter of the umbilical vein (UV) is 0.43 cm. **B,** The pulsed Doppler waveform of the intra-abdominal umbilical vein. The maximal average velocity is 17.6 cm/sec. The mean velocity (17.6/2) is 8.8 cm/sec.

during atrial systole, this may be reflected in the umbilical vein waveform as "notching," which can be observed with severe intrauterine growth restriction, cardiac insufficiency associated with fetal hydrops, fetuses with obstructive right ventricular anomalies, and fetuses with late decelerations recorded during labor.[2]

Quantitative Assessment of the Doppler Waveform

Studies in normal fetuses have demonstrated the following: (1) the mean velocity increases slightly or is constant throughout pregnancy; (2) blood flow (ml/min) increases with gestational age or may show a slight decrease with gestational age; and (3) flow, when corrected for fetal weight (mg/ml/kg), remains constant.[3-5]

Recent studies, however, have demonstrated the clinical utility of measuring umbilical venous flow in fetuses and found the following: decreased flow with intrauterine growth restriction and fetal distress in labor, increased flow with fetal anemia, and hydrops secondary to infection.[6,7] Quantitative flow of the umbilical vein is computed as follows:

$$\text{Umbilical vein flow}_{(\text{mL/min})}$$
$$= \text{vessel cross-sectional area}_{(\text{cm}^2)}$$
$$\times \text{mean velocity}_{(\text{cm/sec})} \times 60 \ _{(\text{sec/min})}$$

To compute the volume flow do the following (see Fig. 41-1):

Step 1. The umbilical vein is imaged with color Doppler ultrasound by directing the ultrasound transducer over the maternal abdominal wall so that the ultrasound beam is parallel or tangential (< 30 degrees) to umbilical venous flow (see Fig. 41-1A).

Step 2. The pulsed Doppler waveform is recorded in centimeters per second (see Fig. 41-1B).

Step 3. The mean velocity is measured. Not all ultrasound machines will compute the mean velocity. However, this can be approximated by measuring the average peak velocity and dividing this by 2. In Figure 41-1 the average peak velocity is 17.6 cm/sec. Therefore the mean velocity is 8.8 cm/sec (17.6/2). The mean velocity has been demonstrated to increase with gestational age until 32 weeks, and then slightly decrease after 38 weeks (Fig. 41-2, Table 41-1).[5,8]

Step 4. The ultrasound transducer is redirected over the abdominal wall so that the umbilical vein is imaged perpendicular or tangential to the ultrasound beam. The diameter is measured from the inner wall to inner wall in centimeters using the B-mode image or the boundary of the color Doppler, if the color Doppler settings do not overlap the B-mode image of the vessel (see Fig. 41-1A). In Figure 41-1A the umbilical vein diameter is 0.43 cm. The diameter of the umbilical vein increases with gestational age (Fig. 41-3, Table 41-2).

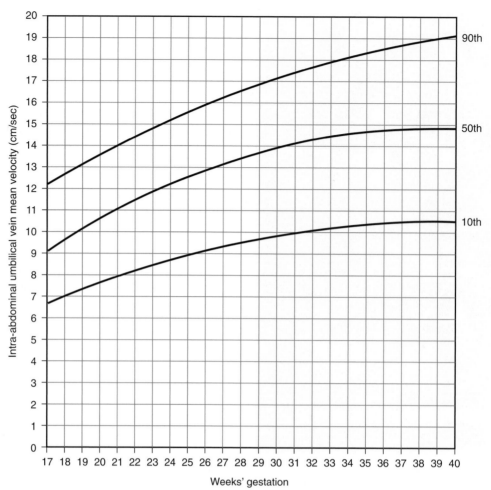

Figure 41-2
The umbilical vein mean velocity is computed directly from the ultrasound machine. If this function is not available, it can be computed by dividing the average peak velocity by 2.[8]

Table 41-1	Intra-abdominal vein mean velocity (cm/sec)						
	Mean Velocity (cm/sec)				**Mean Velocity (cm/sec)**		
Gestation (wks)	**10th Percentile**	**50th Percentile**	**90th Percentile**	**Weeks Gestation**	**10th Percentile**	**50th Percentile**	**90th Percentile**
17	6.65	9.06	12.16	29	9.61	13.66	16.79
18	6.97	9.58	12.63	30	9.77	13.88	17.08
19	7.28	10.07	13.09	31	9.91	14.08	17.35
20	7.58	10.54	13.53	32	10.03	14.26	17.60
21	7.87	10.98	13.96	33	10.14	14.41	17.83
22	8.13	11.40	14.37	34	10.24	14.53	18.05
23	8.39	11.80	14.76	35	10.32	14.63	18.26
24	8.63	12.17	15.14	36	10.39	14.71	18.45
25	8.85	12.52	15.50	37	10.44	14.77	18.62
26	9.07	12.84	15.85	38	10.48	14.79	18.78
27	9.26	13.13	16.18	39	10.50	14.80	18.92
28	9.45	13.41	16.50	40	10.51	14.78	19.05

From Kiserud T, Rasmussen S, Skulstad S: Blood flow and the degree of shunting through the ductus venosus in the human fetus. Am J Obstet Gynecol 2000;182:147-153.

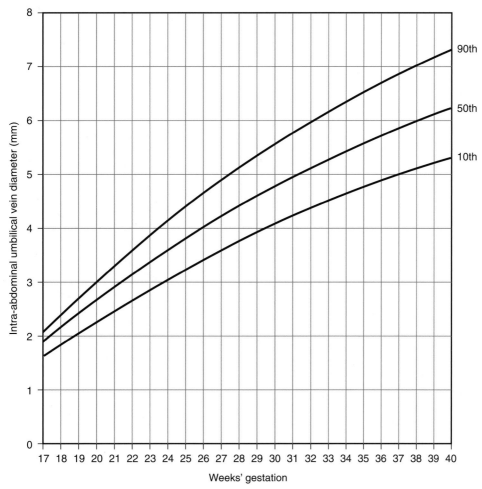

Figure 41-3
The umbilical vein diameter increases with gestational age.[5]

Table 41-2	Intra-abdominal vein diameter (mm)						
	Vein Diameter (mm)				**Vein Diameter (mm)**		
Gestation (wks)	**10th Percentile**	**50th Percentile**	**90th Percentile**	**Weeks Gestation**	**10th Percentile**	**50th Percentile**	**90th Percentile**
17	1.9	1.6	2.1	29	4.6	3.9	5.4
18	2.2	1.9	2.4	30	4.8	4.1	5.6
19	2.4	2.1	2.7	31	5.0	4.2	5.8
20	2.7	2.3	3.0	32	5.1	4.4	6.0
21	2.9	2.5	3.3	33	5.3	4.5	6.2
22	3.2	2.7	3.6	34	5.5	4.6	6.4
23	3.4	2.9	3.9	35	5.6	4.8	6.6
24	3.6	3.1	4.1	36	5.7	4.9	6.7
25	3.8	3.2	4.4	37	5.9	5.0	6.9
26	4.0	3.4	4.7	38	6.0	5.1	7.0
27	4.2	3.6	4.9	39	6.1	5.2	7.2
28	4.4	3.8	5.1	40	6.2	5.3	7.3

From Kiserud T, Rasmussen S, Skulstad S: Blood flow and the degree of shunting through the ductus venosus in the human fetus. Am J Obstet Gynecol 2000;182:147-153.

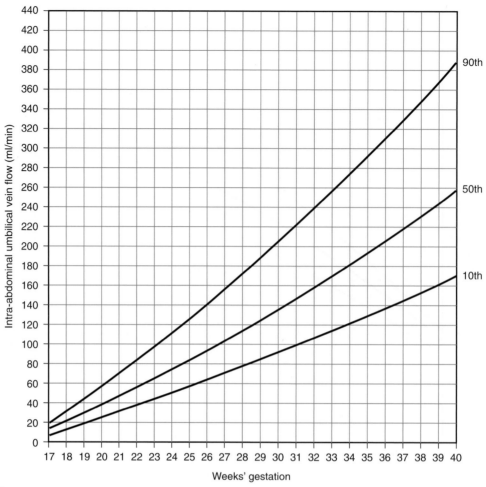

Figure 41-4
The umbilical vein flow increases with gestational age.[5]

Step 5. The umbilical venous flow$_{(mL/min)}$ can be computed using either of the following equations:

$$\text{Volume flow}_{mL/min} = (\text{Vmean}_{cm/sec}) \times (3.14 \times [(\text{Diameter of vessel}_{cm}/2) \times (\text{Diameter of vessel}_{cm}/2)]) \times 60_{sec/min}$$

If the mean velocity is not available then the following equation can be used:

$$\text{Volume flow}_{mL/min} = (\text{peak velocity}_{cm/sec}/2) \times (3.14 \times [(\text{diameter of vessel}_{cm}/2) \times (\text{diameter of vessel}_{cm}/2)]) \times 60_{sec/min}$$

The umbilical venous flow increases with gestational age (Fig. 41-4, Table 41-3).

Using the information from Figure 41-1, the volume flow is computed as follows:

$$\text{Volume flow}_{mL/min} = (17.6_{cm/sec}/2) \times (3.14 \times [(0.43_{cm}/2) \times (0.43_{cm}/2)]) \times 60_{sec/min}$$

$$\text{Volume flow} = 74.9 \text{ mL/min}$$

Once the volume of flow (mm/min) is computed, the examiner can display the flow in one of two ways:

1. Absolute flow for gestational age (see Fig. 41-4; see Table 41-3).
2. Flow per kilogram of estimated fetal weight (Fig. 41-5, Table 41-4).

Figure 41-6 is a proposed clinical sheet that the examiner can use when following a patient at risk for intrauterine growth restriction.

Table 41-3	Intra-abdominal vein flow (ml/min)						
	Venous Flow (ml/min)				**Venous Flow (ml/min)**		
Gestation (wks)	**10th Percentile**	**50th Percentile**	**90th Percentile**	**Weeks Gestation**	**10th Percentile**	**50th Percentile**	**90th Percentile**
17	6	12	16	29	83	122	187
18	12	20	29	30	90	133	203
19	18	28	41	31	97	144	220
20	24	36	54	32	104	156	237
21	30	45	68	33	112	167	255
22	36	54	81	34	119	179	272
23	42	63	96	35	127	191	290
24	49	72	110	36	135	203	309
25	55	82	125	37	143	216	328
26	62	91	140	38	151	229	347
27	69	101	155	39	159	242	366
28	76	112	171	40	167	255	386

From Kiserud T, Rasmussen S, Skulstad S: Blood flow and the degree of shunting through the ductus venosus in the human fetus. Am J Obstet Gynecol 2000;182:147-153.

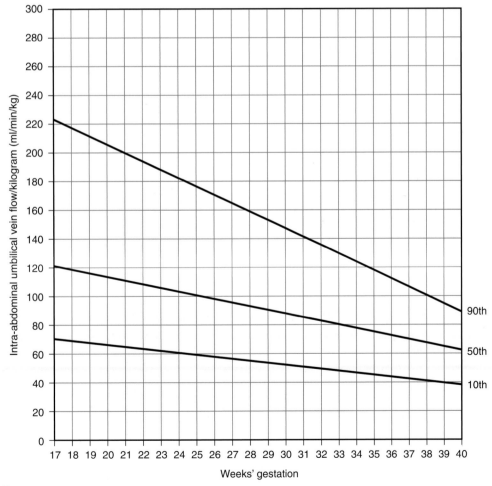

Figure 41-5
The umbilical vein flow per kilogram decreases with gestational age.[5]

Table 41-4	Intra-abdominal vein flow per Kilogram (ml/min/kg)		
	Venous Flow (ml/min/kg)		
Gestation (wks)	**10th Percentile**	**50th Percentile**	**90th Percentile**
17	120	222	71
18	118	216	69
19	115	210	68
20	113	204	67
21	110	199	65
22	108	193	64
23	105	187	62
24	103	181	61
25	100	176	60
26	98	170	58
27	95	164	57
28	93	158	55
29	90	153	54
30	88	147	53
31	85	141	51
32	83	135	50
33	80	130	48
34	78	124	47
35	75	118	46
36	73	112	44
37	70	107	43
38	68	101	41
39	65	95	40
40	63	89	39

From Kiserud T, Rasmussen S, Skulstad S: Blood flow and the degree of shunting through the ductus venosus in the human fetus. Am J Obstet Gynecol 2000;182:147-153.

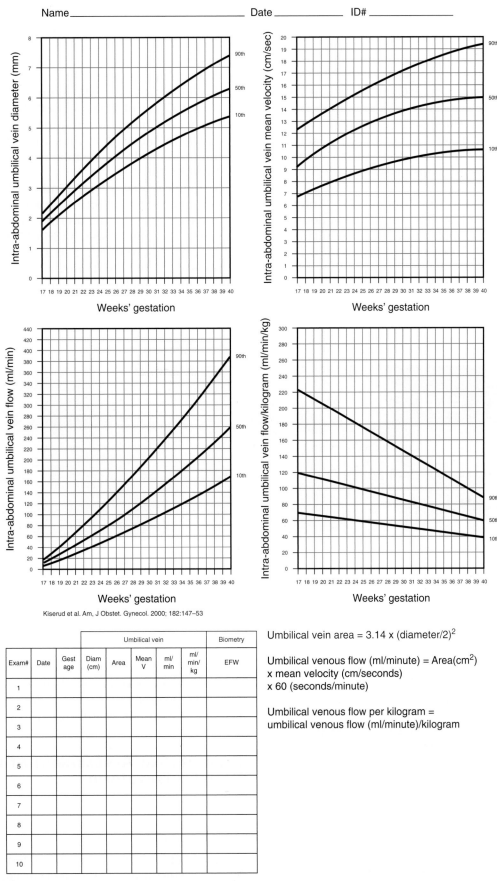

Figure 41-6

Clinical flow sheet. (Redrawn from Kiserud T, Rasmussen S, Skulstad S: Blood flow and the degree of shunting through the ductus venosus in the human fetus. Am J Obstet Gynecol 2000;182:147-153.)

References

1. Rizzo G, Arduini D, Romanini C: Umbilical vein pulsations: a physiologic finding in early gestation. Am J Obstet Gynecol 1992;167:675-677.
2. DeVore GR, Horenstein J: Ductus venosus index: a method for evaluating right ventricular preload in the second-trimester fetus. Ultrasound Obstet Gynecol 1993;3:338-342.
3. Chen HY, Lu CC, Cheng YT: Antenatal measurement of fetal umbilical venous flow by pulsed Doppler and B-mode ultrasonography. J Ultrasound Med 1986;5:319-321.
4. Gerson AG, Wallace DM, Stiller RJ, et al: Doppler evaluation of umbilical venous and arterial blood flow in the second and third trimesters of normal pregnancy. Obstet Gynecol 1987;70:622-626.
5. Kiserud T, Rasmussen S, Skulstad S: Blood flow and the degree of shunting through the ductus venosus in the human fetus. Am J Obstet Gynecol 2000;182:147-153.
6. Hsieh FJ, Chang FM, Huang HC, et al: Umbilical vein blood flow measurement in non-immune hydrops fetalis. Obstet Gynecol 1988;71:188-191.
7. Jouppila P, Kirkinen P: Umbilical vein blood flow in the human fetus in cases of maternal and fetal anemia and uterine bleeding. Ultrasound Med Biol 1984;10:365-370.
8. Barbera A, Galan HL, Ferrazzi E, et al: Relationship of umbilical vein blood flow to growth parameters in the human fetus. Am J Obstet Gynecol 1999;181:174-179.

CHAPTER 42

Greggory R. DeVore

Fetal Intra-Amniotic Umbilical Vein

Introduction

The umbilical cord, free-floating in the amniotic cavity, should be imaged so that the sample volume is placed parallel or slightly tangential to the flow of blood through the umbilical vein.

Qualitative Assessment of the Doppler Waveform

During the first trimester, pulsations in the umbilical vein waveform are normal until the 13th week of gestation.[1] From 13 weeks until term, the normal Doppler waveform of the vein demonstrates continuous, uninterrupted flow (Fig. 42-1).[2] If, however, there is increased resistance to blood flow during atrial systole, this may be reflected in the umbilical vein waveform as "notching," similar to what is observed prior to the 13th week of pregnancy.[3] This change is a more severe form of abnormal ductus venous flow (see Ductus Venosus) observed with severe intrauterine growth restriction or cardiac insufficiency, which can result in fetal hydrops.[4]

Quantitative Assessment of the Doppler Waveform

In the 1980s studies of umbilical vein flow were reported, many of which had large standard deviations (Table 42-1). The reasons for the large standard deviations were attributed to (1) the error in determining the area of the vessel orifice

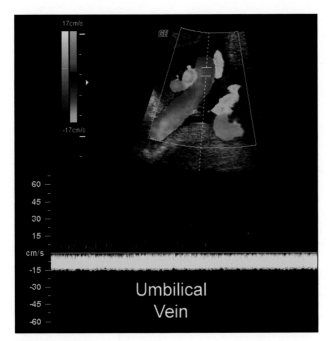

Figure 42-1
The umbilical vein demonstrates continuous flow.

Table 42-1	Umbilical vein flow	
Study	**Mean (ml/min/kg)**	**Standard Deviation**
Gill and Kosoff (1979)[9]	103	—
Eik-Nes et al (1982)[10]	115	36
Van Lierde et al (1984)[11]	117	16
Gill et al (1981)[12]	120	—
Griffin et al (1983)[13]	122	21
Erskine and Ritchie (1985)[14]	125	62

from the real-time or M-mode measurements of the vessel diameter, (2) error in deriving fetal weight from ultrasound measurements, and (3) the error occurring when the angle of the ultrasound beam incident to the vessel is not carefully controlled.[5]

Recent studies, however, have demonstrated the clinical utility of measuring umbilical venous flow in fetuses with intrauterine growth restriction and found that it decreases.[6,7] Quantitative flow of the umbilical vein is computed as follows:

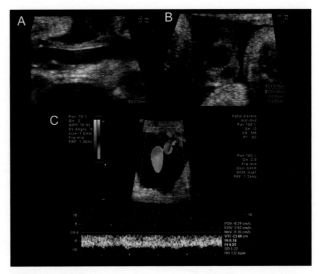

Figure 42-2
A, Longitudinal image of the umbilical vein. This is not the image of choice for measuring umbilical vein diameter because the maximal diameter cannot be determined. **B,** A cross-sectional image of the umbilical vein. The diameter can be accurately measured and the area computed. **C,** The pulsed Doppler of the umbilical vein demonstrating the average maximal peak velocity (8.36 cm/sec). The mean velocity can be computed by dividing the peak velocity (8.35 cm/sec) by 2, which equals a mean velocity of 4.18 cm/sec.

$$\text{Umbilical vein flow}_{(mL/min)} \\ = \text{vessel cross-sectional area}_{(cm^2)} \\ \times \text{mean velocity}_{(cm/sec)} \times 60_{(sec/min)}.$$

Figure 42-2 illustrates B-mode and pulsed Doppler images used for the computation of umbilical vein flow. To compute the volume flow do the following:

Step 1. The umbilical vein is imaged with color Doppler ultrasound by directing the ultrasound transducer over the maternal abdominal wall so that the ultrasound beam is parallel to umbilical vein flow (see Figure 42-2).

Step 2. The pulsed Doppler waveform is recorded in centimeters per second (see Figure 42-2).

Step 3. The mean velocity is measured. Not all ultrasound machines will compute the mean velocity. However, this can be approximated by measuring the average peak velocity and dividing this by 2. In Figure 42-2 the average peak velocity is 8.36 cm/sec. Therefore the mean velocity is 4.18 cm/sec (8.36/2). The mean velocity has been demonstrated to increase with gestational age (Fig. 42-3, Table 42-2).[8]

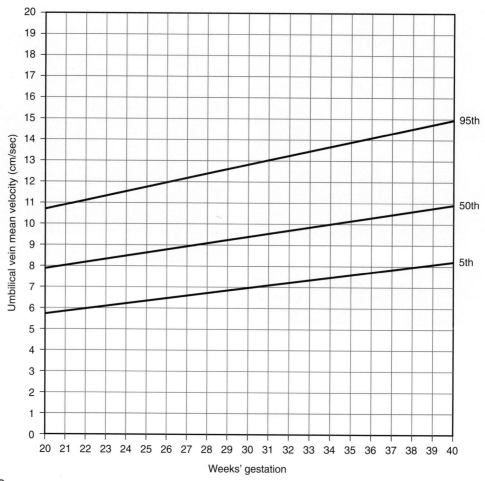

Figure 42-3
The umbilical vein mean velocity is computed directly from the ultrasound machine. If this function is not available, it can be computed by dividing the average peak velocity by 2.[8]

Table 42-2	Umbilical vein mean velocity (cm/sec)						
	Mean Velocity (cm/sec)				**Mean Velocity (cm/sec)**		
Gestation (wks)	**5th Percentile**	**50th Percentile**	**95th Percentile**	**Weeks Gestation**	**5th Percentile**	**50th Percentile**	**95th Percentile**
20	5.70	7.90	10.70	31	7.04	9.67	13.02
21	5.82	8.06	10.91	32	7.17	9.83	13.23
22	5.94	8.22	11.12	33	7.29	9.99	13.44
23	6.07	8.38	11.33	34	7.41	10.16	13.66
24	6.19	8.54	11.54	35	7.53	10.32	13.87
25	6.31	8.71	11.76	36	7.65	10.48	14.08
26	6.43	8.87	11.97	37	7.78	10.64	14.29
27	6.56	9.03	12.18	38	7.90	10.80	14.50
28	6.68	9.19	12.39	39	8.02	10.96	14.71
29	6.80	9.35	12.60	40	8.14	11.12	14.92
30	6.92	9.51	12.81				

From Barbera A, Galan HL, Ferrazzi E, et al: Relationship of umbilical vein blood flow to growth parameters in the human fetus. Am J Obstet Gynecol 1999;181:174-179.

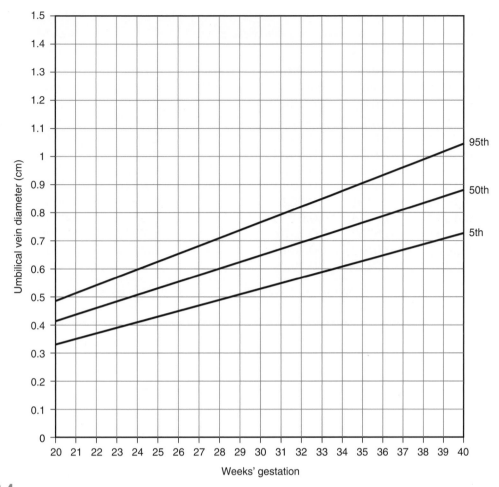

Figure 42-4
The umbilical vein diameter increases with gestational age.[8]

Step 4. The ultrasound transducer is redirected over the abdominal wall so that the umbilical vein is imaged perpendicular to the ultrasound beam. The diameter is measured from the inner wall to the inner wall in centimeters. In Figure 42-2 the umbilical vein diameter is 0.79 cm. The diameter of umbilical vein increases with gestational age (Fig. 42-4, Table 42-3).[8]

Step 5. The umbilical venous flow$_{(mL/min)}$ can be computed using either of the following equations:

$$\text{Volume flow}_{mL/min} = (V\text{mean}_{cm/sec})$$
$$\times (3.14 \times [(\text{diameter of vessel}_{cm}/2)$$
$$\times (\text{diameter of vessel}_{cm}/2)]) \times 60_{sec/min}$$

If the mean velocity is not available, then the following equation can be used:

$$\text{Volume flow}_{mL/min} = (\text{peak velocity}_{cm/sec}/2)$$
$$\times (3.14 \times [(\text{diameter of vessel}_{cm}/2)$$
$$\times (\text{diameter of vessel}_{cm}/2)]) \times 60_{sec/min}$$

The umbilical venous flow increases with gestational age (Fig. 42-5, Table 42-4).

Using the information from Figure 42-2, the volume flow is computed as follows:

$$\text{Volume flow}_{mL/min} = (8.36_{cm/sec}/2)$$
$$\times (3.14 \times [(0.79_{cm}/2) \times (0.79_{cm}/2)]) \times 60_{sec/min}$$

$$\text{Volume flow} = 123 \text{ mL/min}$$

Once the volume of flow (mm/min) is computed, the examiner can display the flow by in one of three ways:

1. Absolute flow for gestational age (see Figure 42-5; see Table 42-4).[8]
2. Flow per kilogram of estimated fetal weight (Fig. 42-6, Table 42-5).[8]
3. Flow per abdominal circumference (Fig. 42-7, Table 42-6).[8]
4. Flow per head circumference (Fig. 42-8, Table 42-7).[8]

Figure 42-9 is a proposed clinical sheet that the examiner can use when following

Text continued on p. 227

Table 42-3	Umbilical vein diameter (cm)						
Gestation (wks)	**Vein Diameter (cm)**			Weeks Gestation	**Vein Diameter (cm)**		
	5th Percentile	50th Percentile	95th Percentile		5th Percentile	50th Percentile	95th Percentile
20	0.3341	0.4093	0.4864	31	0.5475	0.6656	0.7900
21	0.3535	0.4326	0.5140	32	0.5669	0.6889	0.8176
22	0.3729	0.4559	0.5416	33	0.5863	0.7122	0.8452
23	0.3923	0.4792	0.5692	34	0.6057	0.7355	0.8728
24	0.4117	0.5025	0.5968	35	0.6251	0.7588	0.9004
25	0.4311	0.5258	0.6244	36	0.6445	0.7821	0.9280
26	0.4505	0.5491	0.6520	37	0.6639	0.8054	0.9556
27	0.4699	0.5724	0.6796	38	0.6833	0.8287	0.9832
28	0.4893	0.5957	0.7072	39	0.7027	0.8520	1.0108
29	0.5087	0.6190	0.7348	40	0.7221	0.8753	1.0384
30	0.5281	0.6423	0.7624				

From Barbera A, Galan HL, Ferrazzi E, et al: Relationship of umbilical vein blood flow to growth parameters in the human fetus. Am J Obstet Gynecol 1999;181:174-179.

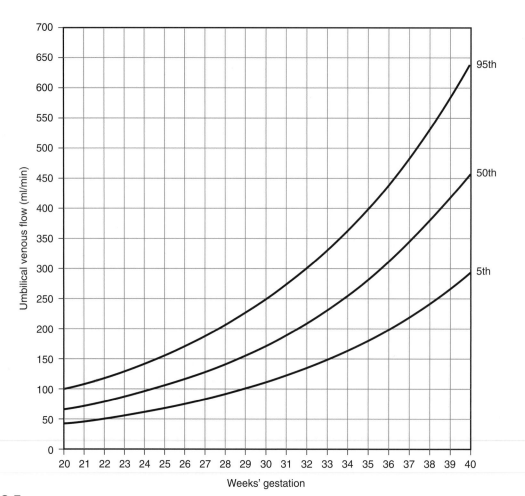

Figure 42-5
The umbilical vein flow increases with gestational age.[8]

Table 42-4	Umbilical vein flow (ml/min)						
	Venous Flow (ml/min)				**Venous Flow (ml/min)**		
Gestation (wks)	**5th Percentile**	**50th Percentile**	**95th Percentile**	**Weeks Gestation**	**5th Percentile**	**50th Percentile**	**95th Percentile**
20	41	65	97	31	120	190	274
21	45	71	107	32	133	209	301
22	49	79	117	33	147	231	331
23	55	87	129	34	162	254	363
24	60	96	142	35	179	281	399
25	67	106	156	36	197	309	438
26	73	116	171	37	218	341	482
27	81	128	188	38	240	376	529
28	90	142	206	39	265	415	581
29	99	156	227	40	293	458	639
30	109	172	249				

From Barbera A, Galan HL, Ferrazzi E, et al: Relationship of umbilical vein blood flow to growth parameters in the human fetus. Am J Obstet Gynecol 1999;181:174-179.

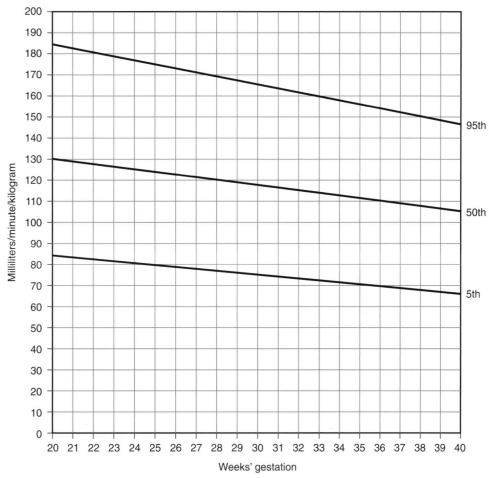

Figure 42-6
The umbilical vein flow per kilogram decreases with gestational age.[8]

Table 42-5	Umbilical vein flow per kilogram (ml/min/kg)						
	Venous Flow (ml/min/kg)				**Venous Flow (ml/min/kg)**		
Gestation (wks)	**5th Percentile**	**50th Percentile**	**95th Percentile**	**Weeks Gestation**	**5th Percentile**	**50th Percentile**	**95th Percentile**
20	84	130	184	31	74	116	163
21	83	129	182	32	73	115	161
22	82	128	180	33	72	114	159
23	81	126	178	34	71	113	158
24	80	125	176	35	70	111	156
25	79	124	175	36	69	110	154
26	78	123	173	37	68	109	152
27	77	121	171	38	68	108	150
28	77	120	169	39	67	106	148
29	76	119	167	40	66	105	146
30	75	118	165				

From Barbera A, Galan HL, Ferrazzi E, et al: Relationship of umbilical vein blood flow to growth parameters in the human fetus. Am J Obstet Gynecol 1999;181:174-179.

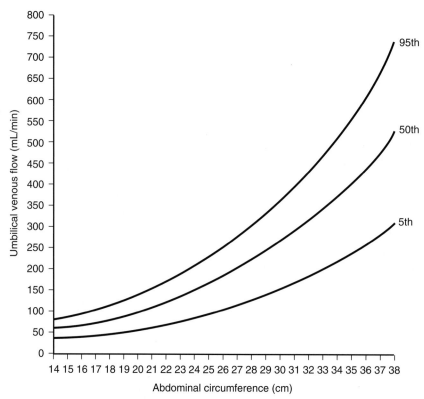

Figure 42-7
The umbilical vein flow by abdominal circumference value increases with gestational age.[8]

Table 42-6	Umbilical vein flow per abdominal circumference (ml/min/abdominal circumference)						
Abdominal Circumference (cm)	Venous Flow (ml/min)			Abdominal Circumference (cm)	Venous Flow (ml/min)		
	5th Percentile	50th Percentile	95th Percentile		5th Percentile	50th Percentile	95th Percentile
14	34	55	81	27	112	188	267
15	37	61	88	28	123	207	293
16	40	67	97	29	135	227	321
17	44	73	106	30	148	249	353
18	49	80	116	31	163	274	387
19	53	88	128	32	179	301	424
20	59	97	140	33	196	331	465
21	64	107	154	34	215	364	510
22	71	117	168	35	236	400	559
23	77	129	185	36	259	439	613
24	85	142	203	37	284	483	673
25	93	156	222	38	312	531	738
26	102	171	244				

From Barbera A, Galan HL, Ferrazzi E, et al: Relationship of umbilical vein blood flow to growth parameters in the human fetus. Am J Obstet Gynecol 1999;181:174-179.

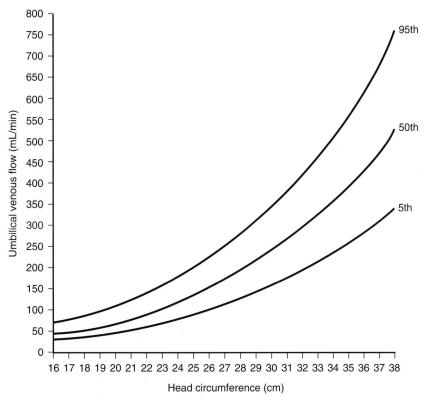

Figure 42-8
The umbilical vein flow by head circumference value increases with gestational age.[8]

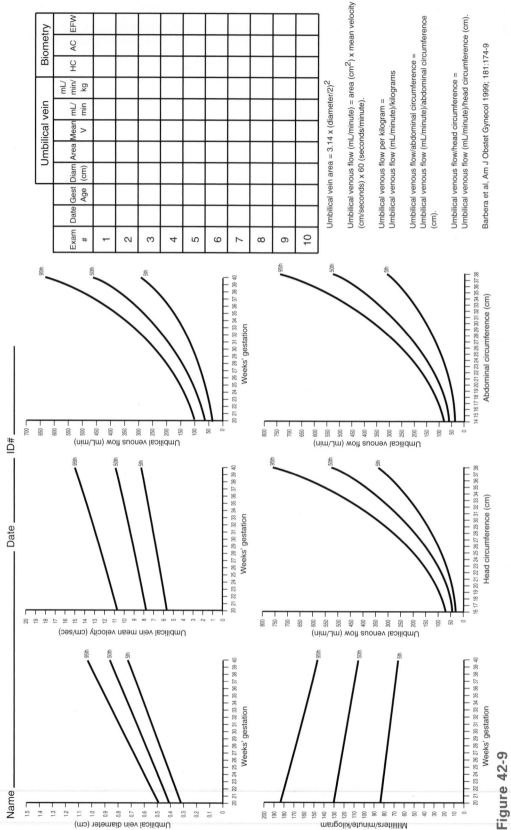

Figure 42-9

Clinical flow sheet. (Redrawn from Barbera A, Galan HL, Ferrazzi E, et al: Relationship of umbilical vein blood flow to growth parameters in the human fetus. Am J Obstet Gynecol 1999;181:174-179.)

Table 42-7	Umbilical vein flow per head circumference (ml/min/head circumference)						
Abdominal Circumference (cm)	Venous Flow (ml/min)			Abdominal Circumference (cm)	Venous Flow (ml/min)		
	5th Percentile	50th Percentile	95th Percentile		5th Percentile	50th Percentile	95th Percentile
16	46	32	71	28	174	115	258
17	52	35	79	29	194	128	288
18	58	39	88	30	217	143	320
19	64	44	98	31	243	159	357
20	72	49	109	32	271	177	397
21	80	54	122	33	302	197	442
22	90	61	135	34	338	219	493
23	100	67	151	35	377	244	549
24	112	75	168	36	421	272	611
25	125	83	187	37	470	302	680
26	140	93	208	38	525	336	758
27	156	103	232				

From Barbera A, Galan HL, Ferrazzi E, et al: Relationship of umbilical vein blood flow to growth parameters in the human fetus. Am J Obstet Gynecol 1999;181:174-179.

a patient at risk for intrauterine growth restriction.

References

1. Rizzo G, Arduini D, Romanini C: Umbilical vein pulsations: a physiologic finding in early gestation. Am J Obstet Gynecol 1992;167:675-677.
2. Gerson AG, Wallace DM, Stiller RJ, et al: Doppler evaluation of umbilical venous and arterial blood flow in the second and third trimesters of normal pregnancy. Obstet Gynecol 1987;70:622-626.
3. Hecher K, Campbell S, Doyle P, et al: Assessment of fetal compromise by Doppler ultrasound investigation of the fetal circulation. Arterial, intracardiac, and venous blood flow velocity studies. Circulation 1995;91:129-138.
4. Gudmundsson S, Huhta JC, Wood DC, et al: Venous Doppler ultrasonography in the fetus with nonimmune hydrops. Am J Obstet Gynecol 1991;164:33-37.
5. DeVore GR, Brar HS, Platt LD: Doppler ultrasound in the fetus: a review of current applications. J Clin Ultrasound 1987;15:687-703.
6. Bellotti M, Pennati G, De Gasperi C, et al: Simultaneous measurements of umbilical venous, fetal hepatic, and ductus venosus blood flow in growth-restricted human fetuses. Am J Obstet Gynecol 2004;190:1347-1358.
7. Rigano S, Bozzo M, Ferrazzi E, et al: Early and persistent reduction in umbilical vein blood flow in the growth-restricted fetus: a longitudinal study. Am J Obstet Gynecol 2001;185:834-838.
8. Barbera A, Galan HL, Ferrazzi E, et al: Relationship of umbilical vein blood flow to growth parameters in the human fetus. Am J Obstet Gynecol 1999;181:174-179.
9. Gill RW, Kossoff G: Pulsed Doppler combined with B-mode imaging for blood flow measurement. Contrib Gynecol Obstet 1979;6:139-141.
10. Eik-Nes SH, Marsal K, Brubakk AO, et al: Ultrasonic measurement of human fetal blood flow. J Biomed Eng 1982;4:28-36.
11. Van Lierde M, Oberweis D, Thomas K: Ultrasonic measurement of aortic and umbilical blood flow in the human fetus. Obstet Gynecol 1984;63:801-805.
12. Gill RW, Trudinger BJ, Garrett WJ, et al: Fetal umbilical venous flow measured in utero by pulsed Doppler and B-mode ultrasound. I. Normal pregnancies. Am J Obstet Gynecol 1981;139:720-725.
13. Griffin D, Cohen-Overbeek T, Campbell S: Fetal and utero-placental blood flow. Clin Obstet Gynaecol 1983;10:565-602.
14. Erskine RL, Ritchie JW: Quantitative measurement of fetal blood flow using Doppler ultrasound. Br J Obstet Gynaecol 1985;92:600-604.

Fetal Ductus Venosus

Introduction

The ductus venosus is a conduit that drains oxygenated blood returning from the placenta via the umbilical vein to the left atrium through the foramen ovale (Fig. 43-1). As a result of the increased velocity of blood flow through the ductus venosus, this vessel can easily be identified using color Doppler ultrasound (Fig. 43-2).[1] Volume flow studies of the ductus venosus have been reported.[2-4] However, analysis of the ductus venosus waveform provides information relating to compliance of the right ventricle and is used clinically.[4-12] During ventricular systole, pressure in the right atrium is lower than the ductus venosus, resulting in forward flow from this vessel into the right atrium through the foramen ovale and into the left atrium. This is represented by the S wave (Fig. 43-3). At the completion of ventricular systole the tricuspid valve opens, allowing blood to flow from the right atrium into the right ventricle during the passive filling of ventricular diastole. This is represented by the D wave (see Figure 43-3). During this phase of the cardiac cycle streaming blood from

the ductus venosus continues, as it did during ventricular systole, to cross the foramen ovale into the left atrium. At the end of the rapid filling phase of diastolic filling, the right atrium contracts against a partially filled right ventricle. During this process the pressure in the left atrium is greater than the right atrium, thus closing the foramen ovale. Because of the stiffness of the right ventricle, there is increased resistance to blood entering the right ventricle. This results in the A wave of the ductus venosus waveform (see Figure 43-3). While the A wave is a normal finding, an increase in ventricular stiffness may result in a larger A wave than normal. The origin of the abnormal A wave resulting from a stiff right ventricle was demonstrated by DeVore and Horenstein[1] in 1993 when they reported that the A wave of the ductus venosus waveform was normal in a fetus with a hypoplastic left ventricle but abnormal in a fetus with a hypoplastic right ventricle. The A wave in a fetus with a hypoplastic right ventricle is the most severe form of a "stiff" right ventri-

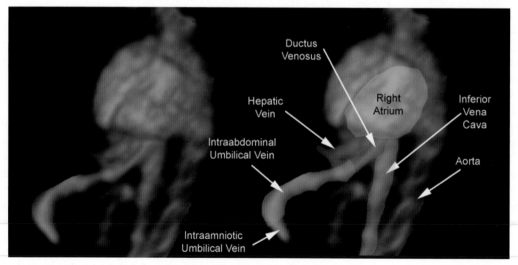

Figure 43-1
This is a three-dimensional B-flow image from a 17-week fetus illustrating the relationships of the venous system, heart, and aorta.

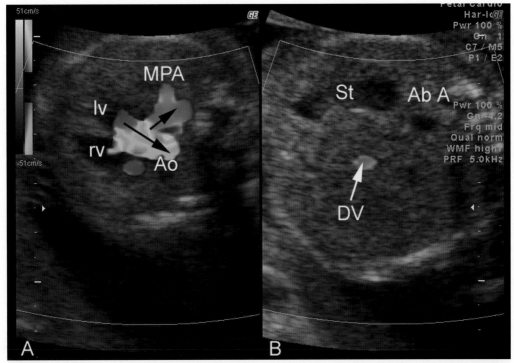

Figure 43-2
Identification of the ductus venosus using color Doppler ultrasound. Because of the increased velocity of the ductus venosus when compared with other vessels within the abdomen, the ductus venosus is easy to identify. One method is to examine the outflow tracts (*A*), using a Doppler setting that does not result in aliasing. In this example, the Doppler velocity is 51 cm/sec. When the abdomen is imaged in a transverse plane (*B*) the ductus venosus "lights up" (*DV*) because of its higher velocity. The other vessels within the abdomen do not "light up" with the color Doppler because of their lower velocity. If, however, the velocity setting were set lower, then the other vessels within the abdomen would become apparent. *Ab A*, abdominal aorta; *Ao*, ascending aorta; *DV*, ductus venosus; *LV*, Left ventricle; *MPA*, main pulmonary artery; *RV*, right ventricle; *St*, stomach.

cle. Under these circumstances, the A wave demonstrates absent or reverse flow during atrial systole.[1] Measurement of an abnormal A wave, therefore, identifies a "stiffer" right ventricle, which has been observed in fetuses with intrauterine growth restriction who may be compromised.[4-11]

Quantitative Assessment of the Ductus Venosus

Several authors have measured blood flow through the ductus venosus concomitant with measurement of blood flow through the intra-abdominal portion of the umbilical vein to determine the net blood flow to the liver.[2,3] Although this may have research implications, it may not be practical for the clinician.

Qualitative Assessment of the Inferior Vena Cava

Investigators have focused primarily on the relationships between the three velocity components (S, D, a) and the time-average maximal velocity (Tamx) of the ductus venosus waveform. A number of investigators have reported normal individual curves for ductus venosus indices.[1-4,6-8,10,12,13] In 1996 Rizzo et al[12] published their results after studying 209 normal fetuses and 89 with growth restriction. They measured six different indices and found that all were significantly different between control and IUGR fetuses. However, when using receiver operator curve analysis to determine which of the venous measurements (inferior vena cava vs. ductus venosus) identified the high-risk fetus, they found that all venous Doppler indices

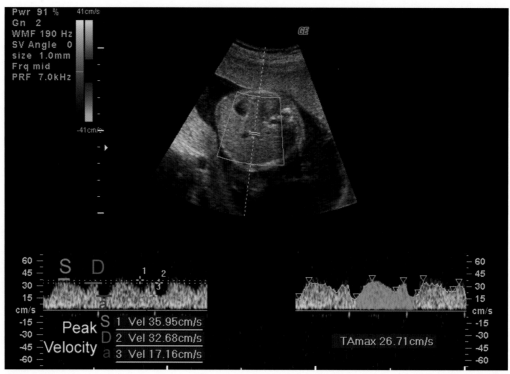

Figure 43-3

Ductus venosus Doppler waveform. The sample volume is placed within the ductus venosus. The Doppler waveform consists of the S (*S*), D (*D*), and a (*a*) waves. The S wave represents ventricular systole, the D wave the early filling phase of ventricular diastole, and the wave atrial contraction. The peak velocity for each of the waveforms is represented as follows: S = 1, D = 2, a = 3. The Tmax (time average maximal velocity) is the area under the waveform (*green overlay*).

Table 43-1	Equations for the ductus venosus[6]			
Index	**Regression Equation**	**Standard Deviation**	**R²**	**P Value**
Preload index	$0.00061 \times GA + 0.5197$	0.1	0.1332	0.0001
Peak velocity index	$-0.0006 \times GA + 0.592$	0.12	0.1582	0.0001
Pulsatility index	$-0.001 \times GA + 0.6625$	0.14	0.1638	0.0001
S/a	$-0.0023 \times GA + 2.2073$	0.50	0.0526	0.0005

GA, Gestational age in weeks. To compute the 95th and 5th percentiles multiply the standard deviation by 1.66.

were associated with acidemia.[12] However, hypoxemia was significantly associated with the preload index (a/S) and S/A ratio of the ductus venosus.[12] In 2003 Baschat[6] evaluated 237 normal fetuses and examined four indices for the ductus venosus. This study demonstrated a linear relationship between the indices and gestational age (Tables 43-1 to 43-5) (Figs. 43-4 to 43-7).[6] In 2004 Baschat et al[7] used the same indices to determine if they could predict fetal acidemia at birth in high-risk fetuses by sampling the umbilical artery following delivery of a nonlaboring patient. They found that although

the inferior vena cava preload index (a/S) had the largest area under the receiver operator curve for predicting fetal academia (pH < 7.2), the ductus venosus indices also had a significant area under the ROC curve for predicting acidemia.[7] The reason this is important is because the examiner may not be able to obtain Doppler waveforms of the inferior vena cava but still can evaluate the ductus venosus. This allows for a versatile approach when examining the high-risk fetus.

Figure 43-8 is a worksheet of Doppler indices that may be useful when examining a high-risk fetus.

Table 43-2 Ductus venosus preload index (a/S)[6]

Gestation (wks)	Pre-Load Index (a/S)		
	5th Percentile	50th Percentile	95th Percentile
20	0.342	0.508	0.674
21	0.341	0.507	0.673
22	0.341	0.507	0.673
23	0.340	0.506	0.672
24	0.339	0.505	0.671
25	0.339	0.505	0.671
26	0.338	0.504	0.670
27	0.338	0.504	0.670
28	0.337	0.503	0.669
29	0.336	0.502	0.668
30	0.336	0.502	0.668
31	0.335	0.501	0.667
32	0.335	0.501	0.667
33	0.334	0.500	0.666
34	0.333	0.499	0.665
35	0.333	0.499	0.665
36	0.332	0.498	0.664
37	0.332	0.498	0.664
38	0.331	0.497	0.663
39	0.330	0.496	0.662
40	0.330	0.496	0.662

Table 43-3 Ductus venosus peak velocity index (S-a)/D[6]

Gestation (wks)	Peak Velocity Index (S-a)/D		
	5th Percentile	50th Percentile	95th Percentile
20	0.381	0.580	0.779
21	0.380	0.579	0.779
22	0.380	0.579	0.778
23	0.379	0.578	0.777
24	0.378	0.578	0.777
25	0.378	0.577	0.776
26	0.377	0.576	0.776
27	0.377	0.576	0.775
28	0.376	0.575	0.774
29	0.375	0.575	0.774
30	0.375	0.574	0.773
31	0.374	0.573	0.773
32	0.374	0.573	0.772
33	0.373	0.572	0.771
34	0.372	0.572	0.771
35	0.372	0.571	0.770
36	0.371	0.570	0.770
37	0.371	0.570	0.769
38	0.370	0.569	0.768
39	0.369	0.569	0.768
40	0.369	0.568	0.767

Table 43-4 Ductus venosus pulsatility index (S-a)/Tamx[6]

Gestation (wks)	Pulsatility Index (S-a)/Tamx		
	5th Percentile	50th Percentile	95th Percentile
20	0.410	0.643	0.875
21	0.409	0.642	0.874
22	0.408	0.641	0.873
23	0.407	0.640	0.872
24	0.406	0.639	0.871
25	0.405	0.638	0.870
26	0.404	0.637	0.869
27	0.403	0.636	0.868
28	0.402	0.635	0.867
29	0.401	0.634	0.866
30	0.400	0.633	0.865
31	0.399	0.632	0.864
32	0.398	0.631	0.863
33	0.397	0.630	0.862
34	0.396	0.629	0.861
35	0.395	0.628	0.860
36	0.394	0.627	0.859
37	0.393	0.626	0.858
38	0.392	0.625	0.857
39	0.391	0.624	0.856
40	0.390	0.623	0.855

Table 43-5 Ductus venosus S/a[6]

Gestation (wks)	S/a		
	5th Percentile	50th Percentile	95th Percentile
20	1.331	2.161	2.991
21	1.329	2.159	2.989
22	1.327	2.157	2.987
23	1.324	2.154	2.984
24	1.322	2.152	2.982
25	1.320	2.150	2.980
26	1.318	2.148	2.978
27	1.315	2.145	2.975
28	1.313	2.143	2.973
29	1.311	2.141	2.971
30	1.308	2.138	2.968
31	1.306	2.136	2.966
32	1.304	2.134	2.964
33	1.301	2.131	2.961
34	1.299	2.129	2.959
35	1.297	2.127	2.957
36	1.295	2.125	2.955
37	1.292	2.122	2.952
38	1.290	2.120	2.950
39	1.288	2.118	2.948
40	1.285	2.115	2.945

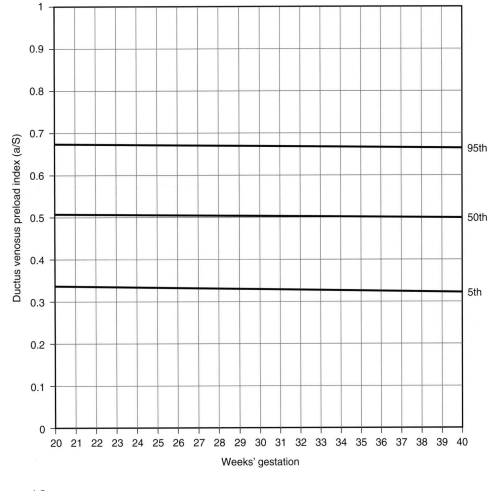

Figure 43-4
Preload index of the ductus venosus. To compute this index, divide the a wave peak velocity by the S wave peak velocity.

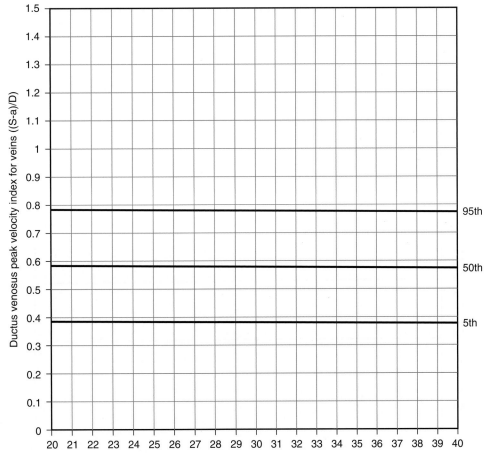

Figure 43-5
Peak velocity index of the ductus venosus. To compute this index subtract the a wave velocity from the S wave velocity and then divide the value by the D wave velocity.

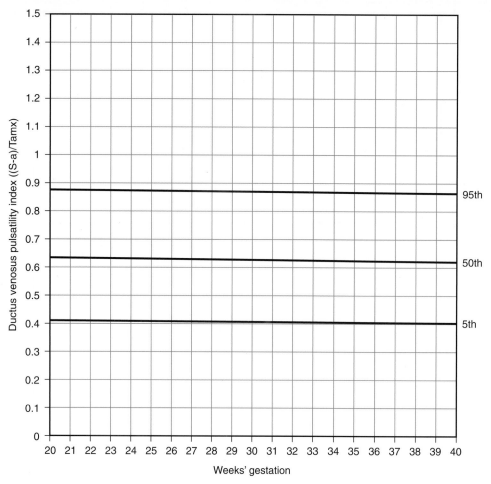

Figure 43-6
Pulsatility index of the ductus venosus. To compute this index subtract the a wave velocity from the S wave velocity and then divide this value by the time average mean velocity.

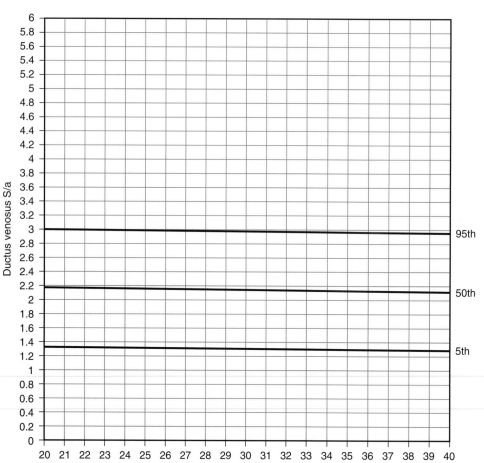

Figure 43-7
S/a of the ductus venosus. To compute this index subtract the S wave velocity from the a wave.

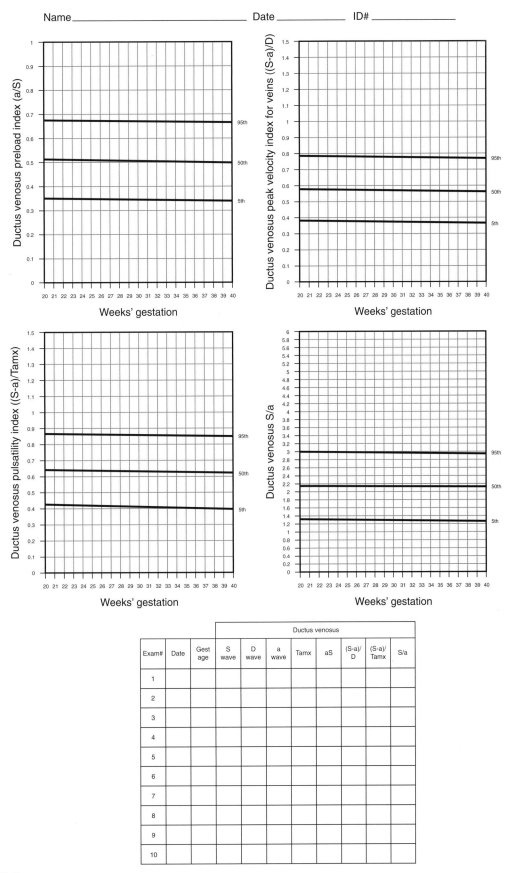

Figure 43-8
Patient flow sheet.

References

1. DeVore GR, Horenstein J: Ductus venosus index: a method for evaluating right ventricular preload in the second-trimester fetus. Ultrasound Obstet Gynecol 1993;3:338-342.

2. Bellotti M, Pennati G, De Gasperi C, et al: Simultaneous measurements of umbilical venous, fetal hepatic, and ductus venosus blood flow in growth-restricted human fetuses. Am J Obstet Gynecol 2004;190:1347-1358.

3. Kiserud T, Rasmussen S, Skulstad S: Blood flow and the degree of shunting through the ductus venosus in the human fetus. Am J Obstet Gynecol 2000;182:147-153.

4. Bahlmann F, Wellek S, Reinhardt I, et al: Reference values of ductus venosus flow velocities and calculated waveform indices. Prenat Diagn 2000;20:623-634.

5. Baschat AA, Gembruch U, Harman CR: The sequence of changes in Doppler and biophysical parameters as severe fetal growth restriction worsens. Ultrasound Obstet Gynecol 2001;18:571-577.

6. Baschat AA: Relationship between placental blood flow resistance and precordial venous Doppler indices. Ultrasound Obstet Gynecol 2003;22:561-566.

7. Baschat AA, Guclu S, Kush ML, et al: Venous Doppler in the prediction of acid-base status of growth-restricted fetuses with elevated placental blood flow resistance. Am J Obstet Gynecol 2004;191:277-284.

8. Hecher K, Campbell S, Doyle P, et al: Assessment of fetal compromise by Doppler ultrasound investigation of the fetal circulation. Arterial, intracardiac, and venous blood flow velocity studies. Circulation 1995;91:129-138.

9. Hecher K, Bilardo CM, Stigter RH, et al: Monitoring of fetuses with intrauterine growth restriction: a longitudinal study. Ultrasound Obstet Gynecol 2001;18:564-570.

10. Rizzo G, Capponi A, Arduini D, Romanini C: Ductus venosus velocity waveforms in appropriate and small for gestational age fetuses. Early Hum Dev 1994;39:15-26.

11. Rizzo G, Capponi A, Arduini D, Romanini C: The value of fetal arterial, cardiac and venous flows in predicting pH and blood gases measured in umbilical blood at cordocentesis in growth retarded fetuses. Br J Obstet Gynaecol 1995;102:963-969.

12. Rizzo G, Capponi A, Talone PE, et al: Doppler indices from inferior vena cava and ductus venosus in predicting pH and oxygen tension in umbilical blood at cordocentesis in growth-retarded fetuses. Ultrasound Obstet Gynecol 1996;7:401-410.

13. Okura I, Miyagi Y, Tada K, et al: The relationship between Doppler indices from inferior vena cava and hepatic veins in normal human fetuses. Acta Med Okayama 2003;57:77-82.

Gynecology

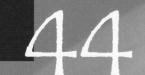

CHAPTER 44

Maria Fogata

Female Pelvic Organ Measurements (Ovaries, Uterus, Endometrium)

Adult Ovaries/Uterus

Introduction

Knowledge of normal measurement of ovaries, uterus, and endometrial stripe is important in detecting gynecologic abnormalities. This chapter reviews the normal measurements of adult ovaries, uterus, and endometrial thickness. Measurements vary depending on menopausal status, age, parity, gravidity, and years since menopause. Endometrial stripe variation in different menstrual cycles and in the postmenopausal period is also discussed. Hormone replacement therapy and tamoxifen effect on endometrium is reviewed.

Adult Ovaries

Materials/Measurements

Cohen et al[1] performed transabdominal pelvic ultrasound using different machines with a 3- to 7-MHz transducer. Tepper et al[2] performed endovaginal ultrasound with an SSD-680 (Aloka Ltd. Tokyo, Japan) and a 5-MHz transducer, while Merz et al[3] used Combison 330 (Kretztechnik, Austria) and a 7.5-MHz endovaginal probe. Cohen et al[1] and Merz et al[3] both studied pre- and postmenopausal patients without ovarian abnormalities, while Tepper et al[2] studied healthy postmenopausal female ovaries.

Ovarian volume was measured using the prolate ellisoid formula—length × width × height × 0.523.[1-3] Table 44-1 shows adult ovarian volume based on menstrual status and age. Table 44-2 lists ovarian volume in postmenopausal women as a function of years since menopause. Table 44-3 shows postmenopausal ovarian volume equal to or less than 5 or greater than 5 years since menopause.

DISCUSSION

Cohen et al[1] noted that ovarian volume significantly differs with menstrual status, with an average adult ovarian volume of 9.8 cm and 5.8 cm³ in menstruating and postmenopausal groups, respectively. Ovarian volume peaked in the 3rd decade of life and declined afterwards. No significant differences were seen between right and left ovaries, presence of uterine myoma, or phase of menstrual cycle.[1] Cohen et al[1] also found out that visualization of ovaries decreases with age from 71% in menstruating patients to 48% in postmenopausal patients.

Tepper et al[2] showed that ovarian volumes decreased from 8.6 cm³ in the first year postmenopausal to 2.2 cm³ after more than 15 years postmenopause. Tepper et al's[2] study showed that both ovaries were visualized in 97% of healthy postmenopausal patients. Merz et al[3] showed small but significant differences in

Table 44-1 Adult ovarian volumes

Age, Decade	Parameter	
	No. of Ovaries	Mean Volume (cm^3 ± SD)
1	19	1.7 ± 1.4
2	83	7.8 ± 4.4
3	308	10.2 ± 6.2
4	358	9.5 ± 5.4
5	206	9.0 ± 5.8
6	57	6.2 ± 5.7
7	44	6.0 ± 3.8
	Menstrual Status	
	No. of Ovaries	Mean Volume (cm^3 ± SD)
Menstruating	866	9.8 ± 5.8
Postmenopausal	100	5.8 ± 3.6

Modified from Cohen HL, Tice HM, Mandel FS: Ovarian volumes measured by US: bigger than we think. Radiology 1990;177:189-192.

Table 44-2 Postmenopausal ovarian volume

Years since menopause	No. of Ovaries	Age Range (Years)	Mean Volume (cm^3 ± SD)
Perimenopause	33	48-54	8.6 ± 2.3
1-2	56	49-57	6.2 ± 2.7
3-4	30	53-58	5.2 ± 1.6
5-6	36	54-59	4.0 ± 1.8
7-8	36	55-60	3.1 ± 1.3
9-10	31	58-63	2.8 ± 2.1
11-12	28	60-74	2.4 ± 1.3
13-14	27	64-68	2.2 ± 1.3
≥15	34	60-78	2.2 ± 1.4

Modified from Tepper R, Zalel Y, Markov S, et al: Ovarian volume in postmenopausal women—suggestions to an ovarian size nomogram for menopausal age. Acta Obstet Gynecol Scand 1995;74:208-211.

Table 44-3 Ovarian volumes based on years since menopause

Years Since Menopause	No. of Ovaries	Mean Volume (cm^3 ± SD)
≤5 years	44	Right 3.4 ± 1.3 Left 3.8 ± 1.6
>5 years	64	Right 2.5 ± 1.3 Left 2.5 ± 1.1

Modified from Merz E, Miric-Tesanic D, Bahlmann F, et al: Sonographic size of uterus and ovaries in pre- and postmenopausal women. Ultrasound Obstet Gynecol 1996;7:38-42.

ovarian volume equal to or less than 5 or greater than 5 years since menopause. No significant differences were seen between left and right ovarian volume in pre- and postmenopausal women.[3]

Adult Uterus

Materials/Measurements

Langlois[4] obtained uterine measurements from 468 pathological reports of hysterectomy specimens, while Platt et al[5] and Merz et al[3] measured uterine size in pre- and postmenopausal patients using real-time ultrasound machines and 3- to 7.5-MHz transducer. The study group did not have more than 1 cm myoma or significant abnormalities. Merz et al's[3] study group did not have hormone replacement treatment.

Langlois[4] obtained uterine size, volume, and weight of hysterectomy specimens and grouped

them on the basis of age, gravidity, and parity, while Platt et al[5] and Merz et al[3] measured uterine size by endovaginal ultrasound and evaluated patients on the basis of menopausal status, parity, and years since menopause. Uterine volume was calculated using the formula: length × width × height × 0.523, where cervix is included in the total length.

Table 44-4 shows adult uterus measurements based on age, gravidity, and parity.[4]

Adult uterine weights are shown on Table 44-5 based on menopausal status, and on Table 44-6 based on parity and years since menopause.[3,5]

Table 44-4 Adult uterine measurements by age, gravidity, and parity

Group	Number of Patients	Linear Measurements (cm ± SD)			Weight (gm)
		Length	Width	Height	
Age					
10-19	3	8.0 ± 0.0	5.0 ± 0.5	2.8 ± 0.7	56.0 ± 13.9
20-29	68	9.2 ± 1.6	5.5 ± 0.8	4.1 ± 0.8	107.0 ± 34.5
30-39	223	9.4 ± 1.5	5.7 ± 1.5	4.1 ± 1.5	114.9 ± 36.1
40-49	114	9.5 ± 1.1	5.9 ± 1.1	4.2 ± 1.1	118.1 ± 44.7
50-59	38	8.1 ± 1.8	5.0 ± 1.2	3.2 ± 1.2	84.3 ± 41.9
60+	15	8.0 ± 1.9	4.5 ± 0.8	2.8 ± 0.8	56.1 ± 20.3
Gravidity					
0	22	7.6 ± 1.4	4.7 ± 0.5	2.8 ± 0.9	61.1 ± 21.6
1	23	8.1 ± 1.4	4.8 ± 1.0	3.3 ± 1.0	82.7 ± 40.0
2-3	138	9.0 ± 1.2	5.5 ± 1.2	3.9 ± 1.2	100.9 ± 36.2
4-5	123	9.4 ± 1.1	5.8 ± 1.1	4.2 ± 1.1	114.7 ± 39.3
6+	155	9.6 ± 1.2	5.9 ± 1.2	4.2 ± 1.2	124.5 ± 38.3
Parity					
0	30	7.7 ± 1.1	4.7 ± 0.5	2.9 ± 1.1	63.2 ± 21.4
1	26	8.6 ± 1.5	5.0 ± 1.0	3.5 ± 1.0	90.4 ± 39.8
2-3	173	9.2 ± 1.3	5.6 ± 1.3	3.9 ± 1.3	104.1 ± 36.0
4-5	115	9.4 ± 1.1	5.8 ± 1.1	4.2 ± 1.1	118.5 ± 42.2
6+	117	9.7 ± 1.1	5.9 ± 1.1	4.2 ± 1.1	125.7 ± 36.9

Modified from Langlois PL: The size of the normal uterus. J Reprod Med 1970;4:220-228.

Table 44-5 Adult uterine weights based on menopausal status

Group	Number of Patients	Weight (g ± SD)
Premenopausal by parity		
0	9	60 ± 20
1	9	109 ± 26
2	18	108 ± 28
3	12	121 ± 35
>4	13	130 ± 35
Total	61	109 ± 37
Group	**Number of Patients**	**Weight (g ± SD)**
Postmenopausal by years since menopause		
0-5	15	84 ± 22
5-10	18	58 ± 21
10-20	19	56 ± 27
>20	24	43 ± 18
Total	76	58 ± 26

Modified from Platt JF, Bree RL, Davidson D: Ultrasound of the normal nongravid uterus: correlation with gross and histopathology. J Clin Ultrasound 1990;18:15-19.

Table 44-6 Uterine measurements by parity and years since menopause

Group Pre-menopause by Parity	UTERINE LENGTH	Uterine Size in cm (SD) CORPUS Length	Width	Height	CERVIX Length	Width	Height
Para 0 (*N* = 52)	7.3 (0.8)	4.4 (0.6)	4.0 (0.6)	3.2 (0.5)	2.9 (0.5)	2.9 (0.5)	2.6 (0.4)
Para 1 (*N* = 50)	8.3 (0.8)	4.9 (0.6)	4.6 (0.5)	3.9 (0.5)	3.4 (0.5)	3.3 (0.5)	2.7 (0.4)
Para ≥ 2 (*N* = 53)	9.2 (0.8)	5.6 (0.9)	5.1 (0.5)	4.3 (0.6)	3.7 (0.6)	3.4 (0.5)	3.0 (0.6)

Group Post-menopause by Years since Menopause	UTERINE LENGTH	Uterine Size in cm (SD) CORPUS Length	Width	Height	CERVIX Length	Width	Height
≤5 years (*N* = 44)	6.7 (0.7)	3.8 (0.5)	3.6 (0.5)	3.1 (0.4)	2.9 (0.4)	2.7 (0.5)	2.4 (0.4)
>5 years (*N* = 64)	5.6 (0.9)	3.3 (0.6)	3.1 (0.5)	2.5 (0.4)	2.4 (0.5)	2.3 (0.4)	2.1 (0.4)

Modified from Merz E, Miric-Tesanic D, Bahlmann F, et al: Sonographic size of uterus and ovaries in pre- and postmenopausal women. Ultrasound Obstet Gynecol 1996;7:38-42.

DISCUSSION

In Platt et al's[5] study the calculated uterine volume correlated with the actual measured volume without statistically significant difference seen. Their study showed that mean uterine density (weight in grams/volume in ml) of 1.03 was not significantly different from 1, so the uterine weight of 1 g is equivalent to 1 ml in volume.[5]

Langlois[4] found increasing uterine weight with increased age and increased gravidity and parity of six or more up to 49 years with decreased uterine weights afterwards. Merz et al[5] showed the parity-related enlargement of uterine size in premenopausal group and decreased uterine size seen in postmenopausal state on the basis of years since menopause.

Adult Endometrial Stripe

Introduction

Measurement of the endometrial thickness is easily performed with ultrasound. Measurement of the endometrial thickness is important to detect a number of benign and malignant endometrial abnormalities.

Materials/Measurements

Endovaginal ultrasound is the best method of measuring the endometrial stripe. A 5 to 7.5 MHz is used and endometrial thickness is measured in the sagittal midline with the calipers placed at the maximal anteroposterior diameter of the echogenic interface of endometrium and inner myometrium[6,7] (Fig. 44-1). If there is fluid in the endometrial cavity, only the sum of the double endometrial layer (anterior and posterior) is included for the measurements, excluding the fluid[6] (Fig. 44-2).

The reproducibility of the endometrial thickness by transvaginal ultrasound was studied by Delisle et al[7] and Bredell et al.[6] Delisle et al[7] found excellent reproducibility of endometrial stripe measurement with 95% intraobserver agreement and 94% interobserver agreement.[7] Bredella et al[6] found that reproducibility of endometrial thickness is due to variability in ultrasound measurements and the experience of the examiner. They found that interobserver variation in measuring endometrial stripe varied up to 2 mm among experienced readers and varied up to 18 mm between experienced and inexperienced observers.[6] Common technical errors to avoid are inadequate depth setting with a large field of view and inaccurate caliper placement.[6]

ENDOMETRIUM IN PREMENOPAUSE WOMEN

Materials/Measurments

Endometrium varies in different phases of the menstrual cycle. During menstruation, endometrium is a 1- to 4-mm thin echogenic line.[8,9] In the proliferative phase of the menstrual cycle (day 6 to 14), endometrium thickness is 5 to 7 mm and becomes more echogenic compared with myometrium.[8] In the periovulatory phase, the endometrium becomes multilayered in appearance and measures up to 11 mm.[8] The multilayered appearance is due to bright echogenic central line of apposed endometrial canal, the hypoechogenic band of endometrium and bright echogenic basal layer.[8,9] During the secretory phase of the menstrual cycle (days 15

ENDOMETRIAL THICKNESS

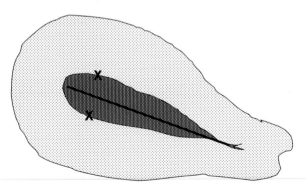

Figure 44-1
Endometrial stripe measurement. Diagram of the uterus in sagittal midline with the central portion of the calipers placed at the maximal endometrial thickness, including both endometrial layers.

ENDOMETRIAL THICKNESS

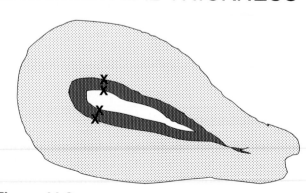

Figure 44-2
Endometrial stripe measurement excluding fluid in the endometrial cavity.

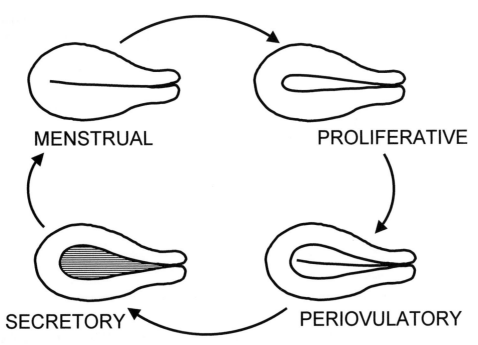

Figure 44-3

Menstrual cycle and endometrium. Endometrium is a thin echogenic 1- to 4-mm line during the menstrual cycle. It becomes thicker, 5 to 7 mm more echogenic during the proliferative phase. On periovulatory cycle, a multiplayer endometrium, up to 11-mm thick is seen. Endometrium is thickest in secretary phase, measuring up to 7 to 14 mm.[8,10]

to 28), the endometrium becomes thicker (7 to 16 mm) and more echogenic.[8,10] Figure 44-3 shows the endometrial stripe variability in the different phases of the menstrual cycle.[8,10]

ENDOMETRIUM IN POSTMENOPAUSE

Materials/Measurements

Many studies have been done on postmenopausal endometrial thickness. Smith-Bindman et al[11] did a literature search of prospective endovaginal ultrasound measurement of endometrial stripe prior to biopsy in postmenopausal patients with vaginal bleeding. A total of 35 studies involving 5892 females were included in the study with a mean age of 61 years.[11] Lin et al,[12] Levine et al,[13] and Karlsson et al[15] also studied postmenopausal endometrium using

endovaginal ultrasound. Lin et al[12] and Levine et al[13] studied 112 and 120 asymptomatic self-referred postmenopausal patients older than 50 years old, 1 year postmenopause. Karlsson et al[15] evaluated the endometrial stripe of 1168 postmenopausal bleeding patients (mean age of 64) before endometrial curettage.[14]

Endovaginal ultrasound was used to measure endometrial thickness. Lin et al[12] and Levine et al[13] excluded endometrial cavity fluid from the endometrial stripe measurement, while Karlsson et al[15] did not exclude the endometrial fluid. Table 44-7 shows endometrial thickness in asymptomatic postmenopausal patients as studied by Lin et al[12] and Levine et al.[13] Table 44-8 shows endometrial thickness of postmenopausal patients with vaginal bleeding with biopsy correlation.[14,15]

DISCUSSION

Smith-Bindman et al[11] in their literature search of endometrial thickness by endovaginal ultrasound found that using a 5-mm threshold to define abnormal endometrium, 96% (95% confidence interval) of women with cancer had

abnormal endovaginal ultrasound, while 92% (95% confidence interval) of women with endometrial disease (cancer, polyp, atypical hyperplasia) had an abnormal result.[11] Smith-Bindman et al[11] also noted that postmenopau-

Table 44-7	Endometrium in asymptomatic postmenopausal women		
Study Group	**No. of Patients**	**Mean (mm) ± SD**	**Range**
Lin			
No hormone	58	5.2 ± 4.5	0.1-25
Unopposed estrogen	10	6.8 ± 5.3	0.1-14
Continuous estrogen & progesterone	9	5.3 ± 1.7	2-7
Sequential estrogen & progesterone	35	6.6 ± 3.9	0.1-17
Levine			
No hormone	61	5.0 ± 2.9	1-18
Unopposed estrogen	7	6.6 ± 4.0	1-13
Continuous estrogen & progesterone	15	6.2 ± 2.4	1-13
Sequential estrogen & progesterone	40	8.3 ± 3.9	1-18

Note: A measurement of 0.1 mm was used to indicate that endometrium was not visible.
Modified from Lin MC, Gosink BB, Wolf SI, et al: Endometrial thickness after menopause: effect of hormone replacement. Radiology 1991;180:427-432; and Levine D, Gosink BB, Johnson LA: Change in endometrial thickness in postmenopausal women undergoing hormone replacement therapy. Radiology 1995;197:603-608.

Table 44-8	Endometrium in postmenopausal patients with vaginal bleeding		
Biopsy Results	**No. of Patients**	**Mean (mm) ± SD**	**Range**
Atrophy	667	3.9 ± 2.5	1-22
Hormonal effect	77	7.8 ± 4.0	2-28
Endometrial polyp	140	12.9 ± 8.1	2-53
Endometrial cancer	114	21.1 ± 11.8	5-68
Hyperplasia	112	12.0 ± 6.0	2-72
Other	19	15.1 ± 7.9	7-35

Modified from Keats TE, Sistrom C: Atlas of Radiologic Measurement, 7th ed. St Louis, Mosby, 2001.

sal patients with vaginal bleeding with a 10% pretest probability of endometrial cancer would have a 1% cancer probability following a normal endovaginal ultrasound.[11] They concluded that endovaginal ultrasound has a high sensitivity for detecting endometrial disease and can identify postmenopausal women with vaginal bleeding who are unlikely to have significant endometrial disease so that endometrial sampling may be unnecessary. Karlsson et al[15] also used 5 mm as the cut-off value, below which the risk of endometrial abnormality is low (5.5%). They also suggested refraining from curettage when endometrial stripe is equal to or less than 4 mm.[15] Therefore correct caliper placement for endometrial thickness and reproducibility of measurement is clinically important. Delisle et al,[7] however, advised that single value of stripe be interpreted with caution when found to be within 1 mm of the cut-off value. Endometrial stripe measurement should also be correlated with the overall clinical picture before deciding the patient's measurement. Levine et al[13] proposed an algorithm for postmenopausal management on the basis of endometrial thickness, women's symptoms (bleeding or not bleeding), and use of hormone (Fig. 44-4)[14]. Note that this proposed flow chart may be modified on the basis of the patients' complete clinical picture.

In addition to hormone replacement therapy, other reported factors affecting endometrium variability in postmenopausal endometrium include years since menopause, tamoxifen use, body weight and BMI, and being Japanese.[16-21] Warming et al,[16] in his endovaginal study of 1182 asymptomatic postmenopausal group, showed that endometrial thickness varies with years since menopause with a mean of 2 to 3 mm during the first 5 years since menopause and then decreases by 0.03 mm per year ($P <$ 0.01). From 5 to 13 years since menopause endometrium stripe remained stable with a

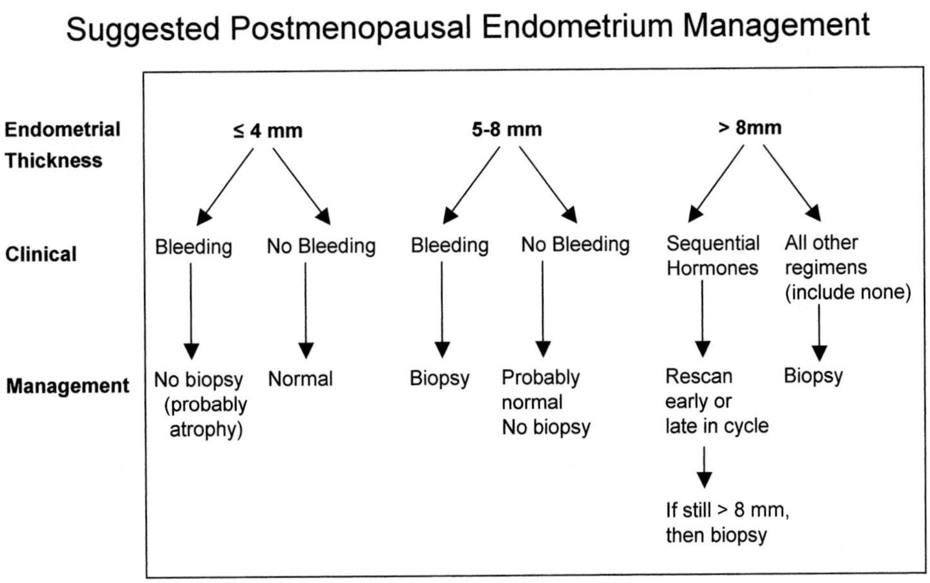

Suggested Postmenopausal Endometrium Management

Figure 44-4
Suggested postmenopausal endometrium management. (From Levine D, Gosink BB, Johnson LA: Change in endometrial thickness in postmenopausal women undergoing hormone replacement therapy. Radiology 1995;197:603-608, Figure 5.)

mean of 1.8 mm, with a minimal increase of 0.01 mm per year (P < 0.05) thereafter.[16]

Ascher et al[17] did a review study on tamoxifen-induced endometrium changes. Tamoxifen is an antiestrogen used as adjuvant chemotherapy in women with breast carcinoma but with contradictory estrogenic effects on female genital symptoms, with increased incidence of subendometrial cysts, hyperplasia, polyps, and endometrial carcinoma.[18] Ascher et al[17] and Lahti et al[19] noted that endometrial thickness in postmenopausal patients taking tamoxifen is greater (9 to 13 mm) compared with untreated postmenopausal patients (4 to 5.4 mm). But since up to 50% of women on tamoxiphen develop endometrial abnormalities within 6 to 36 months of treatment, Ascher et al[17] conservatively chose 4 mm as the upper limit of normal endometrial thickness for these patients. This cut-off value may be modified on the basis of the patient's overall clinical presentation.

Adolph et al,[20] in his study of 300 asymptomatic postmenopausal women, showed that endometrial thickness (>4 mm) is associated with greater body weight and body mass index (BMI).

Tsuda et al[21] studied endometrial thickness differences between occidental and Oriental postmenopausal women and found 3 mm to be the cut-off thickness for detecting endometrial abnormalities in screening Japanese women.

Laifer-Narin et al[22] studied 180 pre- and postmenopausal patients who underwent endovaginal ultrasound and hysterosonogram for abnormal vaginal bleeding showed that 14% of patients showed abnormality (polyp, submucosal myoma) on hysterosonogram, despite normal-appearing endometrium on endovaginal ultrasound. Laifer-Narin et al[22] suggested that patients with abnormal vaginal bleeding should have hysterosonogram, despite normal endovaginal ultrasound findings.

References

1. Cohen HL, Tice HM, Mandel FS: Ovarian volumes measured by US: bigger than we think. Radiology 1990;177:189-192.
2. Tepper F, Zalel Y, Markov S, et al: Ovarian volume in postmenopausal women-suggestions to an ovarian size nomogram for menopausal age. Acta Obstet Gynecol Scand 1995;74:208-211.
3. Merz E, Miric-Tesanic D, Bahlmann F, et al: Sonographic size of uterus and ovaries in pre and postmenopausal women. Ultrasound Obstet Gynecol 1996;7:38-42.
4. Langlois PL: The size of the normal uterus. J Reprod Med 1970;4:220-228.
5. Platt JF, Bree RL, Davidson D: Ultrasound of the normal nongravid uterus: correlation

with gross and histopathology. J Clin Ultrasound 1990;18:15-19.

6. Bredella MA, Feldstein VA, Filly RA, et al: Measurement of endometrial thickness at US in mulicenter drug trials: value of central quality assurance reading. Radiology 2000; 217:516.

7. Delisle MF, Villeneuve M, Boulvain M: Measurement of endometrial thickness with transvaginal ultrasonography: is it reproducible? J Ultrasound Med 199817:481-484.

8. Nalaboff KM. Pellerito JS, Ben-Levi E: Imaging the endometrium: disease and normal variants. Radiographics 2001;21: 1409-1424.

9. Hall DA, Yoder IC Ultrasound evaluation of the uterus. In Callen PW (eds). Ultrasonography in obstetrics and gynecology, 3rd ed. Philadelphia, Saunders, 1994, pp 586-614.

10. McGahan JP, Goldberg BB: Diagnostic Ultrasound: A Logical Approach. Philadelphia, Lippincott-Raven, 1998.

11. Smith-Bindman R, Kerlikowske K, Feldstein VA, et al: Endovaginal ultrasound to exclude endometrial cancer and other endometrial abnormalities. JAMA 1998;280:510-517.

12. Lin MC, Gosink BB, Wolf SI, et al: Endometrial thickness after menopause: effect of hormone replacement. Radiology 1991;180: 427-432.

13. Levine D, Gosink BB, Johnson LA: Change in endometrial thickness in postmenopausal women undergoing hormone replacement therapy. Radiology 1995;197:603-608.

14. Keats TE, Sistrom C: Atlas of Radiologic Measurement. 7th ed. St Louis, Mosby, 2001.

15. Karlsson B, Granberg S, Wikland M, et al: Transvaginal ultrasonography of the endometrium in women with postmenopausal bleeding-a Nordic multicenter study. Am J Obstet Gynecol 1995;172:1488-1494.

16. Warming L, Ravn P, Skouby S, Christiansen C: Measurement precision and normal range of endometrial thickness in a postmenopausal population by transvaginal ultrasound. Ultrasound Obstet Gynecol 2002;20:492-495.

17. Ascher SM, Imaoka I, Lage JM: Tamoxifen-induced uterine abnormalities: the role of imaging. Radiology 2000;214:29-38.

18. Hann LE, Giess CS, Bach AM, et al: Endometrial thickness in tamoxifen-treated patients: correlation with clinical and pathologic findings. AJR Am J Roentgenol 1997;168:657-661.

19. Lahti E, Blanco G, Kauppila A, et al: Endometrial changes in postmenopausal breast cancer patients receiving tamoxifen. Obstetrics & Gynecology 1993;81:660-664.

20. Andolf E, Dahlander K, Aspenberg P: Ultrasonic thickness of the endometrium correlated to body weight in asymptomatic postmenopausal women. Obstetrics & Gynecology 1993;82:936-940.

21. Tsuda H, Kawabata M, Kawabata K, et al: Differences between occidental and oriental postmenopausal women in cutoff level of endometrial thickness for endometrial cancer screening by vaginal scan. Am J Obstet Gynecol 1995;172:1494-1495.

22. Laifer-Narin S, Ragavendra N, Parmenter EK, Grant EG: False-normal appearance of the endometrium on conventional transvaginal sonography: comparison with saline hysterosonography. AJR Am J Roentgenol 2002;178:129-133.

PART

5

Pediatric
Measurements

CHAPTER 45

Rebecca Stein-Wexler

Level of the Conus Medullaris in the Newborn Spine

Introduction

Ultrasound provides an excellent screening tool in infants younger than 3 months with syndromes that place them at risk for spinal dysraphism and in those with the following cutaneous findings: atypical dimples, flat lesions (hemangiomas, cutis aplasia), raised lesions (hairy patches, skin tags/tails), and multiple cutaneous stigmata.[1] Although ultrasound can miss small lipomas of the filum terminale and dermal sinus tracts,[2] most authors support its use as a primary screening tool for tethered cord and spinal dysraphism.[3] In older infants, ossification of dorsal elements obscures portions of the cord, though screening may be successful up to 6 months. Children with covered neural tube defects can be evaluated indefinitely.

Materials/Measurements

The patient is positioned prone, neutral, or gently flexed over a pillow, and two-dimensional spinal ultrasound is performed with a 7.5- to 10-MHz linear probe in sagittal and axial planes. Vertebral level is readily determined by counting up from the lumbosacral junction, the point of transition from the relatively straight lumbar spine to the gently kyphotic sacral vertebrae[4] (Fig. 45-1). It is also possible to count from S5, which is the last large ossified vertebra. Anatomical variants of the lumbosacral spine occur in approximately 7% of patients, influencing the accuracy of both these counting methods.[5] Alternatively, T12 can be assessed by finding the ossified 12th rib, but hypoplastic ribs can be difficult to differentiate from transverse processes, and the incidence of uni- or bilateral 13th ribs is approximately 11%,[6] more than the incidence of lumbosacral anomalies.

DISCUSSION

Conventional wisdom holds that the conus medullaris ascends during the first few months of life from the L3 level to L2/3 or above. However, in a study of 184 MRIs in children newborn to 20 years old, Wilson and Prince[7] found no significant difference in level of the conus, which ranged from T12 to L3.[7] The mean conus level was the L1/2 intervertebral disk space, with two standard deviations including a range from T12 through the L2/3 intervertebral disk.

If the conus does not actually ascend after 40 weeks' gestational age, how significant is its ascent prior to that time; i.e., in the third trimester when premature infants may be imaged? Several authors have addressed this question, with varying results. Wolf et al[8] found a significant difference in conus level in evaluating 59 preterm infants (30 to 39 postmenstrual weeks [PMW]), compared with 55 term infants. Of the preterm group, approximately 65% had the conus at or above L2, 33% from L2/3 to L3, and approximately 2% at L3/4, whereas the term cohort had approximately 94% terminating at or above L2, approximately 4% at L2/3, and 2% at L4. Of the term group, 53% were at L1/2. These results substantiate the commonly held notion that the conus typically ascends to the L1/2 interspace by the 40th PMW and that a conus as low as L2/3 can be considered normal in term neonates. By contrast, in premature infants a conus at L3 would appear to be potentially normal. In a study that included even

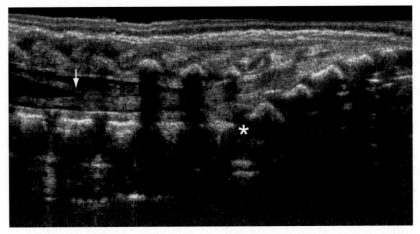

Figure 45-1
Sagittal composite image of the lumbosacral spine demonstrating lumbosacral transition (*) and tip of conus (white arrow).

younger premature infants, Beek et al[9] found that the cord ascends approximately one vertebral level during the third trimester, from the L2/3 interspace at 27 to 29 PMW, to L2 at 30 to 33 PMW, and then to L1/2 in older infants, with no significant trend within the older age group. Hill and Gibson[10] found minimal (0.25 vertebral bodies') ascent from 33 to 42 PMW.

Conflicting data from Sahin et al[11] found no significant difference in conus level between preterm and term infants, with the conus at or above the L2/3 interspace. These authors conclude that in both groups of patients a conus below the L2/3 interspace should be considered abnormal. diPietro[12] found no significant difference in conus level in infants younger than 2 months of age compared with older children, with almost all terminating at or above the mid-L2 level.

Thus in normal infants, a conus as low as the L2/3 interspace may be dismissed, but the L3 vertebral level is more controversial. In a study of adult cadavers, 2% had a conus at L3,[13] and Wilson and Prince[7] found one normal 3-year-old with a conus at L3. But in the cohort of patients with surgically proved tethering, two had a conus as high as L3.[7] By contrast, Hill and Gibson[10] found a conus termination of mid-L3 in 3 of 103 normal infants, at 37 and at 39 PMW.

Taking these papers together, a conus level as low as the L2/3 interspace should be considered normal and a level at L3 probably abnormal. Below L3 is clearly abnormal (Table 45-1). The conus ascends by as much as one vertebral body level during the earlier part of the third trimester, and thus a low conus in a very premature infant may normalize by what would be

Table 45-1	Conus level and filum thickness correlated with clinical significance
Conus level	**Significance**
L2	Normal
L2/3 disk	Normal
L3	Probably abnormal
L3/4 disk	Abnormal
Filum thickness	**Significance**
≤2 mm	Normal
>2 mm	Abnormal

the end of the first trimester. Little, if any, ascent occurs after this time.

Occasionally, a spinal cord can be tethered but terminate at a normal level. This can be suggested if the normal pulsatile motion of the nerve roots of the cauda equina is not observed and also if the filum terminale is positioned relatively posteriorly within the thecal sac. In addition, the configuration of the filum terminale is important, as a thickened filum terminale, measuring more than 2 mm, is considered abnormal and may be associated with tethering or a lipoma.[14]

References

1. Dick EA, de Bruyn R: Ultrasound of the spinal cord in children: its role. Eur Radiol 2003;13:552-562.

2. Kriss VM, Desai NS: Occult spinal dysraphism in neonates: assessment of high-risk cutaneous stigmata on sonography. Am J Roentgenol 1998;171:1687-1692.

3. Rohrschneider WK, Forsting M, Darge K, et al: Diagnostic value of spinal US: comparative study with MR imaging in pediatric patients. Radiology 1996;200:383-388.

4. Beek FJA, van Leeuwen MS, Bax NMA, et al: A method for sonographic counting of the lower vertebral bodies in newborns and infants. AJNR 1994;15:445-449.

5. Ford LT, Goodman FG: X-ray studies of the lumbosacral spine. South Med J 1966;59:1123-1128.

6. Southworth JD, Bersack SR: Anomalies of the lumbosacral junction in five hundred and fifty individuals without symptoms referable to the low back. Am J Roentgenol 1950;64:624-634.

7. Wilson DA, Prince JR: MR imaging determination of the location of the normal conus medullaris throughout childhood. Am J Roentgenol 1989;152:1029-1032.

8. Wolf S, Schneble F, Troger J: The conus medullaris: time of ascendance to normal level. Pediatr Radiol 1992;22:590-592.

9. Beek FJ, de Vries LS, Gerards LJ, et al: Sonographic determination of the position of the conus medullaris in premature and term infants. Neuroradiology 1996;38:(suppl 1):S174-S177.

10. Hill CAR, Gibson PJ: Ultrasound determination of the normal location of the conus medullaris in neonates. Am J Neuroradiol 1995;16:469-472.

11. Sahin F, Selcuki M, Ecin N, et al: Level of conus medullaris in term and preterm neonates. Arch Dis Child Fetal Neonatal Ed 1997;77:F67-F69.

12. diPietro MA: The conus medullaris: normal US findings throughout childhood. Radiology 1993;188:149-153.

13. Reimann AF, Anson BJ: Vertebral level of termination of the spinal cord with report of a case of sacral cord. Anat Rec 1944;88:127-138.

14. Fitz CR, Harwood-Nash DC: The tethered conus. Am J Roentgenol 1970;125:515-523.

CHAPTER 46

Rebecca Stein-Wexler

Measurements of Extra-axial Fluid in the Neonatal Head

Introduction

High-frequency linear array transducers allow exquisitely detailed depiction of fluid over the high convexities, and the question often arises of how much fluid is normal. Excessive fluid may denote atrophy, benign extra-axial fluid of infancy, or pathologic collections.

Materials/Methods

With the patient supine, a high frequency (10- to 12-MHz) linear array transducer is placed over the anterior fontanelle with copious intervening coupling gel. Care must be taken not to compress the fontanelle, as extra-axial fluid is readily distorted and compressed.[1] Three measurements can be determined: craniocortical width (CCW), which measures the distance between the inner table of the calvarium and the surface of the adjacent cortex; sinocortical width (SCW), which measures the distance from the wall of the superior sagittal sinus to the cortical surface; and interhemispheric width (IHW), which measures the widest horizontal distance between the hemispheres across the interhemispheric fissure (Fig. 46-1).

If color Doppler is applied, cortical veins can be recognized coursing through subarachnoid fluid between gyri and calvarium, whereas if the fluid is subdural in location the veins are displaced away from the calvarium.[2]

DISCUSSION

Normal values have been determined for premature infants, term infants, infants up to 1 year

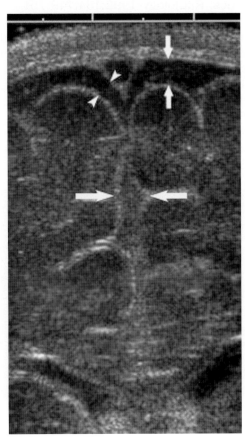

Figure 46-1
Coronal high-resolution image obtained at anterior fontanelle demonstrating CCW (small white arrows), SCW (white arrowheads), and IHW (large white arrowheads).

of age, and those with macrocrania, as shown in Table 46-1.

In a study of preterm infants aged 24 to 36 gestational weeks, Armstrong et al[3] found the SCW to measure less than 3.5 mm. These authors found a general trend toward an increase in the SCW with advancing age at birth, with the SCW increasing on average 0.02 mm per week. A similar but more impressive trend was seen in the amount of subarachnoid fluid as premature infants mature in the extrauterine environment, with SCW increasing 0.2 mm per week. There was no significant difference in head circumference between the two groups, so these findings suggest that decreased brain growth occurs in the extrauterine environment.

Frankel et al[4] studied predominantly term neonates and found CCW to be more reliable than SCW. The CCW ranged from 0 to 3.3 mm, with the mean being 1.6 ± 0.8 mm.[4]

Libicher and Troger[5] evaluated 89 normal infants between 1 and 364 days of age, averaging 105 days, using a 5-MHz transducer. The SCW measured between 0.4 and 3.3 mm, CCW between 0.3 and 6.3 mm, and IHW between 0.5 and 8.2 mm. They found no significant difference between sides (<1 mm). Using the 95% as a cutoff, they recommend 3 mm as the upper limit of normal for SCW, 4 mm as the upper limit of normal for CCW, and 6 mm as the upper limit of normal for IHW.

The ultrasonographer is often requested to evaluate the infant with macrocrania. Fessell et al[6] studied 38 neurologically normal children whose occipital frontal circumference was

Table 46-1	Normal extra axial fluid measurements in infants		
Age	CCW	SCW	IHW
24-36 week premature		<3.5 mm	
Term	<3.3 mm		
<1 year	<4 mm	<3 mm	<6 mm
Macrocrania	<10 mm	<10 mm	

>95%; on follow-up 36 remained neurologically normal, whereas one developed transient head lag that resolved and the other developed stuttering, neither clearly of neurologic etiology. These authors found extra-axial fluid at either SCW or CCW measured less than 10 mm.

References

1. Thomson GD, Teele RL: High-frequency linear array transducers for neonatal cerebral sonography. Am J Roentgenol 2001;176: 995-1001.
2. Chen CY, Chou TY, Zimmerman RA: Pericerebral fluid collection: differentiation of enlarged subarachnoid spaces from subdural collections with color Doppler US. Radiology 1996;201:389-392.
3. Armstrong DL, Bagnall C, Harding JE, et al: Measurement of the subarachnoid space by ultrasound in preterm infants. Arch Dis Child Fetal Neonatal Ed 2002;86:F124-F126.
4. Frankel DA, Fessell DP, Wolfson WP: High resolution sonographic determination of the normal dimensions of the intracranial extraaxial compartment in the newborn infant. J Ultrasound Med 1998;17:411-415.
5. Libicher M, Troger J: US measurement of the subarachnoid space in infants: normal values. Radiology 1992;184:749-751.
6. Fessell DP, Frankel DA, Wolfson WP: Sonography of extraaxial fluid in neurologically normal infants with head circumference greater than or equal to the 95th percentile for age. J Ultrasound Med 2000;19:443-447.

CHAPTER 47

Rebecca Stein-Wexler

Correlation of Cerebellar Measurements and Gestational Age in Neonates

Introduction

Measurement of cerebellar width is an accepted method for determining gestational age in the fetus, and data are now available that allow correlation of vermis and cerebellar body measurements with gestational age in premature neonates as well. Essentially all premature infants undergo cranial ultrasonography as a routine part of their care, and therefore this provides an excellent means of determining gestational age in premature infants without requiring any unusual or additional handling or stress.

Materials/Methods

A 5- to 7-MHz transducer is directed over the anterior fontanelle. A sagittal midline image demonstrates the cerebellar vermis (Fig. 47-1), and vertical length, as well as circumference and area, are readily determined with the help of built-in computer software. Cerebellar body measurements are obtained from a single posterior coronal image (Fig. 47-2) that includes the quadrigeminal plate cistern, also via the anterior fontanelle, and measurements are similarly manipulated.

An alternative approach is via the mastoid (junction of parieto-occipital and lambdoid sutures), just behind the pinna of the ear (Fig. 47-3). A 5- to 7-MHz transducer can be used, but resultant measurements may differ when evaluated with this approach.[1]

DISCUSSION

Cerebellar measurements have been found to increase as a linear function of gestational age between 25 and 41 weeks.[2] These investigators found vermis measurements to be more accurate than those of the cerebellar body, especially in extremely premature neonates, and cerebellar body width was the least meaningful dimension. They suggest the following simple correlation of vermian area with gestational age: 1 cm at 25 weeks, 2 cm at 30 weeks, 3 cm at 35 weeks, and 4 cm at 40 weeks. More precise values are found in Table 47-1.

More recent work on cerebellar body width[3] has found excellent correlation with gestational age (Table 47-2). These authors found cerebellar width much simpler to determine than vermian or cerebellar area or circumference, and they support employing this single value to determine gestational age. They also evaluated neonates small for gestational age, finding that in all, except those with microcephaly, cerebellar diameter correlated fairly well with gestational age.

When evaluated from the mastoid, transverse cerebellar width also shows excellent correlation with gestational age,[1] but the cerebellar measurements for a given age do appear to be smaller when taken from this vantage point (Fig. 47-4).

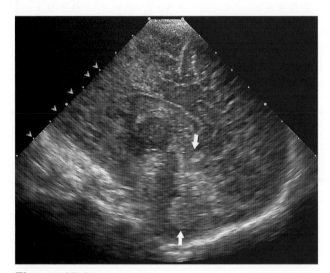

Figure 47-1
Sagittal midline image through anterior fontanelle demonstrates cerebellar vermis (*white arrows*).

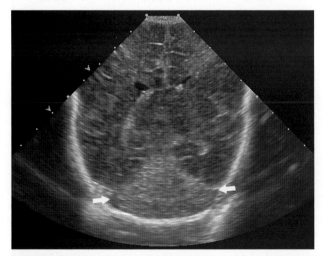

Figure 47-2
Posterior coronal image through anterior fontanelle demonstrates cerebellar body (*white arrows*).

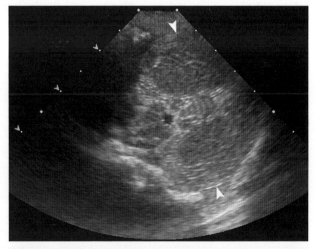

Figure 47-3
Oblique axial image through mastoid demonstrates cerebellar body (*white arrowheads*).

Table 47-1	Gestational age, vermis area, and cerebellar circumference (via anterior fontanelle)[2]				
	Vermis Area (cm)		**Cerebellar Circumference (cm)**		
Gestational Age (wks)	**Mean**	**95% CI**	**Mean**	**95%**	
25	1.07	0.8-1.3	6.88	6.4-7.3	
26	1.27	1.0-1.5	7.21	6.8-7.6	
27	1.46	1.3-1.7	7.53	7.2-7.9	
28	1.66	1.5-1.8	7.87	7.5-8.2	
29	1.86	1.7-2.0	8.19	7.9-8.5	
30	2.05	1.9-2.2	8.52	8.3-8.8	
31	2.25	2.1-2.4	8.85	8.6-9.1	
32	2.45	2.3-2.6	9.18	8.9-9.4	
33	2.64	2.5-2.8	9.50	9.3-9.7	
34	2.84	2.7-3.0	9.83	9.6-10.1	
35	3.03	2.9-3.2	10.16	9.9-10.4	
36	3.23	3.1-3.4	10.49	10.2-10.8	
37	3.43	3.2-3.6	10.82	10.5-11.1	
38	3.62	3.4-3.8	11.14	10.8-11.5	
39	3.82	3.6-4.0	11.47	11.1-11.9	
40	4.02	3.8-4.3	11.80	11.4-12.2	
41	4.21	3.9-4.5	12.12	11.7-12.6	

CI, Confidence interval.

Table 47-2	Measurements of transverse cerebellar diameter (cm) against gestational age in AGA neonates (via anterior fontanellae)[3]					
Gestational Age (wks)	**n**	**Mean**	**Standard deviation**	**10th percentile**	**50th percentile**	**90th percentile**
24-35	9	4	0.24	3.5	3.9	4.3
26-27	12	3.98	0.25	3.8	4	4.4
28	17	4.3	0.35	3.9	4.3	4.7
29	9	4.46	0.21	4	4.5	4.8
30	12	4.59	0.27	4.3	4.55	5
31	18	4.68	0.3	4.3	4.65	5.2
32	29	4.77	0.35	4.3	4.8	5.2
33	34	5.04	0.26	4.7	5	5.4
34	41	5.14	0.32	4.8	5.1	5.6
35	23	5.22	0.36	4.82	5.2	5.6
36	23	5.49	0.25	5.2	5.5	5.8
37	11	5.49	0.32	5.3	5.5	5.9
38	16	5.86	0.18	5.5	5.9	6
39	28	5.89	0.2	5.6	5.9	6.2
40	33	6	0.21	5.7	6	6.2
41-42	19	6	0.2	5.7	6	6.3

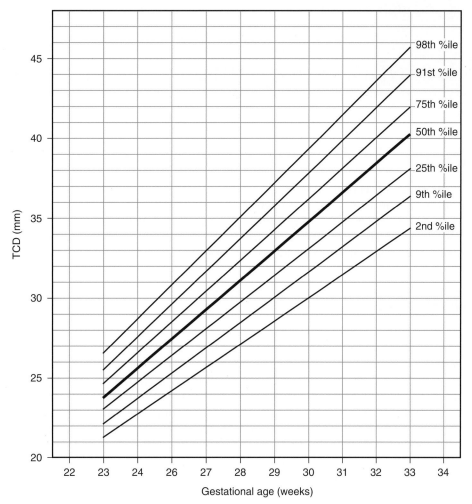

Figure 47-4
Graph displaying transverse cerebellar width assessed via mastoid versus gestational age.[1]

References

1. Davies MW, Swaminathan M, Betheras FR: Measurement of the transverse cerebellar diameter in preterm neonates and its use in assessment of gestational age. Australas Radiol 2001;45:309-312.

2. Co E, Raju TN, Aldana O: Cerebellar dimensions in assessment of gestational age in neonates. Radiology 1991;181:581-585.

3. Makhoul IR, Goldstein I, Epelman M, et al: Neonatal transverse cerebellar diameter in normal and growth-restricted infants. J Matern Fetal Med 2000;9:155-160.

Neonatal Cerebral Ventricles

Introduction

Accurate determination of ventricular size is essential, especially in the preterm infant who is at increased risk for intraventricular hemorrhage and resultant hydrocephalus, and in infants with other etiologies of ventriculomegaly. With the advent of three-dimensional computer-assisted volume rendering, actual ventricular volumes can be determined, and in the future this should provide greater accuracy.

Materials/Methods

For the transtemporal approach, axial-oblique images are obtained with a 3- to 7-MHz sector transducer in a plane approximately 15 degrees oblique to the canthomeatal line. The bodies of the lateral ventricles are readily demonstrated, and hemispheric width is measured from the midline echogenic falx to the echogenic inner table of the skull (Fig. 48-1). The lateral ventricular width is measured from the echogenic lateral wall of the ventricle to the falx, as the medial wall is often not readily identified. However, this technique is rarely employed.[1] Most measurements are now obtained through the anterior fontanelle.

When measurements are acquired through the anterior fontanelle, both sagittal and oblique coronal images are obtained, demonstrating frontal horns, ventricular bodies, posterior lateral ventricles, and third and fourth ventricles as desired. Again a 3- to 7-MHz sector transducer is employed.

DISCUSSION

LATERAL VENTRICLES—TRANSTEMPORAL APPROACH

Johnson et al[1] found the mean lateral ventricular width at the mid-body from a transverse transtemporal approach to be similar for premature and term infants, 1.1 cm for term (range 0.9 to 1.3), and 1 cm for premature infants (range 0.5 to 1.3). The ratio of ventricular width to hemispheric width was also similar; 28% in term and 31% in premature infants. This is consistent with the lateral ventricular ratio found by Garrett et al[2] (0.24 to 0.34). However, this ratio may be inaccurate, in part because of difficulties in determining hemispheric width because of the cranial vault curvature.[3] In addition, medial wall displacement toward the midline can precede displacement of the lateral wall, but this is often difficult to evaluate.[3] Therefore this measurement is rarely used.

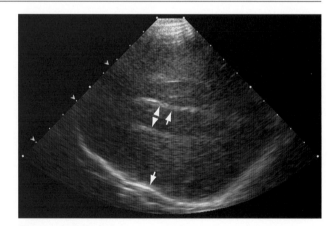

Figure 48-1
Transtemporal oblique-axial image of lateral ventricles, demonstrating lateral ventricular width (*white arrowheads*) and interhemispheric width (*white arrows*).

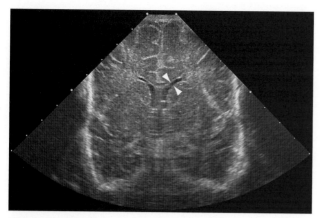

Figure 48-2
Coronal image of ventricular width (*white arrowheads*) of anterior horns of lateral ventricles at level of foramen of Monroe, obtained via anterior fontanelle.

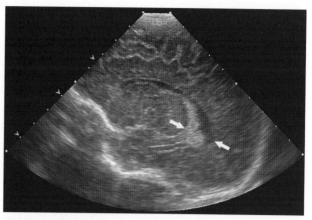

Figure 48-3
Parasagittal image obtained through anterior fontanelle demonstrating atrium and occipital horn of lateral ventricle (*white arrows*).

Table 48-1	Ventricular size determined from anterior fontanelle approach		
Anterior horn width at foramen of Monroe[5]		<3 mm	Premature and term
Atrium and occipital horn of lateral ventricle[5]		8.7-24.7 mm	Premature
Third ventricle[4]		0-2.6 mm	Premature

LATERAL VENTRICLES—ANTERIOR FONTANELLE

From the anterior fontanelle approach, several investigators have evaluated the width of the anterior horn of the lateral ventricle at the level of the foramen of Monroe in the coronal plane, just anterior to the choroid plexus (Fig. 48-2). Davies et al[4] found this measured 0 to 2.9 mm in premature infants, consistent with Perry et al[5], who found a normal width to be less than or equal to 3 mm in both term and preterm infants. According to London et al[6], a normal width is up to 2.5 mm, similar to Liao et al's[7] finding of the normal range being 1.3 to 2.3 mm. It is commonly held that 4 to 6 mm constitutes mild dilatation, 7 to 10 mm moderate, and greater than 10 mm marked dilatation.[8] However, in addition to evaluating measurements, it is essential to note the configuration of the frontal horn, which should be triangular; furthermore, the ventricular walls should be thin.[9]

However, there is also significant interest in scanning the atria of the lateral ventricles, as the posterior portions of the ventricles seem to dilate first with hemorrhagic hydrocephalus.[1,2,10]

Davies et al[4] evaluated the distance between the posterior aspect of the thalamus and tip of the occipital horn on parasagittal scans in premature infants younger than 33 weeks (Fig. 48-3), finding a range of 8.7 to 24.7 mm, with no evidence of size correlating with gestational age.[4] Evaluation of sequential measurements thus allows perception of developing subtle ventriculomegaly, but the range of normal in this area is too great to allow detection of mild initial hydrocephalus by this method. Saliba et al[11] measured the area of the lateral ventricle at mid-body level slightly posteriorly, just before the atria diverge, finding that the area of this region grows linearly with advancing age in premature infants.

Table 48-1 summarizes ventricular size determined via the anterior fontanelle including evaluation of the anterior horn of the lateral ventricle, atrium and occipital horn of the lateral ventricle, and third ventricle.

Several additional issues merit discussion. Asymmetry of the lateral ventricles is common, occurring in approximately 40% to 70% of patients.[7,9] However, this asymmetry is of questionable significance. Ventricular enlargement is sometimes attributed to dependent positioning, but Davies et al[4] found head position had no effect on which ventricle was larger. Ichihashi et al[12] found that the left lateral ventricle is usually the larger, with only a weak correlation with head position.

Another question that has been raised concerns ventricular growth. This issue appears to be more controversial. The fluid content of the ventricular system may increase during the first week as a result of increased CSF production because of changes from fetal low pressure to neonatal high pressure.[11] Liao et al[7] found the lateral span of the lateral ventricles increases linearly with gestational age, but that the frontal horn diameter at level of caudate nucleus (discussed above) does not. Perry et al[5] found that the actual fluid content (ventricular width) of the lateral ventricles is similar in premature and term infants. Employing three-dimensional volume rendering, Csutak et al[13] found a trend toward increased ventricular volume at birth with greater prematurity, but a similar trend was also found in infants at 2 to 6 months post-40 weeks, with the smallest volume at approximately 35 to 45 weeks gestational age. Levene[14] also showed general ventricular enlargement with prematurity.

Another issue commonly encountered concerns complete ventricular effacement (slitlike ventricles). Some have questioned whether this may result from edema, but Patel et al[15] found that 28% of normal premature infants, like term infants,[16] had complete lateral ventricular effacement. Therefore additional findings must be sought, such as altered parenchymal echogenicity or indistinct sulci and fissures, before raising concern for brain edema in the setting of ventricular effacement.

THIRD VENTRICLE

Davies et al[4] measured the third ventricle's transverse diameter in premature infants, finding normal values of 0 to 2.6 mm. Garrett et al[2] evaluated the third ventricle in the transverse plane, finding a maximal width of 5 mm.

References

1. Johnson ML, Mack LA, Rumack cm, et al: B-Mode echoencephalography in the normal and high risk infant. Am J Roentgenol 1979;133:375-381.

2. Garrett WJ, Kossoff G, Warren PS: Cerebral ventricular size in children. Radiology 1980; 136:711-715.

3. Fiske CE, Filly RA, Callen PW: Sonographic measurement of lateral ventricular width in early ventricular dilation. J Clin Ultrasound 1981;9:303-307.

4. Davies MW, Swaminathan M, Chuang SL, et al: Reference ranges for the linear dimensions of the intracranial ventricles in preterm neonates. Arch Dis Child Fetal Neonatal Ed 2000;82:F218-F223.

5. Perry RNW, Bowman ED, Murton LJ, et al: Ventricular size in newborn infants. J Ultrasound Med 1985;4:475-477.

6. London DA, Carroll BA, Enzmann DR: Sonography of ventricular size and germinal matrix hemorrhage in premature infants. Am J Roentgenol 1980;135:559-564.

7. Liao MF, Chaou WT, Tsao LY, et al: Ultrasound measurements of the ventricular size in newborn infants. Brain Dev 1986;8:262-268.

8. Goldberg BB, Kurtz AB: Ultrasound measurements of the central nervous system. In Atlas of Ultrasound Measurements. Chicago, Year Book Medical Publishers, 1990, p 20.

9. Enriquez G, Correa F, Lucaya J, et al: Potential pitfalls in cranial sonography. Pediatr Radiol 2003;33:110-117.

10. Brann BS, Qualls C, Wells L, et al: Asymmetric growth of the lateral cerebral ventricle in infants with posthemorrhagic ventricular dilation. J Pediatr 1991;118:108-112.

11. Saliba E, Bertrand P, Gold F, et al: Area of lateral ventricles measured on cranial ultrasonography in preterm infants: reference range. Arch Dis Child 1990;65:1029-1032.

12. Ichihashi K, Iino M, Eguchi Y, et al: Difference between left and right lateral ventricular sizes in neonates. Early Hum Dev 2002; 68:55-64.

13. Csutak R, Unterassinger L, Rohrmeister C, et al: Three-dimensional volume measurement of the lateral ventricles in preterm and term infants: evaluation of a standardized computer-assisted method in vivo. Pediatr Radiol 2003;33:104-109.

14. Levene M: Measurement of the growth of the lateral ventricles in pre-term infants with real-time ultrasound. Arch Dis Child 1981;56:900-904.

15. Patel MD, Cheng AG, Callen PW: Lateral ventricular effacement as an isolated sonographic finding in premature infants: prevalence and significance. Am J Roentgenol 1995;165:155-159.

16. Winchester P, Brill PW, Cooper R, et al: Prevalence of "compressed" and asymmetric lateral ventricles in healthy full-term infants: ultrasound diagnosis. Am J Roentgenol 1986;146:471-475.

CHAPTER 49

Diane Babcock

Pediatric Patients: Miscellaneous Measurement (Thyroid, Thymus, and Testis)

Introduction

In this chapter measurements of structures in the pediatric patient, not covered in other chapters, are reviewed. The thyroid gland and testis are obtained in a similar technique as in the adult patient.

Thyroid Gland

INTRODUCTION

The normal thyroid gland is located in the neck and is composed of two large lobes to the right and left of the trachea and an isthmus connecting the two inferiorly. The thyroid gland may arrest in descent and be located in a sublingual midline location.

MATERIALS/MEASUREMENTS

Scans are performed with the patient supine and the neck extended. A linear transducer using the highest frequency that will provide adequate penetration of the organ is used. A stand-off pad may be used in older patients. Measurements of both the right and left thyroid lobes are done in transverse, anteroposterior, and superior-caudal dimensions[1,2] (Fig. 49-1). Similar measurements of the isthmus may be made. The volume of each lobe and isthmus is calculated using the formula for a prolate ellipsoid (H × W × L × 0.523). The sums for both lobes and isthmus (if available) are added.

DISCUSSION

Tables 49-1 and 49-2 compare normal thyroid gland volume and thickness as a function of body height.[1,2] Thyroid volume in normal term neonates has also been measured[3,4] (Table 49-3) and ranges from 472 to 1430 mm^3. There is no significant correlation with birth weight.[3]

In the pediatric patient the thyroid gland may be measured in patients with suspected goiter. Its echogenicity is also evaluated, and findings compared with thyroid function test.[5] The thyroid gland may also be evaluated in patients with suspected ectopic sublingual thyroid, particularly searching for presence of the gland in the normal location.

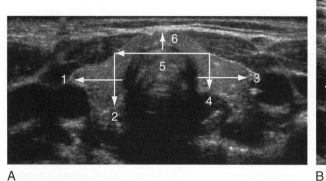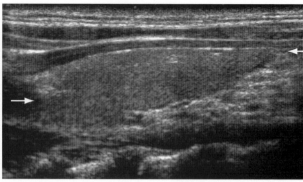

A   B

Figure 49-1
Thyroid Gland
A, Transverse and **B,** longitudinal views. AP and width measurements of both lobes and the isthmus are made on the transverse view. Superior-caudal measurement is made on the longitudinal view. 1 = transverse; 2 = AP of right lobe; 3 = transverse; 4 = AP of left lobe; 5 = transverse; and 6 = AP of isthmus. Superior-caudal dimensions (*arrowheads*).

Table 49-1	The volume of the thyroid gland and thickness of each lobe as a function of body height			
Height (cm)	**n**	**Volume* (cm³)**	**RLT* (cm)**	**LLT* (cm)**
99	16	2.3 ± 0.7	0.8 ± 0.17	0.8 ± 0.18
100-109	34	3.3 ± 1.0	0.8 ± 0.19	0.8 ± 0.21
110-119	35	4.1 ± 1.1	0.9 ± 0.17	0.9 ± 0.19
120-129	45	4.9 ± 1.1	0.9 ± 0.18	0.9 ± 0.20
130-139	36	6.3 ± 2.0	0.9 ± 0.25	1.0 ± 0.25
140-149	42	7.4 ± 2.2	1.0 ± 0.23	1.0 ± 0.23
150-159	59	8.5 ± 2.3	1.1 ± 0.23	1.0 ± 0.24
160	20	10.9 ± 2.5	1.2 ± 0.24	1.2 ± 0.25

LLT, left lobe thickness; RLT, Right lobe thickness.
*Mean ± one standard deviation.
From Ueda D: Normal volume of the thyroid gland in children. J Clin Ultrasound 1990;18:455-462.

Thymus Gland in the Infant

INTRODUCTION

The thymus gland can be easily visualized and measured in neonates and infants up to about 2 years of age.[5] In older children the thymus is relatively smaller and the sternum more ossified, precluding optimum visualization of the mediastinal structures. Adam and Ignotus[6] have reported visualization of the thymus up to 8 years of age.

MATERIALS/MEASUREMENTS

Scans are performed with the patient supine and neck extended. Linear, convex, or sector transducers may be used as needed to image around the sternum. Images are obtained in transverse and longitudinal plane through the maximum size of the thymus gland (Fig. 49-2). The maximum length, width, and AP dimensions are measured.

The thymic index (a sonographic estimate of thymic volume) has been defined as the product of the area (in square centimeters) on longitu-

Table 49-2	Normal dimensions of the thyroid gland as a function of height from neonates to adolescence, and those as a function of corrected gestational weeks in premature neonates

Corrected gestational weeks	No. of Subjects (Male:Female)	Mean ± one standard deviation	
		Thickness (cm)	Width (cm)
30-33	5 (14:1)	0.8 ± 0.1	1.1 ± 0.3
33-37	19 (13:6)	1.1 ± 0.3**	1.4 ± 0.3*
Height (cm)			
45-50	42 (20:22)	1.4 ± 0.2**	1.7 ± 0.2**
50-70	42 (27:15)	1.4 ± 0.1	1.8 ± 0.2
70-90	8 (6:2)	1.4 ± 0.1	1.9 ± 0.1
90-100	8 (3:5)	1.4 ± 0.1	1.8 ± 0.2
100-110	34 (12:22)	1.5 ± 0.3	2.1 ± 0.3
110-120	35 (20:15)	1.7 ± 0.3	2.3 ± 0.3
120-130	45 (23:22)	1.8 ± 0.4	2.4 ± 0.3
130-140	36 (21:15)	1.9 ± 0.5	2.7 ± 0.2
140-150	42 (20:22)	2.1 ± 0.4	2.8 ± 0.3
150-160	59 (25:34)	2.2 ± 0.4	2.8 ± 0.4
160-170	16 (14:2)	2.4 ± 0.4	3.0 ± 0.4

*Compared with 30-33 weeks: *p < 0.05.*
***p < 0.01.*
From Ueda D, et al: Pediatric Radiology 1992;22:102-105.

Table 49-3	Ultrasound measurements of the thyroid gland in 100 healthy newborn infants within the first week of life

	Male infants (n = 49)		Female infants (n = 51)		All infants	
	Mean (SD)	Range	Mean (SD)	Range	Mean (SD)	Range
Length (cm)	R 1.99 (0.22)	1.6-2.5	1.88 (0.26)	0.9-2.5	1.94 (0.24)	0.9-2.5
	L 1.96 (0.21)	1.6-2.4	1.92 (0.27)	0.9-2.4	1.94 (0.24)	0.9-2.4
Breadth (cm)	R 0.87 (0.17)	0.5-1.4	0.86 (0.13)	0.6-1.2	0.87 (0.15)	0.5-1.4
	L 0.89 (0.14)	0.6-1.3	0.88 (0.17)	0.6-1.4	0.89 (0.16)	0.6-1.4
Depth (cm)	R 0.96 (0.12)	0.7-1.3	0.97 (0.20)	0.6-2.0	0.97 (0.16)	0.6-2.0
	L 0.91 (0.13)	0.7-1.2	0.99 (0.20)	0.7-1.9	0.95 (0.17)	0.7-1.9
Volume (ml)	R 0.84 (0.24)	0.3-1.4	0.78 (0.22)	0.5-1.7	0.81 (0.23)	0.3-1.7
	L 0.79 (0.19)	0.4-1.3	0.84 (0.29)	0.4-1.7	0.82 (0.24)	0.4-1.7
Total volume (ml)	1.63 (0.37)	0.7-2.4	1.61 (0.44)	1.0-3.3	1.62 (0.41)	0.7-3.3

The length, breadth, depth, and volume are given for each lobe along with the combined volume of the two lobes (L, left lobe; R, Right lobe).
From Perry RJ, Hollman AS, et al: Ultrasound of the thyroid gland in the newborn: normative data. Arch Dis Child Fetal Neonatal Ed 2002;87:F209-F211.

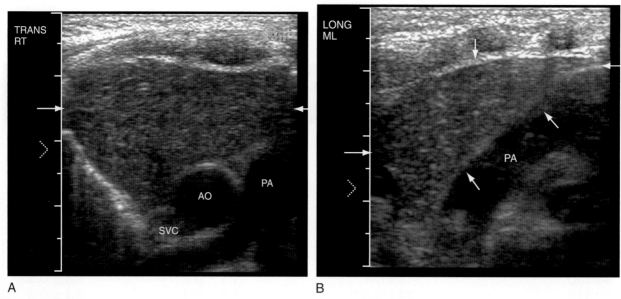

A   B

Figure 49-2
Thymic index determination.
A, Transverse image showing transverse diameter (*arrows*). **B,** Longitudinal image with perimeter (*arrows*) traced for area determination. The thymic index was defined as the product of these two measurements. *AO,* aorta; *PA,* Pulmonary artery; *SVC,* superior vena cava.
(From Hasselbalch H, Nielsen MB, Jeppesen D, et al: Sonographic measurement of the thymus in infants. Eur Radiol 1996;6:700-703.)

dinal scan of the largest lobe and the transverse diameter (in centimeters) of both lobes.[5] It can be used to estimate thymic volume in the infant.[7] Area is measured by tracing its perimeter. The thymic index has been shown to correlate well with thymic weight and volume in a postmortem study.[5]

DISCUSSION

The thymus gland may be asymmetric, with one lobe larger than the other. AP and longitudinal measurements of right and left lobes versus age have been reported (Fig. 49-3).[6] From 2 to 8 years of age the mean AP and longitudinal measurements were 1.4 and 2.5 for the right lobe and 1.4 and 2.9 for the left lobe.[6] Hasselbalch et al have published the thymic index by age, weight, and feeding status (Table 49-4).[7-10] The thymic index correlates with the weight in the healthy newborn.[7] It increases from birth to 4 and 8 months of age and then decreases.[9] It tends to be greater in breast-fed infants.[10] Extremely preterm infants initially had a very low thymic index, but when healthy they reached the normal range.[8]

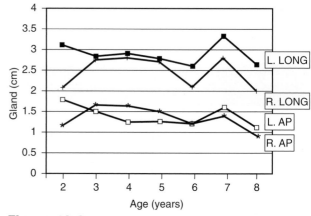

Figure 49-3
Graph shows mean anteroposterior (AP) and longitudinal (long) measurements in centimeters of right (R) and left (L) lobes of thymus plotted against ages of the 50 subjects in this study. (From Adam EJ, Ignotus PI: Sonography of the thymus in healthy children: frequency of visualization, size, and appearance. Am J Roentgenol 1993;161:153-155.)

Table 49-4	Thymic index from birth to 2 years by age and feeding status					
	Birth	**4 MO**	**8 MO**	**10 MO**	**12 MO**	**24 MO**
Median	11.8 (8.3-13.6)	25.7	29.0	18.9	17.3	21.2
Overall mean	11.9	26.3	26.6	18.9	18.3	21.1
Exclusively breast-fed infants		36.34 (27.6-56.1)	27.41 (23.7-36.9)	23.52 (18.4-35.9)	17.7 (14.5-37.4)	22.2 (20.1-29.6)
Partially breast-fed infants		26.50 (20.3-27.6)	23.76 (14.4-29.6)	16.53 (12.4-17.8)	21.0 (12.4-25.8)	19.7 (11.0-24.1)
Exclusively formula-fed infants		18.89 (14.4-28.3)	28.99 (23.5-40.0)	17.33 (13.7-23.6)	16.5 (8.7-25.3)	21.6 (16.8-21.0)
Feeding status p values		0.0002	0.5387	0.0140	0.4662	0.4218

5th and 95th percentiles are given in parentheses.
From Hasselbalch H, Ersboll AK, Jeppesen DL, Nielsen MB: Thymus size in infants from birth until 24 months of age evaluated by ultrasound. A longitudinal prediction model for the thymic index. Acta Radiol 1999;40:41-44.

Although the size of the thymus gland may be measured, more often sonography is requested to determine if a mediastinal mass is normal thymus or an abnormal mass. The infant thymus has a typical sonographic appearance of multiple branching linear echogenic structures representing connective tissue septa and slightly heterogeneous parenchyma. The echogenic medulla and relatively hypoechoic cortices may be differentiated with high-frequency transducers.[11]

Pediatric Testis

INTRODUCTION

In the pediatric patient, testicular volume is routinely measured and evaluated for symmetry.

MATERIALS/MEASUREMENTS

Scans are performed in transverse and longitudinal planes using high-frequency linear transducers. The scrotum may be supported with a towel, and a stand-off pad may be used. If the testes are not identified within the scrotum, the inguinal area up to the peritoneal cavity is imaged for a nondescended testis. Longitudinal, transverse, and AP dimensions are obtained (Fig. 49-4). Testicular volume is determined

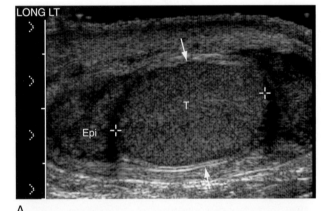

A

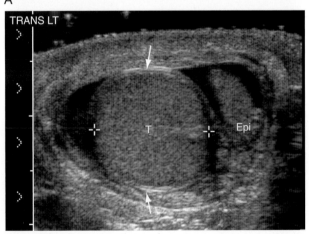

B

Figure 49-4
Testis measurements:
A, Longitudinal and **B,** transverse scans. Long axis (+), width (+), and AP dimension (*arrowheads*) measured. *T,* Testis, *Epi,* epididymis.

Table 49-5	Testicular volumes, mean ± SE, during the first 6 months of life													
	Age (mo)													
	Birth		**1**		**2**		**3**		**4**		**5**		**6**	
Size	**L**	**R**	**L**	**R**	**L**	**R**	**L**	**R**	**L**	**R**	**L**	**R**	**L**	**R**
Mean	1.10	1.10	1.80	1.60	2.00	2.05	2.05	1.95	1.85	1.80	1.75	1.70	1.55	1.50
SD	0.14	0.10	0.11	0.10	0.12	0.09	0.15	0.11	0.13	0.13	0.11	0.11	0.13	0.07
Significance			L	←	P < 0.001		→		P < 0.05					
			R	←	P < 0.0025				P < 0.001					

From Cassorla FG, et al: Testicular volume during early infancy. J Pediatr 1981;99:742-743.

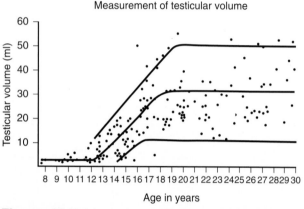

Measurement of testicular volume

Figure 49-5
The effect of chronological age on testicular volume. (From Rundle AT, Sylvester PE: Measurement of testicular volume. Its application to assessment of maturation, and its use in diagnosis of hypogonadism. Arch Dis Child 1962;37:514-517.)

Table 49-6	Testicular volumes in 348 adolescents	
Sex maturity	**Volume (cm³)**	
rating*	**Left testis**	**Right testis**
1	Mean 4.76	Mean 5.20
	SD 2.76	SD 3.86
2	Mean 6.4	Mean 7.08
	SD 3.16	SD 3.89
3	Mean 14.58	Mean 14.77
	SD 6.54	SD 6.1
4	Mean 19.8	Mean 20.45
	SD 6.17	SD 6.79
5	Mean 28.31	Mean 30.25
	SD 8.52	SD 9.64

*Mean of genital and pubic hair ratings.
From Daniel WA Jr, et al: Testicular volumes of adolescents. J Pediatr 1982;101:1010-1012.

using the formula for a prolate ellipsoid: volume = length × width × height × 0.523.

Normal testicular size in newborns[12] (Table 49-5) and compared with age[13] has been reported. The volume increases at puberty, usually beginning around 12 years of age, reflecting the hormonal status (Fig. 49-5). Other authors have reported testicular volume versus sexual development stage[14] (Table 49-6).

DISCUSSION

Testicular volume is routinely measured but of limited clinical use because the organ is easily palpable if located within the scrotum. An undescended testis may not be palpable, and measurement becomes more important. The undescended testis is often smaller. Testicular volume may also be important on sequential examinations in patients with significant varicoceles. Lack of normal growth may be used as an indication for surgical correction.

References

1. Ueda D: Normal volume of the thyroid gland in children. J Clin Ultrasound 1990;18: 455-462.
2. Ueda D, Mitamura R, Suzuki N, et al: Sonographic imaging of the thyroid gland in congenital hypothyroidism. Pediatr Radiol 1992; 22:102-105.
3. Vade A, Gottschalk ME, Yetter EM, et al: Sonographic measurements of the neonatal

thyroid gland. J Ultrasound Med 1997;16:
395-399.

4. Perry R.J, Hollman AS, Wood AM, et al:
Ultrasound of the thyroid gland in the new-
born: normative data. Arch Dis Child Fetal
Neonatal Ed 2002;87:F209-F211.

5. Hasselbalch H, Nielsen MB, Jeppesen D,
et al: Sonographic measurement of the thymus in infants. Eur Radiol 1996;6:700-703.

6. Adam EJ, Ignotus PI: Sonography of the
thymus in healthy children: frequency of
visualization, size, and appearance. Am J
Roentgenol 1993;161:153-155.

7. Hasselbalch H, Jeppesen DL, Ersboll AK,
et al: Sonographic measurement of thymic
size in healthy neonates. Relation to clinical
variables. Acta Radiol 1997;38:95-98.

8. Hasselbalch H, Jeppesen DL, Ersboll AK,
et al: Thymus size in preterm infants evaluated by ultrasound. A preliminary report.
Acta Radiol 1999;40:37-40.

9. Hasselbalch H, Jeppesen DL, Ersboll AK,
et al: Thymus size evaluated by sonography.

A longitudinal study on infants during the
first year of life. Acta Radiol 1997;38(2):
222-227.

10. Hasselbalch H, Ersboll AK, Jeppesen DL, et
al: Thymus size in infants from birth until
24 months of age evaluated by ultrasound.
A longitudinal prediction model for the
thymic index. Acta Radiol 1999;40:41-44.

11. Han BK, Suh YL, Yoon HK: Thymic ultrasound. I. Intrathymic anatomy in infants.
Pediatr Radiol 2001;31:474-479.

12. Cassorla FG, Golden SM, Johnsonbaugh
RE, et al: Testicular volume during early
infancy. J Pediatr 1981;99:742-743.

13. Rundle AT, Sylvester PE: Measurement of
testicular volume. Its application to assessment of maturation, and its use in diagnosis of hypogonadism. Arch Dis Child 1962;
37:514-517.

14. Daniel WA Jr, Feinstein RA, Howard-Peebles
P, et al: Testicular volumes of adolescents.
J Pediatr 1982;101:1010-1012.

CHAPTER 50

Diane Babcock

Pediatric Pylorus

Introduction

Hypertrophic pyloric stenosis (HPS) is an idiopathic condition in which the antropyloric
portion of the stomach becomes abnormally
thickened, resulting in obstruction to gastric
emptying. It affects young infants in the 2- to
10-week age group. The patients are normal at
birth and develop nonbilious vomiting as the
muscle hypertrophies and gastric outlet obstruction progresses. Both ultrasound and upper GI
can be used to diagnose the condition. Sonography has the advantage of using nonionizing
radiation and of directly imaging the thickness
of the pyloric muscle.[1]

Materials/Measurements

Scans are performed with the patient supine
or right side down decubitus position. A high-
frequency linear transducer is used (Fig. 50-1).

The patient is examined before and after oral
feeding with a clear liquid such as glucose
water. Real-time observation of gastric empty-

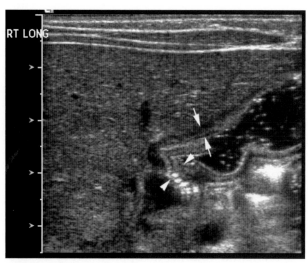

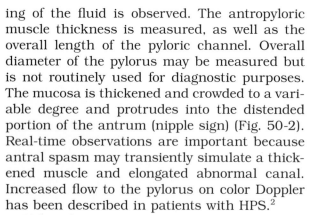

Figure 50-1
Normal pylorus. Scan through the long axis of the antrum (*A*) and pylorus. Pyloric muscle thickness is measured as a hypoechoic layer between the serosa and echogenic submucosa (*arrows*). Pyloric channel length is measured (*arrow*). D, Duodenal bulb.

ing of the fluid is observed. The antropyloric muscle thickness is measured, as well as the overall length of the pyloric channel. Overall diameter of the pylorus may be measured but is not routinely used for diagnostic purposes. The mucosa is thickened and crowded to a variable degree and protrudes into the distended portion of the antrum (nipple sign) (Fig. 50-2). Real-time observations are important because antral spasm may transiently simulate a thickened muscle and elongated abnormal canal. Increased flow to the pylorus on color Doppler has been described in patients with HPS.[2]

Although many measurement criteria have been described (Tables 50-1 and 50-2),[1-3] a muscle thickness of greater than 4 mm and a pyloric channel length greater than 17 mm are considered abnormal (see Fig. 50-2), measurements between 3 and 4 mm as gray zone, and measurements less than 2 mm as normal (see Fig. 50-1).

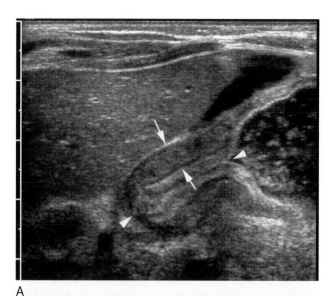

A

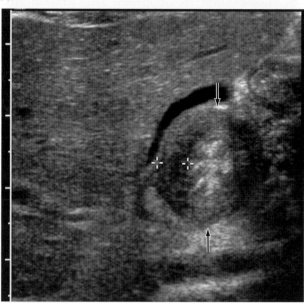

B

Figure 50-2
Hypertrophic pyloric stenosis. **A,** Longitudinal scan demonstrates thickened hypertrophic muscle layer (arrows) and elongated pyloric channel (*arrow*). **B,** Transverse image demonstrates thickened hypertrophic muscle (+) surrounding echogenic submucosa. Pylorus AP dimension measured from serosa to serosa (*arrow*).

DISCUSSION

Patients with hypertrophic pyloric stenosis generally present between 1 and 2 months of age with new onset of projectile vomiting. Ultrasound can be used accurately to diagnose or exclude pyloric stenosis. Occasional patients will be in the gray zone in muscle thickness and may require further imaging with upper GI or a follow-up examination if symptoms persist. If the clinical history is not highly suggestive of hypertrophic pyloric stenosis, an upper GI can

Table 50-1	Measurements of pyloric muscle thickness				
			MUSCLE THICKNESS		
Reference	**Category**	**No.**	**Mean ± SD**	**Range**
Stunden[1]	No HPS	88	1.6 ± 0.4	1.0-3.0
	HPS	112	3.4 ± 0.7	3.0-5.0
Blumhagen[2]	No HPS	210	1.8 ± 0.4	1.0-3.0
	HPS	108	4.8 ± 0.6	3.5-6.0
Lund Kofoed[3]	Control	34	3.5 ± 1.0	2.0-6.0
	No HPS	5	4.1 ± 1.5	3.0-6.0
	HPS	29	6.4 ± 1.1	5.0-10.0
Westra[4]	Control	28		1.0-3.0
	No HPS	25		1.0-3.0
	HPS	22	4.8 ± 0.1	3.0-7.0
Davies[5]	No HPS	10	2.1 ± 0.6	1.0-3.0
	HPS	15	4.3 ± 0.63	3.0-5.6
van der Schouw[6]	No HPS	45	2.6 ± 0.17	
	HPS	60	5.3 ± 0.31	
Hernandez-Schulman[7]	Spasm	7	2.04 ± 0.45	1.3-2.7
	HPS	66		3.0-7.0
Hallan[8]	Control	92	2.0	1.0-3.0
	No HPS	26	2.4	1.5-3.5
	HPS	21	4.0	2.5-5.5
Cohen[9]	Spasm-maximal	34	0.9 ± 1.0	0.0-2.9
	Spasm-maximal	34	3.8 ± 1.0	1.5-6.0
	HPS	37	5.3 ± 0.9	3.0-7.7
Combined (with refs 8 or 9)	No HPS	355	1.9 ± 0.42	1.0-6.0
Combined	HPS	352	4.8 ± 0.69	2.5-10.0

All measurements are in millimeters. Mean ± standard deviation and ranges are given except for Hallam, which are median values, and van der Schouw (mean ± standard error). HPS, Hypertrophic pyloric stenosis; spasm, pylorospasm.
From Keats TE, Sistrom C: Atlas of Radiologic Measurement, 7th ed. St Louis, Mosby, 2001, pp 1-623.

Table 50-2	Measurements of pyloric channel length				
			Channel Length		
Reference	**Category**	**No.**	**Mean ± SD**	**Range**
Stunden[1]	No HPS	88	8.3 ± 2.5	5.0-14.0
	HPS	112	22.3 ± 2.3	18.0-28.0
Blumhagen[2]	No HPS	210	11.3 ± 3.2	5.0-22.0
	HPS	108	17.8 ± 2.6	11.0-25.0
Westra[4]	Control	28	11.6 ± 2.0	8.0-15.0
	No HPS	25	13.0 ± 2.5	9.0-17.0
	HPS	22	19.5 ± 3.1	15.0-26.0
Davies[5]	No HPS	10	10.0 ± 2.4	6.0-12.5
	HPS	15	17.4 ± 2.8	12.0-22.7
van der Schouw[6]	No HPS	45	7.9 ± 0.92	
	HPS	60	18.8 ± 0.53	
Hernandez-Schulman[7]	Spasm	7	12.3 ± 0.15	10.0-14.0
	HPS	66		12.0-30.0
Cohen[9]	Spasm-maximal	34	3.5 ± 3.7	0.0-15.0
	Spasm-maximal	34	14.4 ± 4.7	3.4-27.0
Combined (with refs 8 or 9)	HPS	37	22.5 ± 3.6	14.0-31.0
Combined	No HPS	378	10.4 ± 2.7	5.0-22.0
	HPS	420	20.0 ± 2.5	10.0-31.0

All measurements are in millimeters. Mean ± standard deviation and ranges are given except for van der Schouw (mean ± standard error). HPS, Hypertrophic, stenosis; spasm, pylorospasm.
From Keats TE, Sistrom C: Atlas of Radiologic Measurement, 7th ed. St Louis, Mosby, 2001, pp 1-623.

be performed instead, as other causes of vomiting, such as gastroesophageal reflux and midgut volvulus, can also be diagnosed.

Although the length of the hypertrophic channel and muscle thickness are measured, the overall morphology of the canal and real-time observations are important. The measurable muscle thickness may vary during the examination, and HPS is diagnosed when the muscle thickness is 3 mm or more throughout the examination. The intervening lumen of the pylorus is filled with crowded and redundant mucosa. Gastric peristaltic activity may be increased and fails to distend the preduodenal portion of the stomach.

References

1. Hernanz-Schulman M: Infantile hypertrophic pyloric stenosis. Radiology 2003;227:319-331.
2. Hernanz-Schulman M, Zhu Y, Stein SM, et al: Hypertrophic pyloric stenosis in infants: US evaluation of vascularity of the pyloric canal. Radiology 2003;229:389-393.
3. Keats TE, Sistrom C: Atlas of Radiologic Measurement, 7th ed. St Louis, Mosby, 2001, pp 1-623.

CHAPTER 51

Diane Babcock

Pediatric Kidneys

Introduction

In the pediatric patient, renal length is routinely measured on all examinations. Renal length is compared with normal charts versus age, height, or weight and with prior studies to evaluate for interval growth.

Materials/Measurements

Images of the kidneys are obtained with convex or linear transducers using the highest frequency that will penetrate the structure (Fig. 51-1). In the pediatric patient the kidneys are imaged in both the supine and prone positions. The supine image allows optimal visualization of the upper pole, but the lower pole may be obscured by bowel gas. The echogenicity of the kidney can also be compared with the adjacent liver and spleen. The prone image allows optimal visualization of the lower pole of the kidney, but the upper pole may be obscured by overlying ribs or aerated lungs in the costophrenic angle.

Measurement is made in craniocaudal dimension (see Fig. 51-1). The maximum renal length obtained on either the supine or prone images is used and is plotted against age. In cases where the patient is unusually tall or short for age, the renal length may be plotted against patient height or weight.

Kidney volume may be determined by obtaining a transverse image through the mid-kidney and measuring AP and transverse dimensions through the mid-kidney (see Fig. 51-1). The volume formula for an ellipsoid is used: kidney volume = length × width × height × 0.523.

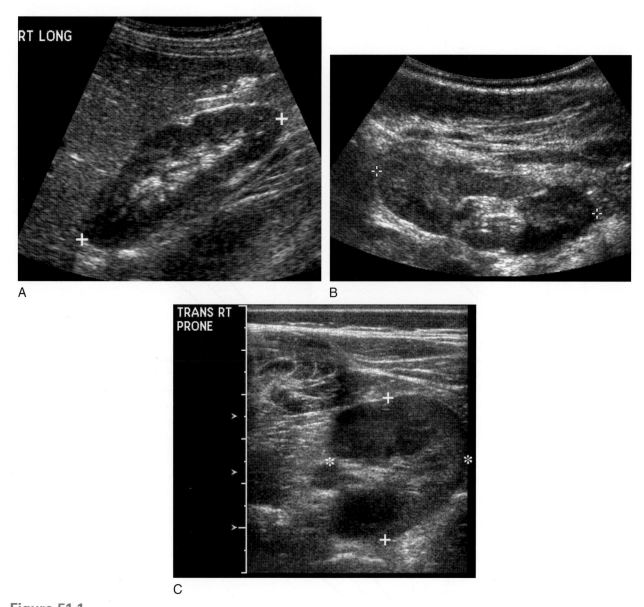

Figure 51-1
Renal length.
A, Longitudinal supine and **B,** Longitudinal prone scans. Measurement is made in maximum craniocaudal dimension (+). **C,** Transverse prone scan through mid-kidney measuring AP (+) and transverse (*) dimensions.

DISCUSSION

Several references are available for normal renal size including length and volume[1-4] (Figs. 51-2 to 51-4, Tables 51-1 and 51-2). Table 51-1 correlates renal length with the average age from birth to 19 years. There was a gradual increase in the mean renal length with age to a near plateau as an older teenager. Similar data are correlated with body height in centimeters and age in months in Tables 51-2 and 51-3.

Data on normal renal length versus gestational age and birth weight in newborn infants, including premature infants, have also been published[5,6] (Fig. 51-5, Table 51-4). The data in Table 51-4 are collected for premature infants with body weights up to 3000 g. Renal length increases with maturity to a range between 4.4 and 5.5 cm for the near-term infant. Similar data are obtained in the chapter on fetal renal length.

Compensatory renal growth of a single functioning kidney occurs in utero, and this relative size increase continues throughout infancy and

Text continued on p. 274

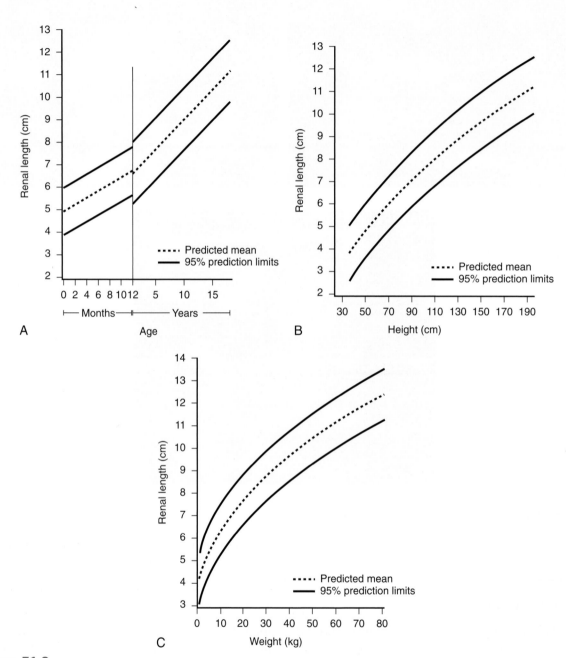

Figure 51-2
Renal length versus **(A)** age, **(B)** height and **(C)** weight. (From Han BK, Babcock DS: Sonographic measurements and appearance of normal kidneys in children. Am J Roentgenol 1985;145:611-616.)

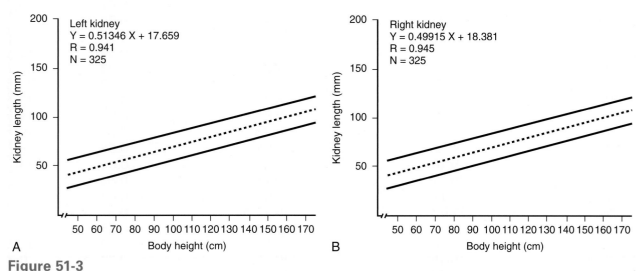

Figure 51-3
Length of both kidney related to body height. Mean values and the 95% regions of tolerance are determined by routine statistical analysis of 325 children. (From Dinkel E, Ertel M, Dittrich M, et al: Kidney size in childhood. Sonographical growth charts for kidney length and volume. Pediatr Radiol 1985;15:38-43.)

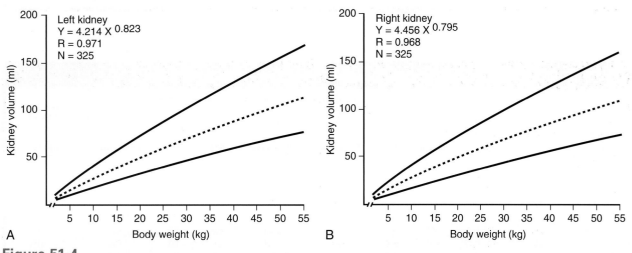

Figure 51-4
Volume of left and right kidney correlated to body weight. Median values and the 95% regions of tolerance are determined by statistical analysis of 325 children. Regression line and tolerance limits were computed after logarithmic transformation of volume and weight and then retransformed. There is only a slight difference between the left and right kidneys. (From Dinkel E, Ertel M, Dittrich M, et al: Kidney size in childhood. Sonographical growth charts for kidney length and volume. Pediatr Radiol 1985;15:38-43.)

Table 51-1 — Summary of grouped observations—mean renal length

Average Age*	Interval*	Mean Renal Length (cm)	SD	n
0 mo	0-1 wk	4.48	0.31	10
2 mo	1 wk-4 mo	5.28	0.66	54
6 mo	4-8 mo	6.15	0.67	20
10 mo	8 mo-1 yr	6.23	0.63	8
$1\frac{1}{2}$	1-2	6.65	0.54	28
$2\frac{1}{2}$	2-3	7.36	0.54	12
$3\frac{1}{2}$	3-4	7.36	0.64	30
$4\frac{1}{2}$	4-5	7.87	0.50	26
$5\frac{1}{2}$	5-6	8.09	0.54	30
$6\frac{1}{2}$	6-7	7.83	0.72	14
$7\frac{1}{2}$	7-8	8.33	0.51	18
$8\frac{1}{2}$	8-9	8.90	0.88	18
$9\frac{1}{2}$	9-10	9.20	0.90	14
$10\frac{1}{2}$	10-11	9.17	0.82	28
$11\frac{1}{2}$	11-12	9.60	0.64	22
$12\frac{1}{2}$	12-13	10.42	0.87	18
$13\frac{1}{2}$	13-14	9.79	0.75	14
$14\frac{1}{2}$	14-15	10.05	0.62	14
$15\frac{1}{2}$	15-16	10.93	0.76	6
$16\frac{1}{2}$	16-17	10.04	0.86	10
$17\frac{1}{2}$	17-18	10.53	0.29	4
$18\frac{1}{2}$	18-19	10.81	1.13	8

From Rosenbaum DM, Korngold E, Teele RL: Sonographic assessment of renal length in normal children. AJR Am J Roentgenol 1984;142:467-469.

Table 51-2 — Longitudinal dimensions of right kidney versus height and age

Body Height (cm)	Subjects No.	Age Range (mo)	Longitudinal Dimensions (mm) of Right Kidney							
			Mean	SD	Minimum	Maximum	Percentile 5th	Percentile 95th	Suggested Limits of Normal Lowermost	Suggested Limits of Normal Uppermost
48-64	50	1-3	50	5.8	38	66	40	58	35	65
54-73	39	4-6	53	5.3	41	66	50	64	40	70
65-78	17	7-9	59	5.2	50	70	52	66	45	70
71-92	18	12-30	61	3.4	55	66	55	65	50	75
85-109	22	36-59	67	5.1	57	77	59	75	55	80
100-130	26	60-83	74	5.5	62	83	65	83	60	85
110-131	32	84-107	80	6.6	68	93	70	91	65	95
124-149	27	108-131	80	7.0	69	96	69	89	65	100
137-153	15	132-155	89	6.2	81	102	82	100	70	105
143-168	22	156-179	94	5.9	83	105	85	102	75	110
152-175	11	180-200	92	7.0	80	107	83	102	75	110

From Konus OL, Ozdemir A, Akkaya A, et al: Normal liver, spleen, and kidney dimensions in neonates, infants, and children: evaluation with sonography. Am J Roentgenol 1998;171:1693-1698.

Table 51-3	Longitudinal dimensions of left kidney versus height and age

Body Height (cm)	Subjects No.	Age Range (mo)	Longitudinal Dimensions (mm) of Left Kidney						Suggested Limits of Normal	
							Percentile			
			Mean	SD	Minimum	Maximum	5th	95th	Lowermost	Uppermost
48-64	50	1-3	50	5.5	38	61	42	59	35	65
54-73	39	4-6	56	5.5	44	66	50	64	40	70
65-78	17	7-9	59	4.6	54	68	54	68	45	75
71-92	18	12-30	66	5.3	54	75	57	72	50	80
85-109	22	36-59	71	4.5	61	77	61	76	55	85
100-130	26	60-83	79	5.9	66	90	70	87	60	95
110-131	32	84-107	84	6.6	71	95	73	93	65	100
124-149	27	108-131	84	7.4	71	99	75	97	65	105
137-153	15	132-155	91	8.9	83	113	84	110	75	115
143-168	22	156-179	96	8.9	83	113	84	110	75	115
152-175	11	180-200	99	7.5	87	116	90	110	80	120

From Schlesinger AE, Hedlund GL, Pierson WP, et al: Normal standards for kidney length in premature infants: determination with US. Work in progress. Radiology 1987;164:127-129.

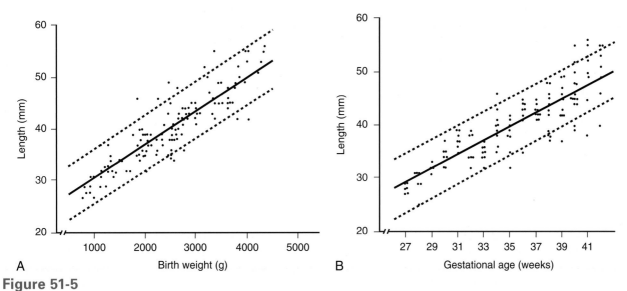

Figure 51-5

Kidney length versus **(A)** (gestational) age and **(B)** birth weight. (From Chiara A, Chirico G, Barbarini M, et al: Ultrasonic evaluation of kidney length in term and preterm infants. Eur J Pediatr 1989;149:94-95.)

Table 51-4 Normal standards for body weight versus kidney length

Body Weight (g)	Kidney Length (mm)*		Body Weight (g)	Kidney Length (mm)*	
	Lower Limit	Upper Limit		Lower Limit	Upper Limit
600	26.4	35.7	1900	36.1	45.4
700	27.2	36.5	2000	36.9	46.2
800	27.9	37.2	2100	37.6	46.9
900	28.7	38.0	2200	38.4	47.7
1000	29.4	38.7	2300	39.1	48.4
1100	30.1	39.5	2400	39.9	49.2
1200	30.9	40.2	2500	40.6	49.9
1300	31.6	41.0	2600	41.3	50.7
1400	32.4	41.7	2700	42.1	51.4
1500	33.1	42.5	2800	42.8	52.2
1600	33.9	43.2	2900	43.6	52.9
1700	34.6	43.9	3000	44.3	53.7
1800	35.1	44.7			

Upper and lower limits are determined from 95% confidence limits.
From Schlesinger AE, Hedlund GL, Pierson WP, et al: Normal standards for kidney length in premature infants: determination with US. Work in progress. Radiology 1987;164:127-129.

Table 51-5 Mean and SD of renal length over fixed age ranges in patients with single functioning kidneys and a group of control subjects[1]

Age Range[a] (wks)	Single Kidney				Control Kidney				P
	Mean Age (wks)	Mean Length (mm)	SD	n	Mean Age (wks)	Mean Length (mm)	SD	n	
0-4	2	51.0	5.8	13	0	44.8	3.1	10	<0.002
5-15	9	56.8	6.3	40	9	52.8	6.6	54	<0.01
17-34	23	62.8	5.6	25	26	61.5	6.7	20	<0.5
34-52	46	69.6	6.8	18	41	62.3	6.3	8	<0.01
53-94	63	71.7	7.9	33	78	66.5	5.4	28	<0.01
103-153	112	78.0	8.0	32	130	73.8	5.4	12	<0.046
156-207	172	79.6	8.2	17	182	73.6	6.4	30	<0.046
208-258	225	86.7	9.5	14	234	78.7	5.0	26	<0.01
260-312	279	91.0	7.9	12	286	80.9	5.4	10	<0.01

[a]*Small gaps in the age ranges are due to the nature of the recall system at our hospital. No data on renal length fell between the intervals.*
From Rottenberg GT, De Bruyn R, et al: Sonographic standards for a single functioning kidney in children. AJR Am J Roentgenol 1996;167:1255-1259.

childhood. Data for length of a single functioning kidney in children have also been reported[7] (Table 51-5). As expected, there is compensatory hypertrophy of the kidney when there is a single kidney. Such increase in length in the range of approximately 1 cm compared with those with two functioning kidneys is outlined in Table 51-5.

References

1. Rosenbaum DM, Korngold E, Teele RL: Sonographic assessment of renal length in normal children. Am J Roentgenol 1984;142:467-469.

2. Konus OL, Ozdemir A, Akkaya A, et al: Normal liver, spleen, and kidney dimensions in neonates, infants, and children: evaluation with sonography. Am J Roentgenol 1998;171:1693-1698.

3. Han BK, Babcock DS: Sonographic measurements and appearance of normal kidneys in children. Am J Roentgenol 1985;145:611-616.

4. Dinkel E, Ertel M, Dittrich M, et al: Kidney size in childhood. Sonographical growth charts for kidney length and volume. Pediatr Radiol 1985;15:38-43.

5. Chiara A, Chirico G, Barbarini M, et al: Ultrasonic evaluation of kidney length in term and preterm infants. Eur J Pediatr 1989;149:94-95.

6. Schlesinger AE, Hedlund GL, Pierson WP, et al: Normal standards for kidney length in premature infants: determination with US. Work in progress. Radiology 1987;164:127-129.

7. Rottenberg GT, De Bruyn R, Gordon I: Sonographic standards for a single functioning kidney in children. Am J Roentgenol 1996;167:1255-1259.

CHAPTER 52

Diane Babcock

Neonatal Adrenal Gland

Introduction

The adrenal gland is relatively prominent in the neonate and is easily visualized with ultrasound. In the older child the adrenal gland is usually not visualized. The gland may be enlarged with congenital adrenal hyperplasia, hemorrhage, or a mass.

Materials/Measurements

The adrenal glands are visualized superior to the kidneys. Longitudinal and transverse images are obtained with a high-frequency convex or sector transducer (Fig. 52-1). From the transverse images through the gland, AP and transverse dimensions are measured.[1] From the longitudinal images the cephalocaudal length is measured from the apex to the midpoint of the base of the gland. Table 52-1[2] lists the adrenal size versus age and the change (decrease) over time expressed as percentage size at the time in question compared with the size at birth.

DISCUSSION

At birth the adrenal gland is relatively large, representing 0.2% to 0.3% of total body weight, compared with 0.001% in adults.[3] There is a linear relationship between body weight and gland lengths in healthy neonates. In premature neonates there is a linear relationship between gestational age and gland size. There is a rapid decrease in adrenal size in the first 10 days of life and continuous decrease in linear dimensions during the first 6 months of life. In addition, the appearance changes as the cortex decreases in size and the echogenicity changes.[1]

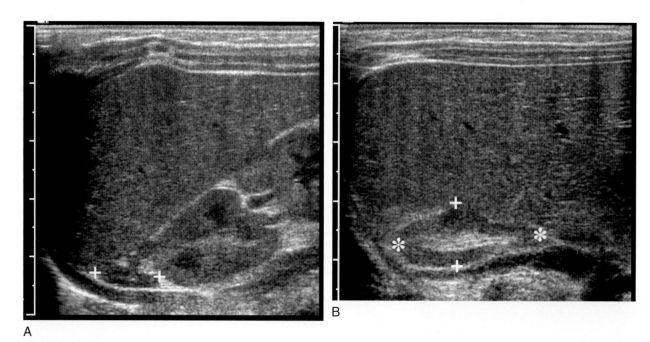

A

B

Figure 52-1
A and **B,** Longitudinal and transverse images are obtained with a high-frequency convex or sector transducer.

Table 52-1	Mean ± SD (mean percentage change ± SD) adrenal measurements in neonates*				
Day	**Transverse**	**Anteroposterior**	**Circumference**	**Area (cm²)**	**Length**
1	17.9 ± 2.7	9.6 ± 2.1	44.5 ± 5.3	1.35 ± 0.3	17.3 ± 1.8
3	14.8 ± 3.3	7.5 ± 2.2	36.7 ± 8.4	0.95 ± 0.5	12.8 ± 3.2
	(84.0 ± 19.9	(78.6 ± 16.9)	(82.4 ± 16.3)	(68.3 ± 24.5)	(73.9 ± 18.7)
5	13.7 ± 2.1	6.9 ± 1.6	33.4 ± 5.1	0.75 ± 0.2	11.4 ± 2.7
	(77.5 ± 11.3)	(62.0 ± 20.6)	(65.2 ± 19.4)	(44.5 ± 29.2)	(51.9 ± 12.6)
11	11.8 ± 2.5	5.9 ± 1.4	28.6 ± 6.1	0.57 ± 0.3	8.9 ± 2.0
	(67.4 ± 17.2)	(62.0 ± 20.6)	(65.2 ± 19.4)	(44.5 ± 19.4)	(51.9 ± 12.6)
21	10.8 ± 1.9	5.6 ± 0.5	25.3 ± 3.9	0.45 ± 0.1	8.2 ± 1.2
	(61.5 ± 13.4)	(61.1 ± 16.3)	(57.8 ± 11.3)	(35.7 ± 13.7)	(47.9 ± 8.0)
42	9.5 ± 1.5	5.7 ± 1.0	23.8 ± 2.8	0.4 ± 0.1	7.7 ± 0.9
	(53.9 ± 11.6)	(61.3 ± 14.8)	(54.4 ± 10.4)	(32.5 ± 11.5)	(45.0 ± 6.4)

*Measurements in millimeters.
From Scott EM, Thomas A, McGarrigle HHG, Lachelin GCL: Serial adrenal ultrasonography in normal neonates. J Ultrasound Med 1990;9:279-283.

References

1. Kangarloo H, Diament MJ, Gold RH, et al: Sonography of adrenal glands in neonates and children: changes in appearance with age. J Clin Ultrasound 1986;14:43-47.

2. Scott EM, Thomas A, McGarrigle HH, et al: Serial adrenal ultrasonography in normal neonates. J Ultrasound Med 1990;9:279-283.

3. Bech K, Tygstrup I, Nerup J: The involution of the foetal adrenal cortex. A light microscopic study. Acta Pathol Microbiol Scand 1969;76:391-400.

CHAPTER 53

Diane Babcock

Pediatric Gallbladder and Biliary Tract

Introduction

The gallbladder may be small with inadequate fasting or biliary atresia. It may dilate with sepsis or Kawasaki's disease. The bile ducts may dilate with obstruction.

Materials/Measurements

Images are obtained in the sagittal and transverse plane using either a convex or sector transducer and the highest frequency that will penetrate the patient. In a study by McGahan et al, younger patients fasted for about 4 hours and older ones 8 hours or more. Length, AP diameter, and width (coronal diameter) of the gallbladder were measured on images that gave greatest dimensions. All measurements were made intraluminally[1] (Fig. 53-1). Table 53-1 lists normal gallbladder dimensions by age.

Gallbladder wall thickness was equal to or less than 3 mm in all pediatric patients.

McGahan et al[1] measured the common hepatic duct on longitudinal scan where it crosses the right portal vein (Fig. 53-2). The lumen increased with age (Table 53-2) but was never greater than 4 mm. Hernanz-Schulman et al[2] measured the common bile duct (CBD) and reported the CBD diameter for children through 13 years of age (Fig. 53-3).

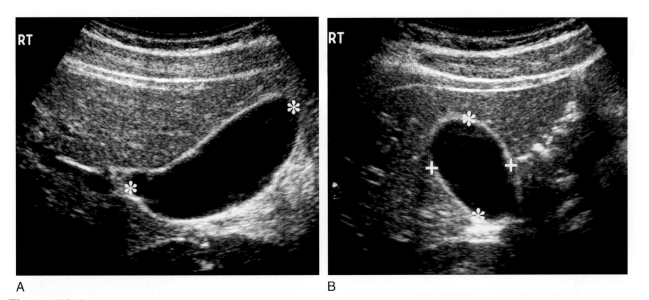

A   B

Figure 53-1

Gallbladder measurements. **A,** Longitudinal scan measuring length (*). **B,** Transverse scan measuring anteroposterior diameter (*) and width (+).

Table 53-1	Sonographic measurement of the normal pediatric gallbladder measurements vs. age							
Age (y)	AP Diameter (cm) Mean	AP Diameter (cm) Range	Coronal Diameter (cm) Mean	Coronal Diameter (cm) Range	Length (cm) Mean	Length (cm) Range	Wall Thickness (mm) Mean	Wall Thickness (mm) Range
0-1	0.9	0.5-1.2	0.9	0.7-1.4	2.5	1.3-3.4	1.7	1.0-3.0
2-5	1.7	1.4-2.3	1.8	1.0-3.9	4.2	2.9-5.2	2.0	None
6-8	1.8	1.0-2.4	2.0	1.2-3.0	5.6	4.4-7.4	2.2	2.0-3.0
9-11	1.9	1.2-3.2	2.0	1.0-3.6	5.5	3.4-6.5	2.0	1.0-3.0
12-16	2.0	1.3-2.8	2.1	1.6-3.0	6.1	3.8-8.0	2.0	1.0-3.0

From McGahan JP, Phillips HE, Cox KL, et al: Sonography of the normal pediatric gallbladder and biliary tract. Radiology 1982;144:873-875.

Table 53-2	Normal sonographic measurement of the normal common hepatic duct sizes vs. age	
Age (y)	Common Hepatic Duct Size (mm) Mean	Common Hepatic Duct Size (mm) Range
0-1	1.3	1.0-2.0
2-5	1.7	1.0-3.0
6-8	2.0	None
9-11	1.8	1.0-3.0
12-16	2.2	1.0-4.0

From McGahan, JP, Phillips HE, Cox KL: Sonography of the normal pediatric gallbladder and biliary tract. Radiology 1982;144:873-875.

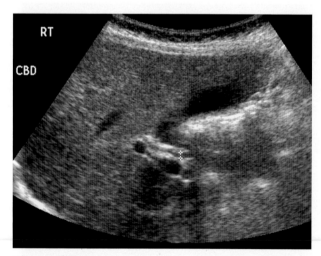

Figure 53-2
Common hepatic duct (+) measured on longitudinal oblique view as it crosses the portal vein.

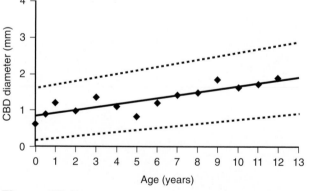

Figure 53-3
Common bile duct (CBD) size in children. *Diamonds,* Mean for age group; *Solid line,* linear regression of CBD diameter versus age; *Dotted lines,* 95% confidence intervals. (From Hernanz-Schulman M, Ambrosino MM, Freeman PC, et al: Common bile duct in children: sonographic dimensions. Radiology 1995;195:193-195.)

DISCUSSION

The gallbladder length is generally less than that of the normal right kidney. An image of the right kidney can be easily obtained for comparison. Nonvisualization or suboptimal visualization of the gallbladder may be because of technical problems, especially in the neonate. When scanning the neonate they should be NPO several hours before scanning to ensure adequate distension of the gallbladder with bile. A small or nonvisualized gallbladder in the neonate may be a useful sign in diagnosing biliary atresia.

An enlarged gallbladder may be identified in pediatric or adult patients who are hospitalized and have not eaten for several days. Gallbladder enlargement may occur with acalculus chole-

cystitis. Pediatric patients with biliary obstruction may have an enlarged or overdistended gallbladder, often called a *Courvoisier gallbladder*. Other etiologies of the enlarged gallbladder include Kawasaki's disease.

References

1. McGahan JP, Phillips HE, Cox KL: Sonography of the normal pediatric gallbladder and biliary tract. Radiology 1982;144:873-875.
2. Hernanz-Schulman M, Ambrosino MM, Freeman PC, et al: Common bile duct in children: sonographic dimensions. Radiology 1995;195:193-195.

CHAPTER 54

Pediatric Liver

Diane Babcock

Introduction

The shape of the normal liver is complex, and therefore it is difficult to measure the volume accurately. The measurement used most often is the cranio-caudal dimension in the midclavicular line.

Materials/Measurements

Scans are performed with the patient supine using the anterior approach in the midclavicular line. Either a convex or sector transducer is used, with the highest frequency transducer that would provide adequate penetration of the organ. Measurement is made from the uppermost portion of the dome of the diaphragm to the inferior tip of the liver[1] (Fig. 54-1). Table 54-1 lists liver lengths by age and body height of the patients.

DISCUSSION

It is difficult to evaluate the size of the liver with a single measurement in a single plane. A volume measurement would be optimal, but not practical to obtain with ultrasound because of patient motion. It is possible with CT or MRI. Overall, liver size is routinely evaluated subjectively without measurement. Measurement can be useful when evaluating change in liver size

Table 54-1	Longitudinal dimensions of right lobe of liver versus height and age									
Subjects			**Longitudinal Dimensions (mm) of Right Lobe of Liver**							
Body Height (cm)	**No.**	**Age Range (mo)**	**Mean**	**SD**	**Minimum**	**Maximum**	**Percentile**		**Suggested Limits of Normal**	
							5th	**95th**	**Lowermost**	**Uppermost**
47-64	53	1-3	64	10.4	45	90	48	82	40	90
54-73	40	4-6	73	10.8	44	92	53	86	45	95
65-78	20	7-9	79	8.0	68	100	70	90	60	100
71-92	18	12-30	85	10.0	67	104	68	98	65	105
85-109	27	36-59	86	11.8	69	109	63	105	65	115
100-130	30	60-83	100	13.6	73	125	77	124	70	125
110-131	38	84-107	105	10.6	81	128	90	123	75	130
124-149	30	108-131	105	12.5	76	135	83	128	75	135
137-153	16	132-155	115	14.0	93	137	95	136	85	140
143-168	23	156-179	118	14.6	87	137	94	136	85	140
152-175	12	180-200	121	11.7	100	141	104	139	95	145

From Konus OL, Ozdemir A, Akkaya A, et al: Normal liver, spleen, and kidney dimensions in neonates, infants, and children: evaluation with sonography. AJR Am J Roentgenol 1998;171:1693-1698.

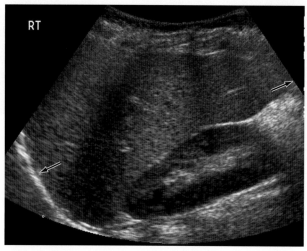

Figure 54-1
Liver length. Longitudinal measurements of liver in midclavicular line. Cranio-caudal dimension from uppermost portion of the dome of the diaphragm to the inferior tip of the liver (*arrows*).

from one study to the next. A prominent Reidel's lobe may be seen and is a normal variant.

Liver size is important with conditions that may cause hepatomegaly. These may include diffuse conditions such as hepatitis, congestive heart failure, or profuse fatty infiltration. A number of uncommon causes of hepatomegaly can cause diffuse enlargement of the liver. In addition to these etiologies, focal multicentric processes such as diffuse metastases may also be etiologies for hepatic enlargement.

Reference

1. Konus OL, Ozdemir A, Akkaya A, et al: Normal liver, spleen, and kidney dimensions in neonates, infants, and children: evaluation with sonography. Am J Roentgenol 1998; 171:1693-1698.

CHAPTER 55

Diane Babcock

Pediatric Pancreas

Introduction

The pancreas may enlarge when inflamed or with masses. It may atrophy in cystic fibrosis and be replaced with fat.

Materials/Measurements

The pancreas is scanned with a convex or sector transducer using the highest frequency that will penetrate the patient. The transverse or oblique plane is used to demonstrate the entire pancreas (Fig. 55-1). The body, head, and tail are measured in AP dimension. Table 55-1[1] lists AP dimensions versus age.

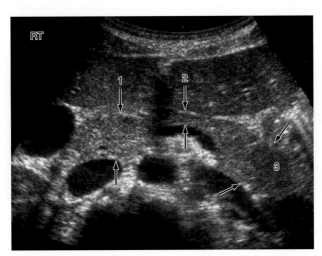

Figure 55-1
Pancreas dimensions. *1*, maximum AP diameter of the head of the pancreas; *2*, maximum AP diameter of the body; *3*, maximum AP diameter of the tail.

Table 55-1	Normal dimensions of the pancreas as a function of age			
		Maximum Anteroposterior Dimensions of Pancreas (cm ± 1 standard deviation)		
Patient Age	**No. of Patients**	**Head**	**Body**	**Tail**
<1 mo	15	1.0 ± 0.4	0.6 ± 0.2	1.0 ± 0.4
1 mo-1 yr	23	1.5 ± 0.5	0.8 ± 0.3	1.2 ± 0.4
1-5 yr	49	1.7 ± 0.3	1.0 ± 0.2	1.8 ± 0.4
5-10 yr	69	1.6 ± 0.4	1.0 ± 0.3	1.8 ± 0.4
10-19 yr	117	2.0 ± 0.5	1.1 ± 0.3	2.0 ± 0.4

From Siegel MJ, Martin WK, Worthington JL. Normal and abnormal pancreas in children: US studies. Radiology 1987;165:15-18.

DISCUSSION

The pediatric pancreas is relatively large and equal in echogenicity to the adjacent left lobe of the liver. With age the pancreas becomes relatively smaller and increases in echogenicity because of fat interposed between the lobules. The normal pancreatic duct is less than 2 mm in diameter.

Enlargement of the pancreas is rare in childhood; it may be secondary to such entities as acute pancreatitis.[2] Ultrasound findings of pancreatitis may be minimal; however, the most common abnormality associated with pancreatitis is an enlarged pancreas. This can be compared with the normal sonography measurements of the pancreas. Decreased echogenicity of the pancreas can occur with pancreatitis. With chronic pancreatitis, the pancreas may appear more hyperechoic, and small calcifications may be identified.[2]

References

1. Siegel MJ, Martin KW, Worthington JL: Normal and abnormal pancreas in children: US studies. Radiology 1987;165:15-18.
2. Berrocal R, Prieto C, Pastor I, Gutierrez J, Al-Assir I: Sonography of pancreatic disease in infants and children. Radiographics 1995; 15:301-313.

CHAPTER 56

Pediatric Portal Vein

Diane Babcock

Introduction

The portal vein may become thrombosed with the development of collateral veins that are small. Prior knowledge of the patency of the portal vein is important with liver transplantation.

Materials/Measurements

Measurements are taken in the supine position, during quiet respiration, 1 to 3 hours after a normal meal. The portal vein is measured in the oblique plane using a convex or sector transducer. The maximum measurement in AP dimension is determined (Fig. 56-1).[1] Figure 56-2 gives portal vein measurement by age, Figure 56-3 by weight.

DISCUSSION

Various factors affect the portal vein size. The portal vein increases slightly in inspiration.

Portal venous flow increases after a meal and decreases with exercise and in the upright

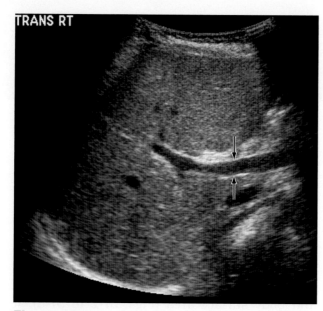

Figure 56-1
Portal vein measurement. Oblique right longitudinal scan of main portal vein. The greatest AP diameter of the vein is measured a few millimeters above the splenomesenteric confluence (*arrows*), near the site where the hepatic artery crosses the portal vein anteriorly.

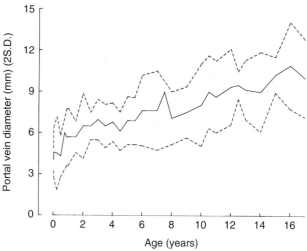

Figure 56-2
Portal venous diameter related to age [in months and years]. Mean (*solid line*) and limits of error (*dashed line*) are shown. (From Patriquin HB, Perrreault G, Grigon A, et al: Normal portal venous diameter in children. Pediatr Radiol 1990;20:451-453.)

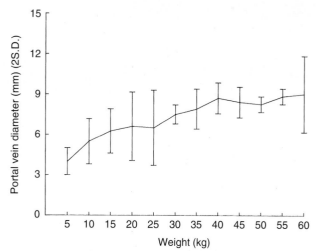

Figure 56-3
Portal venous diameter related to weight. Mean (*solid line*) and limits of error (*dashed line*) are shown. (From Patriquin HB, Perrreault G, Grigon A, et al: Normal portal venous diameter in children. Pediatr Radiol 1990;20:451-453.)

position. The measurement of the portal vein should be done under the standard conditions listed.

Reference

1. Patriquin HB, Perreault G, Grignon A, et al: Normal portal venous diameter in children. Pediatr Radiol 1990;20:451-453.

CHAPTER 57

Diane Babcock

Pediatric Spleen

Introduction

The spleen may enlarge in infectious diseases, anemias, with tumors, and with portal hypertension. It may be small in sickle cell disease and with infarction.

Materials/Measurements

Supine craniocaudal images were obtained through the maximum length of the spleen. Occasionally, right side down oblique scanning was done to better visualize the spleen. The length was measured from the most superomedial to the most inferolateral points (Fig. 57-1).

Konus et al[1] published data on splenic length versus height and age (Table 57-1). Rosenberg et al[2] published data on splenic length versus age (Table 57-2). Megremis et al[3] published data on splenic length versus age, height, weight, and body surface area (Figs. 57-2 to 57-5). It has been reported that the upper normal limit for the spleen/kidney ratio is 1.25.[4]

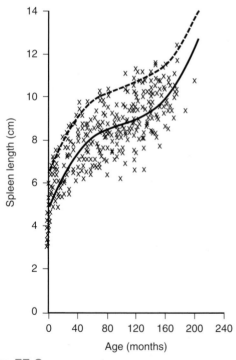

Figure 57-2
Scatterplot shows spleen length plotted against age. Regression curve (*black line*) and approximate 90% upper confidence limit (UCL [*dashed line*]) are also presented. *x*, Individual values. (From Megremis SD, Vlachonikolis IG, Tsilimigaki AM: Spleen length in childhood with US: normal values based on age, sex, and somatometric parameters. Radiology 2004;231:129-134.)

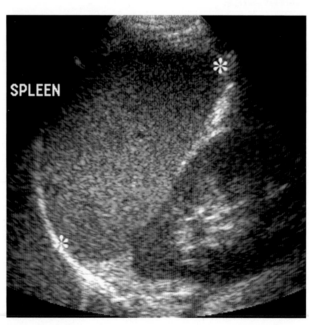

SPLEEN

Figure 57-1
Longitudinal measurement of spleen. Craniocaudal dimension from uppermost portion of the superior medial edge of spleen adjacent to the diaphragm to the inferior tip of the spleen (*).

Table 57-1	Longitudinal dimensions of spleen versus height and age

| Subjects ||| Longitudinal Dimensions (mm) of the Spleen ||||||||
| Body Height (cm) | No. | Age Range (mo) | Mean | SD | Minimum | Maximum | Percentile || Suggested Limits of Normal ||
							5th	95th	Lowermost	Uppermost
48-64	52	1-3	53	7.8	33	71	40	65	30	70
54-73	39	4-6	59	6.3	45	71	47	67	40	75
65-78	18	7-9	63	7.6	50	77	53	74	45	80
71-92	18	12-30	70	9.6	54	86	55	82	50	85
85-109	27	36-59	75	8.4	60	91	61	88	55	95
100-130	30	60-83	84	9.0	61	100	70	100	60	105
110-131	36	84-107	85	10.5	65	102	69	100	65	105
124-149	29	108-131	86	10.7	64	114	70	100	65	110
137-153	17	132-155	97	9.7	72	100	81	108	75	115
143-168	21	156-179	101	11.7	84	120	85	118	80	120
152-175	12	180-200	101	10.3	88	120	88	115	85	120

From Konus OL, Ozdemir A, Akkaya A, et al: Normal Liver, spleen, and kidney dimensions in neonates, infants, and children: evaluation with sonography. AJR Am J Roentgenol 1998;171:1693-1698.

Table 57-2	Age and splenic length in 230 infants and children

| Age (Number) | Length of Spleen (cm) ||||
	10th percentile	Median	90th percentile	Suggested Upper Limit
0-3 mo	3.3	4.5	5.8	6.0
3-6 mo	4.9	5.3	6.4	6.5
6-12 mo	5.2	6.2	6.8	7.0
1-2 yrs	5.4	6.9	7.5	8.0
2-4 yrs	6.4	7.4	8.6	9.0
4-6 yrs	6.9	7.8	8.8	9.5
6-8 yrs	7.0	8.2	9.6	10.0
8-10 yrs	7.9	9.2	10.5	11.0
10-12 yrs	8.6	9.9	10.9	11.5
12-15 yrs	8.7	10.1	11.4	12.0
15-20 yrs				
Female	9.0	10.0	11.7	12.0
Male	10.1	11.2	12.6	13.0

From Rosenberg HK, Markowitz RI, Kolberg H, et al: Normal splenic size in infants and children: sonographic measurements. AJR Am J Roentgenol 1991;157:119-121.

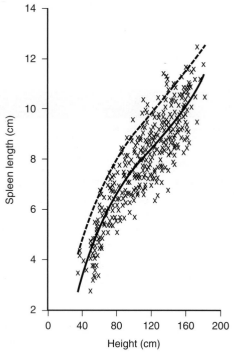

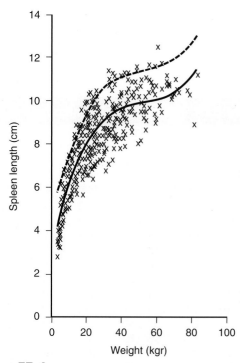

Figure 57-3
Scatterplot shows spleen length plotted against height. Regression curve and approximate 90% UCL are also presented. Keys are the same as for Figure 57-5. (From Megremis SD, Vlachonikolis IG, Tsilimigaki AM: Spleen length in childhood with US: normal values based on age, sex, and somatometric parameters. Radiology 2004;231:129-134.)

Figure 57-4
Scatterplot shows spleen length plotted against weight. Regression curve and approximate 90% UCL are also presented. Keys are the same as for Figure 57-5. (From Megremis SD, Vlachonikolis IG, Tsilimigaki AM: Spleen length in childhood with US: normal values based on age, sex, and somatometric parameters. Radiology 2004;231:129-134.)

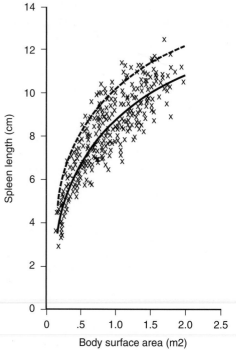

Figure 57-5
Scatterplot shows spleen length plotted against BSA. Regression curve and approximate 90% UCL are also presented. (From Megremis SD, Vlachonikolis IG, Tsilimigaki AM: Spleen length in childhood with US: normal values based on age, sex, and somatometric parameters. Radiology 2004;231:129-134.)

DISCUSSION

Table 57-1 lists spleen lengths by age and body height of the patient. Table 57-2 lists spleen lengths by age and in the 15- to 20-year-old group by gender as well. The best correlation between splenic measurements and patient parameters is for spleen length versus body height. The uppermost limits of normal are slightly greater in Table 57-2.

Scanning of the spleen may be difficult in the pediatric, as well as the adult patient. Subcostal images obtained in the supine position may be easier in pediatric patients with splenomegaly. Breath-holding techniques are best for imaging the spleen, but patient cooperation in the young pediatric patient may be challenging.

Causes of splenomegaly can include infectious etiologies such as mononucleosis or infiltrative diseases such as lymphoma or leukemia. In addition, patients with liver disease who develop portal hypertension may develop splenomegaly. Furthermore, focal abnormalities may cause splenomegaly. These usually have associated sonographic findings.

References

1. Konus OL, Ozdemir A, Akkaya A, et al: Normal liver, spleen, and kidney dimensions in neonates, infants, and children: evaluation with sonography. AJR Am J Roentgenol 1998;171:1693-1698.
2. Rosenberg HK, Markowitz RI, Kolberg H, et al: Normal splenic size in infants and children: sonographic measurements. AJR Am J Roentgenol 1991;157:119-121.
3. Megremis SD, Vlachonikolis IG, Tsilimigaki AM: Spleen length in childhood with US: normal values based on age, sex, and somatometric parameters. Radiology 2004;231:129-134.
4. Loftus WK, Metreweli C: Ultrasound assessment of mild splenomegaly: spleen/kidney ratio. Pediatr Radiol 1998;28:98-100.

CHAPTER 58

Pediatric Lymph Nodes

Diane Babcock

Introduction

Sizes for normal lymph nodes in adults have been published using CT. The same measurements have been applied to ultrasound in children.

Materials/Methods

Scans of the abdomen are performed using convex or longitudinal transducers. Lymph nodes may be detected in many locations including the liver hilum, right lower quadrant, and along the aorta. Maximum short-axis nodal diameter is measured (Fig. 58-1) (Table 58-1).[1]

DISCUSSION

Measurements of lymph nodes may be made in specific diseases or malignancy by sonography to check for enlargement.

Sensitivity and specificity of determining nodal enlargement will depend on which measurements are used as the upper limits of normal

Table 58-1	Threshold estimates for the upper limit of normal short-axis node size			
Region	No. of Patients with Nodes Identified (n = 130)*	Short-Axis Nodal Diameter (mm)+	Tolerance Interval Estimate for Upper Limit of Normal (mm)±	Histographic Estimate for Upper Limit of Normal (mm)
Paracardiac	33 (25.4)	3.9 ± 0.2	6.8 (5.0, 8.0)	8.0
Retrocrural space	64 (49.2)	3.0 ± 0.1	5.0 (5.0, 6.0)	6.0
Gastrohepatic ligament	25 (19.2)	4.1 ± 0.3	6.8 (6.0, 9.0)	8.0
Upper para-aortic (celiac to renal)	58 (44.6)	3.7 ± 0.2	7.0 (6.0, 9.0)	9.0
Lower para-aortic (renal to bifurcation)	130 (100)	3.4 ± 0.1	10.0 (10.0, 11.0)	11.0
Porta hepatis	13 (10.0)	3.2 ± 0.4	6.0 (5.0, 8.0)	7.0
Portacaval space	30 (23.1)	5.3 ± 0.4	8.0 (7.0, 10.0)	10.0

*Numbers in parentheses are percentages.
+Mean plus or minus standard deviation.
± Confidence interval is 90% and is given in millimeters in parentheses.
From Dorfman RE, Alpern MB, Gross BH, Sandler MA: Upper abdominal lymph nodes: criteria for normal size determined with CT. Radiology 1991;180:319-322.

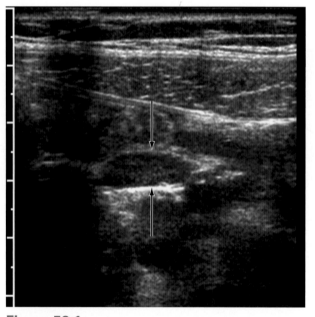

Figure 58-1
Lymph node dimensions. Scan of lymph node in right lower abdomen. *Arrowheads* demonstrate short-axis measurements.

of the short-axis of node size. For instance, if a lower value such as 7 mm is used as the upper limit of normal for a paraaortic node, the sensitivity of this value may be quite high. However, the specificity may be lower than if measurement number such as 9 to 10 mm is picked as the upper limit of normal. If the upper value is used, specificity will increase, but sensitivity will decrease.

Common causes for pediatric abdominal lymphadenopothy could include infectious etiologies or malignancies such as lymphoma or metastases. There are a number of other etiologies for node enlargement in the pediatric abdomen.

Reference

1. Dorfman RE, Alpern MB, Gross BH, et al: Upper abdominal lymph nodes: criteria for normal size determined with CT. Radiology 1991;180:319-322.

Diane Babcock

Pediatric Urinary Bladder

Introduction

Two measurements are used for evaluating the urinary bladder: volume and wall thickness.

Materials/Measurements

Bladder volume is determined on midline longitudinal, and transverse views of the urinary bladder when maximally distended. Images are obtained with a convex transducer using the highest frequency that will penetrate the patient (Fig. 59-1). Harmonic imaging may be useful to minimize artifacts. Because the bladder varies in shape, various formulas have been suggested to calculate its volume.[1] A correction coefficient has been calculated and published on the basis of bladder shape using the formula volume = height × weight × depth × correction coefficient

$(K)^2$ (Table 59-1). Bladder capacity may be compared with normal data obtained during radionuclide cystography[3] (Table 59-2).

Bladder wall thickness is determined with a maximally distended bladder in sagittal plane. The posterior inferior wall is measured (see Fig. 59-1). It can also be measured in the transverse plane lateral to the trigone. Normal measurements are reported for both full and empty bladder. Normal measurement for a full bladder is up to 3 mm and for an empty bladder up to 5 mm.[4]

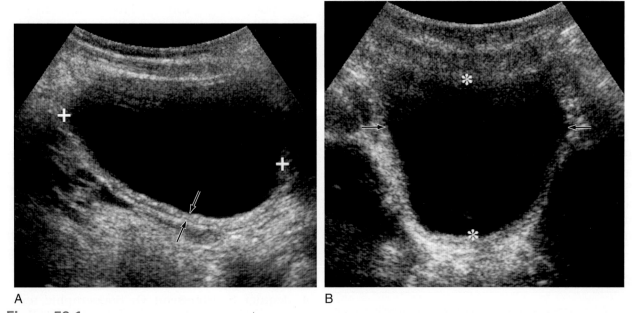

A   B

Figure 59-1
Bladder volume. **A,** Longitudinal midline and **B,** Transverse scans. Length (+), width (*arrows*), and AP dimension (*) measured at inner wall. Bladder wall thickness (*arrowheads*) measured at posterior wall.

Table 59-1 Correction coefficient for bladder volume

Bladder Shape	Correction Coefficient k	S.E. of k	Pearson's r	P	Mean percentage error ± SD
Whole sample—	0.66	0.011	0.927	<0.01	19.19 ± 9.59
regardless of shape	0.561	0.013	0.940	<0.01	5.10 ± 8.30
Round	0.923	0.012	0.982	<0.01	5.53 ± 6.86
Cuboid	0.802	0.006	0.992	<0.01	3.09 ± 3.52
Ellipsoid	0.623	0.007	0.988	<0.01	7.71 ± 8.66
Triangular	0.749	0.048	0.976	<0.01	15.18 ± 17.21
Undefined					

From Kuzmic AC, Brkljacic B, Ivankovic D: The impact of bladder shape on the ultrasonographic measurement of bladder volume in children. Pediatr Radiol 2003;33:530-534.

Table 59-2 Pediatric bladder volumes

Age (yr)	Mean −2 SD	Mean −1.68 SD	Mean +2 SD	Mean	SD	Age (yr)
<1	21	34	189	105	42	<1
1-2	54	72	274	164	55	1-2
2-3	85	104	321	203	59	2-3
3-4	99	121	379	239	70	3-4
4-5	114	136	390	252	69	4-5
5-6	121	145	417	269	74	5-6
6-7	126	150	430	278	76	6-7
7-8	125	152	457	291	83	7-8
8-9	145	172	481	313	84	8-9
9-10	171	197	499	335	82	9-10
10-11	168	198	540	354	93	10-11
11-12	180	212	576	378	99	11-12
12-13	203	233	579	391	94	12-13
13-14	181	219	661	421	120	13-14
Girls 13-14	194	232	666	430	118	Girls 13-14
Boys 13-14	122	162	622	371	125	Boys 13-14
n = 5165						

Modified from Treves ST, Zurakowski D, Bauer SB, et al: Functional bladder capacity measured during radionuclide cystography in children. Radiology 1996;198:269-272.

DISCUSSION

Both the bladder volume and wall thickness are affected by the degree of bladder distention. Spurious measurements can be obtained with a less than fully distended bladder. The thickness of the bladder wall may be increased with inflammation or muscular hypertrophy.

References

1. Hakenberg OW, Ryall RL, Langlois SL, et al: The estimation of bladder volume by sonocystography. J Urol 1983;130:249-251.

2. Kuzmic AC, Brkljacic B, Ivankovic D: The impact of bladder shape on the ultrasonographic measurement of bladder volume in children. Pediatr Radiol 2003;33:530-534.

3. Treves ST, Zurakowski D, Bauer SB, et al: Functional bladder capacity measured during radionuclide cystography in children. Radiology 1996;198:269-272.

4. Jequier S, Rousseau O: Sonographic measurements of the normal bladder wall in children. AJR Am J Roentgenol 1987;149:563-566.

Diane Babcock

CHAPTER 60

Pediatric Appendix

Introduction

The appendix is a common site of inflammation in the pediatric patient. Both ultrasound and CT are used for imaging the patient with suspected appendicitis.

Materials/Measurements

Graded compression technique, as described by Puylaert,[1] of the right lower quadrant is performed using a high-frequency linear transducer. Left-side-down oblique or decubitus positioning may be helpful, especially in larger patients, when looking for a retrocecal appendix.

The appendix is recognized as a structure emanating from the cecum. It may be draped over the right iliac vessels, anterior to the iliopsoas muscle, or retrocecal in location. Measurement of the maximum diameter (serosa to serosa) is performed in either longitudinal or transverse plane to the appendix (Fig. 60-1). A maximum diameter of 6 mm or less in the normal patient is used in pediatric patients, as well as adults.[2] Other criteria for appendicitis include noncompressability of the appendix and focal tenderness in the area. Secondary findings include hypervascular wall at color Doppler, increased echogenicity of the adjacent mesenteric fat, fluid in the appendiceal lumen, and visualization of an appendicolith.[1,3,4] Ancillary findings include complex mass in the right lower quadrant, free fluid in the pelvis, and mesenteric adenopathy.

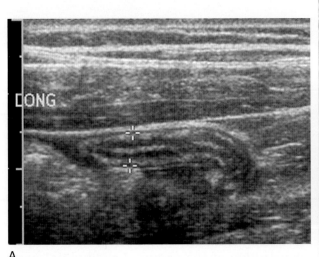
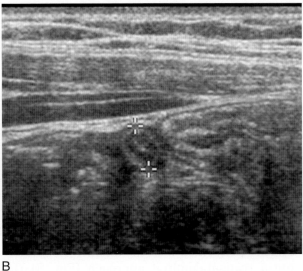

A   B

Figure 60-1
Calipers indicate maximum diameter of the appendix from serosa to serosa performed in longitudinal (**A**) and transverse (**B**) planes.

DISCUSSION

Ultrasound is generally considered the preferable imaging technique in the pediatric patient because it uses nonionizing radiation. It can also be used in the female patient to evaluate the pelvic organs for other pathology causing the symptoms. CT has been used commonly at some institutions in spite of ionizing radiation because it is less operator dependent and the normal appendix can be visualized more easily, especially in patients with even a mild amount of body fat.[3,4] When a complication of appendicitis, such as perforation with abscesses, is suspected, CT is used. The entire abdomen and pelvis can be evaluated for multiple sites of loculated fluid collections potentially needing drainage.

An age-related difference in mean maximum mural thickness (1/2 diameter when compressed) has been shown by Simonovsky[2]; however, it is not statistically significant. He concluded that in children younger than 6 years, the mural thickness should be regarded as normal only when it is less than 3 mm.

References

1. Puylaert JB: Acute appendicitis: US evaluation using graded compression. Radiology 1986;158:355-360.
2. Simonovsky V: Normal appendix: is there any significant difference in the maximal mural thickness at US between pediatric and adult populations? Radiology 2002;224:333-337.
3. Sivit CJ, Siegel MJ, Applegate KE, et al: When appendicitis is suspected in children. Radiographics 2001;21:247-262; questionnaire 288-294.
4. Applegate KE, Sivit CJ, Salvator E, et al: Effect of cross-sectional imaging on negative appendectomy and perforation rates in children. Radiology 2001;220:103-107.

CHAPTER 61

Diane Babcock

Pediatric Uterus

Introduction

The uterine size and endometrial thickness are measured routinely during pediatric pelvic examinations.

Materials/Measurements

Scans are performed with the bladder distended using a transabdominal approach (Fig. 61-1). Endovaginal examinations are occasionally performed in adolescents. Either a convex or linear transducer is used, using the highest-frequency transducer that will provide adequate penetration of the organs. Longitudinal measurement is made from the tip of the fundus to the tip of the cervix. AP measurement is made on a longitudinal scan through the body of the

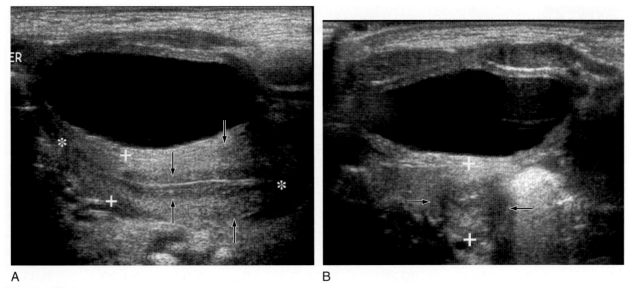

Figure 61-1
Uterine measurements. **A,** Longitudinal and **B,** transverse scans of the neonatal uterus. Longitudinal measurement is from the tip of the fundus to the tip of the cervix (*). AP (+) and transverse measurements (*arrowheads*) are made through the body of the uterus. AP measurements of the body of the uterus (+) and cervix (*arrows*) are determined on longitudinal view. Endometrial stripe measured to include both the hypoechoic and echogenic portions of the endometrium (*arrowheads*).

Table 61-1	**Uterine diameters and volume***					
			Uterine Diameters (mm)			**Uterine Volume (cm³)**
						By Chronologic Age	**By Bone Age**
Age (yr)	**No. of Patients**	**TUL Mean SD**	**COAP Mean SD**	**CEAP Mean SD**	**COAP/ CEAP Mean SD**	**Mean SD**	**Mean SD**
2	7	33.1 ± 4.4	7.0 ± 3.4	8.3 ± 2.0	0.84 ± 0.29	1.98 ± 1.58	1.76 ± 0.72
3	8	32.4 ± 4.3	6.4 ± 1.3	7.6 ± 2.2	0.89 ± 0.29	1.63 ± 0.81	1.80 ± 0.74
4	15	32.9 ± 3.3	7.6 ± 1.8	8.6 ± 1.8	0.90 ± 0.22	2.10 ± 0.57	1.97 ± 0.74
5	7	33.1 ± 5.5	8.0 ± 2.8	8.4 ± 1.6	0.95 ± 0.18	2.36 ± 1.39	2.19 ± 1.16
6	9	33.2 ± 4.1	6.7 ± 2.9	7.5 ± 1.8	0.86 ± 0.18	1.80 ± 1.57	1.65 ± 0.93
7	9	32.3 ± 3.9	8.0 ± 2.2	7.7 ± 2.5	1.08 ± 0.26	2.32 ± 1.07	2.81 ± 1.44
8	11	35.8 ± 7.3	9.0 ± 2.8	8.4 ± 1.7	1.05 ± 0.20	3.12 ± 1.52	2.70 ± 1.43
9	11	37.1 ± 4.4	9.7 ± 3.0	8.8 ± 2.0	1.10 ± 0.24	3.70 ± 1.62	2.69 ± 1.83
10	13	40.3 ± 6.4	12.8 ± 5.3	10.7 ± 2.6	1.17 ± 0.31	6.54 ± 3.78	4.66 ± 3.03
11	13	42.2 ± 5.1	12.8 ± 3.1	10.7 ± 2.6	1.22 ± 0.26	6.66 ± 2.87	6.24 ± 3.07
12	6	54.3 ± 8.4	17.3 ± 5.3	14.3 ± 5.2	1.23 ± 0.16	16.18 ± 9.15	8.88 ± 3.65
13	5	53.8 ± 11.4	15.8 ± 4.5	15.0 ± 2.4	1.03 ± 0.15	13.18 ± 5.64	15.55 ± 5.98

*As determined by ultrasonography in 114 girls from age 2 to 13. CEAP, anteroposterior diameter of the cervix; COAP, anteroposterior diameter of the corpus; TUL, Total uterine length.
From Orsini L.F, Salardi S, Pilu G, et al: Pelvic organs in premenarcheal girls: real-time ultrasonography. Radiology 1984;153:113-116.

uterus. The endometrial stripe is measured to include both the hypoechoic and echogenic portions of the endometrium. The AP diameters of the corpus (COAP) and the cervix (CEAP) are measured in cases with precocious puberty. Transverse measurement is made on a transverse scan. Tables 61-1 through 61-3[1-3] list uterine diameters and volumes by age. Uterine volumes are determined by the formula for a prolate ellipsoid (volume = L × H × W × 0.523).

Table 61-2   Uterine and ovarian volume according to chronologic age (*n* = 133)

Age (yr)	Uterine Volume (cm³)				Ovarian Volume (cm³)			
	No.	Mean	SD	Median	No.	Mean	SD	Median
1	8	0.91	0.40	0.91	3	0.26	0.12	0.24
2	14	1.30	0.68	1.10	10	0.38	0.11	0.38
3	18	1.26	0.44	1.22	13	0.37	0.11	0.32
4	14	1.48	0.79	1.35	14	0.46	0.14	0.47
5	10	1.81	0.44	1.77	10	0.52	0.22	0.49
6	14	1.84	1.09	2.03	12	0.65	0.23	0.70
7	12	2.27	1.23	2.41	11	0.59	0.25	0.47
8	8	2.07	1.38	1.55	8	0.69	0.30	0.65
9	7	3.43	1.08	2.97	6	0.93	0.23	0.95
10	6	3.50	2.70	2.50	5	1.15	0.18	0.70
11	12	4.63	2.70	3.85	11	1.12	0.43	1.21
12	7	10.92	5.27	9.94	7	1.88	1.56	1.37
13	3	16.15	10.78	14.56	3	2.94	1.30	3.03
Mean		2.87	3.68	1.75	113	0.77	0.73	0.56

From Herter LD, Golendziner E, Flores JA, et al: Ovarian and uterine sonography in healthy girls between 1 and 13 years old: correlation of findings with age and pubertal status. AJR Am J Roentgenol 2002;178:1531-1536.

Table 61-3   Uterine and ovarian volume in relation to age

Age	No.	Uterine volume	No.	Ovarian volume
0-1 mo	15	3.4 (1.2)	6	0.5 (0.4)
3 mo[a]	7	0.9 (0.2)	4	0.4 (0.1)
1 yr	19	1.0 (0.2)	6	0.5 (0.2)
3 yr	26	1.0 (0.3)	17	0.7 (0.4)
5 yr	26	1.0 (0.3)	13	0.7 (0.5)
7 yr	28	0.9 (0.3)	15	0.8 (0.6)
9 yr	18	1.3 (0.4)	12	0.6 (0.4)
11 yr	16	1.9 (0.9)	10	1.3 (1.0)
13 yr	8	11.0 (10.5)	8	3.7 (2.1)
15 yr	15	21.2 (13.5)	9	6.7 (4.8)

Values are the mean (SD) in milliliters.
[a] This group comprises girls aged between 1.01 and 3 months. The remaining groups are analogous.
From Haber HP, Mayer EI: Ultrasound evaluation of uterine and ovarian size from birth to puberty. Pediatric Radiology 1994;24:11-13.

DISCUSSION

The uterus varies in size and appearance depending on the child's age. In the newborn the uterus is relatively large, and the endometrium is relatively thick due to the influence of maternal hormones[3,4] (see Fig. 61-1). After about 6 months, the uterus becomes less prominent and assumes its prepubertal shape with the fundus smaller than the cervix. The prepubertal uterus has a spade-shaped configuration. The endometrial cavity is seen as a thin echogenic line, and a hypoechoic endometrium may be seen around it. As the child nears puberty, the uterine fundus becomes relatively larger until it assumes a postpubertal shape. The endometrium is thin until puberty, when it thickens and changes appearance with the menstrual cycle.

References

1. Orsini LF, Salardi S, Pilu G, et al: Pelvic organs in premenarcheal girls: real-time ultrasonography. Radiology 1984;153:113-116.
2. Herter LD, Golendziner E, Flores JA, et al: Ovarian and uterine sonography in healthy girls between 1 and 13 years old: correlation of findings with age and pubertal status. AJR Am J Roentgenol 2002;178:1531-1536.
3. Haber HP, Mayer EI: Ultrasound evaluation of uterine and ovarian size from birth to puberty. Pediatr Radiol 1994;24:11-13.
4. Nussbaum AR, Sanders RC, Jones MD: Neonatal uterine morphology as seen on real-time US. Radiology 1986;160:641-643.

CHAPTER 62

Pediatric Ovary

Diane Babcock

Introduction

The ovaries are routinely measured as part of the pediatric female pelvis ultrasound examination.

Materials/Measurements

The ovaries appear as oval structures usually on either side of the uterus. Occasionally they are visualized above the uterus and even above the bladder. The examination is performed with a distended bladder by transabdominal approach. The height, width, and length are measured (Fig. 62-1), and the ovarian volume determined by the formula for a prolate ellipsoid (volume = $0.523 \times L \times H \times W$). Several authors have published the normal measurements (Tables 62-1 to 62-4).[1-5]

Table 62-1 Ovarian volume by decade of life

Decade	Mean Volume (cm³)	Standard Deviation	No. of Ovaries	95% Confidence Interval (cm³)*
1	1.7	1.4	19	0.2-4.9
2	7.8	4.4	83	1.7-18.5
3	10.2	6.2	308	2.6-23.1
4	9.5	5.4	358	2.6-20.7
5	9.0	5.8	206	2.1-20.9
6	6.2	3.6	57	1.6-14.2
7	6.0	3.8	44	1.0-15.0

*Calculated on the basis of cube root values, then transformed back to cubic centimeters.
From Cohen HL, Tice HM, Mandel FS, et al: Ovarian volumes measured by US: bigger than we think. Radiology 1990;177:189-192.

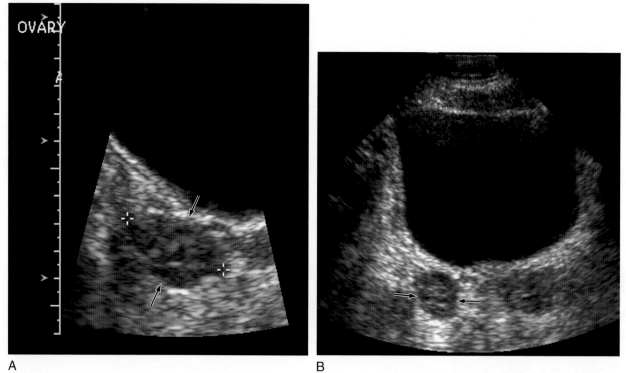

A

B

Figure 62-1

Ovary measurements. **A,** Longitudinal and **B,** transverse scans. Length and AP measurements are performed on longitudinal view. Width is measured on transverse view. Small cysts can frequently be seen in pediatric patients.

Table 62-2	Ovarian volumes in girls 1 day to 24 months old

| | | | Ovarian Volume (cm³) | |
| | | No. of Ovaries | | 95% Confidence |
Age Group	No. of Patients	Imaged	Mean (SD)	Interval
1 day to 3 mo	34	34	1.06 (0.96)	0.03-3.56
4-12 mo	21	34	1.05 (0.67)	0.18-2.71
13-24 mo	22	30	0.67 (0.35)	0.15-1.68

Note: Volumes are based on measurements made on sonograms.
From Cohen HL, Shapiro MA, Mandel FS, et al: Normal ovaries in neonates and infants: a sonographic study of 77 patients 1 day to 24 months old. AJR Am J Roentgenol 1993;160:583-586.

Table 62-3	Ovarian volume*

| | | Ovarian Volume (cm³) | |
Age (yr)	No. of Patients	By Chronologic Age Mean SD	By Bone Age Mean SD
2	5	0.75 ± 0.41	0.78 ± 0.38
3	6	0.66 ± 0.17	0.64 ± 0.18
4	14	0.82 ± 0.36	1.00 ± 0.45
5	4	0.86 ± 0.02	0.95 ± 0.52
6	9	1.19 ± 0.36	1.05 ± 0.65
7	8	1.26 ± 0.59	1.23 ± 0.47
8	10	1.05 ± 0.50	1.29 ± 0.33
9	11	1.98 ± 0.76	1.35 ± 0.71
10	12	2.22 ± 0.69	1.47 ± 0.56
11	12	2.52 ± 1.30	2.45 ± 0.86
12	6	3.80 ± 1.40	3.10 ± 1.29
13	4	4.18 ± 2.30	4.38 ± 2.74

*As determined by ultrasonography in 101 girls from age 2 to 13 years.
From Orsini LF, Salardi S, Pilu G, et al: Pelvic organs in premenarcheal girls: real-time ultrasonography. Radiology 1984;153:113-116.

Table 62-4	**Cysts seen per premenarchal year**				
Age (yr)	**No. of Patients**	**No. of Ovaries Imaged**	**No. (%) of Ovaries with Cysts**	**Cyst Size Range (mm)**	**No. (%) of Ovaries with Macrocysts***
2	14	17	12 (71)	2-9	0 (0)
3	12	20	12 (60)	3-17	4 (20)
4	11	11	9 (82)	3-12	1 (9)
5	11	21	17 (81)	2-14	4 (19)
6	9	12	8 (67)	2-10	1 (8)
7	2	2	2 (100)	6-7	0 (0)
8	17	30	21 (70)	2-15	3 (10)
9	7	13	8 (62)	3-7	0 (0)
10	7	11	7 (64)	2-6	0 (0)
11	2	3	2 (67)	5-7	0 (0)
12	9	15	8 (53)	3-15	2 (13)

* The numbers of patients with macrocysts were 4, 1, 3, 1, 2, and 2 for ages 3, 4, 5, 6, 8, and 12 years, respectively.
From Cohen HL, Eisenberg P, Mandel F, et al: Ovarian cysts are common in premenarchal girls: a sonographic study of 101 children 2-12 years old. AJR Am J Roentgenol 1992;159:89-91.

DISCUSSION

The ovary is relatively easy to visualize in the pediatric female pelvis. Small cysts are seen in more than 80% of patients older than 5 years of age (mean <7.5 mm). Cysts are also frequently seen in infants (see Table 62-4).[6]

References

1. Cohen HL, Tice HM, Mandel FS: Ovarian volumes measured by US: bigger than we think. Radiology 1990;177:189-192.
2. Cohen HL, Shapiro MA, Mandel FS, et al: Normal ovaries in neonates and infants: a sonographic study of 77 patients 1 day to 24 months old. AJR Am J Roentgenol 1993;160: 583-586.
3. Haber HP, Mayer EI: Ultrasound evaluation of uterine and ovarian size from birth to puberty. Pediatr Radiol 1994;24:11-13.
4. Herter LD, Golendziner E, Flores JA, et al: Ovarian and uterine sonography in healthy girls between 1 and 13 years old: correlation of findings with age and pubertal status. AJR Am J Roentgenol 2002;178:1531-1536.
5. Nussbaum AR, Sanders RC, Jones MD: Neonatal uterine morphology as seen on real-time US. Radiology 1986;160:641-643.
6. Cohen HL, Eisenberg P, Mandel F, et al: Ovarian cysts are common in premenarchal girls: a sonographic study of 101 children 2-12 years old. AJR Am J Roentgenol 1992; 159:89-91.

CHAPTER 63

Newborn Hip

Introduction

The femoral head and acetabulum are composed in large part of cartilage that is not visible on x-ray. During the first 4 months of life sonography is the primary imaging modality used because the cartilage is readily visible.

Materials/Measurements

Both the American College of Radiology and the American Institute of Ultrasound in Medicine have adopted a standard ultrasound examination of the neonatal hip that includes a coronal image with the hip in neutral position (Method of Graf) and a transverse image with the hip flexed with and without performing stress maneuver.[1-4] These basic views may be supplemented with additional views. Scans are performed with a high-frequency linear transducer using the highest frequency that will penetrate the body part.

The coronal view is performed with the infant in lateral decubitus position with the hip in a neutral position of approximately 30 degrees of flexion.[1-2] The echogenic line of the ilium is parallel with the transducer. The medial aspect of the bony acetabular roof is clearly identified as an echogenic bright spot. The labrum is visualized superior laterally (Fig. 63-1). Measurements are made solely on this coronal view, and the transverse view is performed to assess movement of the femoral head with stress (Barlow) maneuver.

Using the Graf technique, the alpha angle is measured. A baseline is drawn paralleling the iliac bone. A line is drawn parallel to the bony, acetabular roof. The alpha angle is measured between these two lines. A beta angle may be measured by drawing a third line parallel to the cartilaginous roof between the promontory and labrum. The beta angle is measured between this line and the baseline ilium line. Figure 63-2 shows these measurements.

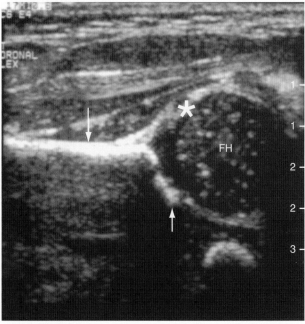

Figure 63-1
Coronal (Graf) view of infant hip. Scan is performed from the lateral aspect of the hip. Echogenic line of ilium (*arrow*). Medial aspects of bony, acetabular roof (*arrowhead*). Echogenic labrum (*). FH, Femoral head.

DISCUSSION

Normal values of alpha and beta angles have been reported from 0 to 6 months of age[5] (Table 63-1). A classification scheme as devised by Graf for types I to IV has been reported. Type I is a normal, mature hip. Type II is an immature hip. Type III is a subluxed hip. Type IV is a dislocated hip[6,7] (Table 63-2). Patients are followed during treatment to assess development of normal, acetabular morphology.

The size of the cartilaginous femoral head can be measured as well. The transverse diameter of the femoral head can be evaluated for symmetry (Fig. 63-3). Normal size versus age has been reported (Fig. 63-4).[8]

Acetabular coverage of the femoral head may be evaluated by measuring the distance between the ilial baseline and acetabular floor line and the maximum width of the femoral head (Fig. 63-5). Recommended cut-off values for normal femoral head coverage have been published by Morin et al[9] and Holen et al[10] (Table 63-3).

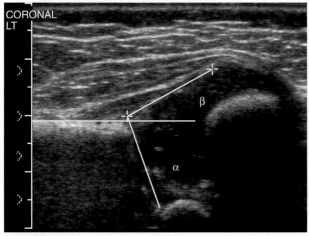

Figure 63-2
Coronal (Graf) view with angles. Alpha angle is measured between baseline ilium line and line drawn parallel to bony, acetabular roof. Beta angle is measured between baseline and line parallel to cartilaginous roof between the bony promontory and labrum.

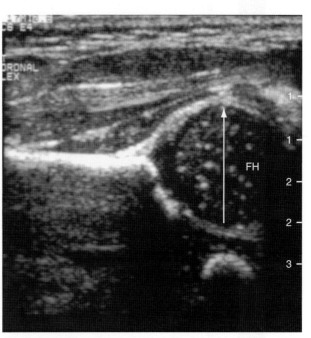

Figure 63-3
Diameter of femoral head measured on coronal view. *FH*, Femoral head.

Table 63-1	Mean values ± SD for angles alpha and beta vs. chronological age (*n* = 600)	
Age (mo)	**Alpha (x ± s)**	**Beta (x ± s)**
0	61.1 ± 3.17	57.6 ± 4.90
1	62.2. ± 3.12	52.6 ± 5.04
2	62.8 ± 2.23	50.3 ± 3.61
3	64.6 ± 2.23	48.0 ± 3.84
4	65.0 ± 2.02	45.5 ± 3.08
5	65.5 ± 2.28	46.1 ± 4.28
6	65.2 ± 1.98	43.6 ± 3.21
Global 0-4 mo	r = +0.946	r = −0.957
	4 = +0.984	
	r = −0.984	

From Zieger, M, Schulz RD: Ultrasonography of the infant hip. III: Clinical application. Pediatr Radiol 1987;17:226-232.

Table 63-2 Synopsis of sonographic hip types, recommended description, and clinical management

Sonographic Type	Bony Modeling	Bony Promontory	Cartilage Roof Triangle	Alpha Angle	Beta Angle	Therapeutic Consequences
Mature hip						
Ia	Good	Angular	Narrow, extending far over the femoral head	>60°	<55°	No therapy
Ib	Good	Slightly rounded	Stubby, extending short distance over crown of femoral head	>60°	>55°	
No age limits						
Immature hip						
IIa (+) (physiological, appropriate for age)	Satisfactory	Rounded	Broad, covering crown of head	50°–59°	>55°	No therapy; follow-up
IIa (−) (maturational deficit)	Deficient	Rounded	Broad, covering crown of the head	50°–59°	>55°	Abduction device, follow-up (borderline cases)
Younger than 3 months of age				50°–59°		
Delayed osseous development						
IIb	Deficient	Rounded	Broad, covering crown of the head	43°–49°	>55°	Abduction device
More than 3 months of age						
Critical zone hip						
IIc	Deficient/ highly deficient	Rounded	Broad, still covering the head	43°–49°	<77°	Abduction device
No age limits				<43°		
Decentering hip						
D (IId)	Highly deficient	Rounded-off/ flattened	Displaced	<43°	>77°	Like eccentric hips
Eccentric hip						
IIIa	Poor	Flattened	Displaced, devoid of echoes	<43°	>77°	Reduction-abduction splint (eventually plaster cast)
IIIb	Poor	Flattened	Displaced, echogenic		>77°	Inpatient treatment
IV	Poor	Flattened	Trapped between femoral head and ilium		>77°	Inpatient treatment

From Graf R (ed): Guide to Sonography of the Infant Hip: New York, Thieme, 1987.

Table 63-3	Recommended cut-off values for femoral head coverage (%)
Author/Patient Group	**Femoral Head Coverage (%)**
Morin et al	
Normal	<58
Abnormal	≤58
Holen et al	
Normal	>50
Abnormal	≤50

Morin and Holen from clinical studies; Millis from review article.
From Morin C, Harcke HT, MacEwen GD: The infant hip: real-time US assessment of acetabular development. Radiology 1985;157:673-677; and Holen KJ, et al: Ultrasound screening for hip dysplasia in newborns. J Pediatr Orthop 1994;14:667-673.

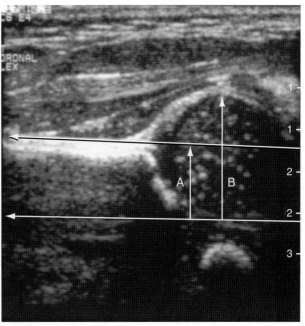

Figure 63-5
Acetabular coverage of femoral head. *A* = Distance between the acetabular apex and the floor; *B* = width of the femoral head. Percentage of coverage = A/B × 100.[9,10]

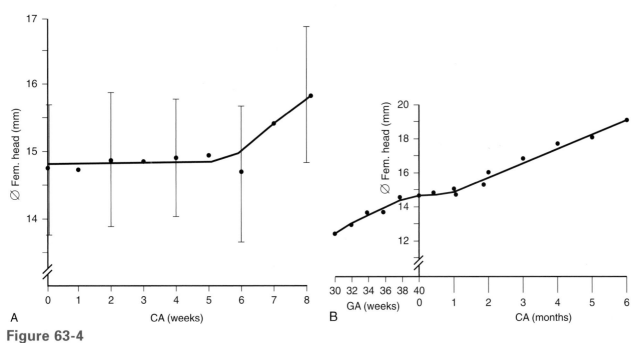

A   CA (weeks)

B   GA (weeks)   CA (months)

Figure 63-4
Diameter of femoral head **(A)** in infants of 40 weeks GA at various chronologic age **(B)** versus age in weeks of GA (until 40) or additional months of CA (up to 6). (From Zieger M, Hilpert S: Ultrasound of the infant hip. IV: Normal development in the newborn and preterm neonate. Pediatr Radiol 1987;17:470-473.)

Ultrasound has become the standard method of evaluation in the infant hip for developmental dysplasia. The standard examinations as accepted by The American College of Radiology and The American Institute of Ultrasound in Medicine are used in North America. Although in some European countries all newborns are examined for hip dysplasia, only those that have increased risks, such as with breech presentations or a strong family history of hip dysplasia, are routinely screened in North America.

References

1. Graf R: The diagnosis of congenital hip-joint dislocation by the ultrasonic Combound treatment. Arch Orthop Trauma Surg 1980; 97:117-133.
2. Graf R: Classification of hip joint dysplasia by means of sonography. Arch Orthop Trauma Surg 1984;102:248-255.
3. ACR Practice Guideline for the Performance of the Ultrasound Examination for Detection of Developmental Dysplasia of the Hip: In ACR Practice Guidelines and Technical Standards Book. 2003, American College of Radiology. p. 597-601.
4. AIUM Practice Guideline for the Performance of the Ultrasound Examination for Detection of Developmental Dysplasia of the Hip: In AIUM Guidelines, American Institute of Ultrasound of Medicine (ed). Maryland, 2003, pp 1-4.
5. Laure I, Zieger M, RD Schulz: Ultrasonography of the infant hip. III. Clinical application. Pediatr Radiol 1987;17:226-232.
6. Graf R (ed): Guide to Sonography of the Infant Hip. New York, Thieme, 1987.
7. Gerscovich EO: A radiologist's guide to the imaging in the diagnosis and treatment of developmental dysplasia of the hip. II. Ultrasonography: anatomy, technique, acetabular angle measurements, acetabular coverage of femoral head, acetabular cartilage thickness, three-dimensional technique, screening of newborns, study of older children. Skeletal Radiol 1997; 26:447-456.
8. Zieger M, Hilpert S: Ultrasound of the infant hip. IV. Normal development in the newborn and preterm neonate Pediatr Radiol 1987; 17:470-473.
9. Morin C, Harcke HT, MacEwen GD: The infant hip: real-time US assessment of acetabular development. Radiology 1985; 157:673-677.
10. Holen KJ, et al: Ultrasound screening for hip dysplasia in newborns. J Pediatr Orthop 1994;14:667-673.

Head and Neck Doppler

Mira L. Katz

CHAPTER 64

Transcranial Doppler Examinations

Introduction

In this chapter measurements used during a transcranial Doppler (TCD) examination are reviewed. The measurements described can be obtained using nonimaging TCD equipment or transcranial color Doppler imaging. TCD is performed with a 2-MHz transducer (Doppler and imaging) using a large sample volume (10 to 15 mm) and assuming a zero-degree angle.

Materials/Methods

INTRACRANIAL ARTERIAL IDENTIFICATION

Four ultrasound windows are used during a complete standard TCD examination to evaluate the intracranial arteries.[1] The four approaches are (1) transtemporal; (2) transorbital; (3) suboccipital; and (4) submandibular. The identification of the intracranial arteries from each ultrasound window is based on the following: depth of the sample volume, angle of the transducer, blood flow direction relative to the transducer, spatial relationship of one artery to another, and the traceability of an artery's anatomic route. The intracranial arteries evaluated from each approach, the depth range, and the direction of blood flow relative to the ultrasound transducer are listed in Table 64-1.

MEAN VELOCITY AND PULSATILITY INDEX

During TCD examinations, mean velocity and pulsatility index are the parameters reported. Mean velocities calculated during TCD examinations are based on the time average of the outline velocity (maximum velocity envelope). The velocity envelope is a trace of the peak velocities as a function of time. The mean velocity (Fig. 64-1) can be calculated using the following formula:

$$\frac{\left(\begin{array}{l}\text{peak systolic velocity} - \\ \text{end-diastolic velocity}\end{array}\right)}{3} + \text{end-diastolic velocity}$$

The pulsatility index (P.I.) is a reflection of the resistance that is encountered with each cardiac cycle. Damped blood flow distal to an obstruction will have a decreased P.I., and Doppler signals obtained proximal to a high resistance (i.e., increased intracranial pressure) will have an increased P.I. Pulsatility index can be calculated using the following formula:

$$\text{pulsatility index} = \frac{\text{systolic velocity} - \text{diastolic velocity}}{\text{mean velocity}}$$

NORMAL INTRACRANIAL ARTERIAL VELOCITIES

Mean velocities (cm/sec) are reported for TCD examinations because this parameter is less affected by changes of central cardiovascular factors (i.e., heart rate, peripheral resistance, etc.) than systolic or diastolic values, thereby diminishing interindividual variations.[2,3] The normal values for the intracranial arterial velocities in the average adult are listed in Table 64-1. Differences between intracranial arterial velocities are more important than the absolute values recorded from an individual. Side-to-side asymmetry in velocities should be minimal (<30%) for normal vessels and undisturbed anatomy of the circle of Willis.[2,4]

Intracranial arterial velocities are increased in children compared with adults. For example, in a child who is 9 years old, the mean velocity

Table 64-1	Intracranial arterial identification criteria			
Window	**Artery**	**Depth (mm)**	**Mean Velocity (cm/sec)**	**Blood Flow Direction (relative to transducer)**
Transtemporal	Middle cerebral	30-67	62 ± 12	Toward
	Anterior cerebral	60-80	50 ± 11	Away
	Terminal–internal carotid	60-67	39 ± 9	Toward
	Posterior cerebral	55-80	39 ± 10	Toward
	Posterior communicating	60-75	36 ± 15	Toward, away
Transorbital	Ophthalmic	40-60	21 ± 5	Toward
	Internal carotid siphon	60-80	47 ± 14	Bidirectional, away, toward
Subocciptal	Vertebral	40-85	38 ± 10	Away
	Basilar	≥80	41 ± 10	Away
Submandibular	Internal carotid	35-70	37 ± 9	Away

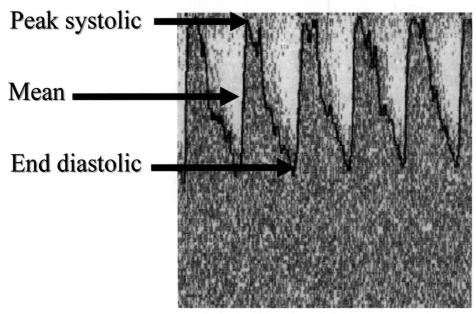

Figure 64-1
The Doppler signal from a middle cerebral artery. Arrows point to the peak systolic, mean, and end-diastolic velocities.

of the middle cerebral artery is approximately 95 cm/sec compared with 62 cm/sec in an adult. Additionally, when performing TCD examinations in children, a smaller sample volume size (6 mm) usually provides good quality Doppler signals and is helpful when trying to isolate the small intracranial arteries.

PHYSIOLOGIC FACTORS

Several physiologic factors affect the intracranial arterial velocities recorded during a TCD examination and are summarized in Table 64-2. It is important to recognize that many parameters are involved in the accurate interpretation of TCD data. Some general interpretation guidelines (Table 64-3) are helpful; however, each patient must be considered individually because of the variety of physiologic factors that affect the intracranial arterial velocities.

LIMITATIONS OF TCD EXAMINATIONS

The limitations of the TCD examination are summarized in Table 64-4. Experience is the

Table 64-2 | Physiologic factors affecting a TCD examination

Parameter	TCD examination
Age[5,6]	Lower intracranial arterial velocities are reported with increasing age
Gender[7]	Penetration of the temporal bone is more difficult in females No significant difference in intracranial arterial velocities between males and females
Race	Penetration of the temporal bone is more difficult in African Americans
Hematocrit[8,9]	Intracranial arterial velocities increase in the presence of anemia (Hct < 30%)
Carbon dioxide reactivity[10,11]	A deficiency of CO_2 in the blood causes a decrease in MCA mean velocity and an increase in the MCA pulsatility index
Heart rate and cardiac output[12]	Cardiac arrhythmias will be reflected in the TCD recording Changes due to cardiac output not associated with hemodilution have little effect on CBF if autoregulation is intact Velocities should be relatively independent of small changes in cardiac output
Fever	A fever increases cerebral blood flow by approximately 10% for every degree of temperature When a patient has a fever, intracranial arterial velocities will be increased compared with their baseline velocities

Table 64-3 | Transcranial Doppler interpretation guidelines

- Document and compare Doppler spectral waveforms (mean velocity) from the anterior and posterior circulation, and from the right and left sides
- Document and compare Doppler spectral waveforms configuration (pulsatility index, upstroke time)
- Consider the status of the extracranial vessels
- Document the patient's age, medical history, risk factors, symptoms, and current medications
- Obtain available laboratory values (hematocrit, intracranial pressure, blood pressure, heart rate, cardiac output)
- Establish institutional diagnostic criteria for the various clinical applications
- Be aware of the limitations of the TCD examination

key factor for obtaining reliable, consistent TCD examinations. Knowledge of the limitations should reduce errors associated with the interpretation of TCD results.

DISCUSSION

TCD interpretation criteria for each clinical setting vary, and each institution must establish institutional diagnostic criteria for the various clinical applications.[1] Interpretation criteria for several common TCD clinical applications are listed in Table 64-5. Despite growth in

Table 64-4	Limitations of the transcranial Doppler examination

- Operator experience
- Improper instrument control settings
- An uncooperative patient or patient movement
- Absent or poor transtemporal window
- Anatomic variations
- Arterial misidentification
- Distal branch disease
- Distal basilar artery is not accessible
- Misinterpretation of collateral channels or vasospasm as a stenosis
- Displacement of arteries by an intracranial mass

Table 64-5	Clinical applications

Stenosis[13-15]	Focal increase (>25%) of velocity Absolute velocity varies with each patient Mean velocity of >80 cm/sec is the threshold causing concern for anterior circulation (>50% diameter reduction) Mean velocity of >70 cm/sec is the threshold causing concern for posterior circulation (>50% diameter reduction)
Occlusion[16]	Limited to the MCA because of inadequate temporal windows, anatomic variation, and congenital aplasia or severe hypoplasia MCA occlusion is suspected if Doppler signal is absent and there are good-quality Doppler signals from the uninvolved ipsilateral intracranial arteries
Collateral pathways[17]	Three collateral pathways can be documented: —Anterior communicating (hemisphere to hemisphere): increase in contralateral ACA velocity, turbulent Doppler signal with increased velocity at midline, reversal of blood flow direction in the ipsilateral ACA —Posterior communicating (anterior to posterior): increased velocity —Ophthalmic artery (internal to external carotid): increased velocity, reversal of blood flow direction, change from high to low resistance signal
Vasospasm[18,19]	Increase in velocity: —MCA: 100-120 cm/sec correlates with mild vasospasm —MCA: 120-200 cm/sec correlates with moderate vasospasm —MCA: >200 cm/sec correlates with severe vasospasm A negative study does not exclude vasospasm
Sickle cell disease[20,21]	For MCA and t-ICA: —Normal: <170 cm/sec —Conditional: 170-199 cm/sec —Abnormal: ≥200 cm/sec

experience and technical improvements, the clinical usefulness of TCD remains controversial.[22] TCD is not useful as a routine screening test as part of the cerebrovascular evaluation because the incidence of intracranial disease is low and because of the technical challenges associated with the examination.

References

1. Katz ML, Alexandrov AV: A Practical Guide to Transcranial Doppler Examinations. Littleton, Colo, 2003, Summer Publishing.

2. Hennerici M, Rautenberg W, Sitzer G, Schwartz A: Transcranial Doppler ultrasound for the assessment of intracranial arterial flow velocity. Part 1. Examination technique and normal values. Surg Neurol 1987;27:439-448.

3. Aaslid R: The Doppler principle applied to measurement of blood flow velocity in cerebral arteries. In Aaslid R (ed): Transcranial Doppler Sonography. Chapter 3. New York, Springer-Verlag, 1986, pp 22-38.

4. Sorteberg W, Langmoen IA, Lindegaard K-F, Nornes H: Side-to-side differences and day-to-day variations of transcranial Doppler parameters in normal subjects. J Ultrasound Med 1990;9:403-409.

5. Arnolds BJ, von Reutern G-M: Transcranial Doppler sonography. Examination technique and normal reference values. Ultrasound Med Biol 1986;12:115-123.

6. Ringelstein EB, Kahlscheuer B, Niggemeyer E, Otis SM: Transcranial Doppler sonography: anatomical landmarks and normal velocity values. Ultrasound Med Biol 1990;16:745-761.

7. Halsey JH: Effect of emitted power on waveform intensity in transcranial Doppler. Stroke 1990;22:1573-1578.

8. Brass LM, Pavlakis SG, DeVivo D, et al: Transcranial Doppler measurements of the middle cerebral artery. Effect of hematocrit. Stroke 1988;19:1466-1469.

9. Ameriso SF, Paganini-Hill A, Meiselman HJ, Fisher M: Correlates of middle cerebral artery blood velocity in the elderly. Stroke 1990;21:1579-1583.

10. Huber P, Handa J: Effect of contrast material, hypercapnia, hyperventilation, hypertonic glucose and papaverine on the diameter of the cerebral arteries. Angiographic determination in man. Invest Radiol 1967;2:17-32.

11. Markwalder T-M, Grolimund P, Seiler RW, et al: Dependency of blood flow velocity in the middle cerebral artery on end-tidal carbon dioxide partial pressure—a transcranial ultrasound Doppler study. J Cereb Blood Flow Metab 1984;4:368-372.

12. Bouma GJ, Muizelaar JP: Relationship between cardiac output and cerebral blood flow in patients with intact and with impaired autoregulation. J Neurosurg 1990;73:368-374.

13. de Bray J-M, Joseph P-A, Jeanvoine H, et al: Transcranial Doppler evaluation of middle cerebral artery stenosis. J Ultrasound Med 1988;7:611-616.

14. Baumgartner RW, Mattle HP, Schroth G: Assessment of = 50% and <50% intracranial stenoses by transcranial color-coded duplex sonography. Stroke 1999;30:87-92.

15. Arenillas JF, Molina CA, Montaner J, et al: Progression and clinical recurrence of symptomatic middle cerebral artery stenosis: a long-term follow-up transcranial Doppler ultrasound study. Stroke 2001;32:2898-2904.

16. Kaps M, Damian MS, Teschendorf U, Dorndorf W: Transcranial Doppler ultrasound findings in middle cerebral artery occlusion. Stroke 1990;21:532-537.

17. Babikian V, Sloan MA, Tegeler CH, et al: Transcranial Doppler validation pilot study. J Neuroimaging 1993;3:242-249.

18. Sloan MA, Burch CH, Wozniak MA, et al: Transcranial Doppler detection of vertebrobasilar vasospasm following subarachnoid hemorrhage. Stroke 1994;25:2187-2197.

19. Harders AG, Gilsbach JM: Time course of blood velocity changes related to vasospasm in the circle of Willis measured by transcranial Doppler ultrasound. J Neurosurg 1987;66:718-728.

20. Adams R, McKie V, Hsu L, et al: Prevention of a first stroke by transfusions in children with sickle cell anemia and abnormal results on transcranial Doppler ultrasonography. N Engl J Med 1998;339:5-11.

21. Kwiatkowski JL, Hunter JV, Smith-Whitley, Katz ML, et al: Transcranial Doppler ultrasonography in siblings with sickle cell disease. Br J Haematol 2003;121:932-938.

22. Sloan MA, Alexandrov AV, Tegeler CH, et al: Assessment: transcranial Doppler ultrasonography. Report of the therapeutics and technology assessment subcommittee of the American Academy of Neurology. Neurology 2004;62:1468-1481.

CHAPTER 65

Temporal Arteritis Ultrasound Findings

Introduction

As the name implies, temporal arteritis is an inflammatory involvement of the affected arteries. This arterial inflammation can be seen with either polymylagia rheumatica or giant cell arteritis, and the relationship between these two disorders was not widely accepted until Paulley and Hughes,[1] who were among the first to recognize their association in 1960.

Polymyalgia rheumatica is an inflammatory condition of unknown cause and is strongly suggestive when a patient complains of persistent pain for at least 1 month with aching and morning stiffness in the neck, shoulder girdle, and pelvic girdle that lasts at least 30 minutes and an increase in the erythrocyte sedimentation rate to at least 40 mm per hour.[2,3]

Giant cell arteritis is a chronic vasculitis of large- and medium-sized vessels and usually involves the cranial branches of the arteries originating from the aortic arch. Systemic symptoms are observed in about half of the patients.[4,5]

A headache is probably the most frequent symptom and occurs in two thirds of patients.[4,6] Pain is frequently marked and tends to be located over the temporal or occipital areas but may be less well defined.[7] The frontal or parietal branches of the superficial temporal arteries may be thickened, nodular, tender, or occasionally erythematous.[7]

If the diagnosis of extracranial giant cell arteritis is suspected, arteriography, computed tomography (CT), and magnetic resonance angiography are all required diagnostic tests for the medium to large arteries of the body. On arteriography, the typical finding is bilateral stenosis or occlusion of the subclavian, axillary, and proximal brachial arteries, and these arteries have a smooth, tapered appearance. The best imaging technique to detect aortic aneurysms or dissections is CT or MRI. The finding of a thickened aortic wall on CT or MRI is a direct indication of inflammation of the aortic wall (Fig. 65-1) and thus active disease.[8]

Materials/Methods

SONOGRAPHIC STUDIES

Giant cell arteritis affecting the smaller temporal arteries usually requires a biopsy of the temporal artery. Several studies have emphasized the diagnostic potentialities of color duplex ultrasound in giant cell arteritis.[9-13] Biopsy remains the gold standard for the diagnosis of giant cell arteritis.[14] However, Schmidt et al[10,15] in 1997 and 2003 suggested that a "dark halo" (edema of the arterial wall) around the vessel is strongly related to the acute phase of the disease and suggested that high-frequency, duplex sonography of the temporal arteries can be used in the diagnosis of temporal arteritis and polymyalgia rheumatica (Fig. 65-2).

SONOGRAPHIC IMAGING

Because the temporal artery and its branch arteries are small, modern, high-frequency, linear-array transducers should be used for maximum resolution. Frequencies above 7.5 MHz are commonly employed in temporal artery evaluation. To begin the ultrasound examination, as completely and continuously as possible using an axial scanning plane, start by identifying the main stem of the superficial temporal artery as it courses in front of the tragus (Fig. 65-3). Usually the main stem bifurcates into the frontal and parietal branches on a level with the top of the auricle. There can be anatomical variance; however, the most common bifurcation (94%) is the branching described earlier. If the patient complains of occipital or nuchal headache, it is necessary to examine the occipital artery, which is found over the mastoid processus.[16] Imaging of the occipital artery may be difficult as it is tortuous distally, and, superfi-

cially, scalp hair may not allow good transducer skin contact. The occipital artery is approximately 4 cm lateral to the external occipital protuberance. The longitudinal plane should also be used, particularly for color Doppler interrogation.

DIAGNOSTIC CRITERIA

Although no commonly accepted criteria exist for the exact definition of a halo measurement, its thickness has been reported to lie between 0.3 and 1.2 mm, while a recent publication proposed a thickness of 1 mm or more for diagnosing a halo.[10,14] Rienhard et al,[16] when describing a "halo," used an observed, circumferential, dark, hypoechoic zone around the perfused lumen with a thickness of at least one quarter that of the perfused lumen.

Sensitivity and specificity values when comparing an ultrasound halo with a biopsy are reported as values of 40% to 86% and 78% to 100%, respectively.[12,14,17] The positive predictive value (PPV) and the negative predictive value (NPV) of ultrasound when compared with biopsy in one study found 96% PPV and 58% NPV,[16] where other studies found a poor PPV (equal to or less than 50% of the halo sign).[12,14]

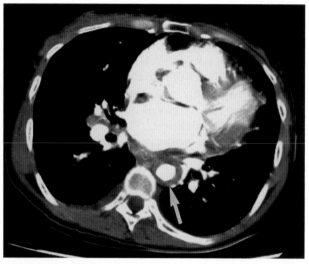

Figure 65-1
Computed tomography image of thickened aortic wall (*arrow*) seen in a patient with arteritis.

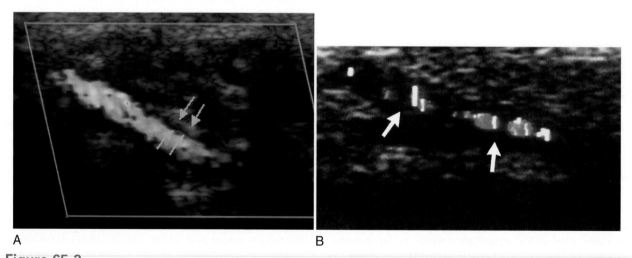

A   B

Figure 65-2
Color Doppler ultrasound evaluation of a normal temporal artery **(A)** displaying "wall to wall" blood flow. Note "thin" arterial wall (*double arrows*). Abnormal temporal artery **(B)** illustrated by hypoechoic, dark halo most likely reflecting edema of the vessel wall. Narrowed color Doppler flow seen centrally (*arrows*). (Image **B** from Schmidt WA, Kraft HE, Vorpahl K, et al: Color duplex ultrasonography in the diagnosis of temporal arteritis. N Engl J Med 1997;337:1336-1342.)

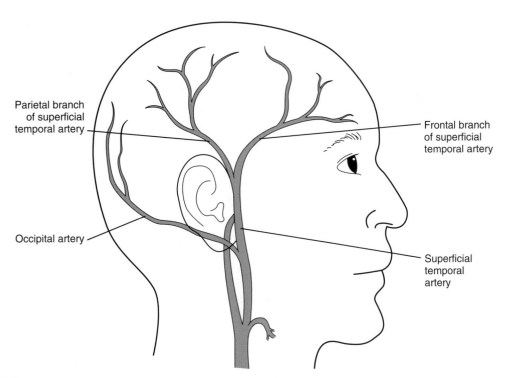

Figure 65-3
Anatomy of the superficial temporal artery and its branches.

Table 65-1	Possible pitfalls in sonographic diagnosis of temporal arteritis
Pitfall	**Comment**
Focus setting	A sole hypoechoic area at the near wall of the vessel observed with the focus setting too deep and *not* at the vessel depth
Color intensity/ sensitivity	Risk of under- or overdiagnosis with the color gain/pulse repetition frequency being too high or too low
Bifurcation halo	Hypoechoic perivascular zone at the ramification into the frontal and parietal rami, observed in nearly half of patients, with the possible causes: (1) lack of a coaxial plane with vessels protruding from the two-dimensional plane, (2) atheromatous plaques, and (3) physiological flow perturbations with no or negative flow components resulting in no color flow signal
Accompanying vein	No or slow flow in the vein accompanying the common superficial temporal artery can appear as a perivascular dark zone

Modified from Reinhard M, Schmidt D, Hetzel A: Color-coded sonography in suspected temporal arteritis—experiences after 83 cases. Rheumatol Int 2004;24:340-346.

DISCUSSION

Diagnostic ultrasound scanning techniques vary from institution to institution and because ultrasound examination is one of the most user-dependent modalities, misinterpretations can be made without proper scanning technique. Reinhard et al,[16] in search of the "halo sign" during his study of 83 patients suspected of having temporal arteritis, discovered some possible pitfalls (Table 65-1).

Schmidt et al[10] felt that sonography could be used in the diagnosis and treatment of temporal arteritis or polymyalgia rheumatica as follows:

1) Patients with typical clinical signs of temporal arteritis and a dark halo on ultrasonography may be treated without a biopsy, unless there is a reason to suspect another form of vasculitis.

2) Patients with strong clinical evidence of temporal arteries who have only stenoses or occlusion or no abnormalities on ultrasonography should still undergo biopsy.

3) Patients with clinical signs of polymyalgia rheumatica who have no symptoms of temporal arteritis but have abnormal findings on ultrasonography (a halo, stenosis, or occlusion) should undergo biopsy and be treated with a higher initial dose of corticosteroids to protect against blindness, at least until the biopsy results are known.

4) Ultrasonography should be particularly helpful in patients with equivocal clinical evidence of temporal arteritis.

In conclusion, ultrasound examination may prove to be a useful, noninvasive, diagnostic tool for the detection of temporal arteritis without the need, in some cases, for an arterial biopsy. Standardization of the ultrasound technique, combined with large patient studies, is necessary to prove the efficacy of this technique.

References

1. Paulley JW, Hughes JP: Giant-cell arteritis, or arteritis of the aged. BMJ 1960;2:1562-1567.

2. Healey LA: Long-term follow-up of polymyalgia rheumatica: evidence for synovitis. Semin Arthritis Rheum 1984;13:322-328.

3. Chuang TY, Hunder GG, Ilstrup DM, Kurland LT: Polymyalgia rheumatica: a 10-year epidemiologic and clinical study. Ann Intern Med 1982;97:672-680.

4. Salvarani C, Macchioni PL, Tartoni PL, et al: Polymyalgia rheumatica and giant cell arteritis: a 5-year epidemiologic and clinical study in Reggio Emilia, Italy. Clin Exp Rheumatol 1987;5:205-215.

5. Calamia KT, Hunder GG: Clinical manifestations of giant cell (temporal) arteritis. Clin Rheum Dis 1980;6:389-403.

6. Huston KA, Hunder GG, Lie JT, Kennedy RH, Elveback LR: Temporal arteritis: a 25-year epidemiologic, clinical, and pathologic study. Ann Intern Med 1978;88:162-167.

7. Salvarani C, Cantini F, Boiardi L, Hunder GG: Polymyalgia rheumatica and giant-cell arteritis. N Engl J Med 2002;347:261-271.

8. Stanson AW: Imaging findings in extracranial (giant cell) temporal arteritis. Clin Exp Rheumatol 2001;18:(suppl 20):S43-S48.

9. Schmidt WA, Kraft HE, Volker L, et al: Colour Doppler sonography to diagnose temporal arteritis. Lancet 1995;345:866.

10. Schmidt WA, Kraft HE, Vorpahl K, Volker L, Gromnica-Ihle EJ: Color duplex ultrasonography in the diagnosis of temporal arteritis. N Engl J Med 1997;337:1336-1342.

11. Hunder GG, Weyand cm: Sonography in giant-cell arteritis. N Engl J Med 1997;337:1385-1386.

12. Nesher G, Shemesh D, Mates M, Sonnenblick M, Abramowitz HB: The predictive value of the halo sign in color Doppler ultrasonogrpahy of the temporal arteries for diagnosing giant cell arteritis. J Rheumatol 2002;29:1224-1226.

13. Le Sar CJ, Meier GH, De Masi RJ, et al: The utility of color duplex ultrasonography in the diagnosis of temporal arteritis. J Vasc Surg 2002;36:1154-1560.

14. Salvarani C, Silingardi M, Ghirarduzzi A, et al: Is duplex ultrasonography useful for the diagnosis of giant-cell arteritis? Ann Intern Med 2002;137:323-238.

15. Schmidt D, Hetzel A, Renhard M, Auw-Haedrich C: Comparison between color duplex ultrasonography and histology of the temporal artery in cranial arteritis (giant cell arteritis). Eur J Med Res 2003;8:1-7.

16. Reinhard M, Schmidt D, Hetzel A: Color-coded sonography in suspected temporal arteritis—experiences after 83 cases. Rheumatol Int 2004;24:340-346.

17. Schmid R, Hermann M, Yannar A, Baumgartner RW: Color duplex ultrasound of the temporal artery: replacement for biopsy in temporal arteritis [German]. Ophthalmologica 2002;216:16-21.

Mark E. Lockhart
Lincoln L. Berland

CHAPTER 66

Internal Carotid Artery Doppler

Introduction

Carotid Doppler measurements usually attempt to quantitate the severity of carotid stenosis to assess the risk for a subsequent stroke. However, velocity criteria for stenosis have varied substantially among institutions. Responding to this problem, the Society of Radiologists in Ultrasound convened an interdisciplinary consensus conference in 2002 and developed a revised set of criteria to guide institutions that do not have internally validated criteria. This chapter will review these consensus criteria and will address when the criteria should be applied.

Since the landmark North American Symptomatic Carotid Endarterectomy Trial (NASCET), European Carotid Surgery Trial, and Asympto-matic Carotid Atherosclerosis Study (ACAS) trials in the early 1990s, noninvasive detection of internal carotid artery (ICA) stenosis has helped guide the need for surgery to reduce the subsequent risk of stroke. NASCET demonstrated that surgery is better than medical management for ICA stenosis greater than 70%.[1] The ACAS trial showed a similar benefit in asymptomatic patients with at least 60% stenosis.[2] Although other techniques have been applied, the NASCET method for calculating the severity of stenosis has become the standard. This uses one minus the diameter of the stenotic segment of the proximal ICA divided by the diameter of the normal ICA beyond the carotid bulb.[1]

Materials/Measurements

Technique

The patient is placed in a comfortable position with the head slightly extended and turned away from the side being investigated. A high-frequency linear transducer (at least 5 to 7 MHz) is necessary to provide satisfactory resolution. The carotids are superficial, and their sonographic interrogation is rarely limited by depth.

Although the sonographic grading of stenosis is primarily determined by flow criteria and waveforms (Fig. 66-1), visualizing vessel lumen narrowing often aids diagnostic confidence for cases in which Doppler criteria are equivocal or confusing. For example, normal Doppler velocities with abnormally dampened waveforms associated with severe intimal plaques may permit an accurate diagnosis of high-grade stenosis.

With color Doppler, the color flow within a normal vessel should fill the lumen and be free of color aliasing. For spectral Doppler, the angle of insonation should be as close to 60 degrees as possible, but always 60 degrees or less, to limit artifactual variability of velocity measurements. In patients with greater than 50% stenosis, one study suggests that serial examinations should use a similar angle of insonation to limit measurement variability.[3] Attention to the direction of flow can prevent interpretative errors. Calculations should be performed from an arterial waveform with strong signal characteristics. The peak systolic velocity (PSV) is the highest velocity in the cardiac cycle (Fig. 66-2). End-diastolic velocity (EDV) is measured at the point immediately prior to the next systolic upstroke, rather than the lowest point on the cardiac cycle. When transient reversal of flow occurs, the EDV may be considered to equal zero. The internal carotid to common carotid artery (ICA/CCA) ratio is calculated as the PSV of the highest velocity in the proximal ICA divided by the PSV of the distal CCA.

The primary objective of carotid Doppler ultrasound is to differentiate stenoses that exceed the threshold for surgery or stenting from those that may be more safely followed with serial ultrasound examinations. The subcategorization of low-grade stenosis has shown

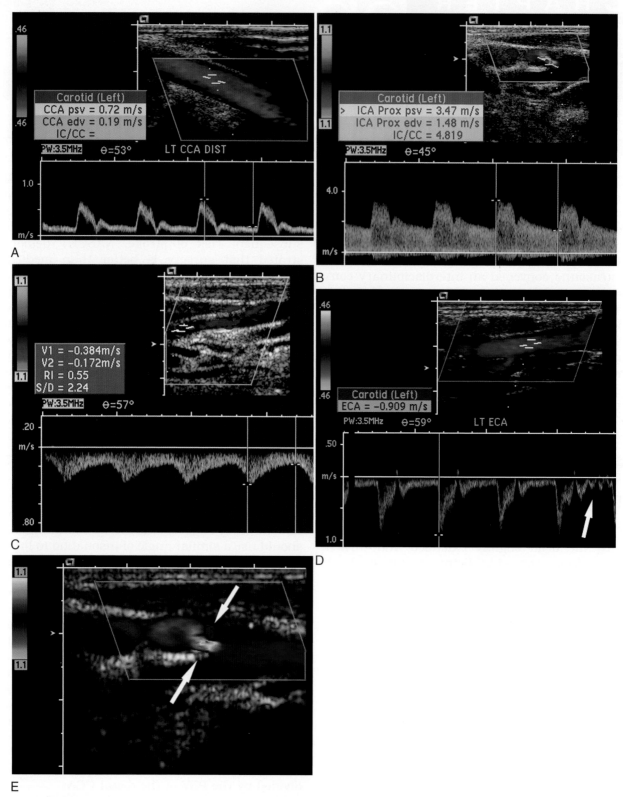

Figure 66-1

Expected waveforms of severe proximal ICA stenosis.

A, Duplex Doppler evaluation includes the common carotid artery showing normal, mildly high resistance flow without turbulence or aliasing. **B,** The ICA demonstrates turbulent flow with elevated PSV. **C,** In the distal ICA, there is delayed systolic acceleration "tardus" with low velocity peak flow "parvus," consistent with poststenotic flow pattern. **D,** Mild internalization of the ECA is present with low-resistance flow. Note the reverberation associated with temporal tap maneuver (*arrow*). **E,** Longitudinal color Doppler visually demonstrates the stenosis in the ICA (*arrows*) indicated by the spectral findings.

Table 66-1	Internal carotid artery stenosis doppler criteria[5]		
Severity of Stenosis	**PSV**	**EDV**	**ICA/CCA**
Normal	<125	<40	<2.0
Less than 50%	<125	<40	<2.0
50-69%	125-230	40-100	2.0-4.0
>70% less than near occlusion	>230	>100	>4.0
Near occlusion	Variable	Variable	Variable
Total occlusion	None	N/A	N/A

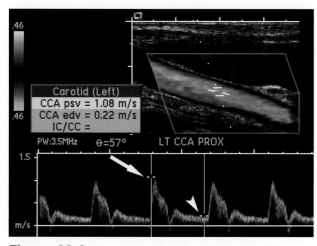

Figure 66-2

Measurement calculations of carotid arterial waveform.
Spectral Doppler of the CCA shows homogenous color and good spectral signal. The first point of measurement (*arrow*) at the highest velocity flow is the PSV. The second point of measurement (*arrowhead*), immediately prior to the next waveform, represents the EDV.

Table 66-2	Clinical situations in which consensus velocity criteria are not validated
Common carotid stenosis	
Previous carotid endarterectomy	
Ipsilateral carotid stenting	
Contralateral carotid occlusion	
Tandem ipsilateral carotid stenoses	

more variation in threshold criteria than have criteria for higher grades of stenosis. Many algorithms have purported to differentiate stenosis by increments of as little as 10%, with poor accuracy and reproducibility.[4] The SRU consensus criteria acknowledge the inability of ultrasound to so finely subcategorize ICA stenosis, especially when the stenosis is less than 50%.[5]

DOPPLER PARAMETERS

The PSV is the most widely validated and accepted criterion for the primary determination of ICA stenosis (Table 66-1). Two "additional parameters" were cited by the consensus panel to assist diagnosis when the primary parameter was equivocal. The ratio of the PSV in the ICA to the CCA is useful, and an elevated end-diastolic velocity also correlates with higher degrees of stenosis.[5] While other velocity criteria and other ratios, such as the EDV ratio of the ICA/CCA, have been proposed as useful, the panel did not recommend them.

Although the consensus criteria are useful for evaluating native proximal internal carotid arteries, they do not apply directly to any other location within the carotid or vertebral system or to patients with prior CEA or stenting (Table 66-2). Markedly elevated velocities are qualitatively useful to identify stenoses in these patients, but they cannot be reliably quantified. Systolic velocities in carotid stents are usually higher than those in native carotid arteries,[6-8] so using proximal ICA criteria would overestimate the severity of disease. Also, occlusion or high-grade stenosis of one carotid artery may elevate the velocities within the remaining patent ICA and lead to overestimation of the degree of stenosis.[9] This effect has been validated by findings of reduced peak systolic velocities after CEA or stenting of the contralateral carotid.[10-12]

DISCUSSION

Sonographers and sonologists should be alert to specific pitfalls. For example, a nearly occluded ICA may be erroneously interpreted as having a stenosis of less than 50% if the ECA is mistaken for the CCA and the first ECA branch point is misidentified as the carotid bulb. Likewise, an ECA stenosis may be mistaken as an ICA stenosis. In these cases, the "temporal tap" maneuver can help to identify the true ECA.[13] Gentle tapping of the temporal artery in the preauricular region will be transmitted to the external carotid artery and will be visualized on spectral Doppler of the ECA as small repetitive peaks. There will be significantly less transmission to the ICA.

Reversal of flow in the ECA may help diagnose occlusion of the CCA. In such a case, the ICA is usually supplied by retrograde flow from the ECA collateral flow from the ophthalmic arteries.[14]

Current standards were developed by correlating ultrasound findings with conventional angiography as the reference standard. However, conventional angiography may underestimate the severity of stenosis.[15-17] An ideal reference standard has not yet been established. However, carotid ultrasound has been established to have a role in strategies to prevent strokes.

The sensitivity, specificity, and accuracy of carotid ultrasound depend on the threshold criteria that are selected. PSV criterion of 260 cm/sec by Moneta et al[20] correlated with sensitivity 84%, specificity 94%, and accuracy 90%. Later work by Carpenter et al[19] chose a PSV threshold of 210 cm/sec for 70% ICA stenosis, yielding a sensitivity 94%, specificity 77%, and accuracy 83%. Another study by Huston et al[18] for 70% stenosis using PSV 230 cm/sec had sensitivity 86%, specificity 90%, and accuracy 89%. In the studies by Moneta et al[20] and Huston et al,[18] EDV and ratio criteria were also included as diagnostic criteria.[18-20]

References

1. North American Symptomatic Carotid Endarterectomy Trial Collaborators: Beneficial effect of carotid endarterectomy in symptomatic patients with high grade carotid stenosis. N Engl J Med 1991;325:445-453.

2. Executive Committee for the Asymptomatic Carotid Atherosclerosis Study: Endarterectomy for Asymptomatic Carotid Artery Stenosis. J Am Med Assoc 1995;273:1421-1428.

3. Logason K, Bärlin T, Jonsson ML, et al: The importance of Doppler angle of insonation on differentiation between 50-69% and 70-99% carotid artery stenosis. Eur J Vasc Endovasc Surg 2001;21:311-313.

4. Grant EG, Duerinckx AJ, El Saden SM, et al: Ability to use duplex US to quantify internal carotid arterial stenoses: fact or fiction. Radiology 2000;214:247-252.

5. Grant EG, Benson CB, Moneta GL, et al: Carotid artery stenosis: grayscale and Doppler ultrasound diagnosis. Society of Radiologists in Ultrasound Consensus Conference. Ultrasound Q 2003;19:190-198.

6. Lal BK, Hobson RW II, Goldstein J, et al: Carotid artery stenting: is there a need to revise ultrasound velocity criteria? J Vasc Surg 2004;39:58-66.

7. Robbin ML, Lockhart ME, Weber TM, et al: Carotid artery stents: early and intermediate follow-up with Doppler US. Radiology 1997;205:749-756.

8. Ringer AJ, German JW, Guterman LR, et al: Follow-up of stented carotid arteries by Doppler ultrasound. Neurosurgery 2002;51:639-643.

9. Fujitani RM, Mills JL, Wang LM, et al: The effect of unilateral internal carotid arterial occlusion upon contralateral duplex study: criteria for accurate interpretation. J Vasc Surg 1992;16:459-467.

10. Abou-Zamzam AM Jr, Moneta GL, Edwards JM, et al: Is a single preoperative duplex scan sufficient for planning bilateral carotid endarterectomy. J Vasc Surg 2000;31:282-288.

11. Henderson RD, Steinman DA, Eliasziw M, et al: Effect of contralateral carotid artery stenosis on carotid ultrasound velocity measurements. Stroke 2000;31:2636-2640.

12. Sachar R, Yadav JS, Roffi M, et al: Severe bilateral carotid stenosis. The impact of ipsilateral stenting on Doppler-defined contralateral stenosis. J Am Coll Cardiol 2004;43:1358-1362.

13. Budorick NE, Rojratanakiat W, O'Boyle MK, et al: Digital tapping of the superficial temporal artery: significance in carotid duplex sonography. J Ultrasound Med 1996;15:459-464.

14. Belkin M, Mackey WC, Pessin MS, et al: Common carotid artery occlusion with patent internal and external carotid arteries: diagnosis and surgical management. J Vasc Surg 1993;17:1019-1027.

15. Elgersma O, Buijs PC, Wüst AF, et al: Maximum internal carotid arterial stenosis: assessment with rotational angiography versus conventional intraarterial digital subtraction angiography. Radiology 1999;213:777-783.

16. Porsche C, Walker L, Mendelow D, et al: Evaluation of cross-sectional luminal morphology in carotid atherosclerotic disease by use of spiral CT angiography. Stroke 2001;32:2511-2515.

17. Pan XM, Saloner D, Reilly LM, et al: Assessment of carotid artery stenosis by ultrasonography, conventional angiography, and magnetic resonance angiography: correlation with ex vivo measurement of plaque stenosis. J Vasc Surg 1995;21:82-88.

18. Huston J III, James EM, Brown RD Jr, et al: Redefined duplex ultrasonographic criteria for diagnosis of carotid artery stenosis. Mayo Clin Proc 2000;75:1133-1140.

19. Carpenter JP, Lexa FJ, Davis JT: Determination of duplex Doppler ultrasound criteria appropriate to the North American Symptomatic Carotid Endarterectomy Trial. Stroke 1996;27:695-699.

20. Moneta GL, Edwards JM, Papanicolaou G, et al: Screening for asymptomatic internal carotid artery stenosis: duplex criteria for discriminating 60% to 99% stenosis. J Vasc Surg 1995;21:989-994.

CHAPTER 67

Mark E. Lockhart
Lincoln L. Berland

Vertebral Artery Doppler

Introduction

There have been considerably fewer studies of vertebral artery than of internal carotid artery flow. Yet the vertebral artery waveforms offer a window into basilar arterial flow, and vertebral artery abnormalities may reflect vertebrobasilar artery insufficiency.

Materials/Methods

TECHNIQUE

The vertebral arteries are imaged as part of a complete sonographic evaluation of the extracranial arterial system. The vertebral artery usually arises as a branch of the subclavian artery. In the longitudinal plane of the CCA, the transducer is angled posteriorly to locate the vertebral artery. Color Doppler may help to localize the vessel. If a vertebral artery is not visualized, occlusion may be suspected, although hypoplasia, or rarely unilateral vertebral artery atresia, may occur.

WAVEFORM ANALYSIS

Analyzing waveform morphology will lead to diagnosing most disturbances of vertebral circulation. With vertebral artery stenosis, the

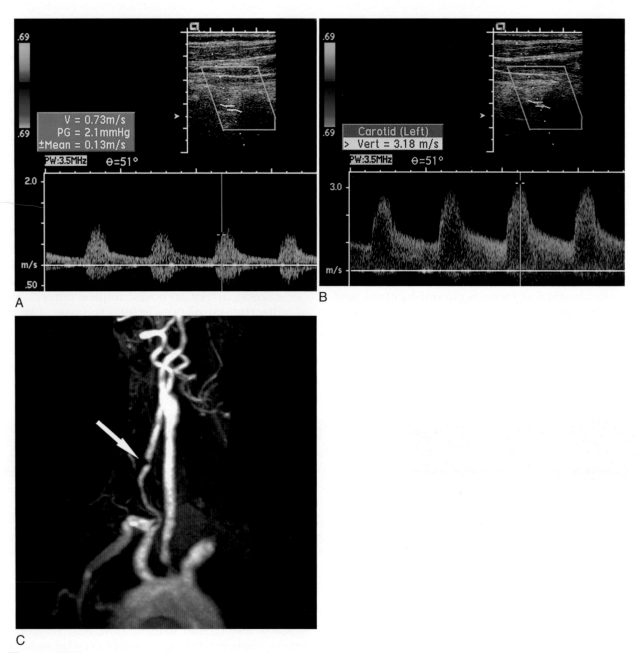

Figure 67-1
Vertebral artery stenosis.
A, Longitudinal duplex Doppler shows normal peak systolic velocity (PSV) in the proximal vertebral artery.
B, Elevated PSV and turbulence are present at the vertebral artery stenosis beyond the vertebral artery origin.
C, Magnetic resonance angiogram of the neck shows focal high-grade stenosis in the proximal vertebral artery (*arrow*).

peak velocity and the characteristics of the waveform depend on the point of interrogation relative to the point of narrowing (Fig. 67-1). Turbulence is often present at the point of stenosis. The resistance in the normal vertebral artery is normally low, with moderate end-diastolic flow. The resistance may be elevated

with downstream vertebral or basilar artery stenosis. High intracranial pressure from edema may also elevate the resistance. Although high-resistance flow in the vertebral artery has been suggested to indicate distal vertebral artery stenosis or occlusion, this finding is neither sensitive nor specific.[1] If high-grade vertebral artery

Table 67-1	Correlation of vertebral arterial waveform categories and severity of stenosis of the ipsilateral proximal subclavian artery[3]
Vertebral Waveform Category	**Mean Percent Subclavian Stenosis**
Type 1	45%
Type 2	53%
Type 3	72%
Type 4	78%

Table 67-2	Normal vertebral artery parameters		
Parameter	**Mean**	**Range**	**Reference**
PSV in midneck	20-60 cm/sec	10-100	8-11
PSV at origin	64 cm/sec	30-100	12
Diameter	3.5 mm	3-5.5	9,13,14

stenosis or occlusion is beyond the posterior inferior communicating artery (PICA) branch, then the vertebral flow may still have diastolic flow.[2]

The flow in the vertebral artery may be reversed to supply blood to the arm in cases of proximal subclavian artery stenosis—the "subclavian steal." However, the symptomatic syndrome is uncommon, and complete flow reversal is not highly sensitive for symptomatic stenosis.

Both color and spectral Doppler may help to accurately identify flow direction, which is the primary finding with subclavian steal. However, abnormal vertebral artery tracings may be associated with subclavian steal physiology prior to the development of symptoms.[3] Different vertebral artery waveforms have been correlated with the likelihood of subclavian stenosis (Table 67-1). To identify the following waveform types, accentuated depression of mid-systolic flow should be distinguished from the normal diastolic notch found later in the cardiac cycle. In a type 1 vertebral waveform, the vertebral artery, mid-systolic depression does not extend below the level of the end diastolic velocity (Fig. 67-2). This may occasionally be a normal variant. A type 2 waveform demonstrates decreased flow at mid-systole at or below the level of the EDV. A type 3 waveform has transient cessation of flow at mid-systole. A type 4 waveform has transient reversal of flow at mid-systole.[3]

Specific maneuvers may be performed to convert a type 1 to 2 waveform into a type 3 to 4 pattern or even to complete reversal of vertebral flow.[3] A blood pressure cuff is inflated above systolic blood pressure to temporarily occlude flow. When the cuff is deflated, the transient ischemia in the arm lowers the flow resistance and may accentuate vertebral artery abnormal waveforms. Demonstrating these increased changes confirms the presence of the subclavian steal.

Multiple tracings of arterial waveforms are obtained with duplex Doppler with preferred angles of insonation of 60% or less. Normal vertebral artery parameters have been defined (Table 67-2). Several sonographic criteria have been described for vertebral artery stenosis.[1,4-6] If there is a focal elevation of the PSV above normal limits, greater than in the adjacent portion of the vessel, it suggests a vertebral artery stenosis of at least 50%.[7] At the origin of the vertebral artery, a PSV greater than 100 cm/sec suggests stenosis.[8-14]

DISCUSSION

With carotid evaluation, angles of insonation of less than 60% are suggested to optimize reproducibility of velocity calculations, but velocity is less important in vertebral artery examination, so the angle of insonation is less critical. Severe carotid stenosis or occlusion may cause a compensatory increase in the PSV of the ipsilateral or contralateral vertebral artery.[15] However, the normal PSV of the vertebral artery varies widely. Some substantially abnormal vertebral waveforms may become evident before symptoms occur, and some subtle distortions of the vertebral waveforms may never become symptomatic.

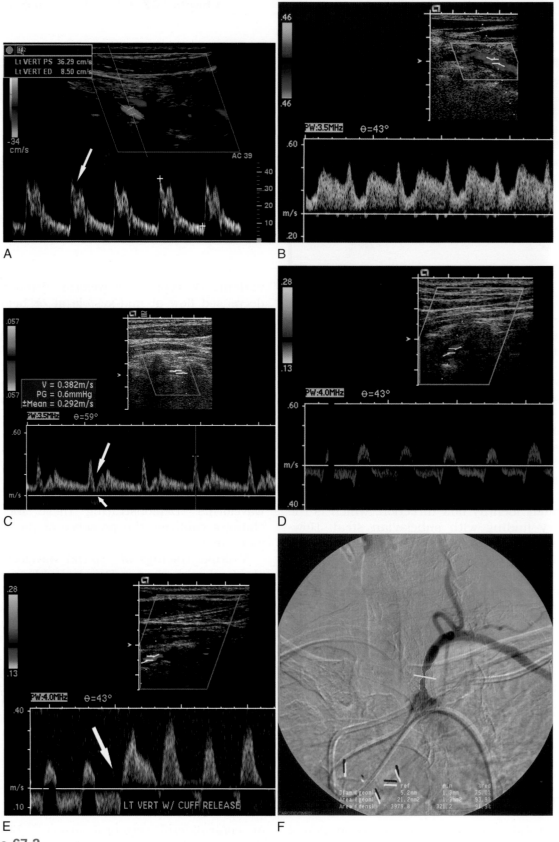

Figure 67-2

Abnormal vertebral artery waveform categories on spectral Doppler.
A, Type 1 waveform has small mid-systolic decrease (*arrow*) with a trough velocity greater than the EDV. **B,** Type 2 has mid-systolic notch equal to or below the level of the EDV. **C,** Type 3 has transient cessation of flow (*arrows*) (to the baseline) without reversal. **D,** Type 4 waveform has temporary reversal of flow. **E,** After release of pressure cuff maneuver (*arrow*) in (D), there is conversion of type 4 waveform to complete reversal of vertebral flow. **F,** Conventional arteriogram shows computer-automated calculation of severity of the proximal subclavian stenosis that yielded the type 4 waveform in **(D)**.

References

1. Nicolau C, Gilabert R, Chamorro A, et al: Doppler sonography of the intertransverse segment of the vertebral artery. J Ultrasound Med 2000;19:47-53.
2. Saito K, Kimura K, Nagatsuka K, et al: Vertebral artery occlusion in duplex color-coded ultrasonography. Stroke 2004;35:1068-1072.
3. Kliewer MA, Hertzberg BS, Kim DH, et al: Vertebral artery Doppler waveform changes indicating subclavian steal physiology. AJR Am J Roentgenol 2000;174:815-819.
4. Kimura K, Yasaka M, Moriyasu H, et al: Ultrasonographic evaluation of vertebral artery to detect vertebrobasilar axis occlusion. Stroke 1994;25:1006-1009.
5. Bartels E, Flügel KA: Evaluation of extracranial vertebral artery dissection with duplex color-flow imaging. Stroke 1996;27:290-295.
6. Bendick PJ, Jackson VP: Evaluation of the vertebral arteries with duplex sonography. J Vasc Surg 1986;3:523-530.
7. Ackerstaff RG, Grosveld WJ, Eikelboom BC, et al: Ultrasonic duplex scanning of the prevertebral segment of the vertebral artery in patients with cerebral atherosclerosis. European J Vasc Surg 1988;2:387-393.
8. Sidhu PS: Ultrasound of the carotid and vertebral arteries. Br Med Bull 2000;56:346-366.
9. Zwiebel WJ: Ultrasound vertebral examination. In Introduction to Vascular Ultrasonography, 4th ed. Philadelphia, WB Saunders Company, 2000, pp 167-176.
10. Trattnig S, Hubsch P, Schuster H, et al: Color-coded Doppler imaging of normal vertebral arteries. Stroke 1990;21:1222-1228.
11. Seidel E, Eicke BM, Tettenborn B, et al: Reference values for vertebral artery flow volume by duplex sonography in young and elderly adults. Stroke 1999;30:2692-2696.
12. Kuhl V, Tettenborn B, Eicke BM, et al: Color-coded duplex ultrasonography of the origin of the vertebral artery: normal values of flow velocities. J Neuroimaging 2000;10:17-21.
13. Matula C, Trattnig S, Tschabitscher M, et al: The course of the prevertebral segment of the vertebral artery: anatomy and clinical significance. Surg Neurol 1997;48:125-131.
14. Bartels E, Fuchs HH, Flügel KA: Duplex ultrasonography of vertebral arteries: examination, technique, normal values, and clinical applications. Angiology 1992;43(3 Pt 1):169-180.
15. Nicolau C, Gilabert R, Garcia A, et al: Effect of internal carotid artery occlusion on vertebral artery blood flow. J Ultrasound Med 2001;20:105-111.

PART

7

Head and Neck

Ophthalmic Ultrasound: Axial Length Measurements

Introduction

The A-scan was first used in ophthalmology in the late 1950s.[1] It was used to determine axial length measurements, as well as to aid in the diagnosis of ophthalmic pathologic conditions. The ultrasonic axial length was first used in 1974 to calculate intraocular lens powers. Since that time, these scans have become routine in the preoperative testing of a patient for cataract surgery. Axial length measurements are also used to monitor infants and children with glaucoma of childhood.

The B-scan was introduced to ophthalmology soon after the A-scan. Early A- and B-scanning was performed with an immersion system. In the late 1970s, a portable A- and B-scan unit was developed using a contact B-scan. Ophthalmic B-scanning became more popular as a diagnostic tool due to the ease of use.

The B-scan is requested by the ophthalmologist when there is no view of the retina. Common causes for this are hemorrhage, mature cataract, corneal scarring, and trauma. The B-scan is used to rule out the presence of a retinal detachment, intraocular tumor, choroidal detachment, posterior rupture, and other vitreoretinal conditions (Fig. 68-1).

Materials/Measurments

ANATOMY OF THE EYE IN RELATION TO THE A-SCAN

With the A-scan, the axis of the sound waves appears as a horizontal line on the oscilloscope. As the sound waves are emitted from the probe and interface the various acoustic structures, vertical deflections on the oscilloscope baseline appear. The locations, size, and number of echo spikes identify the acoustic structures involved.[2]

In the normal eye, the cornea, anterior and posterior lens capsules, vitreoretinal interface, sclera, and orbital fat produce clear, identifiable echo spikes. The anterior chamber, the lens interior, and the vitreous cavity produce no echo return and, therefore, are seen as baseline.

A parallel beam in a 10-MHz transducer is used. The axial length is determined as the distance from the corneal spike to the vitreoretinal interface. The probe must be aligned to assured axiality along the visual axis. This is accomplished by adjusting the probe until all spikes are at their maximum height. The retinal and corneal spike should be equal.

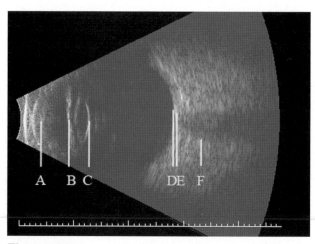

Figure 68-1

B-scan of normal eye. *A* = probe interface and cornea; *B* = anterior lens capsule; *C* = posterior lens capsule; *D* = retina; *E* = sclera; *F* = orbital fat.

TISSUE VELOCITY

The tissue velocities are dependent on the medium. The anterior chamber, from the cornea to the anterior lens echo, is measured at 1532 m/sec. The lens, from the anterior lens echo to the posterior lens echo, is measured at 1641 m/sec. The vitreous, extending from the posterior lens spike to the retina, is measured at 1532 m/sec. In an aphakic eye, without a lens, the entire measurement would be determined at 1532 m/sec.[3]

AXIAL LENGTH METHODS

Axial length measurements may be performed with applanation or immersion methods. Applanation involves placing the biometry probe directly on the corneal surface. The initial spike on the A-scan image is the probe interface and cornea, followed by the anterior lens surface, posterior lens surface, retina, sclera, and orbital fat echoes (Fig. 68-2).

A disadvantage to this method is compression of the cornea. When testing with applanation, particular attention is paid to the anterior chamber depth (ACD), the measurement from the cornea to the anterior lens spike. The longest ACD measurement indicates the best scan.

Immersion A-scanning involves the placement of a scleral shell on the eye. The shell is filled with saline. The probe is aligned along the visual axis of the eye for measurement. With immersion, the initial echo spike represents the interface of the probe and the water bath. The anterior and posterior corneal echo spikes are separate (Fig. 68-3). The immersion method eliminates the problem of corneal compression and has higher reproducibility.

AXIAL LENGTH MEASUREMENTS

Numerous studies have been conducted to investigate the average anterior chamber depth and axial length. As with many organs that change in size with development, there is no one standard of axial length and anterior chamber depth.

Normative pediatric data show axial length ranges of 17.0 to 20.1 mm at birth, 19.1 to 21.9 mm at 6 months, 19.8 to 22.4 mm at 1 year, and 20.5 to 23.1 mm at 2 years of age.[4] Blomdahl[4] found that the average anterior chamber depth in the newborn infants ranged from 2.4 to 2.9 mm with a mean ACD of 2.6 mm. He also measured lens thickness, which ranged from 3.4 to 3.9 mm, with a mean of 3.6 mm.[4]

Studies of axial length measurements indicate a range of average normal values from 23.37 (±0.75) to 23.65 (±1.35) mm in the Western adult population.[5,6] Cross-culturally, the difference may be slight. Yu et al[7] studied normal Chinese adults and found a mean axial length of 23.74 (±1.24) mm.[7]

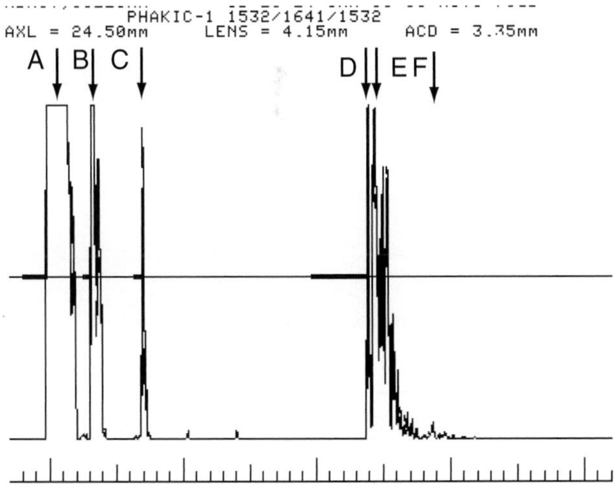

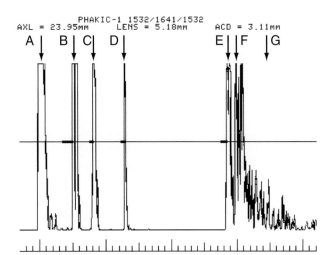

Figure 68-2
Applanation A-scan of normal eye. *A* = probe interface and cornea; *B* = anterior lens capsule; *C* = posterior lens capsule; *D* = retina; *E* = sclera; *F* = orbital fat.

Figure 68-3
Immersion A-scan of normal eye. *A* = probe-waterbath interface; *B* = anterior and posterior cornea; *C* = anterior lens capsule; *D* = posterior lens capsule; *E* = retina; *F* = sclera; *G* = orbital fat.

The mean anterior chamber depth has been measured to be 2.91 (± 0.31) mm.[8]

The lens thickness increases with age. Weekers et al[9] found a normal lens thickness of 3.91 (±0.31) mm for 20- to 29-year olds. This value increased to 4.33 (±0.35) mm for the 40- to 49-year age group, and to 4.87 (±0.66) mm for normal patients in the 6th decade.

DISCUSSION

The axial length is usually stable in normal adult eyes. The anterior chamber depth has a positive correlation to the axial length.[5] Short, or hyperopic, eyes have shorter anterior segments, and longer, myopic eyes have longer anterior chamber depths.

Francois and Goes[5] found the thickness of the lens is independent of the axial length of the eye. As the lens ages, the lens thickens and so correlates positively with age, rather than axial length.

References

1. Gitter K: Ophthalmic ultrasound. In Proceedings of the Fourth International Congress of Ultrasonography in Ophthalmology. St Louis, CV Mosby Co, 1969, pp 1-4, 158-164.
2. Ossoinig K: Echography of the eye, orbit and periorbital region. In Arger PH (ed): Orbit Roentgenology. New York, John Wiley and Sons, 1977.
3. Hoffer KJ: Preoperative cataract evaluation: intraocular lens power calculation. Int Ophthalmol Clin 1982;22:37-75.
4. Blomdahl S: Ultrasonic measurements of the eye in the newborn infant. Acta Ophthalmol 1989;57:1048-1056.
5. Francois J, Goes F: Ultrasonographic study of 100 emmetropic eyes. Ophthalmologica 1977;175:321-327.
6. Hoffer, KJ: Biometry of 7500 cataractous eyes. Am J Ophthalmol 1980;90:360-368.
7. Yu CS, Kao D, Chang CT: Measurement of the length of the visual axis by ultrasonography in 1,789 eyes. Chung Hua Ken Ko Tsa Chih 1979;15:45.
8. Hoffer KJ: Accuracy of ultrasound intraocular lens calculation. Arch Ophthalmol 1981; 99:1819-1823.
9. Weekers R et al: Biometrics of the crystalline lens. In Bellows JG (ed): Cataract and Abnormalities of the Lens. New York, Grune and Stratton, 1980.

CHAPTER 69

Laurence Needleman

Thyroid and Parathyroid

Thyroid Diameter and Volume

INTRODUCTION

Thyroid palpation is a qualitative measure of thyroid size. Scintigraphy is recognized as more accurate than palpation[1] but has been superseded by sonographic measurements.

Measurements are typically obtained to evaluate for thyroid enlargement (goiter). Enlargement is typically defined as greater than the second standard deviation (97th percentile). Mean adult thyroid size is shown in Table 69-1.

MATERIALS/METHODS

Linear measurements have been described by Solbiati et al.[2] Most recent evaluations use thyroid volume to quantify size.

There are two methods to determine volume. The more exact, but more difficult, technique employs recording cross-sections through the gland in short axis and summating these to determine the volume.[1]

The simpler and more common technique uses the volume estimated from a modified rotation ellipsoid. The length, width, and thickness are multiplied together and by a constant. Two constants, approximately 9% different from one another, have been used[3,4] (Table 69-2). Mean adult thyroid volume is shown in Table 69-3.

The study is generally performed with a high-frequency linear transducer. If the length of the gland cannot be captured on a single image, the use of a curved array transducer (Fig. 69-1A) to delineate the borders of the gland is preferable to estimating the length or patching together two images[5,6] (see Fig. 69-1).

The long axis of the gland is determined, and measurement calipers are placed on its caudal and cephalic edge at the longest length of the gland (see Fig. 69-1). The probe is rotated 90 degrees for the short axis. The widest part of the gland is determined, and measurement calipers are placed on the medial and lateral edges of the gland to obtain its width and on the front and back of the gland to measure the anteroposterior dimension (Fig. 69-2). Excess pressure on the neck by the transducer is to be avoided because it may affect measurements.[6]

DISCUSSION

Thyroid volume using the modified ellipsoid formula has an error of 13% to 20%, somewhat greater than the integrated cross-sectional method. Errors increase with increasing gland

Table 69-1	Mean adult thyroid size	
Mean Length (mm)	**Mean Anteroposterior Diameter (mm)**	**Mean Isthmic Thickness (mm)**
40-60	13-18	4-6

From Solbiati L, Charboneau JW, Osti V, et al: The thyroid gland. In Rumack CM, Wilson SR, Charboneau JW (eds): Diagnostic Ultrasound, 3rd ed. St Louis, Elsevier Mosby, 2005, pp 735-770.

Table 69-2	Thyroid volume calculation

1. Calculate volume of each lobe:

$$\text{Volume (ml)} = \text{length} \times \text{width} \times \text{anteroposterior diameter} \times 0.523*$$

2. Calculate the volume from the sum of the two lobes (isthmus is ignored)

*Some investigators use the method of Brunn et al[6-8]:
Volume (ml) = length × width × anteroposterior diameter × 0.479
From Solbiati L, Charboneau JW, Osti V, et al: The thyroid gland. In Rumack CM, Wilson SR, Charboneau JW (eds): Diagnostic Ultrasound, 3rd ed. St Louis, Elsevier Mosby, 2005, p 735-770; Gomez JM, Maravall FJ, Gomez N, et al: Determinants of thyroid volume as measured by ultrasonography in healthy adults randomly selected. Clin Endocrinol (Oxf) 2000;53:629-634.

Table 69-3	Adult thyroid volume*		
Male 50th percentile (ml)	**Male 97th percentile* (ml)**	**Female 50th percentile (ml)**	**Female 97th percentile* (ml)**
9.9	19.1	6.6	10.7

*Based on the following equation: volume of each lobe (ml) = length × width × anteroposterior diameter × 0.523
From Gomez JM, Maravall FJ, Gomez N, et al: Determinants of thyroid volume as measured by ultrasonography in healthy adults randomly selected. Clin Endocrinol (Oxf) 2000;53:629-634.

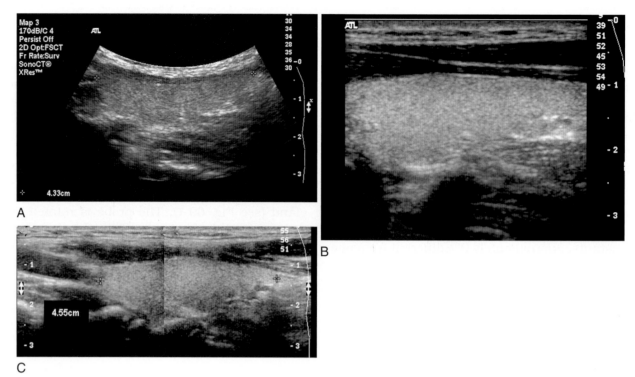

Figure 69-1

A, Long-axis measurement of the thyroid. Because of its length, a curved array was used. **B,** Long-axis view of the thyroid. A measurement is not taken because the cephalic and caudal ends of the thyroid are not included in the image. **C,** Incorrect long-axis measurement of the thyroid. The thyroid is estimated by piecing together two images of the gland. The incorrect length is measured because the two ends do not exactly match up. In this instance, the long-axis measurement should be made from a single image (see image **A**).

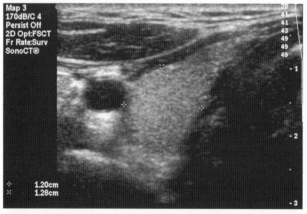

Figure 69-2

Short-axis measurement of the thyroid. The image is perpendicular to the long axis at the widest portion of the gland. Width (distance between the + marks) and anteroposterior measurement (distance between the × marks) are taken from the edges of the gland.

size and the presence of nodules.[6,10] Machine differences are generally not significant.[6,9]

In adults, men have larger glands than women, but this is mostly due to body weight,[11] particularly lean body mass,[12] rather than age or sex.

In a study of US children, Xu et al[9] found no difference between boys and girls but did find increases with age and body surface area. Volume based on body surface area is superior to age but requires knowing the subject's height and weight.

Pediatric thyroid volume (Tables 69-4 and 69-5) is an important measurement for iodine deficiency disorders. European children have demonstrated larger glands than American children,[8] but some of the differences were a result of differences in how the European data were acquired. This was subsequently corrected in a follow-up article, and the differences in the two groups became less.[6]

Other techniques of measurement have been described but have had limited clinical

Table 69-4	Thyroid volume* in children (volume versus age)					
	Thyroid Volume (ml)					
	7		**8**		**9**	
Age	**50th percentile**	**97th percentile**	**50th percentile**	**97th percentile**	**50th percentile**	**97th percentile**
Volume	3.0	4.7	3.3	5.2	3.7	5.9
	Thyroid Volume (ml)					
	10		**11**		**12**	
Age	**50th percentile**	**97th percentile**	**50th percentile**	**97th percentile**	**50th percentile**	**97th percentile**
Volume	4.1	6.6	4.6	7.3	5.1	8.2

Based on the following equation: volume of each lobe (ml) = length × width × anteroposterior diameter × 0.479
From Xu F, Sullivan K, Houston R, et al: Thyroid volumes in US and Bangladeshi schoolchildren: comparison with European schoolchildren. Eur J Endocrinol 1999;140:498-504.

Table 69-5	Thyroid volume* in children (volume versus body surface area)							
	0.8		**0.9**		**1.0**		**1.1**	
BSA (m²)	**50th percentile**	**97th percentile**	**50th percentile**	**97th percentile**	**50th percentile**	**97th percentile**	**50th percentile**	**97th percentile**
Volume (ml)	2.5	3.8	2.8	4.3	3.1	4.8	3.4	5.3
	1.2		**1.3**		**1.4**		**1.5**	
BSA (m²)	**50th percentile**	**97th percentile**	**50th percentile**	**97th percentile**	**50th percentile**	**97th percentile**	**50th percentile**	**97th percentile**
Volume (ml)	3.7	5.8	4.0	6.2	4.4	6.7	4.7	7.2

Based on the following equation: volume of each lobe (ml) = length × width × anteroposterior diameter × 0.479
From Xu F, Sullivan K, Houston R, et al: Thyroid volumes in US and Bangladeshi schoolchildren: comparison with European schoolchildren. Eur J Endocrinol 1999;140:498-504.

validation.[13,14] Three-dimensional ultrasound may become a more common means to measure thyroid volume in the future.[15,16]

Parathyroid Size

INTRODUCTION

Parathyroid measurements are usually performed in the clinical setting of hypercalcemia or hyperparathyroidism. Most patients have four glands. A normal gland is only occasionally seen, but visualization is not an indication for surgery.[17]

MATERIALS/METHODS

The size of a normal parathyroid is determined by pathology series. Each gland is measured in length, width, and anteroposterior diameter (Fig. 69-3).

DISCUSSION

The diagnosis of parathyroid enlargement is based on size. Adenomas are based on size, shape, and echogenicity. Most adenomas are homogeneously hypoechoic (2% with cystic degeneration). Adenomas are typically oblong,

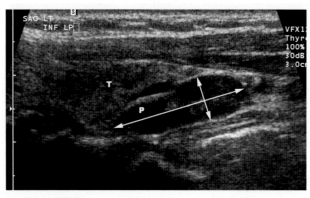

Figure 69-3
Parathyroid adenoma long-axis measurements.
An enlarged parathyroid adenoma (*P*) is seen below
the inferior thyroid (*T*). It is bilobed with a cystic
component superiorly. Measurements are taken
along its greatest length and in the anteroposterior
dimension perpendicular to the length.

sometimes with a bilobed or teardrop shape.
The majority of adenomas are 0.8 to 1.5 cm in
length but can be larger.[17]

References

1. Hegedus L: Thyroid size determined by ultrasound. Influence of physiological factors and non-thyroidal disease. Dan Med Bull 1990;37:249-263.
2. Solbiati L, Charboneau JW, Osti V, et al: The thyroid gland. In Rumack CM, Wilson SR, Charboneau JW (eds). Diagnostic Ultrasound, 3rd ed. St. Louis, Elsevier Mosby, 2005, pp 735-770.
3. Brunn J, Block U, Ruf G, et al: [Volumetric analysis of thyroid lobes by real-time ultrasound (author's transl)]. Dtsch Med Wochenschr 1981;106:1338-1340.
4. Gomez JM, Maravall FJ, Gomez N, et al: Determinants of thyroid volume as measured by ultrasonography in healthy adults randomly selected. Clin Endocrinol (Oxf) 2000;53:629-634.
5. Peeters EY, Shabana WM, Verbeek PA, Osteaux MM: Use of a curved-array transducer to reduce interobserver variation in sonographic measurement of thyroid volume in healthy adults. J Clin Ultrasound 2003; 31:189-193.
6. Zimmermann MB, Molinari L, Spehl M, et al: Toward a consensus on reference values for thyroid volume in iodine-replete schoolchildren: results of a workshop on inter-observer and inter-equipment variation in sonographic measurement of thyroid volume. Eur J Endocrinol 2001;144:213-220.
7. Anonymous: Recommended normative values for thyroid volume in children aged 6-15 years. World Health Organization & International Council for Control of Iodine Deficiency Disorders. Bull World Health Organ 1997;75:95-97.
8. Delange F, Benker G, Caron P, et al: Thyroid volume and urinary iodine in European schoolchildren: standardization of values for assessment of iodine deficiency. Eur J Endocrinol 1997;136:180-187.
9. Xu F, Sullivan K, Houston R, et al: Thyroid volumes in US and Bangladeshi schoolchildren: comparison with European schoolchildren. Eur J Endocrinol 1999;140: 498-504.
10. Hegedus L: Thyroid ultrasound. Endocrinol Metab Clin North Am 2001;30:339-360.
11. Berghout A, Wiersinga WM, Smits NJ, Touber JL: Determinants of thyroid volume as measured by ultrasonography in healthy adults in a non-iodine deficient area. Clin Endocrinol 1987;26:273-280.
12. Wesche MF, Wiersinga WM, Smits NJ: Lean body mass as a determinant of thyroid size. Clin Endocrinol 1998;48:701-706.
13. Sheikh M, Doi SA, Sinan T, Al-Shoumer KA: Technical observations on the assessment of thyroid volume by palpation and ultrasonography. J Ultrasound Med 2004;23:261-266.
14. Szebeni A, Beleznay E: New simple method for thyroid volume determination by ultrasonography. J Clin Ultrasound 1992;20: 329-337.
15. Ng E, Chen T, Lam R, et al: Three-dimensional ultrasound measurement of thyroid volume in asymptomatic male Chinese. Ultrasound Med Biol 2004;30:1427-1433.
16. Schlogl S, Werner E, Lassmann M, et al: The use of three-dimensional ultrasound for thyroid volumetry. Thyroid 2001;11:569-574.
17. Huppert BJ, Reading CC: The parathyroid glands. In Rumack CM, Wilson SR, Charboneau JW (eds). Diagnostic Ultrasound, 3rd ed. St. Louis, Elsevier Mosby, 2005, pp 771-794.

Echocardiography

CHAPTER 70

Anita J. Moon-Grady

Echocardiographic Measurements: Introduction

From its initial description more than 50 years ago, ultrasound imaging of the human heart has evolved into one of the most important tools available to the clinician for examining the structure and function of the heart in normal and diseased states. Echocardiography has become a subspecialty within both adult and pediatric cardiology. Application of echocardiography intraoperatively or during cardiac catheterization using transesophageal, intravascular, and intracardiac routes now allows intervention to be actively guided by the echocardiographer. Fetal cardiac ultrasound can detect and diagnose even very complex congenital heart disease in utero and may be used to guide pre- and postnatal therapy. Three- (or "four") dimensional echocardiography, until recently only available via cumbersome off-line analysis, is now available in real-time.

Several ultrasound modalities are currently standard on most commercially available ultrasound systems designed for echocardiography. These include M-mode, two-dimensional sector-scan imaging, and Doppler, including pulsed and continuous wave and color. Each of these three modalities, their applications, normal values, and use in recognizing disease states will be discussed separately, recognizing that in practice a complete echocardiographic examination includes routine use of all modalities and that accurate interpretation involves integration of all of the information obtained.

The transthoracic echocardiographic examination is generally performed with the patient in a recumbent, left lateral decubitus position, though adequate acoustic windows may also be obtained in the supine position, especially in infants and small children. Parasternal transducer positions in several different left intercostal spaces may be necessary. The examination then generally moves to the apical position, defined by the cardiac position rather than the anatomic positioning of the transducer. Subcostal and suprasternal transducer positions are part of the routine examination in children and should also be attempted in the adult population. Doppler examination can and should be performed from a variety of locations to optimize the angle of insonance between the emitted ultrasound beam and the structures of interest.

Traditionally, two-dimensional and Doppler echocardiograms have been recorded on videotape for subsequent analysis, while M-mode tracings have been printed on paper. More recently the use of digital acquisition and storage technology has been leading to the replacement of videotape and paper with digital "movies" and still images.

C H A P T E R **71**

Anita J. Moon-Grady

Echocardiographic Doppler

Introduction

Doppler echocardiography is an essential part of every complete echocardiogram. Its three modalities, pulsed wave, continuous wave, and color (superimposed on a two-dimensional reference image) all rely on basic principles and can be used to obtain important hemodynamic information, but with some limitations. A basic understanding of these principles is necessary in order to properly apply the techniques.

The Doppler principle, which states that the relative motion between a sound source and an observer determines the observed frequency of the sound wave, can be applied to ultrasound reflected waves in tissue and expressed by the following equation:

$$V = (F_d \times c/2)/(\cos\theta \times F_o), \quad \text{(equation 1)}$$

where V is the velocity of the ultrasound target relative to the transducer, F_o is the emitted frequency, F_d is the observed frequency, c is the speed of sound in tissue (1540 cm/sec), and θ is the angle of incidence, assumed to be 0 or 180 degrees such that the cos θ equals 1 (this is a valid assumption until the angle exceeds approximately 20 degrees, at which point angle becomes a substantial factor in the equation).

Velocity is displayed by the ultrasound equipment on the y axis, while direction is generally indicated as toward the transducer equals positive (above the baseline) or away from the transducer equals negative (below the baseline). The velocity of blood can provide information in itself (typical patterns of forward or reverse flow can be recognized during phases of the cardiac cycle), or the velocity information can be used to calculate differences in pressure proximal and distal to the region from which the measurement is taken by application of the Bernoulli principle, which states that the energy lost to a pressure drop across an orifice is related to the energy gained in convective and flow acceleration and in viscous friction:

$$\Delta P = \frac{1}{2}\rho(v_2^2 - v_1^2) + \rho\int_1^2 \frac{dv}{dt}ds + R(v).$$
(equation 2)

where pressure drop ΔP is equal to convective term $1/2\ \rho(v_2^2 - v_1^2)$ plus the sum of inertial effects and viscous losses, $\rho\int_1^2 dv/dtds + R(v)$. In clinical application, contribution from the second part of the equation is assumed to be negligible, and the equation is simplified to

$$\Delta P = \frac{1}{2}\rho(v_2^2 - v_1^2) \quad \text{(equation 3)}$$

The ρ term is a coefficient related to blood density, and assuming that the proximal velocity is negligible compared to the distal velocity (<1.5 m/sec, in general), the equation becomes

$$\Delta P = 4v_2^2 \quad \text{(equation 4)}$$

It should be noted, however, that this simplified Bernoulli equation can only accurately predict actual pressure change if the above assumptions are true; stated alternately, the simplified equation cannot be applied to situations in which proximal velocity is not negligible (such as is seen in multiple level obstruction or in tunnel-like lesions and tubes such as the ductus arteriosus), which may lead to an overestimation of the true gradient from failure to subtract the v_1^2 term. The viscous term $R(v)$ becomes important in nondiscrete narrowings, such as aortopulmonary shunts, ductus arteriosus, tunnel-like subaortic stenosis, and stenotic surgically placed conduits, and exclusion of this term from the equation leads to underestimation of the true gradient. However, for most of the basic applications described later, the simplified Bernoulli equation will suffice.

Three modalities using the Doppler principle are available and will be discussed in the following section. In pulsed-wave Doppler, the operator selects a specific depth along a single scan line at which to sample blood velocity. The amplitude of the return velocity is limited by the power and frequency of the transducer, and aliasing will occur above the threshold. Continuous-wave Doppler allows much higher velocities to be recorded, but at the cost of ambiguity in depth of sampling. Color Doppler is essentially pulsed-wave Doppler in a sector scan, with color-coding of pixels superimposed on a two-dimensional reference image (red by convention for velocities toward the transducer, blue away). Aliasing when measured velocity exceeds the Nyquist limit again occurs, and continuous-wave Doppler must again be used for measurement purposes. A fourth Doppler modality, termed tissue Doppler, is pulsed-wave Doppler using different gain and filter settings to display the motion of tissue rather than blood and will be discussed separately. Recommendations for the use of Doppler in echocardiography from the American Society of Echocardiography were published in 2002 and, where applicable, are incorporated here.[1] Normal values compiled from a variety of sources[2-8] are presented in Table 71-1.

Table 71-1	Normal Doppler values in children and adults
Sampling site	**Normal range**
Superior vena cava	0.28-1.5 m/sec
Tricuspid valve	
Peak E	0.41-0.84 m/sec
Peak A	0.2-0.6 m/sec
E/A	0.6-2.6
Right ventricular outflow	
Below pulmonary valve	0.4-1.05 m/sec
Pulmonary valve	0.5-1.3 m/sec
Main pulmonary artery	0.5-1.1 m/sec
Pulmonary veins	
Peak S	0.3-0.55 m/sec
Peak D	0.4-0.7 m/sec
Mitral valve	
Peak E	0.6-1.3 m/sec
Peak A	0.4-0.6 m/sec
E/A	1.4-2.4 (up to 4 in children)
Deceleration time	160-200 msec
Left ventricular outflow	
Below aortic valve	0.44-1.28 m/sec
Aortic valve	0.75-1.85 m/sec
Ascending aorta	0.6-1.85 m/sec
Descending aorta	0.7-1.6 m/sec

Materials/Methods

PULSED-WAVE DOPPLER (PW)

PW guided by two-dimensional imaging is performed using the acoustic windows previously described to evaluate blood flow velocities and patterns through several anatomic structures. The sample gate is placed in the proximal inferior vena cava, hepatic veins, and superior vena cava from the subcostal sagittal or suprasternal notch positions, in the tricuspid valve at the level of the annulus in diastole or of the leaflet tips, in the right ventricular outflow tract just below and just above the pulmonary valve from the parasternal or subcostal windows, in the proximal branch pulmonary arteries from the parasternal short axis, in the right upper pulmonary vein 2 to 5 mm from the vein-left atrial junction, in the mitral valve at the level of the annulus in diastole or at the level of the leaflet tips, in the left ventricular outflow tract just below and just above the aortic valve, in the ascending and proximal descending aorta from the suprasternal notch, and in the descending thoracic aorta near the level of the diaphragm from the subcostal sagittal view. Additional interrogation, for example, of low-velocity shunt flow as through an atrial septal defect, should be done as indicated, always taking care that the angle of insonance is as parallel to the direction of flow as possible. Normal flow profiles are shown in Figures 71-1 through 71-5, and normal velocities for children and adults compiled from several sources are presented in Table 71-1.[2-8]

Systemic venous flow

Flow in the inferior and superior vena cava varies considerably with respiration. Typically flow is biphasic, with a peak of forward flow in systole (s wave) corresponding with ventricular contraction and a second peak in diastole (d wave) during diastole (see Fig. 71-1). The s and d waves may merge at high heart rates. There is generally a low-velocity reversed peak corre-

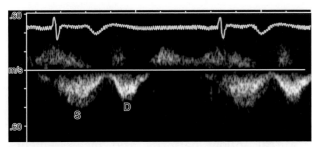

Figure 71-1
Doppler tracing obtained from a normal inferior vena cava. Flow is biphasic, with a peak of forward flow in systole (*S*), corresponding with ventricular contraction, and a second peak in diastole (*D*).

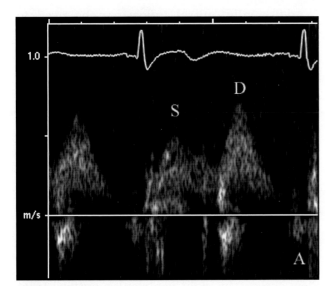

Figure 71-2
Doppler tracing obtained from a normal pulmonary vein. The Doppler sample volume is placed in the right upper pulmonary vein. Flow is biphasic, with a peak of forward flow in systole (*S*), corresponding with ventricular contraction, and a second peak in diastole (*D*). A small amount of reversal of flow during atrial contraction (*A*) may be seen.

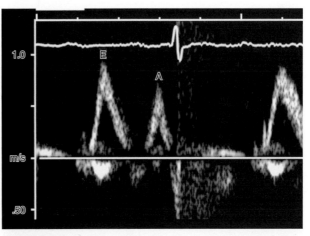

Figure 71-3
Doppler tracing showing flow through a normal mitral valve. The first peak (*E*) corresponds with passive and the second (*A*) wave with atrial contraction.

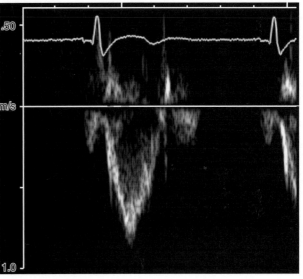

Figure 71-4
Doppler tracing showing flow through a normal pulmonary valve.

sponding with atrial contraction, which may be increased in velocity and duration in disease states including moderate to severe tricuspid regurgitation and right ventricular restrictive physiology.

Pulmonary venous flow
Flow in the pulmonary veins varies less with respiration than in the systemic veins. Typically flow is also biphasic, though more continuous in nature, with a peak of forward flow in systole (s wave) corresponding with ventricular contraction and a second peak in diastole (d wave)

during diastole (see Fig. 71-2). There is generally either no or a very low-velocity, short-duration reversed peak corresponding with atrial contraction (a wave); in disease states the a wave increases in velocity and duration, such as is seen in moderate to severe mitral regurgitation and left ventricular diastolic dysfunction.

Tricuspid valve
Tricuspid valve inflow Doppler varies significantly with respiration. The pattern resembles

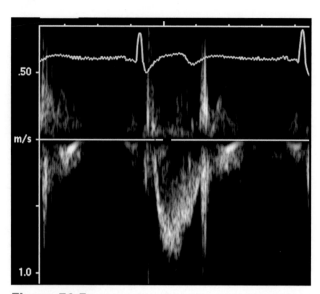

Figure 71-5
Doppler tracing showing flow through a normal aortic valve.

an "M" in diastole, with the first peak (E) corresponding with the passive filling phase of diastole and the second (A) wave with atrial contraction. The peak velocities can be recorded and compared with normal, and their ratio (E/A) is generally around 1.6 at end-expiration. The ratio is normally reversed in fetuses and neonates. The E and A waves may merge at high heart rates.

Tricuspid regurgitation may be present; however, the velocity generally exceeds the limit by PW, and changing to continuous-wave Doppler is necessary (see in the following sections). Mild tricuspid regurgitation can be detected in many subjects and can be a normal finding.[9]

Mitral valve

Mitral valve inflow Doppler does not vary significantly with respiration (<10%)[10] except in the presence of increased pericardial pressure, such as in tamponade or in other disease states. The normal pattern (see Fig. 71-3), similar to that of the tricuspid inflow, resembles an "M" in diastole, with the first peak (E) corresponding with the passive filling phase of diastole and the second (A) wave with atrial contraction. The peak velocities can be recorded and compared with normals, and their ratio (E/A) is generally 1.4 to 2.4 at end-expiration, though it may be normal up to 4 in children.[2,3] The ratio is also normally reversed in fetuses and neonates.

Again, the E and A waves may merge at high heart rates.

Additional useful measurements that can be made include A wave duration, time from peak E to the return after E to baseline (deceleration time (DT), normal <220 msec[11,12]), and the time for the E to reach peak (acceleration time).

Mitral inflow patterns and measurements have been studied extensively as indices of left ventricular diastolic function and, when abnormal, can be combined with tissue Doppler measurements (TDI, DTI) in a comprehensive evaluation of the patient with heart failure (Fig. 71-6).

Additionally, mitral inflow can be used to estimate valve area (MVA) in the presence of valve stenosis (Fig. 71-7). The time for pressure estimate from the E wave to decline to half of its peak value (pressure half-time, P1/2) is determined. The formula

$$MVA\ (cm^2) = 220/P_{1/2}\ (msec)\quad (equation\ 5)$$

has been shown to correlate well with MVA calculated at catheterization[13] in adults but has not been validated in children and should be used with caution in patients with combined mitral stenosis and insufficiency and in the presence of aortic insufficiency.[14]

Pulmonary valve

Flow across the right ventricular outflow tract and pulmonary valve is usually laminar with a single forward peak in systole (see Fig. 71-4). Trivial pulmonary insufficiency may be seen in many patients and is a normal finding.[9] When present, the spectral envelope of insufficiency peaks rapidly in early diastole and declines linearly throughout diastole. The velocity at end-diastole can be used in estimating pulmonary artery diastolic pressure by adding an estimate of right atrial mean pressure to the pressure estimated by the simplified Bernoulli equation.[15]

Aortic valve

Flow across the left ventricular outflow tract and aortic valve is laminar with a single forward peak in systole (see Fig. 71-5). Aortic insufficiency may be seen in many patients but is generally not considered normal. The velocity of the insufficiency jet generally exceeds the range detectable with PW and must be examined with continuous-wave Doppler.

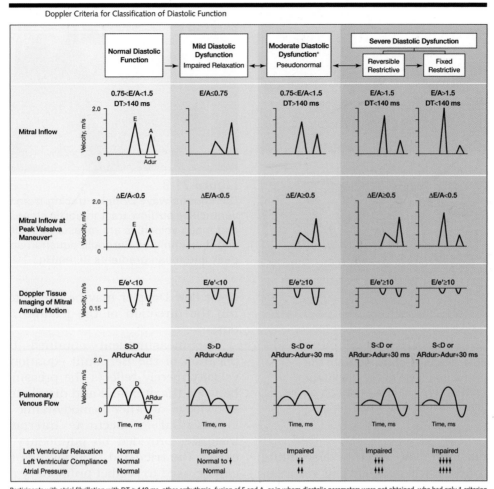

Doppler Criteria for Classification of Diastolic Function

Participants with atrial fibrillation with DT >140 ms, other arrhythmia, fusion of E and A, or in whom diastolic parameters were not obtained, who had only 1 criterion suggesting moderate or severe diastolic dysfunction, or in whom diastolic parameters were borderline and suggestive of but not diagnostic of abnormality were classified as having indeterminate diastolic function. E, peak early filling velocity; A, velocity at atrial contraction; DT, deceleration time; Adur, A duration; ARdur, AR duration; S, systolic forward flow; D, diastolic forward flow; AR, pulmonary venous atrial reversal flow; e', velocity of mitral annulus early diastolic motion; a', velocity of mitral annulus motion with atrial systole; DT, mitral E velocity deceleration time.
*Corrected for E/A fusion.[40]

Figure 71-6
Doppler criteria for classification of diastolic function. (From Redfield MM, Jacobsen SJ, Burnett JC Jr, et al: Burden of systolic and diastolic ventricular dysfunction in the community: appreciating the scope of the heart failure epidemic. JAMA 2003;289:194-202. Copyright © 2003 American Medical Association. All rights reserved.)

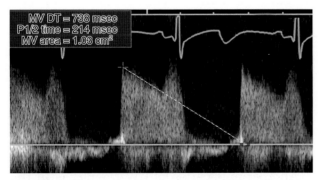

Figure 71-7
Doppler tracing in mitral stenosis. The pressure half-time method for valve area calculation is demonstrated.

Aorta

Flow profiles in the ascending and descending aorta should appear similar to the flow seen in the left ventricular outflow tract and should not exceed about 1.5 m/sec in systole (though it may be somewhat higher in the presence of high-output states such as fever and anemia), with cessation of flow in diastole. Examination of the descending aortic signal can alert the examiner to serious pathology, such as coarctation of the aorta (with low-velocity, late-peaking velocity distal to the obstruction, Fig. 71-8A), aortic insufficiency, or aortopulmonary connections such as patent ductus arteriosus (with

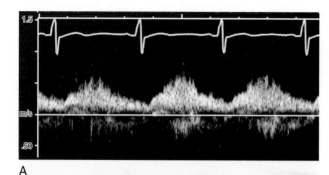

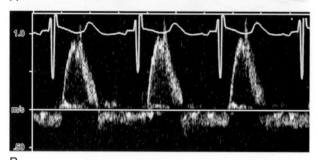

B

Figure 71-8
Abnormal Doppler tracings obtained from the descending aorta at the level of the diaphragm, showing flow pattern typical in coarctation of the aorta (**A**) and aortic insufficiency (**B**).

retrograde diastolic flow in the descending aorta, Fig. 71-8B). Early diastolic flow reversal, however, is a normal finding.

CONTINUOUS-WAVE DOPPLER (CW)

CW is used to record and measure high-velocity blood flow. The most commonly encountered flows of this nature include tricuspid regurgitation, mitral regurgitation, aortic insufficiency, and flow across ventricular septal defects. Additional uses for CW include evaluation of degree of obstruction in aortic, pulmonary, and mitral stenosis; detection of coarctation of the aorta; and estimation of pulmonary artery pressure. Measurement of peak and mean velocity can be performed using the outer border of the spectral envelope (Fig. 71-9) and the simplified Bernoulli equation applied, squaring the velocity and multiplying by 4 to yield pressure gradient in mmHg. Optimal alignment of the cursor with the blood flow jet may be difficult to determine; multiple sites of interrogation (for instance, subcostal, apical, and suprasternal for interrogation of the aortic valve) should be investigated, and the highest obtainable gradient reported.

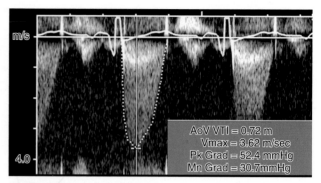

Figure 71-9
Continuous-wave Doppler tracing from the left ventricular outflow tract in aortic stenosis. The peak and mean velocities are measured as demonstrated, and the simplified Bernoulli equation applied to give peak and mean gradients in mmHg.

Color flow Doppler may be useful for determining the direction of the jet and aligning the cursor.

The measurement obtained by the application of the Bernoulli equation to the CW velocity merely reflects the pressure difference between the proximal and distal structure, and knowledge of other hemodynamic information is essential for accurate interpretation. For instance, provided no pulmonary obstruction exists, the tricuspid regurgitation (TR) velocity can be used to predict pulmonary artery systolic pressure[16] by adding an estimate of right atrial pressure to the difference between right atrium and right ventricle (pulmonary artery pressure = right ventricle − right atrium (TR) + right atrium pressure). Provided there is no aortic outflow obstruction and the systolic blood pressure is known (which should then equal left ventricular pressure in systole), the right ventricular pressure can be calculated from a ventricular septal defect (VSD) velocity as systolic blood pressure − VSD pressure drop (left ventricle to right ventricle). More complex information can be gleaned from additional measurements; however, care must be taken to avoid violating the assumptions made in using the simplified Bernoulli equation—pulmonary artery pressure estimates made from measuring the velocity across a surgical shunt or patent ductus arteriosus, for example, may be invalid due to the long tubular nature of these connections.

Another application of CW Doppler is in the measurement of degree of aortic insufficiency. Because normal aortic diastolic pressure usually exceeds left ventricular diastolic pressure

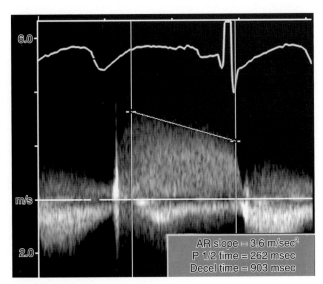

Figure 71-10
Continuous-wave Doppler tracing demonstrating severe aortic insufficiency.

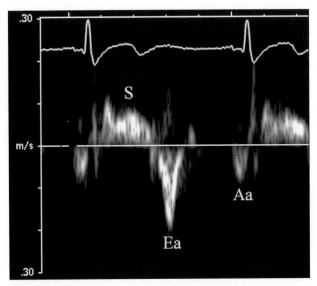

Figure 71-11
Tissue Doppler pattern obtained from the lateral mitral valve annulus. Note the systolic positive deflection (*S*) and two negative peaks in diastole, *Ea* and *Aa*, corresponding to early diastolic filling and atrial contraction, respectively.

throughout diastole, the pressure half-time (P1/2), defined as the time in milliseconds for the pressure gradient at onset diastole to decline to half its original value will be rapid (<400 msec)[11] in severe insufficiency (as the aortic and ventricular pressures quickly move toward equalization) and slow in mild insufficiency (Fig. 71-10).

COLOR DOPPLER

Color Doppler examination of all of the structures noted in the PW Doppler section should be performed. A common use of color Doppler is in estimating the severity of valvular regurgitation. Though the width of the regurgitant jet and the area which it occupies in the receiving chamber (right atrium for tricuspid regurgitation) have been used in grading severity, care should be taken in inferring any more information.[17] Even when following a single patient with serial studies, we see that inherent characteristics of the Doppler signal that depend on sample depth, the power and frequency of the transducer, as well as variations in the volume, pressure, and geometry of the receiving chamber, can lead to underestimates of regurgitation severity.

TISSUE DOPPLER IMAGING (DTI, TDI)

Recently, an additional Doppler modality has been gaining acceptance in the routine evalua-tion of ventricular diastolic function. Termed tissue Doppler (TDI, DTI), it involves using the pulsed-wave Doppler capability of the ultrasound equipment with adjustments in machine settings (manual or as a preset option), which decrease gain and filter settings to display tissue motion rather than blood (Fig. 71-11). The sample volume, or gate, is increased to 3 to 5 mm and placed in various standard positions, including the medial and lateral annulus of the mitral or tricuspid valve or in various positions in the left ventricular myocardium. The examination is most frequently performed from the apical four-chamber view. The normal, observed Doppler pattern is similar to the mitral or tricuspid inflow pattern. There is a systolic positive deflection, termed S. During diastole there are two negative peaks, Ea and Aa (or E' and A'), corresponding to early diastolic filling and atrial contraction, respectively. Normal values for the mitral annular velocities vary somewhat among authors, but in general Ea ranges from 15 to 17 cm/sec (up to 23 in children), Aa from 3.8 to 8 cm/sec, and the ratio of transmitral E/Ea is less than 10 (and indicates normal left atrial pressure), while an E/Ea ratio of more than 15 has been found to be highly specific for elevation in left atrial pressure.[3,18-20]

DISCUSSION

PULSED-WAVE DOPPLER IN EVALUATION OF SYSTOLIC FUNCTION AND VOLUME FLOW/SHUNTS

Properly obtained, the information contained in the PW spectral envelope can be used to calculate volume flow through a structure if the cross-sectional area (or diameter) is obtained from two-dimensional imaging. Figure 71-12 illustrates this concept for the aortic valve. The PW signal is traced at the outer edge of the brightest (modal) portion of the signal, and using the software package built into the ultrasound system the velocity-time integral (VTI) is derived. Volume flow is the product of VTI and cross-sectional area as $\pi (D/2)^2$, and, in this case, represents the stroke volume of the left ventricle. Provided there is no valvular regurgitation, stroke volume and cardiac output (the product of stroke volume and heart rate) can be estimated from flows across the pulmonary, tricuspid, or mitral valves as well. If valvular regurgitation is present, the regurgitant volume or fraction can be calculated as the remainder of the total antegrade flow across the diseased valve minus the normal antegrade flow across any other normal valve in the heart, provided no shunts exist. If instead there is evidence of a shunt lesion, the relative ratio of pulmonary to systemic blood flow (Qp:Qs) can be calculated as the ratio of the flow across the right ventricular outflow tract to the left ventricular outflow tract.[21] These methods are not applicable in the presence of stenoses.

Though some studies have shown good correlation with cardiac catheterization-derived measures,[1,22,23] in practical application large estimation errors are generated with small errors in measurement, and correlation with true flows and comparisons among patients are difficult to make reliably; however, due to the relative constant valve diameter in any given adult patient, the method may be useful in serial assessment of function, using a single constant measurement of diameter.

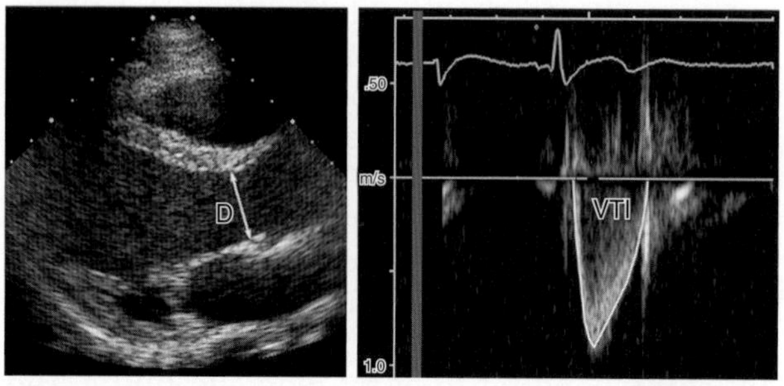

DOPPLER IN ESTIMATION OF SEVERITY OF STENOSIS AND VALVE AREAS

Transvalvular Gradients

The use of Doppler-derived estimates of transvalvular gradients has dramatically reduced the need for cardiac catheterization in the longitudinal follow-up of patients with valvular stenoses. Several studies have shown excellent correlation of Doppler with catheter-derived measurement,[1,22,23] obviating the need for catheterization in many of these patients. However, an important distinction should be made when interpreting the noninvasively derived data in the light of natural history studies based on catheterization-derived data. The basic distinction is in the parameter being measured, and some confusion arises due to lack of understanding that catheterization and Doppler echocardiography are in fact evaluating a different physiologic phenomenon.[24] Doppler allows estimation of the peak instantaneous gradient across an obstruction, while cardiac catheterization techniques, by simultaneous or pullback measurement, will generally be interpreted by reporting the peak-to-peak gradient (Fig. 71-13). The peak instantaneous gradient is generally higher than the peak-to-peak, and, in fact, large "errors" in measurement can be generated–though not true "errors," but rather misinterpretation of accurate data. For this reason it has become common practice, especially in pediatrics, to report both peak and mean gradients across a stenotic valve; the mean will be lower and more closely approximates the catheterization-derived measurement.

Figure 71-12
Demonstration of estimation of volume flow through the aortic valve. The diameter (*D*) of the aortic annulus is measured from the parasternal long-axis view. The velocity-time integral (*VTI*) is obtained by tracing the outer edge of the modal velocity from the Doppler tracing obtained from the apical four-chamber view with the sample volume in the left ventricular outflow tract just below the aortic valve. Stroke volume is then calculated as $VTI \times \pi (D/2)^2$.

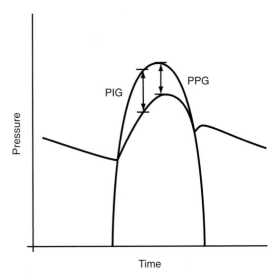

Figure 71-13

Illustration demonstrating the difference in measurement of peak-to-peak gradient (PPG) and peak instantaneous gradient (PIG). The peak instantaneous gradient is generally higher than the peak-to-peak.

Valve Areas

The method most commonly used to estimate valve area noninvasively is the use of the continuity equation. The principle simply stated is that the stroke volume remains the same when measured proximal to the valve or through the stenotic valve itself; therefore the method outlined above for determining volume flow, VTI × CSA (cross-sectional area; $\pi (D/2)^2$), is applied to, for example, the left ventricular outflow tract (LVOT) for measurement of VTI and diameter; then the maximal velocity across the aortic valve is integrated, VTI_{max}, allowing for calculation of valve area:

$$\text{Valve area} = (VTI_{lvot} \times CSA_{lvot})/VTI_{max}$$
$$\text{(equation 6)}$$

Normal aortic valve area indexed to body surface area is 1.3 to 2 cm^2/m^2; an area of 0.8 to 1.3 cm^2/m^2 is considered mild stenosis, 0.51 to 0.8 cm^2/m^2 moderate stenosis, and less than 0.5 cm^2/m^2 severe stenosis.[25] Although the use of the continuity equation has been validated in pediatric population,[26,27] these criteria are not generally applied to children.

The application of the continuity equation to the mitral valve has also been validated in adults with mitral stenosis. The method is generally valid provided there is no significant valvular regurgitation.

Another widely used method for calculating mitral valve area was first suggested by Hatle et al[13] and uses the rate of pressure decay in the early part of diastole in the formula

$$\text{Mitral valve area} = 220/P_{1/2} \quad \text{(equation 7)}$$

Normal mitral valve area in the adult is 4 to 6 cm^2 or 2.4 to 3.6 cm^2/m^2. Mild mitral stenosis equates with a valve area of 1.2 to 2.4 cm^2/m^2, moderate 0.6 to 1.2 cm^2/m^2, and severe less than 0.6 cm^2/m^2 (see Fig. 71-5).[28] These measurements are indexed to body surface area for adults and are not generally applied to the pediatric population.

In-depth discussion of analysis of color Doppler information, including the use of proximal isovelocity surface area (PISA) for calculation of orifice size and volume flows, is outside the scope of this text; interested readers are referred to texts specifically devoted to echocardiography.

PULSED WAVE AND TISSUE DOPPLER IN EVALUATION OF DIASTOLIC FUNCTION

There has been a recent explosion in the clinical and research use of a combination of Doppler-derived indices for evaluation of diastolic function. The general premise lies in the physiology of the cardiac events that comprise diastole. In brief, diastole consists of four distinct phases: isovolumic relaxation, early rapid filling, diastasis, and atrial contraction. Doppler examination of the mitral inflow and pulmonary venous velocities and of the motion of the mitral annulus in diastole can give information about ventricular diastolic filling, including rate of ventricular relaxation, the driving force across the valve, and the compliance of the left ventricle. An overview of the data obtained and the alterations seen in various states of dysfunction is presented in Figure 71-6.[19] The complexities involved in interpretation of the data, including effects of alterations in preload, are beyond the scope of this text. The interested reader is referred to any one of several recent review articles on the subject.[19,29]

References

1. Quinones MA, Otto CM, Stoddard M, et al: Recommendations for quantification of Doppler echocardiography: a report from

the Doppler Quantification Task Force of the Nomenclature and Standards Committee of the American Society of Echocardiography. J Am Soc Echocardiogr 2002;15:167-184.

2. O'Leary PW, Durongpisitkul K, Cordes TM, et al: Diastolic ventricular function in children: a Doppler echocardiographic study establishing normal values and predictors of increased ventricular end-diastolic pressure. Mayo Clin Proc 1998;73:616-628.

3. Kapusta L, Thijssen JM, Cuypers MH, et al: Assessment of myocardial velocities in healthy children using tissue Doppler imaging. Ultrasound Med Biol 2000;26:229-237.

4. Hatle L, Angelsen B: Doppler Ultrasound in Cardiology. Philadelphia, Lea & Febiger, 1985.

5. Goldberg BB, Kurtz AB (eds): Atlas of Ultrasound Measurements. Chicago, Year Book Medical Publishers, 1990;58-67.

6. Garson A, Bricker JT, McNamara DG (eds): The Science and Practice of Pediatric Cardiology, 2nd ed. Philadelphia, Lea & Febiger, 1990;826.

7. Gardin JM, Henry WL, Savage DD, et al: Echocardiographic measurements in normal subjects: evaluation of an adult population without clinically apparent heart disease. J Clin Ultrasound 1979;7:439-447.

8. Benjamin EJ, Levy D, Anderson KM, et al: Determinants of Doppler indexes of left ventricular diastolic function in normal subjects (the Framingham Heart Study). Am J Cardiol 1992;70:508-515.

9. Kostucki W, Vandenbossche JL, Friart A, et al: Pulsed Doppler regurgitant flow patterns of normal valves. Am J Cardiol 1986;58:309-313.

10. Riggs TW, Snider AR: Respiratory influence on right and left ventricular diastolic function in normal children. Am J Cardiol 1989;63:858-861.

11. Braunwald E: Heart disease: A Textbook of Cardiovascular Medicine, 5th ed. Philadelphia, Saunders, 1997.

12. Feigenbaum H: Echocardiography, 5th ed. Philadelphia, Lea & Febiger, 1994;675-677.

13. Hatle L, Angelsen B, Tromsdal A: Noninvasive assessment of atrioventricular pressure half-time by Doppler ultrasound. Circulation 1979;60:1096-1104.

14. Nakatani S, Masuyama T, Kodama K, et al: Value and limitations of Doppler echocardiography in the quantification of stenotic mitral valve area: comparison of the pressure half-time and the continuity equation methods. Circulation 1988;77:78-85.

15. Ge Z, Zhang Y, Ji X, et al: Pulmonary artery diastolic pressure: a simultaneous Doppler echocardiography and catheterization study. Clin Cardiol 1992;15:818-824.

16. Stephen B, Dalal P, Berger M, et al: Noninvasive estimation of pulmonary artery diastolic pressure in patients with tricuspid regurgitation by Doppler echocardiography. Chest 1999;116:73-77.

17. Zhang J, Shiota T, Shandas R, et al: Effects of adjacent surfaces of different shapes on regurgitant jet sizes: an in vitro study using color Doppler imaging and laser-illuminated dye visualization. J Am Coll Cardiol 1993;22:1522-1529.

18. Firstenberg MS, Levine BD, Garcia MJ, et al: Relationship of echocardiographic indices to pulmonary capillary wedge pressures in healthy volunteers. J Am Coll Cardiol 2000;36:1664-1669.

19. Khouri SJ, Maly GT, Suh DD, et al: A practical approach to the echocardiographic evaluation of diastolic function. J Am Soc Echocardiogr 2004;17:290-297.

20. Garcia MJ, Ares MA, Asher C, et al: An index of early left ventricular filling that combined with pulsed Doppler peak E velocity may estimate capillary wedge pressure. J Am Coll Cardiol 1997;29:448-454.

21. Silverman NH: Pediatric echocardiography. Baltimore, Williams & Wilkins, 1993.

22. Huntsman LL, Stewart DK, Barnes SR, et al: Noninvasive Doppler determination of cardiac output in man. Clinical validation. Circulation 1983;67:593-602.

23. Lewis JF, Kuo LC, Nelson JG, et al: Pulsed Doppler echocardiographic determination of stroke volume and cardiac output: clinical validation of two new methods using the apical window. Circulation 1984;70:425-431.

24. Currie PJ, Seward JB, Reeder GS, et al: Continuous-wave Doppler echocardiographic assessment of severity of calcific aortic stenosis: a simultaneous Doppler-catheter correlative study in 100 adult patients, Circulation 1985;71:1162-1169.

25. Gutgesell HP, French M: Echocardiographic determination of aortic and pulmonary valve areas in subjects with normal hearts. Am J Cardiol 1991;68:773-776.

26. Wendel H, Teien D, Human DG, et al: Non-invasive estimation of aortic valve areas in children with aortic stenosis. Acta Paediatr Scand 1990;79:1112-1115.

27. Bengur AR, Snider AR, Meliones JN, et al: Doppler evaluation of aortic valve area in children with aortic stenosis. J Am Coll Cardiol 1991;18:1499-1505.

28. Braunwald E: Heart disease: A Textbook of Cardiovascular Medicine. Philadelphia, W.B. Saunders, 1992.

29. Ommen SR: Echocardiographic assessment of diastolic function. Curr Opin Cardiol 2001;16:240-245.

CHAPTER 72

Anita J. Moon-Grady

Echocardiographic M-Mode

Introduction

M-mode echocardiography was the first method of ultrasound interrogation of the human heart to develop clinical usefulness. The advantage of M-mode lies in its temporal resolution, typically 1000-3000 frames per second, which far exceeds that of two-dimensional displays and allows for greater precision in measurement of structures in motion. M-mode remains the mainstay of standard measurement of left ventricular size and function, as well as for the measurement of wall thickness and diameters of left-sided heart structures. It is also useful for precision measurement of time intervals, even at the high heart rates in infants and children, because of its high resolution. Although originally produced as tracings from non-"imaging" transducers, in practice most ultrasound systems now have the capability to display a two-dimensional image on which the M-mode cursor pathway is displayed for the purpose of obtaining an appropriate sample during M-mode acquisition. Therefore, for the purposes of this chapter, two-dimensional guiding reference images are presented with the discussion of the technique.

M-mode–derived measurements and the normal value ranges in nondisease states have been fairly well established.[1-12] Standardization of the M-mode examination has been mostly successful since the original recommendations of the American Society of Echocardiography in 1978.[13] The following represents in large part a summary of these recommendations with additional attention given to the special pediatric population. What follows is a detailed account with regards to the most common measurements obtained using this technique. It is meant to be complete, yet not exhaustive. Where available, both adult and pediatric measurement normal values are given (Table 72-1, Fig. 72-1).

Materials/Methods

Measurements are made from three standard echocardiographic tracings. All are obtained using the left parasternal window. Figure 72-2 shows a two-dimensional, parasternal long-axis reference image with the three standard scan line cursor positions. Figure 72-3 shows corresponding short-axis reference images with the same scan lines, as well as the M-mode tracing obtained at each site. Best reproducibility is obtained with the scan line as perpendicular as possible to the structure being measured; therefore for the left heart structures it is recom-

Table 72-1	M-mode measurement normal values for adults and children

Measurement	Normal range
Aortic root	2.0-3.7 cm
Left atrium	1.9-4.0 cm
Right ventricle	0.7-2.7 cm
Interventricular septum	0.6-1.2 cm
Left ventricle (diastole)	3.5-5.7 cm
Left ventricle (systole)	1.3-3.0 cm
Left ventricular posterior wall	0.6-1.2 cm
Left ventricular mass	48-103 g/m² (males)
	36-81 g/m² (females)
LVPEP/LVET	0.345 ± 0.036
RVPEP/RVET	0.18 ± 0.3
MVEF slope	70-150 msec
E-point septal separation	<1 cm
Ejection fraction	64-83%
Fractional shortening	28-45% (all)
	35-45% (2 weeks)
	33-43% (2 years)
	31-41% (4 years)
	28-44% (14 years-adult)
VCFc	0.9-1.94 circ/sec

LVPEP/LVET, Left ventricular pre-ejection period to left ventricular ejection time ratio; MVEF, mitral valve E to F slope; RVPEP/RVET, right ventricular pre-ejection period to right ventricular ejection time ratio; VCFc, velocity of circumferential fiber shortening corrected for heart rate.

tion of the movement of the aortic valve leaflets throughout the cardiac cycle and the left atrium and allowing for measurement of the aortic root and left atrial dimension. Because there may be considerable expansion of the aortic root in systole, it is recommended that the measurement be standardized to the end of diastole at the onset of the QRS complex of the electrocardiogram.[13] The aortic root is measured from the leading edge of the anterior M-mode signal to the leading edge of the posterior signal, as noted in Figure 72-4. Left atrial measurement is made at the end of ventricular systole (or at the time of the maximum diameter of the left atrium) and includes the posterior wall of the aorta on the tracing. Examination of the position of the aortic valve closure line in diastole, which may be eccentric in the case of a bicuspid aortic valve, has become less useful as two-dimensional imaging has improved visualization of the valve in its entirety during the cardiac cycle.

Because of its superior temporal resolution, M-mode is especially well suited for the determination of time intervals. These include left ventricular ejection time (LVET), from aortic valve opening to aortic valve closure, and pre-ejection period (LVPEP), from the onset of the QRS to aortic valve opening. LVPEP/LVET ratio, useful though limited in demonstrating left ventricular dysfunction when increased, can be calculated and is relatively age independent.[4,6]

LEFT VENTRICLE AT THE LEVEL OF THE MITRAL VALVE

The second M-mode scan line is slightly more inferior, toward the apex of the heart, displaying the anterior and posterior mitral valve leaflets, and is used for interrogation of the movement of the mitral valve, for assessment of mitral prolapse, and for measurement of a variety of events occurring in diastole. Each inflection on the M-mode tracing of the valve is assigned a letter, A through F, as shown in Figure 72-5, beginning with "A", the peak opening corresponding to the catheter-derived "a" wave associated with atrial contraction. The point of valve closure, when the anterior and posterior leaflet coapt, is termed "C," with "B" (if present) representing a notch in the tracing between A and C. The point in diastole corresponding to early opening of the mitral valve, or early diastolic filling, is labeled "D," and the

mended that the reference image be displayed in short-axis rather than the long-axis (which may result in an unintentional oblique line of interrogation). Because of the slightly more horizontal orientation of the heart in the chest of infants and small children, modification of transducer position may be necessary in these patients. It is important to note, however, that the relative positions of the anatomic features in the reference image should be preserved.

AORTIC ROOT AND LEFT ATRIUM

The first scan line passes the M-mode line of interrogation perpendicularly through the right ventricle, aortic root at the level of and perpendicular to the aortic valve, allowing visualiza-

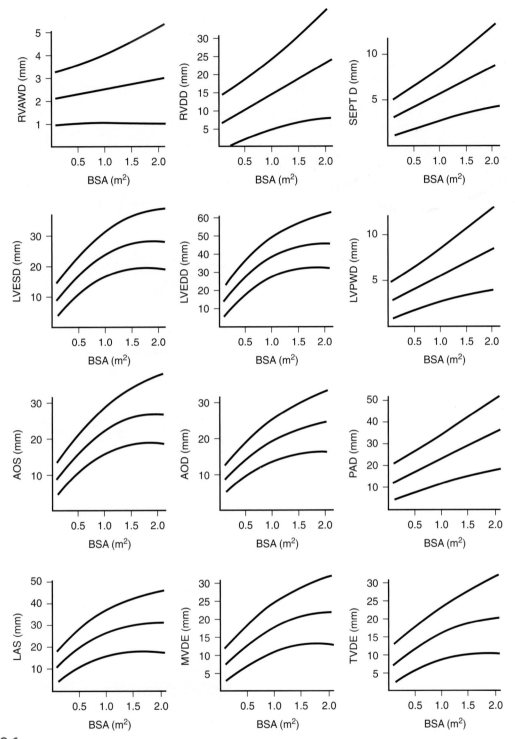

Figure 72-1

Normal ranges for M-mode–derived echocardiographic dimensions in millimeters plotted against body surface area (BSA) in square meters. Mean and 90% tolerance lines are shown. RVAW, Right ventricular anterior wall in diastole; RVDD, right ventricular end-diastolic dimension; SEPT D, interventricular septal thickness at end-diastole; LVESD, left ventricular end-systolic dimension; LVEDD, left ventricular end-diastolic dimension; LVPWD, left ventricular posterior wall thickness at end-diastole; AOS, aorta in systole; AOD, aorta in diastole; PAD, pulmonary artery diameter; LAS, left atrium in systole; MVDE, anterior mitral leaflet excursion; TVDE, tricuspid valve leaflet excursion. (Modified from Silverman NH: Pediatric Echocardiography. Baltimore, Williams & Wilkins, 1993, p 39, Figure 2.4.)

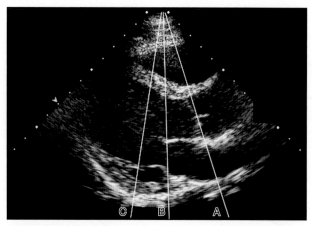

Figure 72-2
Parasternal long-axis reference image with the three standard scan line cursor positions, *A*, *B*, and *C*.

maximum early diastolic deflection is labeled "E." As the valve leaflets again move toward a closed position, prior to the onset of the "a" wave, another deflection point at which the anterior leaflet stops moving rapidly in the posterior direction is termed "F." The slope of the line from E to F is called the "EF slope" and is expressed in mm/sec. E-point-septal separation, the distance in millimeters between the left ventricular side of the interventricular septum at the endocardium and the E point, can also be measured and may be increased in left ventricular dysfunction or in association with dilation of the left ventricle.

RIGHT AND LEFT VENTRICLE AT THE LEVEL OF THE CHORDAL INSERTIONS AND CALCULATED MEASURES OF LEFT VENTRICULAR FUNCTION

The third line of interrogation, again at a perpendicular angle to the chest wall, at the level of the ventricles at the tips of the mitral valve leaflets in the open position, is illustrated in Figure 72-6. Care must be taken to include the right ventricle in the tracing and to avoid any obliquing of the angle of interrogation—on the reference image the left ventricular cavity is as round as possible with the cursor passing midway between the papillary muscles. Clear definition of both the epicardial and endocardial surfaces of the structures to be measured is necessary. From this tracing, measurements

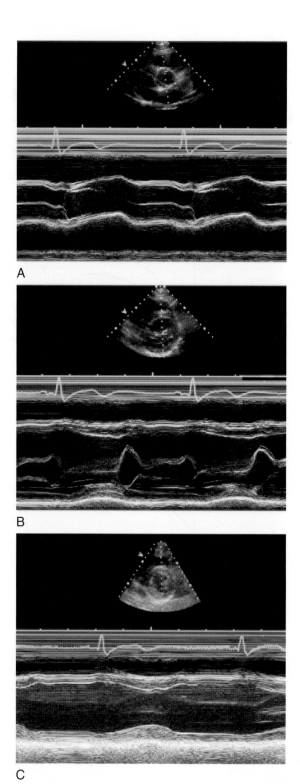

A

B

C

Figure 72-3
Parasternal short-axis reference images with scan lines corresponding to those in Figure 72-2 (**A, B,** and **C**) and the M-mode tracing obtained at each site. For details please see text.

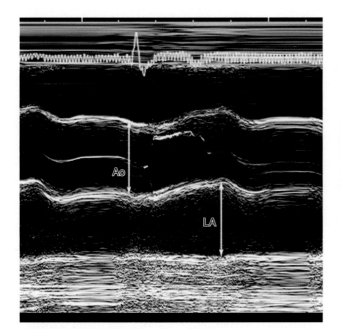

Figure 72-4
M-mode measurements of the aortic root and left atrium. The aortic root is measured at the end of diastole at the onset of the QRS as shown, from the leading edge of the anterior M-mode signal to the leading edge of the posterior signal. Left atrial measurement is made at the end of ventricular systole and includes the posterior wall of the aorta. Ao, Aortic root; LA, left atrial dimension.

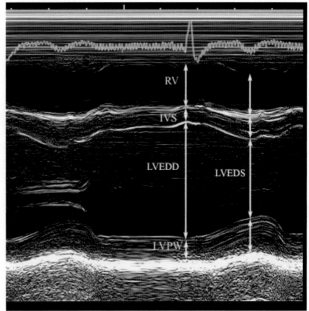

Figure 72-6
M-mode tracing of the right and left ventricles. Shown are the measurements as recommended by the American Society of Echocardiography. Measurements in diastole at the onset of the QRS, as well as systole at the time of peak septal wall motion, are made. IVS, Interventricular septum; LVEDD, left ventricular cavity dimension in diastole; LVEDS, left ventricular cavity dimension in systole; LVPW, left ventricular posterior free wall at end-diastole; RV, right ventricular cavity in diastole.

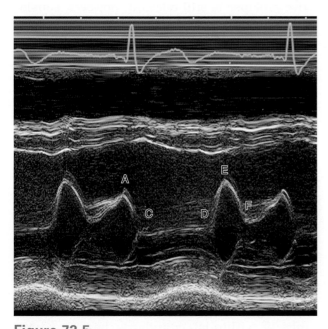

Figure 72-5
M-mode tracings of the left ventricle at the level of the mitral valve. Each inflection on the M-mode tracing of the valve is assigned a letter, labeled A through F, as described in the text.

of the right ventricular anterior wall thickness (RVAW), right ventricular cavity (RV) in diastole, interventricular septum (IVS), left ventricular cavity dimension in diastole and systole (LVEDD, LVEDS), and left ventricular posterior free wall (LVPW) at end-diastole can be made as shown in the figure. Measurements in diastole at the onset of the QRS, as well as systole at the time of peak septal wall motion, are made. Manual or computer-derived calculations of various indices of left ventricular systolic function can then be generated, including fractional shortening

$$FS\% = (LVEDD - LVESD)/LVEDD \times 100$$
$$\text{(equation 1)}$$

and ejection fraction (EF%)

$$EF\% = (LVEDV - LVESV)/LVEDV \times 100$$
$$\text{(equation 2)}$$

which estimates ventricular volume as a prolate ellipsoid of revolution, in which volume is approximately equal to diameter cubed, with or without the Teichholz correction.[14]

Additional derived measurements include velocity of circumferential fiber shortening (VCF) and velocity of circumferential fiber shortening corrected for heart rate (VCFc) (indices of contractility[2,15])

$$VCF = \frac{(LVEDD - LVESD)}{LVEDD} \times LVET$$

(equation 3)

$$VCF_c = \frac{\dfrac{(LVEDD - LVESD)}{LVEDD} \times LVET}{\sqrt{RR}}$$

(equation 4)

Left ventricular mass can also be estimated from M-mode measurements[12]:

$$LV\ mass = 1.04([LVEDD + LVPW + IVSD]^3 - [LVEDD]^3) - 14\ g$$

(equation 5)

DISCUSSION

M-mode was once the mainstay of echocardiographic assessment of cardiac function; however, with the widespread availability of two-dimensional imaging, it has assumed a secondary role due largely to its inherent limitations. Care should be taken when relying on M-mode evaluation. For instance, FS% is a valid assessment of systolic function and can be followed serially in patients only when the short-axis shape of the left ventricle is circular, the ventricle is elliptical, and there are no regional wall motion abnormalities. If these conditions are not met, it is best to evaluate the patient's ventricular systolic function by other methods. Similarly, left ventricular EF%, when extrapolated from the M-mode measurements of left ventricular dimension, is only a valid calculation if the above criteria are satisfied and if the ventricle assumes the shape of a prolate ellipsoid, twice as long as it is wide. In patients with septal flattening, regional wall motion abnormalities, and dilated cardiomyopathies and in normal infants, these conditions do not apply, and ejection fraction must be estimated using two-dimensional methods as described in the following section.

Another M-mode-derived index of systolic function, the systolic time intervals described above, were at one time more broadly used than they are today. Due in large part to the fact, however, that these time intervals are affected by loading conditions (preload, afterload) and heart rate, their use is limited.

The role of M-mode in detection of disease states was also more important at one time than it is now in the age of two- and three-dimensional imaging. There are a variety of M-mode clues to valvular diseases, acquired and congenital, and though few are still clinically relevant, some deserve mention. These include the finding of "flutter" on the aortic or pulmonary valve tracing, which is indicative of either subvalvular obstruction or of the presence of a ventricular septal defect; "flutter" on the mitral valve tracing may be a clue to the presence of aortic insufficiency. Mid-systolic closure of the aortic valve is seen in cases of dynamic subaortic obstruction, and a decreased EF slope on the mitral valve tracing is seen in mitral stenosis.

The use of M-mode in the diagnosis of mitral valve prolapse is still relevant; however, considerable controversy exists regarding the precise application of M-mode and the interpretation of the M-mode and two-dimensional echo findings.[16] In our laboratory, any degree of posterior displacement of the mitral valve during ventricular diastole on the M-mode trace is considered abnormal; however, additional criteria must be fulfilled for a diagnosis of mitral valve prolapse to be made, including prolapse of the posterior leaflet beyond the annulus of the mitral valve, prolapse of the anterior leaflet more than 3 mm above the annulus of the mitral valve, or a combination of these criteria in the presence of mitral regurgitation. For detailed discussion of the diagnosis of mitral valve prolapse, the interested reader is referred to the text by Feigenbaum.[7]

M-mode reproducibility has been demonstrated by multiple authors, although the importance of within-lab standards has also been stressed.[17-19] Although the American Society of Echocardiography defines end-diastole quite clearly as the onset of the QRS complex, one must keep in mind that at high heart rates, such as those seen in neonates and infants, mechanical end-diastole may be later, enough to produce a significant alteration in measurements. Peak systole as defined by the maximal excursion of the interventricular septum will be affected by wall-motion abnormalities and abnormal right ventricular loading conditions, and, in this case, it has been recommended that the maximal posterior wall excursion be used instead in the measurement of the left ventricle. One must be aware that when making such adjustments, either in the measurements at end-diastole or in systole, comparison with normal values must be interpreted with caution.

References

1. Braunwald E: Heart Disease: A Textbook of Cardiovascular Medicine, 5th ed. Philadelphia, Saunders, 1997.
2. Colan SD, Borow KM, Neumann A: Left ventricular end-systolic wall stress-velocity of fiber shortening relation: a load-independent index of myocardial contractility. J Am Coll Cardiol 1984;4:715-724.
3. Goldberg BB, Kurtz AB (eds): Atlas of Ultrasound Measurements. Chicago, Year Book Medical Publishers, 1990;47.
4. Silverman NH: Pediatric Echocardiography. Baltimore, Williams & Wilkins, 1993;35-52.
5. Garson A, Bricker JT, McNamara DG (eds): The Science and Practice of Pediatric Cardiology, 2nd ed. Philadelphia, Lea & Febiger, 1990;821-825.
6. Gutgesell HP, Paquet M, Duff DF, et al: Evaluation of left ventricular size and function by echocardiography. Results in normal children. Circulation 1977;56:457-462.
7. Feigenbaum H: Echocardiography, 5th ed. Philadelphia, Lea & Febiger, 1994;658-668.
8. Gardin JM, Henry WL, Savage DD, et al: Echocardiographic measurements in normal subjects: evaluation of an adult population without clinically apparent heart disease. J Clin Ultrasound 1979;7:439-447.
9. Henry WL, Ware J, Gardin JM, et al: Echocardiographic measurements in normal subjects. Growth-related changes that occur between infancy and early adulthood. Circulation 1978;57:278-285.
10. Huwez FU, Houston AB, Watson J, et al: Age and body surface area related normal upper and lower limits of M mode echocardiographic measurements and left ventricular volume and mass from infancy to early adulthood. Br Heart J 1994;72:276-280.
11. Daniels SR, Meyer RA, Liang YC, et al: Echocardiographically determined left ventricular mass index in normal children, adolescents and young adults. J Am Coll Cardiol 1988;12:703-708.
12. Devereux RB, Reichek N: Echocardiographic determination of left ventricular mass in man. Anatomic validation of the method. Circulation 1977;55:613-618.
13. Sahn DJ, DeMaria A, Kisslo J, et al: Recommendations regarding quantitation in M-mode echocardiography: results of a survey of echocardiographic measurements. Circulation 1978;58:1072-1083.
14. Teichholz LE, Kreulen T, Herman MV, et al: Problems in echocardiographic volume determinations: echocardiographic-angiographic correlations in the presence or absence of asynergy. Am J Cardiol 1976;37:7-11.
15. Colan SD: Nonlinearity of left ventricular end-systolic wall stress-velocity of fiber shortening relation. J Am Coll Cardiol 1994;24:1178-1180.
16. Krivokapich J, Child JS, Dadourian BJ, et al: Reassessment of echocardiographic criteria for diagnosis of mitral valve prolapse. Am J Cardiol 1988;61:131-135.
17. de Leonardis V, Cinelli P: Evidence of no interobserver variability in M-mode echocardiography. Clin Cardiol 1986;9:324-326.
18. Crawford MH, Grant D, O'Rourke RA, et al: Accuracy and reproducibility of new M-mode echocardiographic recommendations for measuring left ventricular dimensions. Circulation 1980;61:137-143.
19. Pietro DA, Voelkel AG, Ray BJ, et al: Reproducibility of echocardiography. A study evaluating the variability of serial echocardiographic measurements. Chest 1981;79:29-32.

Two-Dimensional Echocardiography

Introduction

Despite its clear temporal resolution advantage, M-mode has largely given way to two-dimensional imaging. Measurements made from two-dimensional images may be less prone to error due to unintentional oblique imaging. Estimations of area, volume, and mass, as well as percent area and volume changes, made from the two-dimensional images, are likely to be more accurate because there is less dependence on geometric assumption than with M-mode determination of the same measurements.

Methods and standards for two-dimensional measurements have been developed for adult and pediatric patients, and in 1989 the American Society of Echocardiography published recommendations for two-dimensional measurements of the left ventricle.[1] Presented below is a combination of these recommendations for the left ventricle and various other sources for additional important measurements using the two-dimensional technique, along with normal values where available (Table 73-1).[1-6]

Materials/Methods

The standard imaging windows for two-dimensional measurements are the left parasternal and the apical four- and two-chamber views. Again, because of the slightly more horizontal orientation of the heart in the chest of infants and small children, modification of transducer position may be necessary in these patients. It is important to note, however, that the relative positions of the anatomic features in the reference image should be preserved. Additional imaging from the subcostal (coronal and sagittal) and suprasternal notch positions complements the examination.

Because of difficulty in discerning gray-white interface on two-dimensional images, convention prefers the use of the sharp demarcation between cavity and endocardium for measurement purposes. Therefore the endocardium-cavity interface is used rather than the leading edge, as for M-mode.[1]

tal view. The apical four-chamber is preferred, rotating to the apical two-chamber for the left atrium. In this combination of images, the maximal and mid-cavity superoinferior and anterolateral right atrial dimensions and superoinferior, mediolateral, and anteroposterior left atrial dimensions can be determined. The measurement is generally done at the end of systole, defined as the frame prior to opening of the atrioventricular valve when the atrial dimension is at its largest. It should be noted that the left atrial dimensions determined in this way may not correlate with the left atrial dimension obtained by M-mode, and they are are not interchangeable. Measurements of the interatrial septum, including estimation of the dimension of defects in the septum, are best made from the subcostal coronal and sagittal transducer positions, minimizing dropout artifact by maintaining an interrogation plane nearly perpendicular to the septum.

ATRIA

The right and left atria can be imaged and their dimensions measured from the parasternal long-axis view, from the apex, or in the subcos-

ATRIOVENTRICULAR VALVES

Using two-dimensional imaging, estimation of valve areas by planimetry of a cross-sectional

Table 73-1	Normal two-dimensional echocardiographic measurements
	Range
Aorta	
Annulus	1.4-2.6 cm
Sinuses of Valsalva	2.2-3.6 cm
Ascending	2.1-3.4 cm
Arch	2.0-3.6 cm
Pulmonary artery	
Annulus	1.0-2.2 cm
Main	0.9-2.9 cm
Left atrium	
Anteroposterior (PLAX)	2.3-4.5 cm
Mediolateral (A4C)	2.5-4.5 cm
Superoinferior (A4C)	3.4-6.1 cm
Right ventricle (A4C)	
Minor axis	2.2-4.4 cm
Major axis	6.5-9.5 cm
Left ventricle (A4C)	
Major axis (diastole)	6.9-10.3 cm
Minor axis (diastole)	3.3-6.1 cm
Minor axis (systole)	1.9-3.7 cm
Fractional shortening	27-50%
Left ventricle (PLAX)	
Diameter (diastole)	3.5-6.0 cm
Diameter (systole)	2.1-4.0 cm
Fractional shortening	25-46%
Left ventricle (PSAX)	
Diameter, chordal (diastole)	3.5-6.2 cm
Diameter, chordal (systole)	2.3-4.0 cm
Fractional shortening	27-42%
Diameter, papillary muscle (diastole)	3.5-5.8 cm
Diameter, papillary muscle (systole)	2.2-4.0 cm
Fractional shortening	25-43%
Left ventricular volume, end-diastole	
(modified Simpson's) apical	36-82 ml/m^2
Left ventricular ejection fraction	
(modified Simpson's) apical, male	70 ± 7%
(modified Simpson's) apical, female	65 ± 10%
Left ventricular mass (truncated ellipsoid)	
Male	76 ± 13 g/m^2
Female	66 ± 11 g/m^2

Abbreviations: A4C, apical four-chamber view, PLAX, parasternal long-axis view, PSAX, parasternal short-axis view.

image can be performed but may be unreliable, and valve areas in disease states are best determined by other methods. In pediatric patients with congenital heart disease, however, meaningful, two-dimensional measurements of the diameters of the tricuspid and mitral valves can be made in the apical four-chamber view at the valve annulus at the onset of diastole. Measurement is done at the hinge point of the valve, compared with the established normal for body surface area, and assigned a "Z-score" correlating with the number of standard deviations from the mean the measurement lies (a Z-score of 0 being at the mean for BSA):

$$Z\ value = \frac{\text{measured value} - \text{mean value of a normal population}}{\text{standard deviation of a normal population}}$$

(equation 1)

A comprehensive listing of Z-score nomograms is beyond the scope of this text, but for additional information the reader is referred to several excellent texts.[7-9]

LEFT VENTRICLE

Imaging for performance of two-dimensional measurements of the left ventricle is most often accomplished from the parasternal and apical transducer positions. Measurement at end-diastole is done at or immediately before the initial systolic closure of the mitral valve. End-systole is defined as the time point of or immediately preceding diastolic mitral opening. Note that the mitral valve is closing or closed at both points–end-diastole and end-systole. The onset of the QRS complex can also be used as end-diastole.

Dimensions of the left ventricle can be measured from the apex in the four-chamber view. The length, or major axis of the ventricle, and the width, or minor axis at a point approximately one third of the length of the major axis from the base, can be measured in systole or diastole and compared to published normal values (see Table 73-1). Measurement of the left ventricular chamber can also be done from

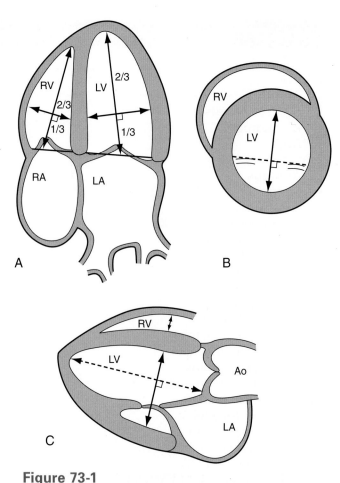

Figure 73-1
Intracardiac dimensions obtained from the apical four-chamber (**A**), parasternal short-axis (**B**), or parasternal long-axis (**C**) views. The major and minor axes of the right and left ventricles are shown, as is the method for measuring annular diameters of the tricuspid and mitral valves from the apical view. Ao, Aorta; LA, left atrium; LV, left ventricle; RA, right atrium; RV, right ventricle. (Modified from Schiller NB, Shah PM, Crawford M, et al: Recommendations for quantitation of the left ventricle by two-dimensional echocardiography. American Society of Echocardiography Committee on Standards, Subcommittee on Quantitation of Two-Dimensional Echocardiograms. J Am Soc Echocardiogr 1989;2: 358-367.)

the parasternal long- (Fig. 73-1C) or short-axis (Fig. 73-1B).[1,4]

The area of the ventricle in the apical four-chamber view can be computed from a tracing of the endocardial surface at end-diastole and end-systole, and the volume estimated by a variety of methods. For estimation of left ven-

LV VOLUME
BY METHOD OF DISKS (MODIFIED SIMPSON'S RULE)

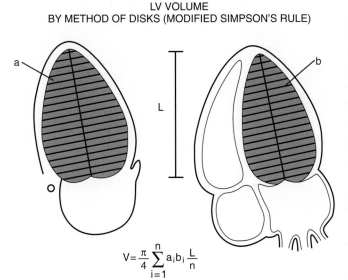

$$V = \frac{\pi}{4} \sum_{i=1}^{n} a_i b_i \frac{L}{n}$$

Figure 73-2
Diagram illustrating the estimation of left ventricular volume using Simpson's biplane method of disk summation. The volume of each disk is calculated from the diameters *a* and *b* in two orthogonal planes and the thickness of the disk (in this example, 1/20 of the length *L*). (Redrawn from Schiller NB, Shah PM, Crawford M, et al: Recommendations for quantitation of the left ventricle by two-dimensional echocardiography. American Society of Echocardiography Committee on Standards, Subcommittee on Quantitation of Two-Dimensional Echocardiograms. J Am Soc Echocardiogr 1989;2: 358-367.)

tricular volume[5,10] and ejection fraction[11] as an index of systolic function, we prefer that the areas in two orthogonal planes be determined and this information applied to the volume estimation using the disk summation method (modified biplane Simpson's rule, Fig. 73-2).[1,12-14] The apical two-chamber view is used to complement the four-chamber view. It should be noted that the two-chamber view does not incorporate the left ventricular outflow tract or the aortic valve for the purposes of the measurement. The endocardium-cavity interface is traced, extending toward the base of the heart to the mitral annulus; however, a straight line from medial to lateral annulus is generally taken rather than attempting to trace the closed mitral leaflets. Done properly, the length of the long axis of the volumes traced should be nearly equal (no more than 20% difference) for the two orthogonal views.

In addition to the M-mode method described in the previous section, myocardial mass can be determined from a two-dimensional measurement of myocardial cross-sectional area from a parasternal, short-axis view at the level of the papillary muscle tips at end-diastole. The epicardial and endocardial surfaces are traced, and computation of the mean wall thickness and myocardial area are performed. If the ventricular major axis in diastole is also known, the left ventricular myocardial volume can be calculated, and, assuming a myocardial specific gravity of 1.05 g/mL, ventricular mass can be calculated. There are several methods for actually calculating the volumes, based on a variety of geometric assumptions[1,6,10,15]; it is important to be aware of which method is used by the computational equipment when making comparisons to normal values.

RIGHT VENTRICLE

Dimensions of the right ventricle can be measured in a manner analogous to those of the left ventricle, from the apex in the four-chamber view, as shown in Figure 73-1A. The length, or major axis of the ventricle, and the width, or minor axis at a point approximately one third of the length of the major axis from the tricuspid valve (usually the widest point of the ventricle), are the standards advocated by some.[1] Less useful is the dimension of the cavity from the parasternal, long-axis view at the level of the chordae tendinae of the left ventricle, as shown in Figure 73-1C. Normal values are presented in Table 73-1.[1,4]

Imaging of the right ventricle throughout the cardiac cycle, as is necessary for assessment of systolic function, is difficult in adults and pediatric patients due to the ventricle's proximity to the sternum and to its irregular shape. Imaging can be easier in the very young patient when done from the subcostal transducer position. Some authors have advocated using this approach to acquire orthogonal views of the right ventricle, from which the ventricular areas may be traced and volumes estimated by application of Simpson's method, described above.[13,16] Care must be taken to use the same long-axis of measurement, from the diaphragmatic surface to the pulmonary valve, in both the coronal and sagittal views, if this method is to be employed (Fig. 73-3).

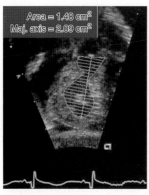
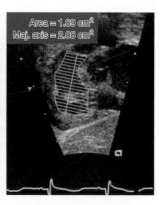

Figure 73-3

Subcostal two-dimensional images demonstrating method for volume measurement of the right ventricle. Shown are two frames, from orthogonal coronal (left) and sagittal (right) planes, at end-diastole. The endocardial border is traced, and the major axis superimposed on the figure. Note that the major axis for both planes extends from diaphragmatic surface to the outflow tract and is approximately equal in both projections.

AORTA

The aortic valve and proximal aorta are best imaged in the parasternal long-axis view. From this image, several measurements can be made, as noted in Figure 73-4. The aortic valve annulus is measured at the onset of systole, in the first frame after valve opening, and is measured at the hinge points of the valve. The aortic root, at the sinuses of Valsalva, can also be measured at the widest point. The ascending aorta is measured at the sino-tubular junction. Additional measurement of the ascending aorta may also be useful in serial examination of patients with aortic disease, and this may be obtained from the parasternal or suprasternal notch positions (Fig. 73-5). In pediatric patients, additional measurements of the transverse aortic arch, between the innominate artery and left

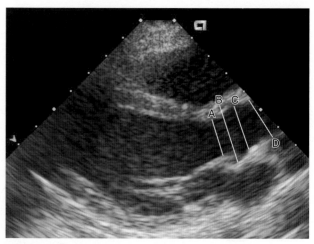

Figure 73-4

Parasternal long-axis image demonstrating measurements of the aortic valve and ascending aorta. The aortic valve annulus (**A**) is measured at the onset of systole, in the first frame after valve opening, and is measured at the hinge points of the valve. The aortic root (**B**), at the sinuses of Valsalva, can also be measured at the widest point. The dimension C represents the sinotubular junction and D the ascending aorta diameter.

carotid artery, and isthmus (region between the left subclavian artery and origin of the ductus arteriosus) may also be made from the suprasternal notch position and are helpful in evaluating the patient with coarctation of the aorta.

PULMONARY ARTERIES

The pulmonary arteries are best imaged in the parasternal short-axis. From this window, measurement of the pulmonary valve annulus, main pulmonary artery, and proximal branch pulmonary arteries can be made (see Fig. 73-5).

DISCUSSION

Once widely used, the area-length method for left ventricular volume estimation is not presented here; though easier conceptually and easier when calculation is being carried out manually, it is not as accurate as the biplane method of Simpson. In practice, the cumbersome mathematical calculations are now performed online by the ultrasound equipment,

obviating the need for simpler methods involving geometric assumptions.

A large part of the discussion regarding two-dimensional echocardiography revolves around the use of echo for volume and function assessment. As noted, it is possible to noninvasively estimate not only volume and mass but also stroke volumes, ejection fraction, and other

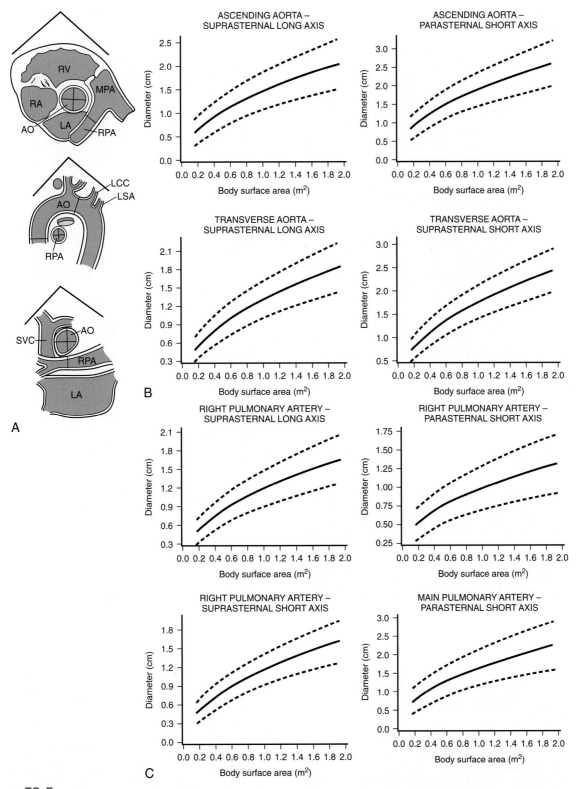

Figure 73-5

Illustration demonstrating measurement of the dimensions of the ascending aorta and main and branch pulmonary arteries (**A**), and normal value curves (**B, C**) showing the relation between measurements and body surface area. The dashed lines are the tolerance limits weighted for body surface area for prediction of normal values for 80% of the future population with 50% confidence. Ao, Aorta; LA, left atrium; LCC, left common carotid; LPA, left pulmonary artery; LSA, left subclavian artery; MPA, main pulmonary artery; RA, right atrium; RPA, right pulmonary artery; RV, right ventricle; SVC, superior vena cava. (Redrawn from Snider AR, Enderlein MA, Teitel DF, Juster RP: Two-dimensional echocardiographic determination of aortic and pulmonary artery sizes from infancy to adulthood in normal subjects. Am J Cardiol 1984;53:218-224, with permission from Excerpta Medica.)

indices of systolic function, as well as regurgitant fraction in both right- and left-heart disease. It has been shown, however, that estimations of left ventricular volumes by the methods described earlier, though accurate and reproducible, tend to underestimate the volume measured by angiography.[17-19] This is thought to be due to a variety of factors, including differences in endocardial definition with radio-opaque contrast within the trabeculations, the exclusion of the papillary muscles from the volume measurement by angiography, and technical difficulties resulting in foreshortening using echocardiographic technique. It is possible that the use of three-dimensional echocardiographic techniques, either with manual definition or using automated border detection, may help resolve some of the issues in measurement of ventricular volumes. This technology, unfortunately, is not yet widely available. At this time, magnetic resonance imaging (MRI) may be the best noninvasive method for determining volumes, especially in the case of the right ventricle, when echo imaging may be inadequate.[20-23]

References

1. Schiller NB, Shah PM, Crawford M, et al: Recommendations for quantitation of the left ventricle by two-dimensional echocardiography. American Society of Echocardiography Committee on Standards, Subcommittee on Quantitation of Two-Dimensional Echocardiograms. J Am Soc Echocardiogr 1989;2:358-367.
2. Shiina A, Tajik AJ, Smith HC, et al: Prognostic significance of regional wall motion abnormality in patients with prior myocardial infarction: a prospective correlative study of two-dimensional echocardiography and angiography. Mayo Clin Proc 1986;61:254-262.
3. Otto CM, Pearlman AS: Textbook of Clinical Echocardiography, 2nd ed. Philadelphia, W.B. Saunders, 1995.
4. Schnittger I, Gordon EP, Fitzgerald PJ, et al: Standardized intracardiac measurements of two-dimensional echocardiography. J Am Coll Cardiol 1983;2:934-938.
5. Wahr DW, Wang YS, Schiller NB: Left ventricular volumes determined by two-dimensional echocardiography in a normal adult population. J Am Coll Cardiol 1983;1:863-868.
6. Helak JW, Reichek N: Quantitation of human left ventricular mass and volume by two-dimensional echocardiography: in vitro anatomic validation. Circulation 1981;63:1398-1407.
7. Garson A, Bricker JT, McNamara DG (eds): The Science and Practice of Pediatric Cardiology, 2nd ed. Philadelphia, Lea & Febiger, 1990.
8. Feigenbaum H: Echocardiography, 5th ed. Philadelphia, Lea & Febiger, 1994.
9. Kirklin JW, Barratt-Boyes BG: Cardiac surgery: morphology, diagnostic criteria, natural history, techniques, results, and indications. New York, Churchill Livingstone, 1993.
10. Byrd BF 3rd, Wahr D, Wang YS, et al: Left ventricular mass and volume/mass ratio determined by two-dimensional echocardiography in normal adults. J Am Coll Cardiol 1985;6:1021-1025.
11. Mickelson JK, Byrd BF 3rd, Bouchard A, et al: Left ventricular dimensions and mechanics in distance runners. Am Heart J 1986;112:1251-1256.
12. Mercier JC, DiSessa TG, Jarmakani JM, et al: Two-dimensional echocardiographic assessment of left ventricular volumes and ejection fraction in children. Circulation 1982;65:962-969.
13. Silverman NH: Pediatric Echocardiography. Baltimore, Williams & Wilkins, 1993.
14. Silverman NH, Ports TA, Snider AR, et al: Determination of left ventricular volume in children: echocardiographic and angiographic comparisons. Circulation 1980;62:548-557.
15. Reichek N, Helak J, Plappert T, et al: Anatomic validation of left ventricular mass estimates from clinical two-dimensional echocardiography: initial results. Circulation 1983;67:348-352.
16. Hiraishi S, DiSessa TG, Jarmakani JM, et al: Two-dimensional echocardiographic assessment of right ventricular volume in children with congenital heart disease. Am J Cardiol 1982;50:1368-1375.
17. Erbel R, Schweizer P, Lambertz H, et al: Echoventriculography–a simultaneous analysis of two-dimensional echocardiography and cineventriculography. Circulation 1983;67:205-215.

18. Schmidt KG, Silverman NH, Van Hare GF, et al: Two-dimensional echocardiographic determination of ventricular volumes in the fetal heart. Validation studies in fetal lambs. Circulation 1990;81:325-333.

19. Starling MR, Dell'Italia LJ, Walsh RA, et al: Accurate estimates of absolute left ventricular volumes from equilibrium radionuclide angiographic count data using a simple geometric attenuation correction. J Am Coll Cardiol 1984;3:789-798.

20. Geva T, Sandweiss BM, Gauvreau K, et al: Factors associated with impaired clinical status in long-term survivors of tetralogy of Fallot repair evaluated by magnetic resonance imaging. J Am Coll Cardiol 2004; 43:1068-1074.

21. Helbing WA, de Roos A: Clinical applications of cardiac magnetic resonance imaging after repair of tetralogy of Fallot. Pediatr Cardiol 2000;21:70-79.

22. Pattynama PM, De Roos A, Van der Wall EE, et al: Evaluation of cardiac function with magnetic resonance imaging. Am Heart J 1994;128:595-607.

23. Rebergen SA, de Roos A: Congenital heart disease. Evaluation of anatomy and function by MRI. Herz 2000;25:365-383.

PART 9

Abdomen Genitourinary

CHAPTER 74

Marijo A. Gillen
Ethan J. Halpern

Adrenal Gland

Introduction

The adrenal glands are paired retroperitoneal organs. The right adrenal gland is located superior to the right kidney, posteromedial to the right lobe of the liver, posterior to the inferior vena cava (IVC), and lateral to the right crus of the diaphragm. The left adrenal gland is located medial and anterior to the superior pole of the left kidney, lateral to the left crus of the diaphragm and the aorta, and posterior to the pancreas and splenic vessels.

Materials/Measurements

LINEAR DIMENSIONS

Adrenal size from conventional anatomy[1] is as follows: normal thickness 2 to 8 mm, length 4 to 6 cm, width 2 to 3 cm, and the average weight 3 to 5 g.

Zappasodi et al[2] measured adrenal glands in 70 normal volunteers and found the thickness of the body to be 0.56 cm, the thickness of the limbs to be 0.28 cm, and the maximum length was 4.2 cm. The maximum width of the body plus the limb is 3.5 cm.

Krebs et al[3] found that the left adrenal measured 2 to 4 cm in length and between 0.9 and 1.4 cm in AP thickness, with the left larger than the right; in pediatric patients the length was found to be less than 2 cm.

Many of the studies showing adrenal size used CT or MRI due to the relative ease of visualizing the adrenals with those modalities. Buck et al[4] measured the adrenal size in 20 patients and found the average measurements shown in Table 74-1.

Karstaedt et al[5] measured adrenal gland size on CT in 200 nonpathologic patients and found the average measurements shown in Table 74-2.

Montangne et al[6] studied 60 random patients on CT, where he defined length as cephalocaudal, width as greatest linear (AP) diameter seen on any single slice, and thickness as the dimension perpendicular to the long axis of the gland or to the limbs. He found the length of the adrenals was between 2 and 4 cm, the width between 2 and 2.5 cm, and the thickness less than or equal to 1 cm.

Vincent et al[7] measured the maximum width of the body and of each limb perpendicular to the long axis of the limb. He felt that measurement of the limbs was important because they contained mostly cortical tissue with minimal medullary tissue. His findings are summarized in Table 74-3.

Table 74-1	Size of normal adrenal glands measured by CT	
Measurement	**R adrenal (cm)**	**L adrenal (cm)**
Height	3.70 ± 0.39	4.32 ± 0.6
Width	1.65 ± 0.30	1.54 ± 0.32
Length	2.68 ± 0.64	2.43 ± 0.79
Diameter	0.55 ± 0.10	0.57 ± 0.12

Modified from Buck J, Reiser U, Heuck F: Computed tomography of the adrenal glands. Europ J Radiol 1982;2: 52-59.

Table 74-2	Normal adrenal-gland measurements	
Side	**Greatest diameter (cm)**	**Thickness (cm)**
R adrenal	2.15 ± 0.46	0.67 ± 0.17
L adrenal	2.28 ± 0.63	0.51 ± 0.11

From Karstaedt N, Sagel SS, Stanley RJ, et al: Computed tomography of the adrenal gland. Radiology 1978;129:723.

Table 74-3 Range of measurements of normal adrenal glands

Side	Max body width (cm)	Medial limb width (cm)	Lateral limb width (cm)
Right	0.61 ± 0.2	0.28 ± 0.08	0.28 ± 0.06
Left	0.79 ± 0.21	0.33 ± 0.09	0.30 ± 0.10

Modified from Vincent JM, Morrison ID, Armstrong P, Reznek RH: The size of normal adrenal glands on computed tomography. Clin Radiol 1994;49:453-455.

Table 74-4 Dimensions of the adrenal glands

Age	Transverse diameter (cm)	Vertical diameter (cm)	Anteroposterior diameter (cm)
Newborn	3.3-3.5 cm	2.3-2.8 cm	1.2-1.3 cm
Adult	3.0-7.0 cm	2.0-3.5 cm	0.3-0.8 cm

From International Commission on Radiological Protection. Task Group on Reference Man. Report of the Task Group on Reference Man. Prepared by the Task Group Committee No. 2. International Commission on Radiologic Protection. New York, Pergamon Press, 1975, pp 202-206.

The findings of the *Report of the Task Group on Reference Man*[8] on adrenal gland dimensions are summarized in Table 74-4.

VOLUME

Other studies measured adrenal gland volume. Amsterdam et al,[9] in a pilot study of 11 healthy volunteers, measured adrenal gland volumes by tracing the CT contours on a workstation; they found the average adrenal gland volume to be $3.5 ± 1.5\,cm^3$.

Rubin and Phillips[10] measured adrenal gland volume on CT and MRI in 10 healthy volunteers by tracing the contours of the adrenal on a workstation. They found the mean volume of the right adrenal to be $2.45 ± 0.74\,cm^3$ on CT and $2.37 ± 0.51\,cm^3$ on MRI. The mean volume of the left adrenal gland was $2.81 ± 0.82\,cm^3$ on CT and $2.53 ± 0.80\,cm^3$ on MRI. The volumes were slightly larger on CT.

According to the *Report of the Task Group on Reference Man*,[8] the mean volume of one adrenal gland is $5.47\,cm^3$ in males (with $0.43\,cm^3$ of medulla and $5.04\,cm^3$ of cortex) and $6.09\,cm^3$ in females (with $0.30\,cm^3$ of medulla and $5.79\,cm^3$ of cortex).

WEIGHT

According to the *Report of the Task Group on Reference Man*,[8] the total weight of both adrenal glands for normal adults, both male and female, is 14 g.

Holmes et al[11] found the mean adrenal weights for both glands was 12 ± 0.28 for males and 10.8 ± 0.33 g for females.

DISCUSSION

The shapes of the adrenal glands are variable; classically the right adrenal gland is triangular and the left is cresentic.[12] Miekos[13] studied 220 cadaver adrenal glands and showed that the shapes have more complexity and variability. On the right he found 61% were pyramidal, 20% were in a birette shape, 9% were in a sandglass, 5% were in a half-moon, 3% were oval, and 2% had a quadrangular shape. On the left he found 63% were semi-lunar, 19% were triangular, 11% were elliptical, and 7% were irregular.

On cross-sectional anatomy, the adrenals appear in a variety of shapes depending on the level at which they are imaged. On the right these include triangular, X, Y, V, K, inverted V, comma, linear, or double line. Shapes on the left are triangular, V, Y, inverted V, inverted Y, linear, crescentic, or reversed L.[4,5,14] Most importantly, the normal adrenal gland demonstrates a concave contour. Any bulge or convexity in the adrenal contour should raise suspicion for an adrenal mass.

On ultrasound, visualizing the adrenals takes experience due to the complexity of the anatomy, the small size, and location of the organs. Using a longitudinal oblique approach on a static compound ultrasound scanner, Sample[15,16] visualized 85% of normal adrenal glands, the right same as the left. Gunther et al[17] used real-time ultrasound with an intercostal approach in both transverse and longitudinal planes and saw the adrenal area, but in only 1 out of 60 patients did he see a normal adrenal gland. Yeh,[18] using a static scanner, visualized 78.5% of normal right adrenal glands and 44% of normal left adrenal glands. Oppenheimeret al,[19] using real-time scanners, visualized the right adrenal in 97% and left adrenal in 83% of newborns. Marchal et al[20] using real-time scanners visualized the right adrenal gland in 92% and left adrenal in 71% of 100 patients.

Krebs et al[3] used the caval-suprarenal line with the patient in a 45° LPO position; the adrenals were visualized in 90% of 50 patients but only 60% of the time with a conventional RPO position. This included visualization 67% of the time with the 15 obese patients included in the study.

Visualization of the right adrenal on ultrasound is best done intercostally, with the patient supine and the transducer in the mid- or anterior axillary line in a coronal plane (Fig. 74-1). The landmarks are the right kidney, right lobe of the liver, and IVC. Visualization of the left adrenal gland is best done intercostally, with the patient in a right lateral decubitus position, imaging in the mid- or posterior axillary line in a coronal plane[2,17,21] (Fig. 74-2). The landmarks are the spleen, left kidney, and aorta.

On ultrasound, the adrenal gland is hypoechoic peripherally, similar to the crus of the diaphragm. In some cases, particularly in children, a central echogenic area is seen, which corresponds to the adrenal medulla. This gives a tri-layered appearance[2,19] (Fig. 74-3). When seen, the three-layered appearance is usually only visualized in the body of the gland and, much less frequently, the limbs. This is consistent with the research of Dobbie and Symington,[22] who showed that the limbs have little medullary tissue.

With real-time ultrasonography, visualization of the adrenal glands is slightly more complex and takes experience with special positioning

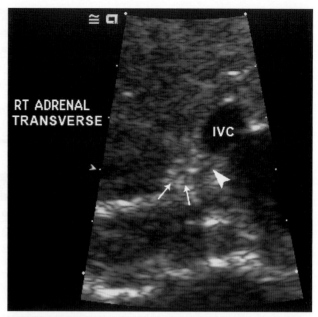

Figure 74-1
Transverse images in an adult showing two limbs of the right adrenal (*arrows*) posterior to the IVC and lateral to the right crus of the diaphragm (*arrowhead*).

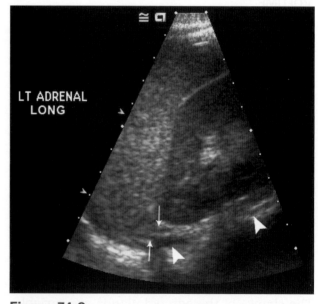

Figure 74-2
Longitudinal image in an adult showing two limbs of the left adrenal (*arrows*) adjacent to the left crus of the diaphragm (*arrowheads*) and superior to the left kidney.

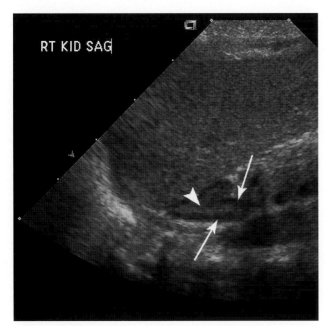

Figure 74-3
Longitudinal neonatal ultrasound showing right adrenal with tri-laminar appearance consisting of outer layers of hypoechoic adrenal cortex (*arrows*) and inner layer of hyperechoic adrenal medulla (*arrowhead*).

of the patient. CT or MRI have standard imaging planes, are operator independent, and less limited by body habitus. Furthermore, CT and MRI are also better suited than ultrasound to identify fatty tissue within an adrenal mass, and thereby confirm the diagnosis of a benign adrenal adenoma. Therefore they are the standard procedures for excluding adrenal abnormalities. Abrams et al[23] compared accuracy of CT and ultrasound for adrenal pathology and found CT to have a sensitivity of 84% and a specificity of 98% with an accuracy of 90%, while ultrasound was reported to have a sensitivity of 79%, specificity of 61%, and accuracy of 70%.

Sonography is preferred in fetuses, children, and pregnant women due to the lack of ionizing radiation. It is also preferred in thin adults, where visualization of the retroperitoneum may be problematic due to a lack of fat, or in circumstances where CT is unavailable.

References

1. Soffer LJ, Soffer LJ, (eds): Disease of the Endocrine Glands. Philadelphia, Lea & Febiger, 1951, pp 189-197.

2. Zappasodi F, Derchi LE, Rizzato G: Ultrasonography of the normal adrenal glands: study using linear array real-time equipment. Br J Radiol 1986;59:759.

3. Krebs CA, Eisenberg RL, Ratcliff S, Jouppi L: Cava-suprarenal line: new position for sonographic imaging of the left adrenal gland. J Clin Ultrasound 1986;14:535-539.

4. Buck J, Reiser U, Heuck F: Computed tomography of the adrenal glands. Eur J Radiol 1982;2:52-59.

5. Karstaedt N, Sagel SS, Stanley RJ, et al: Computed tomography of the adrenal gland. Radiology 1978;129:723.

6. Montagne JP, Kressel HY, Korobkin M, Moss AA: Computed tomography of the normal adrenal glands. AJR Am J Roentgenol 1978;130:963-966.

7. Vincent JM, Morrison ID, Armstrong P, Reznek RH: The size of normal adrenal glands on computed tomography. Clin Radiol 1994;49:453-455.

8. International Commission on Radiological Protection. Task Group on Reference Man. Report of the Task Group on Reference Man. Prepared by the Task Group Committee No. 2. International Commission on Radiologic Protection. New York, Pergamon Press, 1975, pp 202-206.

9. Amsterdam JD, Marinelli DL, Arger P, Winokur A: Assessment of adrenal gland volume by computed tomography in depressed patients and healthy volunteers: a pilot study. Psychiatry Res 1986;21:189-197.

10. Rubin RT, Phillips JJ: Adrenal gland volume determination by computed tomography and magnetic resonance imaging in normal subjects. Investig Rad 1991;26:465-469.

11. Holmes RO, Moon HD, Rinehart JE: A morphologic study of the adrenal gland with correlations of body size and heart size. Am J Pathol 1951;27:724-730.

12. Soffer LJ: The anatomy, morphologic structure, and embryology of the adrenal glands. In Soffer LJ (ed). Disease of the Endocrine Glands. Philadelphia, Lea & Febiger 1951, pp 189-197.

13. Miekos E: Anatomical basis of radiodiagnosis of the adrenal gland. Int Urol Nephrol 1979;11:193-200.

14. Wilms G, Baert A, Marchal G, Goddeeris P: Computed tomography of the normal adrenal

glands: correlative study with autopsy specimens. J Comput Assist Tomogr 1979;3: 467-469.

15. Sample WF: A new technique for the evaluation of the adrenal gland with gray scale ultrasonography. Radiology 1977;124:463-469.

16. Sample WF: Adrenal ultrasonography. Radiology 1978;127:461-466.

17. Gunther RW, Kebel C, Lenner V: Real-time ultrasound of normal adrenal glands and small tumors. J Clin Ultrasound 1984;12: 211-217.

18. Yeh H: Sonography of the adrenal glands: normal glands and small masses. AJR Am J Roentgenol 1980;135:1167-1177.

19. Oppenheimer DA, Carrol BA, Yousem S: Sonography of the normal neonatal adrenal gland. Radiology 1983;146:157-160.

20. Marchal G, Gelin J, Verbeken E, et al: High resolution real-time sonography of the adrenal glands: a routine examination? J Ultrasound Med 1986;5:65-68.

21. Mittelstaedt CA: Abdominal Ultrasound. New York, Edinburgh, London, Melbourne, Churchill Livingstone, 1987, pp 381-394.

22. Dobbie JW, Symington T: The human adrenal gland with special reference to the vasculature. J Endocrinol 1966;34:479.

23. Abrams HL, Siegelman SS, Adams DF, et al: Computed tomography versus ultrasound of the adrenal gland: a prospective study. Radiology 1982;143:121.

CHAPTER 75

Ethan J. Halpern

Renal Measurements

Introduction

The kidneys are paired organs located in the retroperitoneum. One kidney is present along the lateral margin of each psoas muscle. The kidneys serve to filter the blood for waste products and are integral components in several metabolic pathways, including the hormonal pathways that control blood pressure. Normal kidneys are well visualized by ultrasound because the renal cortex is sharply delineated by the renal capsule and differs in echotexture from the surrounding echogenic perinephric fat.

Materials/Measurements

Kidney length is measured along a long axis parallel to the adjacent psoas muscle. The oblique plane of this long axis extends from the more medially located upper pole to the more laterally/anteriorly located lower pole. The angle between the long axis of the kidney and the sagittal plane ranges from 8 to 20 degrees.[1] The variation of this angle produces variability in the renal length measured by x-ray urography.[2] Ultrasound is well suited to define this long axis in real time and can therefore provide more reliable measurement of renal length (Fig. 75-1).

In order to provide an accurate long-axis measurement of the kidney, the sonographer must carefully define both the upper and lower poles. This may be difficult in patients with ectopic/malrotated kidneys, renal scarring, or scoliosis. Measurement of renal length is most accurate when performed on coronal or sagittal views with the patient in supine or decubitus position. Measurements in the prone position

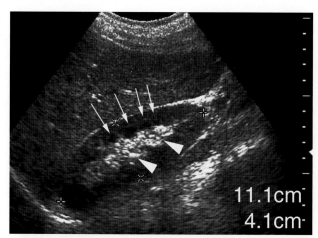

Figure 75-1

Sagittal image of the right kidney imaged through the liver. The kidney consists of three sonographically distinct regions. The renal sinus (*arrowheads*) is the echogenic area in the center of the kidney. The cortex is the bulk of the parenchyma that surrounds the sinus and demonstrates mid-level echotexture. The renal pyramids are visible as subtle hypoechoic foci at regular intervals along the junction between the cortex and the sinus (*arrows*).

below the costal margin. Tissue harmonic imaging is often useful in obese patients.

Determination of renal volume is not generally requested on ultrasound examination. However, measurement of volume may be a more sensitive method for detection of renal abnormalities.[4] Renal volume may be estimated from three orthogonal measurements on the basis of an adjusted ellipsoid formula that is corrected for the actual renal volume by water displacement. Specifically, the volume $V = 0.49 \times L \times W \times AP$, where L is the length of the long axis, W is the width measured at the renal hilum, and AP is the anteroposterior dimension at the hilum (Fig. 75-2).[5] Advances in ultrasound technology that allow volume measurement from a three-dimensional data set provide more accurate estimates of renal volume as compared to two-dimensional measurements in orthogonal planes.[6]

In order to obtain accurate renal measurements, a sonographer must have some familiarity with sonographic anatomy of the kidney. The kidney consists of three sonographically visible areas: the cortex, medullary pyramids, and renal sinus/collecting system (see Fig. 75-1). In the adult, the cortex is isoechoic or slightly hypoechoic relative to liver. The medullary pyramids are triangular structures embedded within the cortex at regular intervals and appearing slightly hypoechoic relative to the cortex. The renal sinus in the center of the kidney is bright due to the presence of sinus fat.

tend to underestimate renal length and should be reserved for situations in which the kidney appears foreshortened on other views.[3] In order to view the upper pole of the kidney, the patient can raise the ipsilateral arm above the head and take a deep breath to move the kidney

DISCUSSION

Sonography of the kidneys is often requested in the setting of reduced renal function. Evaluation of the collecting system and ureteral jets is performed to exclude obstruction as a cause of renal failure. Assessment of renal size is an important part of this examination. Small kidneys are often associated with chronic renal disease, while normal-size kidneys suggest a more acute cause of renal failure. Enlarged kidneys may be associated with an inflammatory/infiltrative process,[7] or renal vein thrombosis.

Interobserver variation in the length of the normal adult kidney is proportionately less than interobserver variation in the measurement of the pediatric kidney. It is less than 1.85 cm in 95% of cases.[8] As noted for children, there is a definite relationship between adult kidney

length and somatometric measurements.[9] Kidney size varies with a number of variables, including patient age, size, sex, and state of hydration. Kidneys tend to be larger in men and tend to decrease in size more rapidly after the age of 60.[10] Sonographic measurements of the adult kidney are 1 to 1.5 cm smaller than those obtained by urography because of the magnification factor with x-rays and the osmotic forces of contrast material. The median adult renal length is 11.2 cm on the left and 10.9 cm on the right side (Table 75-1).[11] The right kidney is often 1 to 2 cm lower than the left kidney. The standard deviation for normal adult renal measurements is approximately 12 to 13 mm for length and 5 to 7 mm for AP and transverse dimensions (Tables 75-2 and 75-3).[12]

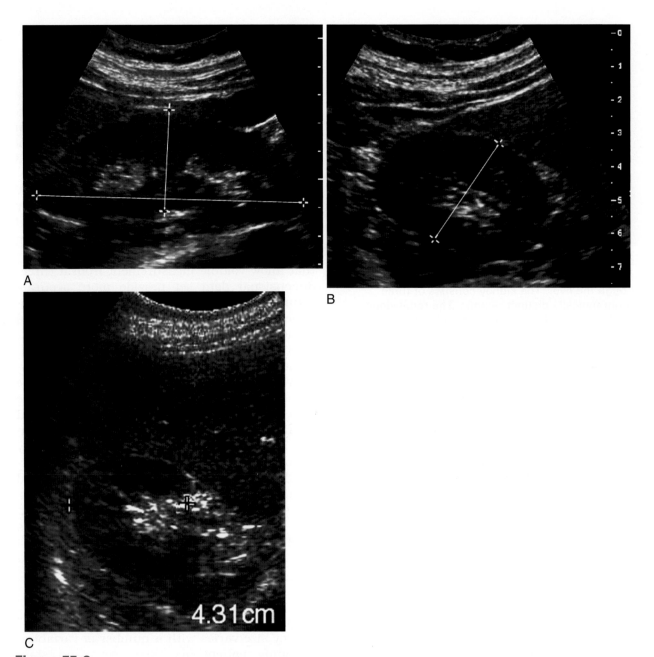

Figure 75-2
Coronal (**A**) and transverse (**B** and **C**) images of a kidney with measurements. The long-axis and transverse measurements may be obtained from the coronal image (**A**). An anteroposterior (AP) diameter is then obtained from a transverse image at the level of the renal hilum (**B**). If the long axis and AP diameter are obtained from a sagittal image, then a transverse diameter can be obtained from the transverse image (**C**). In order to perform volume computations, three perpendicular measurements are required.

In addition to measurements of overall renal size, cortical thickness can be measured when the medullary pyramids are visibly distinct from the cortex. The adult cortex is generally more than 1 cm in thickness over the pyramids. However, measurements of cortical thickness demonstrate greater interobserver and intraob-server variability as compared to other measurements of renal size.[13]

It is quite likely that state-of-the-art three-dimensional sonography (Fig. 75-3) with automated planimetry provides a more accurate assessment of renal volume as compared to three measurements in orthogonal planes with

Table 75-1 Renal size in adults measured with ultrasound

Reference parameter	Decade						
	3	4	5	6	7	8	9
Emamian							
Number	121	144	168	162	70	11	8
Length (L)	11.5 (10.4-12.8)	11.3 (10.3-12.3)	11.3 (10.2-12.5)	11.1 (10.0-12.2)	10.5 (9.4-12.0)	10.2 (9.4-11.0)	9.8 (8.7-10.9)
Length (R)	11.1 (10.1-12.4)	11.2 (10.0-12.3)	11.0 (10.0-12.2)	10.8 (9.5-12.0)	10.4 (9.1-1.8)	9.9 (9.0-10.8)	9.6 (8.5-10.7)
Width (L)	5.9 (5.1-6.6)	5.8 (5.0-6.5)	5.8 (5.3-6.5)	5.8 (5.1-6.5)	5.6 (4.9-6.2)		
Width (R)	5.8 (5.0-6.6)	5.8 (5.2-6.6)	5.8 (5.2-6.4)	5.7 (5.0-6.4)	5.5 (5.0-6.3)		
Miletic							
Number	32	32	42	28	22		
Length (L)	11.5 (10.1-13.0)	11.5 (9.9-13.1)	11.4 (9.5-13.4)	11.3 (10.2-12.4)	10.9 (9.2-12.5)		
Length (R)	11.3 (10.2-12.8)	11.2 (9.7-12.9)	11.2 (9.6-12.8)	11.0 (10.3-11.7)	10.7 (9.3-12.1)		

Emamian SA, Nielsen MB, Pedersen JF, Ytte L: Kidney dimensions at sonography: correlation with age, sex, and habitus in 665 adult volunteers. AJR Am J Roentgenol 1993;160:83-86.

Table 75-2 Right renal dimensions in sample groups of patients examined retrospectively

	Mean (cm)	SD
Length		
Oblique (n = 52)	10.646	1.345
Prone (n = 51)	10.743	1.349
Width*		
Oblique (n = 35)	4.920	0.638
Prone (n = 32)	5.047	0.764
Depth*		
Oblique (n = 19)	3.947	0.812
Prone (n = 9)	4.167	0.507

*, approximate values.
Brandt TD, Neiman HL, Dragowski MJ, et al: Ultrasound assessment of normal renal dimensions. J Ultrasound Med 1982;1:49-52.

Table 75-3 Left renal dimensions in sample groups of patients examined retrospectively

	Mean (cm)	SD
Length		
Oblique (n = 50)	10.130	1.165
Prone (n = 50)	11.096	1.152
Width*		
Oblique (n = 36)	5.303	0.744
Prone (n = 31)	5.300	0.802
Depth*		
Oblique (n = 18)	3.578	0.912
Prone (n = 10)	4.140	0.844

*, approximate values.
Brandt TD, Neiman HL, Dragowski MJ, et al: Ultrasound assessment of normal renal dimensions. J Ultrasound Med 1982;1:49-52.

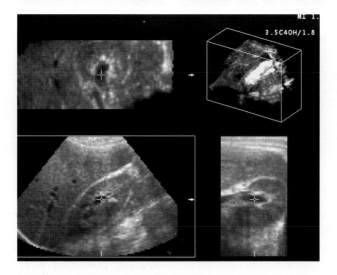

Figure 75-3
Three-dimensional volume acquisition of the right kidney. Images are acquired with a single acquisition and displayed in three orthogonal planes. The images can be rotated to obtain a true long- and short-axis measurement.

volume estimates based upon the prolate ellipse formula. Nonetheless, for most clinical applications, a simple long-axis measurement of renal length is the most appropriate study (see Fig. 75-1).

References

1. Griffiths GJ, Cartwright G, McLachlan MSF: Estimation of renal size from radiographs: is the effect worthwhile? Clin Radiol 1974;26:249-256.
2. Dure-Smith P, McArdle GH: Tomography during excretory urography. Technical aspects. Br J Radiol 1972;45:896-901.
3. De Sanctis JT, Connolly SA, Bramson RT: Effect of patient position on sonographically measured renal length in neonates, infants, and children. AJR Am J Roentgenol 1998; 170:1381-1383.
4. Jones TB, Riddick LR, Harpen, et al: Ultrasonographic determination of renal mass and renal volume. J Ultrasound Med 1983;2: 151-154.
5. Hricak H, Lieto RP: Sonographic determination of renal volume. Radiology 1983;148: 311-312.
6. Partik BL, Stadler A, Schamp S, et al: 3D versus 2D ultrasound: accuracy of volume measurement in human cadaver kidneys. Invest Radiol 2002;37:489-495.
7. Pickworth FE, Carlin JB, Ditchfield MR, et al: Sonographic measurement of renal enlargement in children with acute pyelonephritis and time needed for resolution: implications for renal growth assessment. AJR Am J Roentgenol 1995;165:405-408.
8. Ablett MJ, Coulthard A, Lee RE, et al: How reliable are ultrasound measurements of renal length in adults? Br J Radiol 1995; 68:1087-1089.
9. Miletic D, Fuckar Z, Sustic A, et al: Sonographic measurement of absolute and relative renal length in adults. J Clin Ultrasound 1998;26:185-189.
10. Akpinar IN, Altun E, Avcu S, et al: Sonographic measurement of kidney size in geriatric patients. J Clin Ultrasound 2003; 31:315-318.
11. Emamian SA, Nielsen MB, Pedersen JF, Ytte L: Kidney dimensions at sonography: correlation with age, sex, and habitus in 665 adult volunteers. AJR Am J Roentgenol 1993;160:83-86.
12. Brandt TD, Neiman HL, Dragowski MJ, et al: Ultrasound assessment of normal renal dimensions. J Ultrasound Med 1982;1: 49-52.
13. Emamian SA, Nielsen MB, Pedersen JF: Intraobserver and interobserver variations in sonographic measurements of kidney size in adult volunteers. A comparison of linear measurements and volumetric estimates. Acta Radiol 1995;36:399-401.

CHAPTER 76

Ethan J. Halpern

Prostate and Seminal Vesicle Measurements

Introduction

The prostate gland is the most caudal organ within the male pelvis, located just below the urinary bladder. The seminal vesicles and vasa deferentia are paired structures located just above the base of the prostate and situated slightly posterior to the prostate. On each side of midline, the seminal vesicle and vas deferens join to form an ejaculataory duct that passes through the prostate to enter the urethra at the verumontanum.[1]

Materials/Measurement

Measurement of the seminal vesicles is rarely performed because of the large variation in the size of these organs among individuals. In general, the two seminal vesicles within a particular individual are similar in size. A subjective assessment of seminal vesicle size may be obtained by comparison of the two sides. The seminal vesicles are usually in the range of 2 to 4 cm in long axis. Each seminal vesicle should taper smoothly as it approaches the prostate near the midline. A study using planimetric area measurements of step sections of the seminal vesicles found that the average volume is approximately 13.7 cc.[2]

The prostate gland is very small before puberty, generally measuring less than 5 cc in volume. Under the influence of androgens, the prostate enlarges substantially through the adolescent years and reaches a size of 20 to 30 cc in normal young men.[3] The normal adult prostate maintains its size, unless there is further enlargement related to benign prostatic hyperplasia (BPH).[4]

The normal adult prostate has average dimensions of 33 mm in craniocaudal dimension, 24 mm in anteroposterior dimension, and 39 to 53 mm in transverse dimension.[5] Normal sonographic measurements are reported as 20 to 40 mm in craniocaudal dimension, 21 to 34 mm in anteroposterior dimension, and 39 to 53 mm in transverse dimension, with a volume of 12.9 to 37.1 cc.[6] Because the weight of prostatic tissue is approximately 1 g/cc, the size in cubic centimeters is roughly the same as the weight in grams.

DISCUSSION

In an attempt to simplify the estimation of prostatic size, charts have been devised to estimate the size of the prostate from a single transabdominal measurement of the transverse diameter.[7] However, given the frequently asymmetric nature of BPH, a single diameter measurement is unlikely to provide an accurate estimate of prostate size. As a rough estimate, a single transverse diameter below 4 cm is generally associated with a normal size prostate, while a diameter above 5 cm suggests substantial enlargement.

For those willing to measure the prostate in multiple planes, various techniques and mathematical formulae have been used to estimate the volume of the prostate from three perpendicular measurements.[8-10] Although most clinicians measure the anteroposterior dimension of the prostate from a mid-sagittal image, at least one study has suggested that volume determination may be more accurate when the anteroposterior dimension is measured from a transaxial image.[11] The most commonly employed method for computation of prostate volume is the measurement of three perpendicular diameters (Fig. 76-1) and application of the formula for an ellipsoid or prolate ellipse.[12,13]

Prolate ellipse volume, $V = (\pi/6) \times (L \times W \times H)$

Interexaminer reliability for transrectal measurement of prostate volume can be quite high, with intraclass correlation reported as high as 0.96.[14] Unfortunately, the ellipsoid formula may underestimate the true prostatic volume by as much as 20%.[15] Underestimation of prostate volume by sonographic measurement increases as a function of prostate size.[16] This error is largest when the angle between the transverse plane of the scan and longitudinal axis of the prostate deviates from a true perpendicular.[17,18]

The accuracy of prostate volume estimates can be improved by planimetry, but volume determinations based upon the formula for a prolate ellipse are only marginally inferior to methods based upon a single planimetry measurement.[19] Three-dimensional acquisition of ultrasound images through the prostate may allow more accurate estimates of prostate volume.[20] The use of multiple planimetry measurements with three-dimensional imaging of the prostate can provide superior reproducibility in measurement of prostate volume.[21]

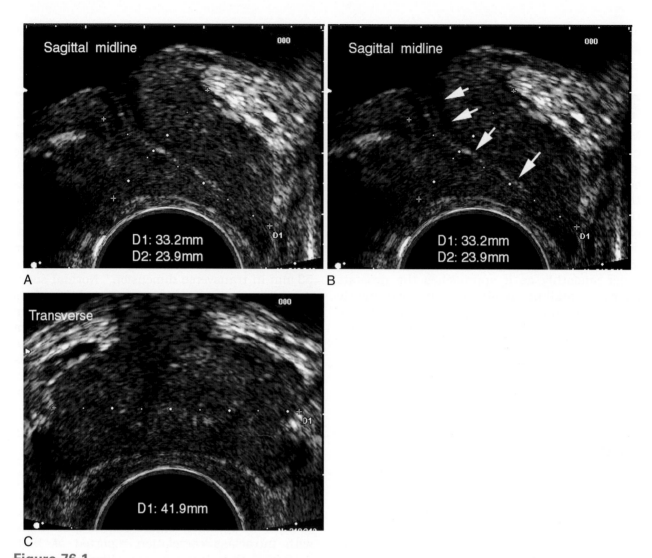

Figure 76-1

Sagittal (**A** and **B**) and transverse (**C**) images of a normal-size prostate. The sagittal midline image is obtained along the course of the urethra (arrows in **B**). The craniocaudal (CC) dimension is measured along the course of the urethra from the base of the prostate to the apex. The anteroposterior dimension is measured as the largest diameter perpendicular to the CC diameter. The transverse diameter is measured at the widest portion of the prostate on a transverse image.

BPH is commonly associated with obstructive urinary symptoms, otherwise known as prostatism. Evaluation and treatment of prostatism requires an assessment of prostatic size. Although the overall size of the gland is measured to quantify macroscopic BPH, the severity of symptoms may not be proportionate to gland size. The presence of hypertrophy of transition zone into the region of the bladder neck, also known as median lobe hypertrophy, should be noted. Because a sonographically visible surgical capsule usually demarcates the transition zone, the transition zone can be measured independently of the overall gland.[22] Ultrasound measurements of transition zone diameters have been found to correlate with severity of bladder outlet obstruction, though this correlation is not adequate for clinical utility.[23] In most clinical practices, only overall measurements of the prostate gland are requested from the ultrasound examination of BPH. In addition to the evaluation of BPH, measurement of the prostate may be used for radiation treatment planning and, when screening for cancer, to correlate prostate volume with prostate specific antigen.[24]

Sonographic assessment of prostate size can be accomplished by either transabdominal or transrectal ultrasound of the prostate. Transabdominal examination is adequate to demonstrate a transverse diameter and to define the base of the prostate.[25] However, transabdominal visualization of the prostate apex may be limited by the symphysis pubis, and transabdominal visualization of the posterior margin may be limited by shadowing from a calcified inner gland. Although early studies described transabdominal measurement of prostatic volume,[26-28] the transrectal approach provides a better sonographic window to the prostate, and it is generally accepted that transrectal scanning with planimetry provides the most reproducible measurements.[29,30]

To conclude, when the goal of imaging the prostate is to demonstrate the presence of enlargement, the accuracy provided by measurement of three perpendicular diameters with transabdominal imaging is probably satisfactory for routine clinical practice.[31] However, when the degree of prostatic enlargement is necessary for preoperative assessment or for post procedural follow-up, transrectal examination is superior. Planimetry with three-dimensional sonography may provide measurements that are slightly more accurate and reproducible, but the additional effort is not generally justified. Although some have advocated magnetic resonance imaging to determine prostatic volume,[32] transrectal ultrasound provides an inexpensive, minimally invasive, and equally accurate method to estimate prostate volume.[33]

References

1. Halpern EJ: Anatomy of the prostate gland. In Halpern EJ, Cochlin DL, Goldberg BB (eds): Imaging of the Prostate. London, Martin Dunitz, 2002;3–15.
2. Ronnberg L, Ylostalo P, Jouppila P: Estimation of the size of the seminal vesicles by means of ultrasonic B-scanning: a preliminary report. Fertil Steril 1978;30:474-475.
3. Leissner KH, Tisell LE: The weight of the human prostate. Scand J Urol Nephrol 1979;13:137-142.
4. Berry SJ, Coffey DS, Walsh PC, Ewing LL: The development of human benign prostatic hyperplasia with age. J Urol 1984;132:474-479.
5. Fornage BD: Normal US anatomy of the prostate. Ultrasound Med Biol 1986;12:1011-1021.
6. Watanabe H, Igari D, Tanahashi Y, et al: Measurements of size and weight of prostate by means of transrectal ultrasonography. Tohoku J Exp Med 1974;114:277-285.
7. Romero-Aguirre CR, Tallada MB, Mayayo TD, et al: Comparative evaluation of prostate size by transabdominal echography, urethral profile and radiology. Journal d Urologie 1980;86:675-769.
8. Myschetzky PS, Suburu RE, Kelly BS Jr, et al: Determination of prostate gland volume by transrectal ultrasound: correlation with radical prostatectomy specimens. Scand J Urol Nephrol Suppl 1991;137:107-111.
9. Yip YL, Chan CW, Li CK, et al: Quantitative analysis of the accuracy of linear array transrectal ultrasound in measurement of the prostate. Br J Urol 1991;67:79-82.
10. Bangma CH, Niemer AQ, Grobbee DE, Schroder FH: Transrectal ultrasonic volumetry of the prostate: in vivo comparison of different methods. Prostate 1996;28:107-110.
11. Park SB, Kim JK, Choi SH, et al: Prostate volume measurement by TRUS using heights obtained by transaxial and midsagittal scanning: comparison with specimen volume following radical prostatectomy. Korean J Radiol 2000;1:110-113.
12. Littrup PJ, Williams CR, Egglin TK, Kane RA: Determination of prostate volume with transrectal US for cancer screening. II. Accuracy of in vitro and in vivo techniques. Radiology 1991;179:49-53.
13. Terris MK, Stamey TA: Determination of prostate volume by transrectal ultrasound. J Urol 1991;145:984-987.
14. Sech S, Montoya J, Girman CJ, et al: Interexaminer reliability of transrectal ultrasound for estimating prostate volume. J Urol 2001;166:125-129.
15. Kimura A, Hirasawa K, Aso Y: Accuracy of ellipsoid method for estimation of prostatic weight. Jpn J Med Ultrasonics 1991;18:620-625.
16. Tong S, Cardinal HN, McLoughlin RF, et al: Intra- and inter-observer variability and reliability of prostate volume measurement via two-dimensional and three-dimensional ultrasound imaging. Ultrasound Med Biol 1998;24:673-681.
17. Kimura A, Kurooka Y, Hirasawa K, et al: Accuracy of prostatic volume calculation in

transrectal ultrasonography. Int J Urol 1995;2:252-256.

18. Dahnert WF: Determination of prostate volume with transrectal US for cancer screening. Radiology 1992;183:625-627.

19. Eri LM, Thomassen H, Brennhovd B, Haheim LL: Accuracy and repeatability of prostate volume measurements by transrectal ultrasound. Prostate Cancer Prostatic Dis 2002;5:273-278.

20. Sehgal cm, Broderick GA, Whittington R, et al: Three-dimensional US and volumetric assessment of the prostate. Radiology 1994; 192:274-278.

21. Tong S, Cardinal HN, McLoughlin RF, et al: Intra- and inter-observer variability and reliability of prostate volume measurement via two-dimensional and three-dimensional ultrasound imaging. Ultrasound Med Biol 1998;24:673-681.

22. Greene DR, Egawa S, Hellerstein DK, Scardino PT: Sonographic measurements of transition zone of prostate in men with and without benign prostatic hyperplasia. Urology 1990;36:293-299.

23. Terris MK, Afzal N, Kabalin JN: Correlation of transrectal ultrasound measurements of prostate and transition zone size with symptom score, bother score, urinary flow rate, and post-void residual volume. Urology 1998;52:462-466.

24. Littrup PJ, Kane RA, Williams CR, et al: Determination of prostate volume with transrectal US for cancer screening. I. Comparison with prostate-specific antigen assays. Radiology 1991;178:537-542.

25. Doebler RW: Transverse prostate measurement obtained using transabdominal ultrasound: possible role in transurethral needle ablation of the prostate. Urology 2000;55: 564-567.

26. Vilmann P, Hancke S, Strange-Vognsen HH, et al: The reliability of transabdominal ultrasound scanning in the determination of prostatic volume. Scand J Urol Nephrol 1987;21:5-7.

27. Henneberry M, Carter MF, Neiman HL: Estimation of prostatic size by suprapubic ultrasonography. J Urol 1979;121:615-616.

28. Walz PH, Wenderoth U, Jacobi GH: Suprapubic transvesical sonography of the prostate: determination of prostate size. Eur Urol 1983;9:148-152.

29. Hastak SM, Gammelgaaard J, Holm HH: Transrectal ultrasonic volume determination of the prostate—a preoperative and postoperative study. J Urol 1982;127:1115-1118.

30. Miyazaki Y, Yamaguchi A, Hara S: The value of transrectal ultrasonography in preoperative assessment for transurethral prostatectomy. J Urol 1983;129:48-50.

31. Hough DM, List A: Reliability of transabdominal ultrasound in the measurement of prostate size. Australas Radiol 1991;35: 358-360.

32. Rahmouni A, Yang A, Tempany cm, et al: Accuracy of in-vivo assessment of prostatic volume by MRI and transrectal ultrasonography. J Comput Assist Tomogr 1992;16: 935-940.

33. Tewari A, Indudhara R, Shinohara K, et al: Comparison of transrectal ultrasound prostatic volume estimation with magnetic resonance imaging volume estimation and surgical specimen weight in patients with benign prostatic hyperplasia. J Clin Ultrasound 1996;24:169-174.

CHAPTER 77

Scrotal Ultrasound Measurements

Eugenio Gerscovich

Introduction

Ultrasound is the imaging modality of choice for the scrotum. Current available commercial equipment combines an excellent anatomical resolution with evaluation of regional vascularity and real time capability.

Technique/Materials

In adults, because of the small size of the scrotum and its contents, the ultrasound examination requires high-resolution, linear array transducers in the frequency range of 6 to 12 MHz. In young children, we prefer the 13 to 15 MHz frequency, which allows optimal resolution and detection of blood flow. Before transducers with that frequency were available, detection of blood flow in the prepubertal testis could not be easily achieved. Occasionally, when examining large scrotums, like those with large hydroceles or masses, we use a curved array 6-MHz transducer to allow us a panoramic view of the pathology but then switch back to linear, higher-frequency transducers for the detailed study. In adults, to elevate and hold the testes anterior to the thighs, we place a towel underneath the scrotum. A second towel holds the penis superiorly. This is not necessary in children. The scanning parameters regarding echogenicity and Doppler flow should be adjusted for the assumed normal side, which is scanned first. In this way, when scanning the side of concern, cases of hypoechogenecity or hyperechogenicity and increased or decreased vascularity will be observed.

Scrotum in the Adult

SCROTUM

The scrotum is a multilayered sac containing the testes and epididymis. The individual layers forming the sac cannot be recognized on ultra-sound. One of the layers is the cremasteric muscle, which is a continuation of the internal oblique muscle of the abdomen and is responsible for the contraction of the scrotum and the upward motion of the testes for protection and temperature regulation. The contraction of the muscle results in changes in scrotal wall thickness, which normally ranges from 2 to 8 mm (Fig. 77-1).[1] We prefer to measure it in the axial plane for more accuracy. The scrotum is divided

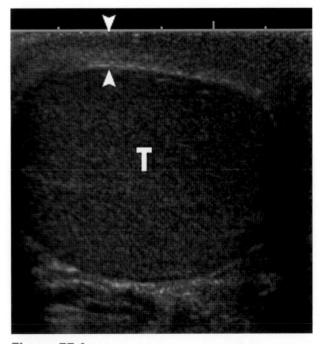

Figure 77-1
Scrotal wall thickness (calipers). T, Testis.

into two symmetrical sacs by a fibrous membrane extending in the anteroposterior plane and called "median raphe." Each sac contains one testis and the corresponding epididymis.

TESTIS

The testes are two paired oval structures with smooth contours and homogeneous medium echogenicity. They are made up of multiple, convoluted, seminiferous tubules divided into lobules, but none are visualized as individual structures on ultrasound. A longitudinal echogenic line is visualized on the posterior aspect of the testis and corresponds to the "mediastinum testis," which is a condensation of fibrous tissue where the arteries, veins, lymphatics, and efferent tubules enter and leave the testis.

The adult size of the testis is in the range of 3 to 5 cm in length (L) and 2 to 3 cm in anteroposterior (AP) and transverse (T) diameters (Table 77-1). When measuring the testis, the operator should have in mind its high mobility and look for the long and short axes of the testis, independent of the patient's body planes (Fig. 77-2). Slight asymmetry between the two testes is within normal limits. Adult volume of

Table 77-1 Normal adult scrotal measurements	
Anatomy	**Measurement (cm)**
Scrotal wall thickness	0.2-0.8
Testis length	3-5
Testis transverse diameter	2-3
Testis anteroposterior diameter	2-3
Epididymal head diameter	0.45-1.5
Epididymal body tail thickness	<0.2-0.5
Testis resistive index	Mean 0.62 (0.48-0.75)
Epididymis resistive index	0.54-0.58
Appendix testis diameter	0.1-0.7
Appendix epididymis diameter	0.3-0.8

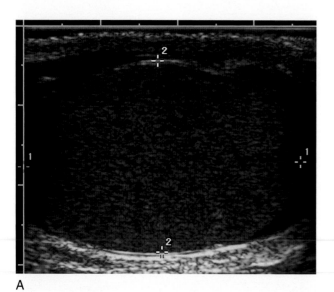

A

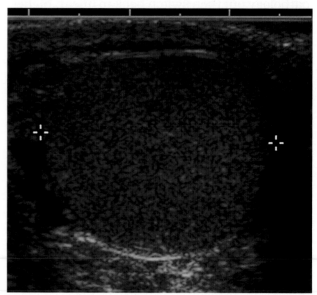

B

Figure 77-2
Testis measurements. **A**, Longitudinal, **B**, transverse.

Table 77-2	Testis size in men younger than 40 years old	
Testis volume	**Mean (cc)**	**Range (cc)**
Right and left testes	16.9 ± 4.7	6.1-26.9
Right testis	17.5 ± 5.8	0-29.8
Left testis	15.85 ± 4.9	5.5-26.6
Student t test, P	0.106	Nonsignificant

From Spyropoulos E, Borousas D, Mavrikos S, et al: Size of external genital organs and somatometric parameters among physically normal men younger than 40 years old. Urology 2002;60:485-489.

the testis is in the range of 15 to 20 cc. The testis is considered an ellipsoid, and its volume is calculated by the equation:

$$\text{Volume} = L \times AP \times T \times 0.52^{2,3}$$

Testis size decreases in elderly men. There are variations in the size of the testes with age and race. For this reason, in an individual patient, it is recommended to use the contralateral testis for comparison.[4] This applies when there is no bilateral pathology. Comparison of size between the right and left testis in men younger than 40 years old showed that the right testis was slightly larger in 65.4% of men, the left was larger in 28.8%, and they were of equal size in 5.8% (Table 77-2).[5]

EPIDIDYMIS

The epididymis receives the efferent tubules from the testis at the upper portion that converge to form a giant, convoluted tubule that makes the epididymis itself. The epididymis rests on the posterolateral aspect of the testis, extending in the superior inferior direction. Its length is approximately similar to that of the testis. The cephalad portion of the epididymis is called "head" or "globus major," the mid portion "body," and the distal "tail" or "globus minor." Normally only the head is visualized on ultrasound. It has an echogenicity similar to the testis and a variable shape that may be pyramidal, crescent, or droplike and measures 0.45 to 1 cm in diameter (Fig. 77-3).[6] As a rule, it does not exceed 1.5 cm. Sometimes the body and tail of the epididymis are visualized with a thickness not exceeding 2 to 5 mm.[2]

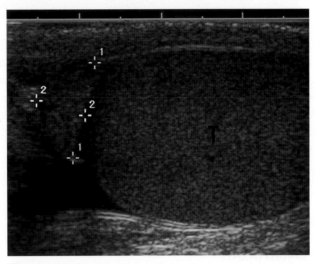

Figure 77-3
Epididymis measurements (calipers). T, Testis.

VASCULARITY

The testis is perfused by the testicular arteries, branches from the aorta. The spectral waveform of flow in the mature testis is of low resistance, similar to other parenchymal arteries. The mean resistive index is 0.62 (0.48 to 0.75).[7] The epididymis is hypovascular as compared to the testis. It is perfused by the deferential artery, branch of the superior vesical artery, and by the cremastric artery, branch of the inferior epigastric artery. In general, the spectral waveform is reported as of high resistancy, but some authors have found this not to be the case. They reported resistive indices in the range of 0.54 to 0.58.[8] The venous drainage from the testis is by small veins originating from the mediastinum testis that converge above the testis to form the pampiniform plexus. These veins are only found

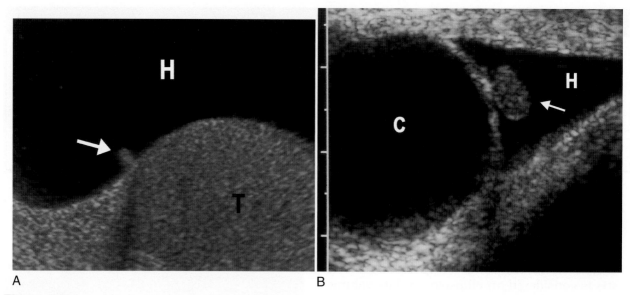

Figure 77-4
A, Appendix testis (*arrow*). T, Testis; H, hydrocele. **B**, Appendix epididymis (*arrow*) originating from the surface of an epididymal cyst (labeled "C"). H, hydrocele.

after a careful search in the region of the upper pole of the testis and above. They are isolated and not exceeding 1.5 mm in caliber. They do not enlarge with a Valsalva maneuver, although they might occassionally show transient retrograde flow on Doppler.[8]

EMBRYOLOGY

Occasionally, in the presence of a hydrocele, two small embryological remnants may be seen in the upper pole of the testis and epididymal head. These are the appendix testis and appendix epididymis, respectively (Fig. 77-4). The appendix testis measures between 1 and 7 mm. It may be seen in up to 92% of patients, being bilateral in 69% of them. The appendix epididymis measures between 3 and 8 mm. It is less frequently seen in about 6% of patients.[10]

Scrotum in the child

TESTIS

At birth, the testis measures approximately 1.5 × 1 cm. In the next 2 to 3 months, it slightly increases in size to a peak of 2 × 1.2 cm. Then, it again slowly decreases until 6 months, when it is smaller than at 2 months, to remain constant until about 6 years with an approximate

volume of 1 to 2 cc (Table 77-3). After that age, it slowly increases in size during the pubescent period. The described change in size is secondary to the changes in the serum levels of follicle-stimulating, lutenizing hormones, and testosterone.[11] The testis of young children is relatively hypoechoic with respect to that of adults. At about 8 to 9 years of age, it progressively increases in echogenicity to reach the adult appearance. This finding correlates with the histologic development of germ cell elements and tubular maturation.[13] The epididymis in children is proportionally larger as compared to the testis in the adult (Fig. 77-5). As the testis grows, the epididymis becomes progressively smaller. Its echogenicity approximates that of the testis.

VASCULARITY

Blood flow in young children with a testis volume under 4 cc (prepubertal) shows a spectral waveform of high resistance with nondetectable diastolic flow, resulting in a resistive index in the range of 1. Peak systolic velocity is also decreased with respect to that of the adult.[14]

The onset of puberty regarding age and velocity of change is extremely variable. For this reason, correlation of testicular size with chronological age is poor. A better association has been found with sex maturity ratings for genital

Table 77-3	Testicular volumes, mean ± SE, during the first 6 months of life													

	Age (mo)													
	Birth		**1**		**2**		**3**		**4**		**5**		**6**	
Side	**L**	**R**	**L**	**R**	**L**	**R**	**L**	**R**	**L**	**R**	**L**	**R**	**L**	**R**
Mean	1.10	1.10	1.80	1.60	2.00	2.05	2.05	1.95	1.85	1.80	1.75	1.70	1.55	1.50
SE	0.14	0.10	0.11	0.10	0.12	0.09	0.15	0.11	0.13	0.13	0.11	0.11	0.13	0.07

Significance

L ← $P < 0.001$ → ————————— $P < 0.05$ —————————

R ← $P < 0.0025$ → ————————— $P < 0.001$ —————————

SE, Standard error.
From Cassorla FG, Golden SM, Johnsonbaugh RE, et al: Testicular volume during early infancy. J Pediatr 1981;99:742-743.

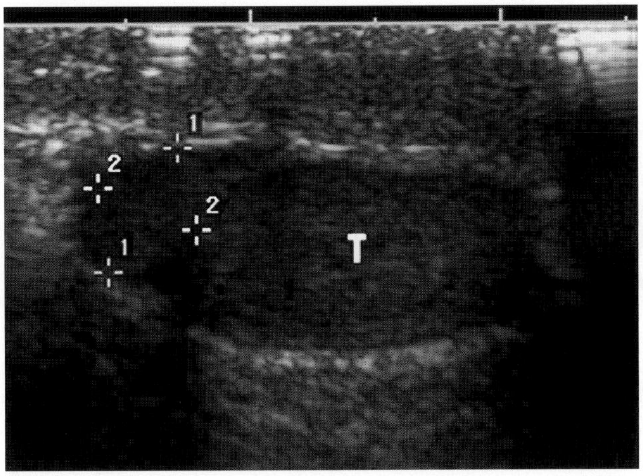

Figure 77-5
Epididymis in a child (calipers). T, Testis.

Table 77-4	Testicular volumes in 348 adolescents	
Sex maturity rating*	**Volume (cc)**	
	Left testis	**Right testis**
1	Mean 4.76	Mean 5.20
	SD 2.76	SD 3.86
2	Mean 6.4	Mean 7.08
	SD 3.16	SD 3.89
3	Mean 14.58	Mean 14.77
	SD 6.54	SD 6.1
4	Mean 19.8	Mean 20.45
	SD 6.17	SD 6.79
5	Mean 28.31	Mean 30.25
	SD 8.52	SD 9.64

*Mean of genital and pubic hair ratings.
From Daniel WA Jr, Feinstein RA, Howard-Peebles P, Baxley WD: Testicular volumes of adolescents. J Pediatr 1982;101:1010-1012.

and pubic hair (Table 77-4). No differences between white and black boys was observed.[15] A difference with Japanese boys was described.[16]

Scrotum in the fetus

TESTIS

The sex of the embryo is genetically determined at the time of fertilization, but the gonads do not acquire male characteristics until the 7th week of development under the influence of the Y chromosome and primordial germ cells. All of this occurs in the genital ridges located in the high posterior region of the future retroperitoneum. The cords of the testis remain solid until puberty, when they acquire a lumen and become the seminiferous tubules. Once the primitive testis, rete testis, and efferent tubules are formed, the testis becomes able to influence the development of the epididymis, seminal vesicle, and ejaculatory duct from the mesonephric duct by the excretion of androgens. Androgens are also responsible for the development of prostate, penis, penile urethra, and scrotal sac. From the original location of the testis in the area adjacent to the posterior abdominal wall, it descends into the scrotum in late pregnancy. It does not happen by active migration but by the fact that the testis is anchored to the scrotum by a nonelastic ligament called "gubernaculum testis." As

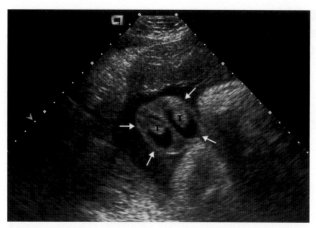

Figure 77-6
Fetal scrotum (*arrows*) in a 32-week pregnancy with descended testes (T).

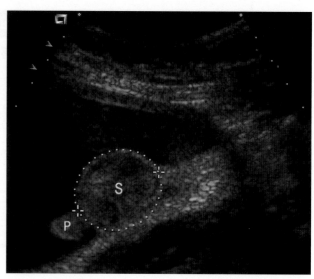

Figure 77-7
Fetal scrotum circumference in a second-trimester pregnancy with, as yet, undescended testicles. S, Scrotum; P, penis.

Table 77-5	Determination of testicular descent according to gestational age in 210 fetuses (excluding fetuses age 14-24 weeks)			
Gestational age (wks)	No. of fetuses	No. of descended testes	One descended testis (in scrotum)	Both testes descended (in scrotum)
25	10	7	2	1*
26	10	1	7	2
27	8	0	1	7
28	10	0	2	8
29	10	0	2	8
30	9	0	1	8
31	10	0	1	9
32	10	0	0	10
33	10	0	1	9
34	8	0	0	8
35	13	0	0	13

*$p < 0.0001$
From Achiron R, Pinhas-Hamiel O, Zalel Y, et al: Development of fetal male gender: prenatal sonographic measurement of the scrotum and evaluation of testicular descent. Ultrasound Obstet Gynecol 1998;11:242-245.

the body of the fetus grows, the testis finds itself progressively lower until it reaches the scrotum.[17]

The earliest time ultrasound has observed the fetal testes descending into the scrotum has been at 25 weeks of gestation (Fig. 77-6). At that gestational age and out of 10 examined fetuses, authors have found one fetus with both testes in the scrotum, two fetuses with only one, and seven fetuses with none (Table 77-5). The same authors have measured the scrotal circumference in utero at different gestational ages (Table 77-6). This is done by drawing an ellipse around the scrotum (Fig. 77-7).[18]

Table 77-6	Scrotal circumference by gestational age and 95% confidence intervals (CI)			
Gestational age (wks)	Number of observations	Predicted values (mm)	Lower 95% CI (mm)	Upper 95% CI (mm)
14-15	20	16.63	16.27	16.99
16-17	17	19.75	19.28	20.21
18-19	14	24.29	23.71	24.87
20-21	20	28.53	27.92	29.15
22-23	21	34.09	33.37	34.80
24-25	20	40.90	40.01	41.78
26-27	18	48.72	47.60	49.84
28-29	20	58.62	57.35	59.88
30-31	19	70.34	68.78	71.90
32-33	20	84.02	82.20	85.83
34-35	18	101.09	98.79	103.39
36-37	3	118.62	103.08	134.15

From Achiron R, Pinhas-Hamiel O, Zalel Y, et al: Development of fetal male gender: prenatal sonographic measurement of the scrotum and evaluation of testicular descent. Ultrasound Obstet Gynecol 1998;11:242-245.

References

1. Hricak H, Filly RA: Sonography of the scrotum. Invest Radiol 1983;18:112-121.
2. Hamm B: Differential diagnosis of scrotal masses by ultrasound. Eur Radiol 1997;7:668-679.
3. Hricak H, Hamm B, Kim B: Imaging of the Scrotum: Textbook and Atlas. New York, Raven Press, 1995.
4. Kass EJ: Evaluation and management of the adolescent with a varicocele. AUA Update Series IX, lesson 1990;12:89-96.
5. Spyropoulos E, Borousas D, Mavrikos S, et al: Size of external genital organs and somatometric parameters among physically normal men younger than 40 years old. Urology 2002;60:485-489.
6. Nashan D, Behre HM, Grunert JH, Nieschlag E: Diagnostic value of scrotal sonography in infertile men: report on 658 cases. Andrologia 1990;22:387-395.
7. Siegel MJ: The acute scrotum. Radiol Clin North Am 1997;35:959-976.
8. Keener TS, Winter TC, Nghiem HV, Schmiedl UP: Normal adult epididymis: evaluation with color Doppler US. Radiology 1997;202:712-714.
9. Petros JA, Andriole GL, Middleton WD, Picus DD: Correlation of testicular color Doppler ultrasound, physical examination, and venography in the detection of left varicoceles in men with infertility. J Urol 1991;145:785-788.
10. Johnson KA, Dewbury KC: Ultrasound imaging of the appendix testis and appendix epididymis. Clin Radiol 1996;51:335-337.
11. Cassorla FG, Golden SM, Johnsonbaugh RE, et al: Testicular volume during early infancy. J Pediatr 1981;99:742-743.
12. Daniel WA Jr, Feinstein RA, Howard-Peebles P, Baxley WD: Testicular volumes of adolescents. J Pediatr 1982;101:1010-1012.
13. McAlister WH, Sisler CL: Scrotal sonography in infants and children. Curr Probl Diagn Radiol 1990;19:201-242.
14. Paltiel HJ, Rupick RC, Babcock DS: Maturation changes in arterial impedance of the normal testis in boys: Doppler sonographic study. AJR Am J Roentgenol 1994;163:1189-1193.
15. Daniel WA Jr, Feinstein RA, Howard-Peebles P, Baxley WD: Testicular volumes of adolescents. J Pediatr 1982;101:1010-1012.
16. Schonfeld WA, Beebe GW: Normal growth and variation in male genitalia from birth to maturity. J Urol 1942;48:759.
17. Langman J: Medical Embryology, 4th ed. Baltimore: Williams & Wilkins, 1981.
18. Achiron R, Pinhas-Hamiel O, Zalel Y, et al: Development of fetal male gender: prenatal sonographic measurement of the scrotum and evaluation of testicular descent. Ultrasound Obstet Gynecol 1998;11:242-245.

CHAPTER 78

Bladder

Ethan J. Halpern

Introduction

The urinary bladder serves as a reservoir for urine between episodes of micturition. As such, the volume of the bladder is constantly changing. Although there is no absolute cutoff for top, normal bladder volume, the maximum capacity of the normal adult bladder is approximately 400 to 500 cc (Fig. 78-1). The normal postvoid residual volume in the adult bladder is below 5 cc in 78% and below 12 cc in 100%.[1]

Materials/Measurements

A number of measurement techniques and mathematical models have been applied to estimate bladder volume. The most basic formula measures only the transverse diameter (see Fig. 78-1) of the bladder and compares the results to a chart.[2] This method provides an estimate of bladder volume to the nearest 50 cc on the basis of a single transverse dimension (Table 78-1).

More precise estimates of bladder volume require measurements of the height, depth, and transverse dimensions of the bladder.

The following is a sampling of formulas that have been proposed and tested for bladder volume. In these formulas, H is the craniocaudal height, W is the transverse width, and D is the anteroposterior depth (Figs. 78-1 and 78-2):

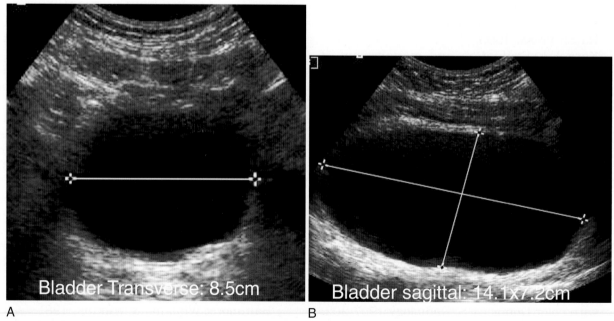

A   B

Figure 78-1

Transverse (**A**) and sagittal (**B**) images of the full bladder. Three perpendicular diameters are measured. A simple estimate of volume based upon the transverse diameter of 8.5 cc suggests that the bladder volume is greater than 200 cc. A more precise estimate based upon all three measurements with the formula for a prolate ellispe (0.52 × 8.5 × 14.1 × 7.2) suggests a volume of 450 cc.

Table 78-1	Predicted bladder volume based upon transverse dimension

Transverse diameter range (cm)	Bladder volume (cc)
1.0-3.5	50
3.5-5.5	100
4.0-6.5	150
5.5-8.0	200

From Henriksson I, Marsal K: Bedside ultrasound diagnosis of residual urine volume. Arch Gynecol 1982;231:129-133.

1. $V = H \times W \times (DT + DL)/2$, where DT is the bladder depth on a transverse image and DL is the bladder depth on a longitudinal image[3]

2. $V = 0.7 \times (H \times W \times D)$, where 0.7 represents an empirical correction factor to compensate for the bladder shape relative to a cuboid structure[4]

3. $V = 12.56 \times (r) \times H$, where r is the radius of transverse dimension[5]

Of the various mathematical models for estimation of bladder volume, the preferred model in many practices is based upon the volume of a prolate ellipse:

$$V = (\pi/6) \times (H \times W \times D)$$

One study compared many of the above formulas and concluded that planimetry was more accurate. Nonetheless, the prolate ellipse, $V = (\pi/6) \times (H \times W \times D)$, was suggested as the preferred method in the clinical environment because of simplicity of use.[14]

DISCUSSION

In an attempt to obtain a more accurate assessment of bladder volume, several authors have used planimetry.[6-8] Prior to the introduction of three-dimensional ultrasound systems, planimetry techniques were very cumbersome. Planimetry was often performed manually with visual assessment of the outline of the bladder on a limited number of ultrasound images. Estimates of bladder volume obtained with limited planimetry are based upon a mathematical model of the bladder shape. More recently, accurate volumetric assessment has been obtained by combining planimetry with three-dimensional ultrasound of the entire bladder (Fig. 78-3).[9,10]

In addition to estimation of bladder volume, ultrasound has also been used to estimate bladder weight. Ultrasound estimates of bladder weight are calculated from the thickness of the bladder wall and the estimated intravesical volume.[11] Good interobserver agreement can be obtained for the estimation of bladder weight.[12] The estimated bladder weight is significantly greater in patients with bladder wall hypertrophy and does correlate with symptoms of bladder outlet obstruction. Although the ultrasound estimate of bladder weight provides a number to quantify bladder mass, measurement of bladder wall thickness is a simpler technique that provides adequate clinical information. Bladder wall thickness above 5 mm is a useful predictor of outlet obstruction (Fig. 78-4).[13] Although ultrasound measurements provide a useful adjunct in the evaluation of bladder dysfunction, no ultrasound techniques can replace a good urodynamic flow study to demonstrate the mechanism of bladder dysfunction.

Measurement of the urinary bladder is commonly requested along with the assessment of urodynamics. Uroflowmetry, a recording of the urinary flow rate throughout micturition, is a commonly used, noninvasive, urodynamic test for the diagnosis of bladder dysfunction. The presence of a significant postvoid residual volume in the bladder is often associated with bladder outlet obstruction (see Fig. 78-2). However, the volume of postvoid residual may not correlate with severity of symptoms and probably does not predict damage to renal parenchyma.

The determination of bladder volume by ultrasound is complicated by variability in the shape of the bladder. The shape of the bladder may be described as round, ellipsoid, cuboid, or triangular in roughly equal proportions of the population.[14] Furthermore, the shape of the bladder will change as it distends with urine. Estimates of bladder volume are further complicated by measurement errors, which are above 50% in some studies.

The measurement of bladder volume is most accurate when the volume is low and generally

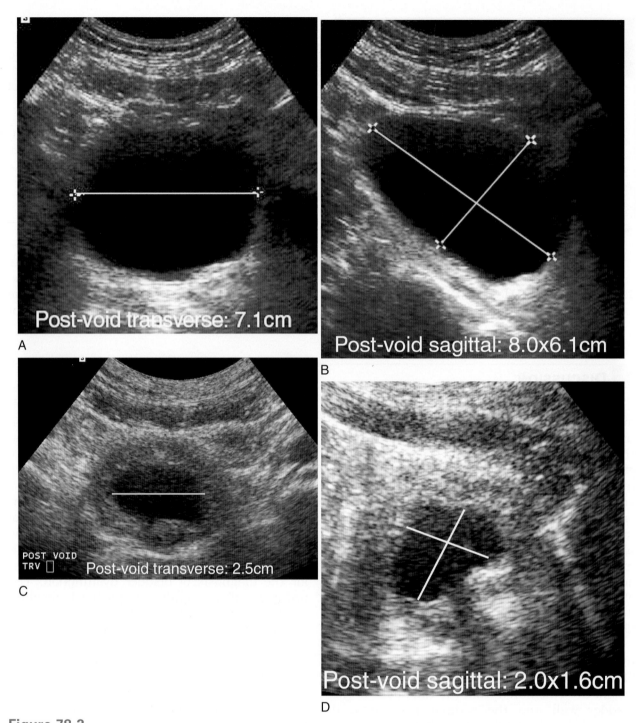

Figure 78-2
Transverse (**A, C**) and sagittal (**B, D**) images of the bladder after voiding. There is an obvious substantial postvoid residual in the bladder depicted in **A** and **B**. The formula for a prolate ellipse (0.52 × 7.1 × 8.0 × 6.1) suggests a volume of 180 cc. A normal postvoid appearance is demonstrated in a different bladder in **C** and **D**. Note the normal, "thickened" appearance of the bladder wall after voiding.

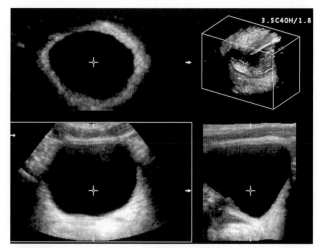

Figure 78-3

Three-dimensional volume imaging of the bladder. Images of the bladder in three orthogonal planes are obtained from a single acquisition. Accurate volumetric assessment of the bladder can be obtained by automated planimetric evaluation of the three-dimensional image volume.

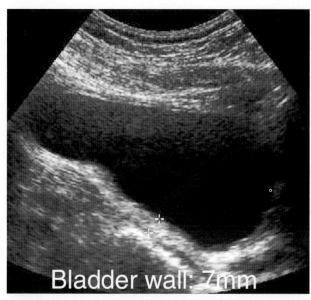

Figure 78-4

Measurement of bladder wall thickness. The wall thickness is measured in a full urinary bladder, preferably with a volume of at least 150 to 200 cc. Measurement of wall thickness will be artificially elevated in an underdistended bladder (as in Figs. 78-2C and 78-2D). In order to obtain an accurate measurement of bladder wall thickness, both the anterior and posterior boundaries of the wall must be well defined. The anterior wall of the bladder is not adequately defined for measurement of thickness in this patient.

most accurate for volumes of less than 50 ml. However, measurement of the absolute volume in the bladder is not usually critical. The major question is whether or not there is a clinically significant postvoid residual, generally taken to mean a residual volume greater than 50 ml.

To conclude the chapter on bladder measurements, one should remember that measurement of the absolute volume in the bladder is not usually critical. The major question is whether or not there is a clinically significant postvoid residual. This assessment requires good communication with the patient, who must attempt to completely empty the bladder. Imaging should be performed immediately after the patient voids so that the bladder does not refill.

References

1. DiMare JR, Fish SR, Harper JM, Politano VA: Residual urine in normal male subjects. J Urol 1963;96:180-181.
2. Henriksson I, Marsal K: Bedside ultrasound diagnosis of residual urine volume. Arch Gynecol 1982;231:129-133.
3. Hakenberg OW, Ryall RL, Langlois SL, Marshall VR: The estimation of bladder volume by sonocystography. J Urol 1983;130:249-251.
4. Poston GJ, Joseph AE, Riddle PR: The accuracy of ultrasound in the measurement of changes in bladder volume. Br J Urol 1983;55:361-363.
5. Espuela Orgaz R, Zuluaga Gomez A, Torres Ramirez C, Martinez Torres JL: Applications of bladder ultrasonography. I. Bladder content and residue. J Urol 1981;125:174-176.
6. Beacock CJ, Roberts EE, Rees RW, Buck AC: Ultrasound assessment of residual urine. A quantitative method. Br J Urol 1985;57:410-413.
7. Holmes JH: Ultrasonic studies of the bladder. J Urol 1987;97:654-663.
8. Pedersen JF, Bartrum RJ Jr, Grytter C: Residual urine determination by ultrasonic scanning. AJR Am J Roentgenol 1975;125:474-478.
9. Riccabona M, Nelson TR, Pretorius DH, Davidson TE: In vivo three-dimensional sonographic measurement of organ volume: validation in the urinary bladder. J Ultrasound Med 1996;15:627-632.

10. Byun SS, Kim HH, Lee E, et al: Accuracy of bladder volume determinations by ultrasonography: are they accurate over entire bladder volume range? Urology 2003;62:656-660.

11. Kojima M, Inui E, Ochiai A, et al: Ultrasonic estimation of bladder weight as a measure of bladder hypertrophy in men with infravesical obstruction: a preliminary report. Urology 1996;47:942-947.

12. Naya Y, Kojima M, Honjyo H, et al: Intraobserver and interobserver variance in the measurement of ultrasound-estimated bladder weight. Ultrasound Med Biol 1998; 24:771-773.

13. Manieri C, Carter SS, Romano G, et al: The diagnosis of bladder outlet obstruction in men by ultrasound measurement of bladder wall thickness. J Urol 1998;159: 761-765.

14. Griffiths CJ, Murray A, Ramsden PD: Accuracy and repeatability of bladder volume measurement using ultrasonic imaging. J Urol 1986;136:808-812.

PART 10

Abdomen-Vascular Ultrasound Measurements

Hisham Tchelepi
Edward Grant
Philip W. Ralls

CHAPTER 79

Doppler Ultrasound Measurements in the Liver

Introduction

Spectral and color Doppler are an integral part of abdominal sonography. This includes, but is not limited to, the following organs: liver, kidneys, pancreas, and spleen. The concepts described below are based on our in-house techniques and protocols used in the evaluation of patients with a wide spectrum of diseases within the liver.

Materials/Measurements

LIVER

In the liver the portal and hepatic veins are routinely and systematically evaluated. The hepatic arterial system is mainly evaluated in patients with liver transplant.

PORTAL VEINS

The portal venous system evaluation is an integral part of any ultrasound examination of the liver. This is achieved by using both color and spectral Doppler techniques. Color Doppler offers significant advantages over spectral Doppler.[1] Color Doppler passively and automatically displays color-coded flow information superimposed on all or a selected portion of the gray scale image. Flow is visible in real time within the selected region of interest. This is quite different from conventional spectral Doppler, where the operator must actively seek flow by moving the sample volume over the image. If the person scanning does not interrogate an area, flow will not be detected; unexpected flow will be missed. Thus color Doppler sonography provides flow information from a large area, faster, and with less operator dependence than does spectral Doppler.

Color Doppler evaluation includes the splenic vein, main portal vein, and its bifurcation into right and left portal veins within the liver. Color Doppler evaluation is followed up with spectral Doppler. The blood flow within the portal system is normally hepatopetal (toward the liver). The normal spectral Doppler signal in the right and left portal veins shows hepatopetal flow with an almost continuous monophasic pattern. Reversed, hepatofugal, or biphasic flow signifies pathology such as portal hypertension. A biphasic waveform is also seen in tricuspid regurgitation[2] (Fig. 79-1). Many factors influence the

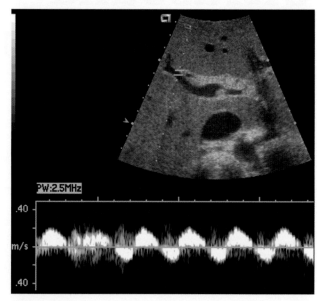

Figure 79-1
This is a sonogram showing spectral Doppler from a portal vein with biphasic pattern in this patient with tricuspid valve regurgitation. Other findings that may support the diagnosis include evidence on gray scale imaging of dilatation of the hepatic veins with or without inferior vena cava (IVC) enlargement.

Table 79-1	Ultrasound, endoscopic, and clinical findings in patients with and without recurrent bleeding		
Parameter	**No rebleeding**	**Rebleeding**	**No Vs. rebleeding**
Number in group	18	12	—
Portal vein velocity (cm/sec)	17.2 ± 11	9.5 ± 9	NS
Portal vein diameter (mm)	13.2 ± 3.9	16.3 ± 6.2	NS
Portosystemic collaterals	83	100	NS
Coronary vein ≥5 mm (%)	22	50	NS
Ultrasound score	3.3 ± 1.5	5.0 ± 1.6	<0.05
Endocopic score	−0.2 ± 0.4	−0.3 ± 0.2	NS
Pugh/Child classification	8.1 ± 2.3	8.9 ± 1.6	NS

Measurements given as mean ± standard deviation. Observations given as percentage. NS, Not significant.
From Schmassmann A, Zuber M, Liver M, et al: AJR Am J Roentgenol 1993;160:41-47.

portal vein waveform–fasting or postprandial state, patient position during the scan, and respiration.[3] Potential confusion can be minimized when color Doppler is combined with spectral Doppler. Many authors have suggested that recording portal vein velocity with spectral Doppler can be of value in patients with and without recurrent upper gastrointestinal bleeding (Table 79-1).[4] Although spectral velocity measurements are not widely used in practice, they have merit in the study of patients with transjugular intrahepatic portosystemic stent shunts (TIPS).[5]

HEPATIC VEINS

The hepatic veins drain blood from the liver into the IVC and from there to the right side of the heart. The normal spectral Doppler pattern seen in these veins is usually multiphasic[6]: (1) antegrade systolic wave resulting from movement of tricuspid annulus toward cardiac apex, (2) retrograde v wave from atrial overfilling, (3) antegrade diastolic wave from tricuspid valve opening, (4) and retrograde a wave from atrial contraction (Fig. 79-2).

The hepatic veins may show abnormalities when studied by both color and spectral Doppler. Abnormalities of hepatic venous flow may be related to obstruction or congestion.[7] Hepatic vein compression by fibrosis in patients with cirrhosis is an example of obstruction. In this situation, the vein may show evidence of aliasing on color Doppler, suggesting stenosis from venous drainage compromise (Fig. 79-3). This will also be reflected in the spectral pattern. On

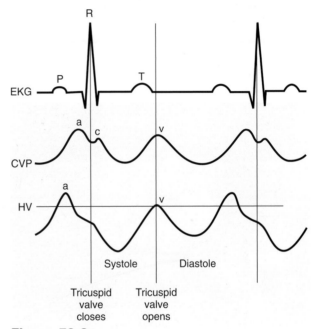

Figure 79-2
Schematic representation shows temporal events of cardiac cycle (EKG) and their relationship to central venous pressure (CVP) tracing and hepatic venous (HV) velocity waveform. Opening and closing of tricuspid valve are indicated.

the other hand, disease processes that affect the right side of the heart will result in congestion and dilatation of the hepatic veins and IVC. Right-sided heart failure with tricuspid regurgitation is an example of this phenomenon. In tricuspid regurgitation the normal multiphasic waveform on spectral Doppler will be replaced with a biphasic wave or even a flat one.[8]

Evaluation of blood flow velocities within the hepatic veins may help establish presence or

Table 79-2 | **Hepatic vein waveform morphologies observed in different populations**

Reference/Group	N	Triphasic (%)	Biphasic (%)	Monophasic (%)
Shapiro[12]	75	68 (91)	Monophasic or	7 (9)
Normal			biphasic	
Roobotom[13]				
Pregnant women				
10-20 wks	25	16 (64)	5 (20)	4 (16)
20-30 wks	25	3 (12)	5 (520)	4 (16)
30-40 wks	25	2 (8)	3 (12)	20 (80)
Bolondi[14]				
Normal controls	65	65 (100)	0	0
Cirrhosis	60	30 (50)	19 (32)	11 (18)
Dietrich[15]				
Normal	75	56 (75)	7 (9)	12 (16)
Chronic HCV	135	64 (47)	23 (17)	48 (36)
Gorka[16]				
Cirrhosis – varices	7	7 (100)	0	0
Cirrhosis + varices	43	18 (42)	13 (30)	12 (28)

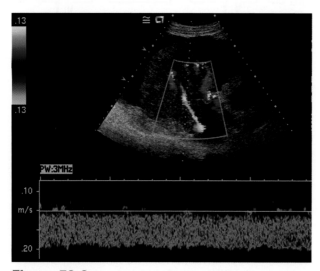

Figure 79-3
Narrowed hepatic vein in cirrhosis. The morphologic distortion caused by cirrhosis often causes compression of hepatic veins, which results in loss of the normal multiphasic waveform. The flattened waveform is similar in appearance to that seen in portal veins.

absence of disease. Such measurements, however, must be evaluated in the context of the color and spectral Doppler patterns. Hepatic vein velocity measurements in different populations are described in Table 79-2.

HEPATIC ARTERY

The usefulness of Doppler sonography of the hepatic artery in patients without transplantation is not well established. One study established a positive correlation between increased arterial flow resistance and portal pressure in intrinsic liver diseases like cirrhosis.[9] Although such results may seem promising, in practical terms, portal hypertension is diagnosed by parameters such as flow reversal within the portal veins or detecting portosystemic collaterals. Others have evaluated the role of hepatic artery Doppler in predicting whether patients with acute viral hepatitis will progress to fulminant liver failure. Tanaka et al[10] found that a high resistive index predicts liver failure with a sensitivity of 84% and a specificity of 94%. CDS sometimes shows conspicuously enlarged and tortuous hepatic arteries in cirrhotic livers. This finding, similar to "corkscrew" arteries seen angiographically, probably occurs because of truncation of arteries from cirrhosis-related liver atrophy, coupled with the increased arterial flow that occurs when portal venous flow decreases. These enlarged hepatic arteries usually have higher velocity (frequency shifts), often with aliasing, compared with normal hepatic arteries. Similarly enlarged arteries may occur with portal thrombosis, portal vein flow reversal, and portosystemic shunts.[11]

Conclusion

Many methods of evaluating the liver vasculature have been suggested. Unfortunately, velocity measurements in normal conditions and in disease vary significantly, often with significant overlap. Thus no widely accepted normal standards for such measurements exist. There are many reasons for this. Factors that influence such measurements include disease severity, presence or absence of venous collaterals, fasting state, and respiratory variations. The most appropriate and reliable method for evaluating vascular abnormalities in the liver remains the pattern of color Doppler and spectral waveform, not velocity measurements.

References

1. Ralls PW: Color Doppler sonography of the hepatic artery and portal venous system. AJR Am J Roentgenol 1990;155:517-525.
2. Abu-Yousef MM: Duplex Doppler sonography of the hepatic vein in tricuspid regurgitation. AJR Am J Roentgenol 1991;156:79-83.
3. Bolondi L, Gandolfi L, Arienti V, et al: Ultrasonography in the diagnosis of portal hypertension: diminished response of portal vessels to respiration. Radiology 1982;142:167-172.
4. Schammasmann A, Zuber M, Livers M, et al: Recurrent bleeding after variceal hemorrhage: predictive value of portal venous sonography. AJR Am J Roentgenol 1993;160:41-47.
5. Fung Y, Glajchen N, Shapiro RS, et al: Portal vein velocities measured by ultrasound: usefulness for evaluating shunt functioning following TIPS placement and TIPS revision. Abdominal Imaging 1998;23:511-514.
6. Abu-Yousef MM: Normal and respiratory variations of the hepatic and portal venous duplex Doppler waveforms with simultaneous electrocardiographic correlation. J Ultrasound Med 1992;11:263-268.
7. Desser TS, Sze DY, Brooke JR: Imaging and intervention in the hepatic veins. AJR Am J Roentgenol 2003;180:1583-1591.
8. Shapiro RS, Stancato-Pasik A, Glajchen N, Zalasin S: Color Doppler applications in hepatic imaging. Clin Imaging 1998;22:272-279.
9. Schneider AW, Kalk JF, Klein CP: Hepatic arterial pulsatility index in cirrhosis:correlation with portal pressure. J Hepatol 1999;30:876-881.
10. Tanaka K, Numata K, Morimoto M, Shirato K: Elevated resistive index in the hepatic artery as a predictor of fulminant hepatic failure in patients with acute viral hepatitis: a prospective study using Doppler ultrasound. Dig Dis Sci 2004;49:833-842.
11. Tchelepi H, Ralls PW, Radin R, Grant E: Sonography of diffuse liver disease. J Ultrasound Med 2002;21:1023-1032.
12. Shapiro RS, Winsburg F, Maldjian C, et al: Variability of hepatic vein Doppler tracings in normal subjects. J ultrasound Med 1993;12:701-703.
13. Roobottom CA, Hunter JD, Weston MJ, et al: Hepatic venous Doppler waveforms: changes in pregnancy. J Clin Ultrasound 1995;23:477-482.
14. Bolondi L, Bassi SL, Giani S, et al: Liver cirrhosis: changes of Doppler waveform of the hepatic veins. Radiology 1991;178:513-516.
15. Dietrich CF, Lee JH, Gottschalk R, et al: Hepatic and portal vein flow pattern in correlation with intrahepatic fat deposition and liver histology in patients with chronic hepatitis C. AJR Am J Roentgenol 1998;171:436-443.
16. Gorka W, Mulla AA, Sebayel MA, et al: Qualitative hepatic venous Doppler sonography vs portal flowmetry in predicting the severity of esophageal varices in hepatitis C cirrhosis. AJR Am J Roentgenol 1997;169:511-515.

Hisham Tchelepi
Edward Grant
Philip W. Ralls

Doppler Ultrasound in the Evaluation of Transjugular Intrahepatic Portosystemic Shunts (TIPS)

Introduction

Color Doppler sonography (CDS) often displays surgical shunts,[1] even when they are unapparent on preliminary gray scale images. Failure to detect color Doppler patency within the anastomosis is the only reliable sign of surgical shunt thrombosis (Fig. 80-1). Secondary signs of shunt thrombosis, such as hepatopedal, intrahepatic, portal flow,[1] may be misleading.[2]

Materials/Methods

Transjugular intrahepatic portosystemic stent shunts (TIPS) can be evaluated with Doppler sonography. Preprocedure evaluation and post-TIPS follow-up is useful. Intraprocedure CDS guidance is occasionally helpful. Low-frequency Doppler (e.g., 2 MHz) is generally best for imaging TIPS patients. Many factors influence stent velocity; most important is respiration, which can lead to a significant decrease in velocity within the stent. Considerable decrease in flow velocity in inspiration compared to quiet respiration has been documented.[3]

TIPS stenosis may result in increased or decreased flow velocity within the stent (Fig. 80-2). A velocity range of 0.9 to 2.0 m/sec in the mid and distal (HV side) stents is considered by many observers to be normal. We do not use the velocity in the proximal stent (PV side) or any of the many other reported flow parameters. These intrastent velocity parameters are fairly sensitive for stent dysfunction, but occasional false positives will result in venography in some patients with normal stents. Some investigators, on the other hand, see merits in measuring velocities within the portal veins following TIPS. The concept stems from the fact that, following TIPS, the velocities within the portal vein will usually increase. Kanterman et al[4] found that a value of greater than 40 cm/sec (42.8 cm/sec) is to be expected. Stenosis of the shunt causes the portal vein velocity to drop. The drop in velocity varies from one institution to another, but it was found that the lowest permissible value should not be less than 30 cm/sec.[5] Any measurement less than this number may indicate shunt malfunction.

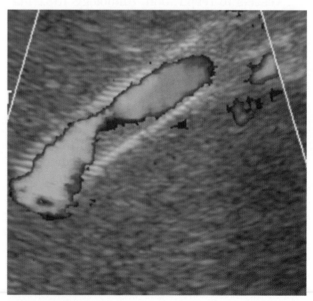

Figure 80-1
Color Doppler sonogram of transjugular intrahepatic portosystemic stent shunt. There is evidence of significant narrowing of the color-filled lumen of the stent, indicating thrombosis.

In the normally functioning stent, blood flow in the native portal veins is almost always toward the stent—thus flow in the left and right portal vein is hepatofugal.[6] A fairly specific, but insensitive, parameter for stent dysfunction is finding flow away from the stent (hepatopetal) in the native portal veins. Occasionally, poor acoustic access, poor Doppler angle, and other technical factors may result in nonvisualization of flow, even when the shunt is patent. Another phenomenon observed, following TIPS, is that blood flow within the hepatic arteries shows evidence of increased velocities. The enlarged

arteries can also be appreciated with CDS. One must be aware of the fact that these enlarged arteries can be easily mistaken for portal vein radicals within the liver if spectral Doppler is not used in the evaluation of these vessels, hence giving false information about flow within the portal veins.[7] In one study the velocity within the hepatic artery was increased from 79 cm/sec before TIPS to 131 cm/sec after the procedure.[8]

Recently the use of new stents, known as covered stents (PTFE stents), has been studied in many centers in the United States and Europe. Initial results indicate that these stents have less tendency to clot and/or stenose as compared to conventional uncovered stents. It has been also suggested that these stents last longer and even improve the overall survival in patients with cirrhosis.[9,10] When studying these stents with sonography, it is crucial to keep in mind that they can only be evaluated 24 to 48 hours or more after TIPS. The reason behind this is simple. These covered stents display significant shadowing secondary to the presence of microbullae embedded inside the expandable PTFE[11] in the first few days after the procedure, which may result in false-positive interpretation of malfunctioning.

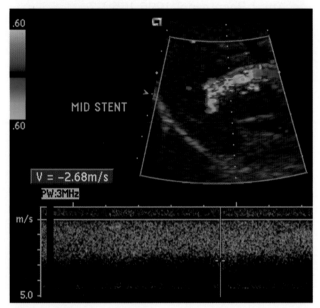

Figure 80-2
High velocity in dysfunctional TIPS stent. Mid-stent velocity is 2.68 m/sec (mps). Velocity exceeding 2 mps or less than 0.9 mps in the mid or distal (HV end) stent usually means stent dysfunction is present.

Conclusion

Doppler of TIPS is a valuable tool that, if used correctly, can minimize the number of both false-positive and false-negative cases of suspected dysfunction. The technique is highly operator dependent with variable sensitivity and specificity from many reputable institutions (Table 80-1).[5] We believe that a positive

Table 80-1	Overall results from the Mallinckrodt Institute of Radiology				
Doppler parameter	**Velocity criterion (cm/sec)**	**Sensitivity (%)**	**Specificity (%)**	**PPV (%)**	**NPV (%)**
Stent velocity	<90 or >190	84	70	82	72
Change in stent velocity	Decrease >40 Increase >60	71	88	89	67
Portal vein velocity	<30	82	77	86	71
Overall impression	Not applicable	92	72	84	86

PPV, Positive predictive value; NPV, negative predictive value.
From Middleton WD, Teefy SA, Darcy MD: Ultrasound Quarterly 2003;19:56-70.

TIPS Doppler must be complemented with venography. On the other hand, a normal Doppler study of the shunt does not appear to need more invasive intervention.

References

1. Ralls PW, Lee KP, Mayekawa DS, et al: Color Doppler sonography of portocaval shunts. J Clin Ultrasound 1990;18:379.

2. Rice S, Lee KP, Johnson MB, et al: Portal venous system after portosystemic shunts or endoscopic sclerotherapy: evaluation with Doppler sonography. AJR Am J Roentgenol 1991;156:85.

3. Kliewer MA, Hertzberg BS, Heneghan JP, et al: Transjugular intrahepatic portosystemic shunts (TIPS): effects of respiratory state and patient position on the measurements of Doppler velocities. AJR Am J Roentgenol 2000;175:149-145.

4. Kanterman RY, Darcy MD, Middleton WD, et al: Doppler sonographic findings associated with TIPS shunt malfunction. AJR Am J Roentgenol 1997;168:467-472.

5. Middleton WD, Teefey SA, Darcy MD: Doppler evaluation of transjugular intrahepatic portosystemic shunts. Ultrasound Quarterly 2003;19:56-70.

6. Lafortune M, Martinet JP, Denys A, et al: Short- and long-term hemodynamic effects of transjugular intrahepatic portosystemic shunts: a Doppler/manometric correlative study. AJR Am J Roentgenol 1995;164:997-1002.

7. Wachsberg RH: Doppler ultrasound evaluation of transjugular intrahepatic portosystemic shunt function: pitfalls and artifacts. Ultrasound Quarterly 2003;19:139-148.

8. Foshager MC, Ferral H, Nazarian GK, et al: Duplex sonography after TIPS shunt: normal hemodynamic findings and efficacy in predicting shunt patency and stenosis. AJR Am J Roentgenol 1995;165:1-7.

9. Bureau C, Garcia-Pagan JC, Otal P, et al: Improved clinical outcome using polytetrafluoroethylene-coated stents for TIPS: results of a randomized study. Gastroenterology 2004;126:469-475.

10. Rossi P, Salvatori FM, Fanelli F, et al: Polytetrafluoroethylene-covered nitinol stent-graft for transjugular intrahepatic portosystemic shunt creation: 3-year experience. Radiology 2004;231:820-830.

11. Otal P, Smayra T, Bureau C, et al: Preliminary results of a new expanded-polytetrafluoroethylene-covered stent-graft for transjugular intrahepatic portosystemic shunt procedures. AJR Am J Roentgenol 2002;178:141-147.

CHAPTER 81

Hisham Tchelepi
Edward Grant
Philip W. Ralls

Doppler Ultrasound Measurements in the Kidney

Introduction

Spectral and color Doppler techniques have an important role in the evaluation of kidney disease. This evaluation includes clinical conditions such as pyelonephritis, ureteral obstruction, renal parenchymal disease, renal vein thrombosis, and renovascular hypertension/renal artery stenosis. Renal artery stenosis (RAS) has been the focus of many investigators because it may result in renal vascular hypertension, a treatable cause of hypertension.[1]

Arteriosclerosis causes two thirds of stenoses; other causes, mainly fibromuscular dysplasia, account for the remaining one third. Sonography of the renal arteries is a noninvasive tool, which is fairly specific and sensitive compared to other more invasive imaging modalities such as angiography, computed tomography and magnetic resonance angiography.[24] The reported sensitivity and specificity of Doppler sonography in the evaluation of RAS vary considerably. Likewise, the technique used to diagnose RAS has varied from one investigator to another. Before discussing the techniques available, one should understand that for RAS to cause hypertension, the stenosis must be hemodynamically significant. The degree of stenosis required to produce RAS-related hypertension has been variously reported from 50% to 70%.

Materials/Measurements

Currently two basic Doppler techniques are available to study RAS. The first approach is direct Doppler of the renal arteries. Sampling near the origin of the renal arteries may appear ideal for this purpose; however, the technique is difficult in most of the cases and limited by factors like the patient's body habitus, anatomic variants in the origin of the renal arteries, and the presence of multiple renal arteries in one or both kidneys. Measurements using this technique (peak systolic velocity [PSV] and renal artery/aorta peak velocity ratio [RAR]) are more accurate than those obtained from intrarenal arteries (acceleration indices).[5] Nevertheless, the limitations mentioned above may compromise this technique. For this reason, direct Doppler techniques are commonly combined with intrarenal measurements to improve diagnostic confidence.[6] The sensitivity and specificity of such techniques vary significantly in the literature (Table 81-1).

The main criteria for diagnosing RAS with direct, renal artery Doppler are: (1) a renal-aortic ratio above 3.5 and (2) PSV greater than 180 to 200 cm/sec (>200 cm/sec indicates stenosis greater than 60%)[7] (Fig. 81-1). Color Doppler is an important part of the study because it can guide placement of the sample volume over the site of a high-velocity jet.

The second technique used is Doppler of the intrarenal arteries. This technique may be less sensitive but is often more practical because it is technically easier and more reliable. Investigators have evaluated many intrarenal Doppler parameters for the diagnosis of RAS. These include acceleration time, acceleration index, resistive index (RI), and pulsatility index (PI). The best Doppler signals for evaluation come from the large segmental or interlobar arteries as they course directly toward the transducer. In this location, signals are the strongest and most reproducible.[13] Before attempting Doppler studies for renal arteries, the operator needs to optimize the Doppler settings to avoid false-positive and false-negative outcomes. Table 81-2 describes the technique of such optimization. Martin et al[14] investigated the role of acceleration time and acceleration index and found 87% sensitivity and 98% specificity. Halpern et al,[10] on the other hand, found that acceleration time is the most important parameter to be measured when RAS is suspected. Acceleration of less than 3 m/sec^2 was considered abnormal. An abnormally shaped, intrarenal artery waveform may indicate RAS. Stavros et al[15,16] found that the loss of the normal ESP is adequate to suggest the diagnosis of RAS and that this finding was better than other calculation methods like peak systolic velocity (PSV) or acceleration time. Many sonologists have adopted this technique in practice with a sensitivity of 95% and specificity of 97%, respectively. To appreciate the importance of this technique, the observer needs to become familiar with the appearance of the normal intrarenal spectral

Table 81-1	Specificity and sensitivity of duplex ultrasound in RAS using direct sampling of the extrarenal arteries	
Study	**Sensitivity**	**Specificity**
Olin, et al[7]	98%	99%
Hoffman, et al[8]	92%	62%
Hansen, et al[9]	93%	98%
Halpern, et al[10]	71%	96%
Spies, et al[11]	93%	92%
Krumme, et al[12]	71%	96%

Note: Please note that the results of these studies relied on different measured variables. References at the end of the chapter are available for in-depth review.

Table 81-2	Suggested criterion to optimize Doppler studies for RAS				
Extrarenal approach	**Transducer**	**Frequency**	**Filter**	**SR**	**DA**
	Sector	Low 2-2.5 MHZ	low*		<60
Intrarenal approach	Sector	3-5 MHZ		fast	<30

*Low to minimize noise from respiration.
SR, Sweep rate; DA, Doppler angle.

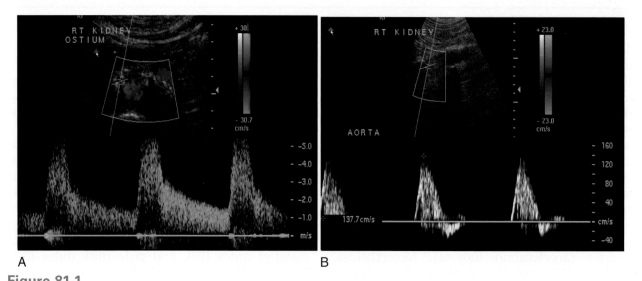

A   B

Figure 81-1

A, Spectral Doppler sonogram of extrarenal artery shows markedly increased velocity (>400 cm/sec) immediately beyond the ostium. **B,** The aortic velocity is 138 cm/sec. The renal-aortic ratio is abnormal.

Doppler waveform (Fig. 81-2). Another finding related to the shape of the Doppler waveform in RAS is the so-called tardus-parvus waveform.[17] This appearance results from the slow rise to the peak systolic velocity distal to the site of stenosis. Identification of the tardus-parvus waveform is diagnostic of RAS (Fig. 81-3A).

Measurements of intrarenal vascular resistance were used in the very beginning of RAS Doppler studies. These measurements were proved inadequate to accurately diagnose RAS because they are influenced by other factors such as underlying intrinsic kidney disease, obstruction, age of the patient, and stiffness of the arteries under study. New studies showed that resistive index (RI) measurements may play a role in the evaluation of revascularization following angioplasty or stenting of the stenosed renal artery.[18,19] Still, this can also be studied using other, more sensitive parameters such as the shape of the waveform, PSV, and renal-aortic ratio (see Fig. 81-3A and B). Another

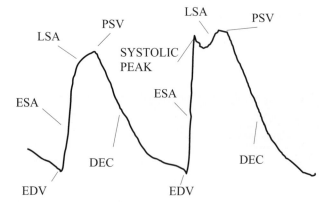

Figure 81-2

Normal intrarenal Doppler signals. The waveform to the right has an early systolic peak (ESP), and the one to the left does not. The general consensus is that both types may be seen in normal subjects. The early systolic acceleration (ESA) is between end-diastole (EDV) and either the ESP or the inflection point at the beginning of the late systolic acceleration (LSA). The deceleration (DEC) and peak systolic velocity (PSV) are also shown.

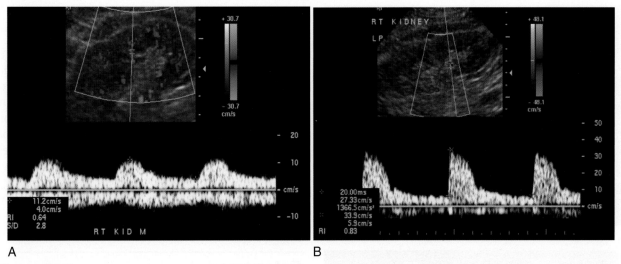

Figure 81-3
A, Tardus-parvus waveforms in a patient with RA stenosis. Note the delayed and dampened upstroke, yielding a rounded appearance to the waveform. **B**, Spectral Doppler from the same patient, immediately after angioplasty, shows a normal appearance. Note the return of a rapid systolic upstroke and a well-defined ESP.

Table 81-3	Cut-off values and performance of Doppler parameters in detecting renal artery stenosis			
Parameter	**Cutoff**	**Sensitivity**	**Specificity**	**Comments**
Maximum velocity	>1.0	0-70%	37-80%	Technically difficult, may miss stenosis in one of multiple arteries
Renal-aortic ratio	>3-3.5	0-70%	37-90%	As above
Resistive index (RI)	<0.6-0.7	50-65%	43-72%	Better discrimination after captopril
RI difference	>5-7	77-100%	92-100%	The side with the low RI is abnormal % stenosis $= 0.6 \times \Delta RI + 57.0$
Acceleration index	<4	—	—	Excellent discrimination of >75% stenosis in children
Early systolic acceleration	<3-4.7	70-90%	35-83%	<3-3.5 most commonly cited
Acceleration time	>0.07-0.12	57-78%	20-91%	>0.07 most commonly cited
Waveform analysis	Only type C = positive; types B & C positive	46-95%	67-100%	Mostly only type C positive

"Positive" in waveform analysis is diagnostic of stenosis.
From Keats TE, Sistrom C: Atlas of Radiologic Measurement, 7th ed. St Louis, Mosby, 2001, p 613.

study showed that RI measurement can predict whether patients with RAS will benefit from stenting.[20,21] According to the study, an RI value of more than 0.8 makes a treatment effect highly unlikely, and these patients should not undergo angioplasty or surgery.

Table 81-3 shows the cutoff values and performance of different Doppler parameters in detecting RAS. Sonography of the renal arteries also found its place during surgical intervention on the renal artery. Doppler assessment of the graft site can identify abnormal flow pattern

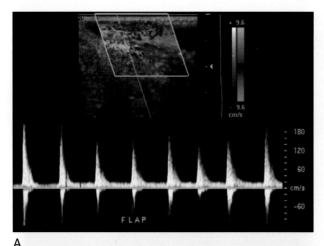

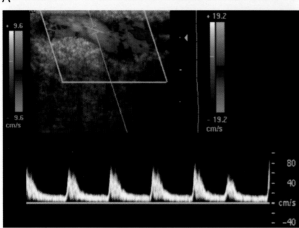

Figure 81-4
Intraoperative sonography. **A,** A strikingly abnormal Doppler waveform is shown at the anastomotic site of a renal bypass graft secondary to intimal flap. **B,** After repair, color and spectral Doppler images show normal findings.

related to the presence of intimal flap (Fig. 81-4A and B).

Doppler sonography may be useful in determining whether or not acute obstruction is present. Increased peripheral resistance (resistive index (RI) > 0.75) supports the presumption that pyelocaliectasis is caused by acute obstruction. Potential pitfalls include increased peripheral resistance related to diffuse renal parenchymal diseases and persistent elevated peripheral resistance after obstruction has been relieved. Resistive index may be normal the first few hours after the onset of obstruction and normal in obstructed patients with chronic renal failure who have significant cortical loss.[22] Peripheral resistance may also be normal in obstructed patients for unexplained reasons.

Conclusion

Doppler sonography is a valuable tool for the assessment and study of renal disease, specifically reno-vasular hypertension secondary to renal arterial stenosis. It has evolved into a technique that is not only appropriate for primary diagnosis but, also, for detection of recurrent stenosis and occlusion following therapeutic intervention. Because of its availability, noninvasiveness, and lower cost, Doppler sonography may be considered the imaging modality of choice to screen patients for RAS.[23]

References

1. Bloch MJ, Basile J: Clinical insights into the diagnosis and management of renovascular disease. An evidence-based review. Minerva Med 2004;95:357-373.
2. Gilles Soulez, Vincent L Oliva, Sophie Turpin, et al: Imaging of renovascular hypertension: respective values of renal scintigraphy, renal Doppler US, and MR angiography. Radiographics 2000;20:1355-1368.
3. De Cobelli F, Venturini M, Vanzulli A, et al: Renal arterial stenosis: prospective comparison of color Doppler US and breath-hold, three-dimensional, dynamic, gadolinium-enhanced MR angiography. Radiology 2000;214:373-380.
4. Voiculescu A, Hofer M, Hetzel GR, et al: Noninvasive investigation for renal artery stenosis: contrast-enhanced magnetic resonance angiography and color Doppler sonography as compared to digital subtraction angiography. Clin Exp Hypertens 2001;23:521-531.
5. van der Hulst VP, van Baalen J, Kool LS, et al: Renal artery stenosis: endovascular flow wire study for validation of Doppler ultrasound. Radiology 1996;200:165-168.
6. Radermacher J, Chavan A, Schaffer J, et al: Detection of significant renal artery stenosis with color Doppler sonography: combining extrarenal and intrarenal approaches to minimize technical failure. Clin Nephrol 2000;53:333-343.
7. Olin JW, Piedmonte MR, Young JR, et al: The utility of duplex ultrasound scanning of the renal arteries for diagnosing significant renal artery stenosis. Ann Intern Med 1995;122:833-838.

8. Hoffmann U, Edwards JM, Carter S, et al: Role of duplex scanning for the detection of atherosclerotic renal artery disease. Kidney Int. 1991;39:1232-1239.

9. Hansen KJ, Tribble RW, Reavis SW: Renal duplex sonography: evaluation of clinical utility. J Vasc Surg 1990;12:227-236.

10. Halpern EJ, Needleman L, Nack TL, East SA: Renal artery stenosis: should we study the main renal artery or segmental vessels? Radiology 1995;195:799-804.

11. Spies KP, Fobbe F, El-Bedewi M, et al: Color-coded duplex sonography for noninvasive diagnosis and grading of renal artery stenosis. Am J Hypertens 1995;8(12 Pt 1): 1222-1231.

12. Krumme B, Blum U, Schwertfeger E, et al: Diagnosis of renovascular disease by intra- and extrarenal Doppler scanning. Kidney Int 1996;50:1288-1292.

13. Lee HY, Grant EG: Sonography in renovascular hypertension J ultrasound Med 2002;21:431-441.

14. Martin RL, Nanra RS, Wlodarczyk J, et al: Renal hilar Doppler analysis in the detectionof renal artery stenosis. J Vas Tech 1991;15:173-180.

15. Stavros AT, Parker SH, Yakes WF, et al: Segmental stenosis of the renal artery: pattern recognition of tardus and parvus abnormalities with duplex sonography. Radiology 1992;184:487-492.

16. Stavros T, Harshfield D: Renal Doppler, renal artery stenosis, and renovascular hypertension: direct and indirect duplex sonographic abnormalities in patients with renal artery stenosis. Ultrasound Q 1994; 12:217-263.

17. Kliewer MA, Tupler RH, Carroll BA, et al: Renal artery stenosis: analysis of Doppler waveform parameters and tardus parvus pattern. Radiology 1993; 189:779-787.

18. Coen G, Moscaritolo E, Catalano C, et al: Atherosclerotic renal artery stenosis: one year outcome of total and separate kidney function following stenting. BMC Nephrol 2004;5:15.

19. Melhem JA, Sharafuddin MD, Carl A, Raboi, MD: Renal artery stenosis: duplex US after angioplasty and stent placement. Radiology 2001;220:168-173.

20. Radermacher J: Echo-Doppler to predict the outcome for renal artery stenosis. J Nephrol 2002;15(Suppl 6):S69-S76.

21. Radermacher J, Chavan A, Bleck J, Vitzthum A, Stoess B, Gebel MJ, Galanski M, Koch KM, Haller H, et al: Use of Doppler ultrasonography to predict the outcome of therapy for renal artery stenosis. N Engl J Med 2001;344:410-417.

22. Platt JF: Duplex Doppler evaluation of native kidney dysfunction: obstructive and nonobstructive disease. AJR Am J Roentgenol 1992;158:1035-1042.

23. Nchimi A, Biquet JF, Brisbois D, et al: Duplex ultrasound as first-line screening test for patients suspected of renal artery stenosis: prospective evaluation in high-risk group. Eur Radiol 2003;13:1413-1419.

Hisham Tchelepi
Edward Grant
Philip W. Ralls

CHAPTER 82

Doppler Ultrasound in the Evaluation of Mesenteric Ischemia

Introduction

There is no definitive information regarding the prevalence of chronic mesenteric ischemia. Asymptomatic stenosis is common. Autopsy data[1] suggests a prevalence of 22% for stenosis of the celiac, 16% for stenosis of the SMA, and 10% for stenosis of the IMA, with much higher prevalence for older individuals. Chronic mesenteric ischemia is generally a disease of middle age to elderly patients who have arteriosclerotic vascular disease. Other causes may be seen in younger individuals, for example, the median arcuate ligament syndrome. Unlike other arteriosclerosis-associated diseases, chronic mesenteric ischemia is more common in women (60% of cases) than men.[2]

The classic symptom of chronic mesenteric ischemia is visceral angina–postprandial pain.

The pain is worst within the first hour after eating and resolves gradually over the next 1 to 2 hours. The severity of pain is related to the quantity and fat content of the meal. Fasting pain is a sign of more severe disease. Weight loss and "food fear" are common. The symptoms, pain, weight loss, and decreased eating, may be mistaken for cancer-related symptoms.[2]

Spectral Doppler is the screening test of choice in evaluating patients with suspected chronic mesenteric ischemia. It can contribute to an expeditious diagnosis. When surgery is planned, however, angiography is indicated.[2] Angioplasty[3] and stenting[4,5] show some promise as therapeutic tools.

Materials/Measurement

Patient preparation for Doppler sonography of the superior mesenteric artery is similar to that for many abdominal examinations. The patient should be on a clear liquid diet 24 hours prior to examination and remain NPO overnight prior to the morning examination. Sector transducers are usually employed to scan these patients. A large footprint curved, linear array transducer may be useful to compress gas and bowel contents out of the overlying gastrointestinal tract, providing acoustic access to the artery. Another benefit of compression is that the transducer is closer to the superior mesenteric artery.

We typically use color Doppler to localize the abdominal aorta and superior mesenteric artery in the transverse plane. After inspection of the anatomy of the celiac and superior mesenteric arteries with color Doppler, a sample volume is placed and spectral Doppler waveforms are obtained. Lower scan angles, as close to 0^B as possible, are beneficial. Lower angles yield a larger Doppler frequency shift and are less prone to error in measuring the velocity. Generally, a low Doppler carrier frequency in the range of 2.5 to 3.5 MHz is used to interrogate the superior mesenteric artery. On occasion, a 5-MHz Doppler may be used. The spectral Doppler scale should be selected so that the waveform encompasses most of the display. Accurate angle correction is important, as the peak systolic velocity is the main criterion used to diagnose significant stenosis.

Sonographic Findings

Peak systolic velocity in the superior mesenteric artery (fasting) generally ranges between 80 and 200 cm/sec. In the fasting state there is

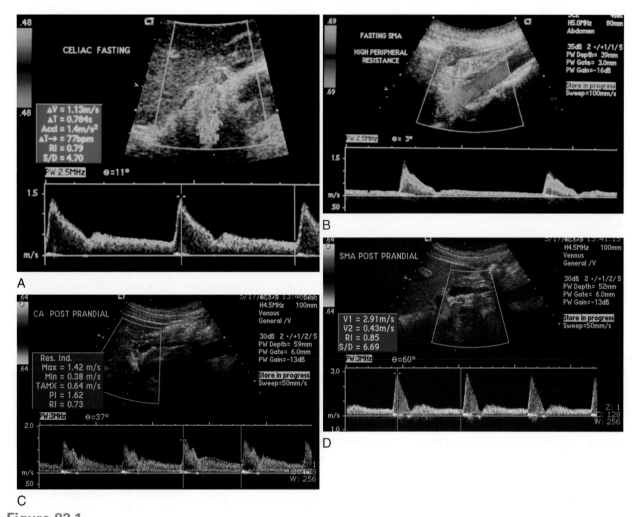

Figure 82-1

Normal celiac and superior mesenteric artery prefasting and postfasting. The fasting sonogram of the celiac artery (**A**) shows a peak velocity of 1.13 m/sec with a considerable amount of diastolic flow, resulting in a resistive index measurement of 0.79. There is less diastolic flow in the fasting sonogram (**B**) of the superior mesenteric artery. Peak velocity in the superior mesenteric artery in this normal individual was 0.93 m/sec, with a resistive index measurement of 0.86.

After eating a meal (in another normal volunteer), the flow pattern changes. In the celiac axis sonogram (**C**), peak velocity has diminished to 1.42 m/sec from 2.0 m/sec when fasting. The resistive index has changed little (0.73 from 0.77 when fasting). Considerable changes have occurred in the superior mesenteric artery postprandially (**D**). There is more diastolic flow and the peak velocity has increased significantly. Peak velocity is now 2.9 m/sec, and resistive index is 0.85 from 0.90. These parameters reflect the increased blood flow required by the superior mesenteric artery circulation after the individual has eaten.

little diastolic flow in the superior mesenteric artery. Peripheral resistance is relatively high (Fig. 82-1). After consumption of food, the blood flow requirements of the gut increase. Postprandially, the superior mesenteric artery dilates, the peak systolic velocity increases, and there is increased diastolic flow (a consequence of lower peripheral resistance). The celiac artery has more diastolic flow than the superior mesenteric artery in fasting patients. Postpran-

dially, celiac axis blood flow decreases and peripheral resistance increases.[6]

The diagnosis of arterial insufficiency in the superior mesenteric artery depends on detecting a stenosis of 70% or greater. Lesions less than this are usually not associated with symptoms, although patients with moderate atherosclerosis are probably at increased risk for acute mesenteric ischemia compared to normals. Significant stenosis in any artery results in

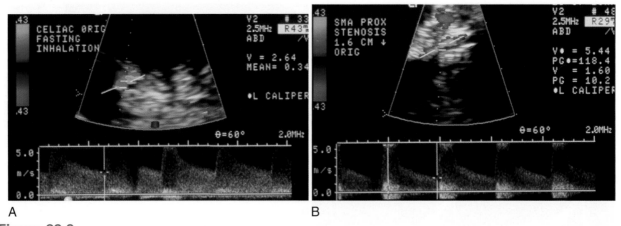

A   B

Figure 82-2

High-grade stenosis of both celiac artery and superior mesenteric artery.
The Doppler sonogram of the proximal celiac artery (**A**) reveals a poststenotic jet in this patient with a high-grade celiac stenosis. Peak velocity is greater than 4 m/sec. The sonogram of the superior mesenteric artery (**B**) also reveals a high-grade stenosis. Peak velocity is slightly greater than 4 m/sec. Direct detection of the poststenotic jet is the best means of identifying stenosis of the celiac and superior mesenteric artery. This patient had moderate to severe mesenteric ischemic symptoms. (Courtesy Myles Kramer.)

Table 82-1	Doppler flow measurements in normal mesenteric, splenic, and common hepatic arteries					
Vessel	**Gender**	**N**	**Diameter (Mm)**	**Velocity (Cm/Sec)**	**Flow (Ml/Min)**	**Flow (Ml/Mm/Kg)**	**Pulsatility index**
SMA	Male	25	6.6 ± 3.7	26.2 ± 7.8	516 ± 183	8.9 ± 2.8	0.85 ± 0.07
	Female	22	5.8 ± 3.1	28.5 ± 6.8	434 ± 136	8.7 ± 2.8	0.85 ± 0.04
	Total	47	6.2 ± 3.6	27.3 ± 7.4	478 ± 166	8.8 ± 2.8	0.85 ± 0.04
SA	Male	15	4.8 ± 2.7	36.1 ± 10.1	398 ± 202	6.8 ± 2.0	0.74 ± 0.10
	Female	6	4.6 ± 2.5	31.0 ± 7.2	301 ± 96	5.9 ± 1.9	0.76 ± 0.08
	Total	21	4.8 ± 2.6	34.6 ± 9.5	370 ± 181	6.5 ± 2.7	0.75 ± 0.09
CHA	Male	12	4.3 ± 2.4	30.3 ± 10.0	267 ± 154	4.7 ± 3.0	0.80 ± 0.05
	Female	6	4.1 ± 2.5	33.7 ± 19.3	226 ± 70	4.6 ± 1.5	0.77 ± 0.07
	Total	18	4.2 ± 2.4	31.3 ± 13.3	254 ± 131	4.7 ± 2.6	0.79 ± 0.05

All measurements given as mean ± standard deviation. mm, Millimeters; ml/min, milliliters per minute; ml/min/kg, milliliters per minute per kilogram body weight; cm/sec, centimeters per second; SMA, superior messentry artery; SA, splenic artery; CHA, common hepatic artery.
From Nakamura T, Moriyasu F, Ban N, et al: Quantitative measurement of abdominal arterial blood flow using image-directed Doppler ultrasonography: superior mesenteric, splenic, and common hepatic arterial blood flow in normal adults. J Clin Ultrasound 1989; 17:261-268.

increased velocity related to the poststenotic jet. Elevated peak velocities are rarely identified in stenoses less than 60% to 70%. Consequently, the most important finding in mesenteric ischemia is elevation of peak systolic velocity. Other changes also occur, including elevation of end-diastolic velocity and less increase in flow velocity in normals in postprandial examinations. Most authorities feel that peak systolic velocity is the only parameter that is useful clinically. Waveform analysis, changes in diasto-lic flow, and preprandial and postprandial comparisons are generally considered to be of lesser clinical usefulness.[7,8]

Moneta et al[9] found that a cutoff level of 275 cm/sec and greater was predictive of a 70% stenosis (Fig. 82-2). In this study the superior mesenteric artery was visualized in 93% of patients. Above the 275 cm/sec cutoff level, sensitivity was 92%, specificity was 96%, positive predictive value was 80, and negative predictive value was 99%. They also found that, unlike renal artery stenosis, the aortic velocity/ superior mesenteric artery ratio is of little clinical usefulness. Table 82-1[10] shows some of the normal variables measured using Doppler sonography in splanchnic vessels.

Conclusion

Spectral Doppler is the screening test used to evaluate patients with suspected mesenteric ischemia. Doppler analysis may help identify those patients who require further evaluation or therapy.

References

1. Jarvinen O, Laurikka J, Sisto T, et al: Atherosclerosis of the visceral arteries. Vasa 1995;24:9-14.
2. Moawad J, Gewertz BL: Chronic mesenteric ischemia. Clinical presentation and diagnosis. Surg Clin North Am 1997;77:357-369.
3. Hackworth CA, Leef JA: Percutaneous transluminal mesenteric angioplasty. Surg Clin North Am 1997;77:371-380.
4. Yamakado K, Takeda K, Nomura Y, et al: Relief of mesenteric ischemia by Z-stent placement into the superior mesenteric artery compressed by the false lumen of an aortic dissection. Cardiovasc Intervent Radiol 1998;21:66-68.
5. Busquet J: Intravascular stenting in the superior mesenteric artery for chronic abdominal angina. J Endovasc Surg 1997;4: 380-384.
6. Lafortune M, Dauzat M, Pomier-Layrargues G, et al: Hepatic artery: effect of a meal in healthy persons and transplant recipients. Radiology 1993;187:391-394.
7. Nicoloff AD, Williamson WK, Moneta GL, et al: Duplex ultrasonography in evaluation of splanchnic artery stenosis. Surg Clin North Am 1997;77:339-355.
8. Gentile AT, Moneta GL, Lee RL, et al: Usefulness of fasting in postprandial duplex ultrasound examinations for predicting high grade superior mesenteric stenosis. Am J Surg 1995;169:476-479.
9. Moneta GL, Yeager RA, Dalman R, et al: Duplex ultrasound criteria for the diagnosis of splanchnic artery occlusion or stenosis. J Vasc Surg 1991;14:511-520.
10. Nakamura T, Moriyasu F, Ban N, et al: Quantitative measurement of abdominal arterial blood flow using image-directed Doppler ultrasonography: superior mesenteric, splenic, and common hepatic arterial blood flow in normal adults. J Clin Ultrasound 1989;17:261-268.

Hisham Tchelepi
Edward Grant
Philip W. Ralls

CHAPTER 83

Doppler Ultrasound Measurements in Abdominal Organ Transplantation

Doppler Ultrasound in Renal Transplantation

INTRODUCTION

Doppler has been used extensively in the evaluation of renal transplants and is perhaps best known for its role in the diagnosis of transplant rejection. The use of Doppler in this diagnosis, however, has largely proven unreliable. Important uses for Doppler do exist in renal transplant and include the evaluation of acute arterial and venous thrombosis, renal artery stenosis, arteriovenous fistulae (AVFs), and obstruction.

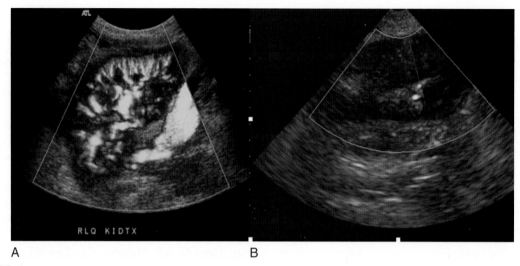

A   B

Figure 83-1

Acute thrombosis renal artery thrombosis. Longitudinal power Doppler image (**A**) at baseline shows normal flow in this renal transplant. Later image (**B**) shows little flow, presumably related to minor collateral pathways. This change is related to acute renal artery thrombosis.

ACUTE VASCULAR COMPLICATIONS

Color Doppler is invaluable in the establishment of vascular integrity in the immediate post operative period.[1] Acute arterial thrombosis may be caused by intimal dissection or severe kinking of the allograft artery. The patient presents with postoperative anuria, and the clinical differential diagnosis includes acute tubular necrosis (ATN), ureteral obstruction, and occasionally hyperacute rejection. Absence of a color/power Doppler signal should be definitive (Fig. 83-1). To be certain that the absence of flow is not technical, one should always identify signal from patent vessels outside the kidney at a similar or greater depth. Segmental infarction may be diagnosed by the focal absence of arterial signals. This is probably done best by using color/power Doppler; infarction will appear as an area without color flow. We have seen the most severe forms of segmental infarction in transplants with two renal arteries in which one was not adequately functioning. In these cases as much as one half of the kidney will be devascularized. The clinical significance of smaller segmental infarctions remains to be further investigated.

Renal vein thrombosis is another possible complication of the immediate postoperative period that can lead to loss of the allograft, as no capsular anastomoses are present to provide collateral drainage. Several sonographic reports have described a characteristic "U-shaped" or plateau-like reversal of arterial flow throughout diastole on spectral Doppler in renal vein thrombosis (Fig. 83-2).[2] Other causes of diastolic flow reversal include acute rejection and ATN, but in these entities, the flow reversal does not tend to be holodiastolic. Color Doppler imaging of the renal vein itself should also be used to confirm the diagnosis.

TRANSPLANT DYSFUNCTION

A widely publicized role for Doppler is the assessment of transplant dysfunction. Aside from hydronephrosis (which is visible on the gray scale examination), the major causes of transplant dysfunction are acute rejection, ATN, and cyclosporin-A nephrotoxicity.

Several gray scale abnormalities (allograft enlargement, compression of the central sinus echo-complex, enlarged hypoechoic pyramids) were suggested as being diagnostic of acute rejection. Unfortunately, these signs are not specific. With the introduction of duplex Doppler, sonography was once again considered in the diagnosis of rejection, based on the theory that acute rejection would cause constriction of the renal vasculature and result in an elevation of the resistive index (RI). Initial investigations were encouraging, but, in subsequent investigations, an unacceptable proportion of patients with acute rejection were found to have normal or near normal flow patterns, and many patients with ATN were shown to have high resistive

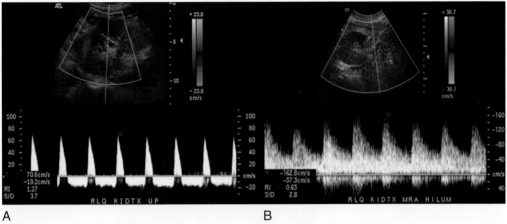

Figure 83-2
Acute renal vein thrombosis—increased peripheral resistance. The intrarenal spectral Doppler tracing (**A**) shows diastolic flow reversal indicative of very high peripheral resistance, a finding often seen in renal vein thrombosis.

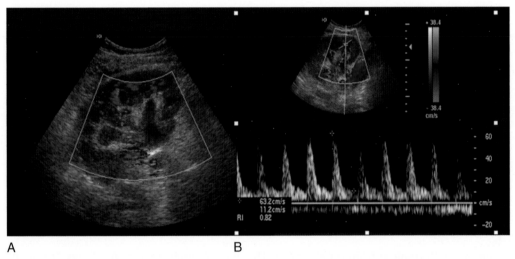

Figure 83-3
Acute ureteral obstruction—increased peripheral resistance. **A,** Hydronephrosis that, while suggestive of obstruction, is not definitive for that diagnosis. The elevated RI (0.83) in (**B**) strongly suggests that the hydronephrosis is obstructive in nature.

indices.[3,4] Despite the lack of specificity and sensitivity, we do tend to obtain an RI as part of our routine evaluation. If more than 0.80, it does imply that the kidney is abnormal (Fig. 83-3).

RENAL ARTERY STENOSIS

This diagnosis is a correctable cause of hypertension and renal dysfunction. Complicating the identification of a stenosed renal artery is the small size of the artery, the difficulty in visualizing and obtaining Doppler signals from the entire vessel, and areas of marked tortuosity. An elevated peak systolic velocity (PSV; in general, we use > 200 cm/sec) is the best known criterion in arterial stenosis (Fig. 83-4),[5] but false positives can occur, probably due to areas where sharp bends in the vessel make adequate angle adjustment impossible. In addition, we commonly find areas of high-speed flow around the anastomosis in the immediate postoperative period. All of the above render the use of simple PSV measurements for the diagnosis of renal artery stenosis nonspecific. We therefore tend to evaluate the peak velocity in the adjacent iliac artery and compare it to that in the renal artery

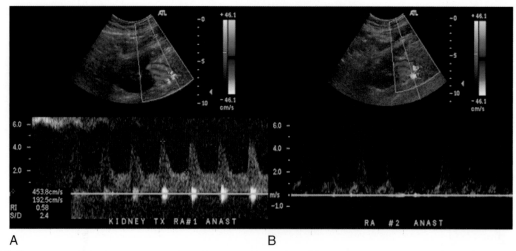

Figure 83-4

Renal artery stenosis. The elevated peak systolic velocity of more than 4 m/sec at the region of the poststenotic jet (**A**) is diagnostic for hemodynamically significant renal artery stenosis in one of the renal arteries. The second anastamosis (**B**) shows normal flow velocity.

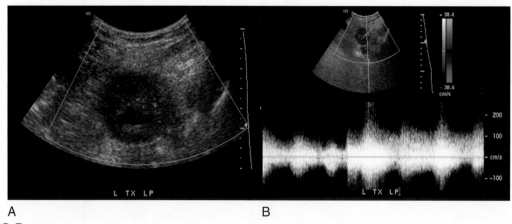

Figure 83-5

Renal arteriovenous malformation from renal biopsy. The color Doppler image (**A**) shows "tissue hum" from the tissue vibration caused by the rapidly flowing blood in the AV fistula. The spectral Doppler tracing (**B**) reveals both arterial and venous signals and disorganized rapid flow.

to determine if there is focal high-speed flow or just systemically increased velocity.[6] Several studies of segmental artery spectral patterns in patients suspected of having renal artery stenosis suggest that alterations in waveform shape (loss of the early systolic peak) increase in acceleration time, and acceleration index may also add specificity in the diagnosis of renal artery stenosis.[7]

POSTBIOPSY ARTERIOVENOUS FISTULAE AND PSEUDOANEURYSMS

Arteriovenous fistulae are usually the result of previous biopsy and are readily identified with color Doppler by demonstrating an area of artifactual color assignment in the renal parenchyma. This artifactual color assignment has been postulated to be secondary to parenchymal tissue vibration around an area of high-speed flow and has been termed a "color Doppler bruit."[8] Further evidence of a renal arteriovenous fistula includes finding a decreased resistive index, increased flow velocities in the feeding artery, and arterialization of the draining venous waveform (Fig. 83-5). Pseudoaneurysm is a rare transplant complication and may be found at the anastomotic site or after biopsy. Color Doppler should be diagnostic and will depict the "yin-yang" appearance seen in pseudoaneurysms elsewhere in the body.

CONCLUSION

Spectral Doppler is a very useful, noninvasive tool in evaluation of renal transplant. Doppler may be used to evaluate acute arterial and venous thrombosis, renal artery stenosis, arteriovenous fistulae, and obstruction.

Doppler Ultrasound in Liver Transplantation

INTRODUCTION

Liver transplantation is now a commonly performed procedure in the United States. This complicated procedure was limited to a few tertiary centers but is now performed in numerous hospitals. Ultrasound with Doppler is a pivotal imaging examination that can diagnose, follow numerous complications, or direct further workup. Although the diagnosis of vascular abnormalities using color-directed Doppler is the basis of most evaluations, careful gray scale examination should be performed to evaluate the hepatic parenchyma for focal lesions, intra- and extrahepatic biliary dilatation, and perihepatic collections such as hematomas and bilomas.

MATERIALS/MEASUREMENTS

Among the vascular complications, hepatic artery thrombosis is the most serious. Hepatic artery thrombosis occurs most frequently in the first weeks following transplantation. The incidence of hepatic artery thrombosis is described as 3% to 12% in adults and 11% to 42% in children.[9] Thrombosis is particularly common in pediatric patients with small arteries or adults with a history of primary biliary cirrhosis where the recipient hepatic artery may be brittle.[10] As complex surgical procedures increase the risk of thrombosis and complicate the sonographic evaluation, knowledge of any unusual vascular anatomy is essential. Hepatic artery reconstruction is variable, and the anastomotic site will depend upon several factors. An end-to-end anastomosis is preferred, but unusual surgical reconstructions may be necessary, including hepatic artery/aortic anastomoses, dual arterial blood supplies, and even synthetic vascular grafts.[11]

Duplex/color evaluation of the hepatic artery is usually initially undertaken in the region of

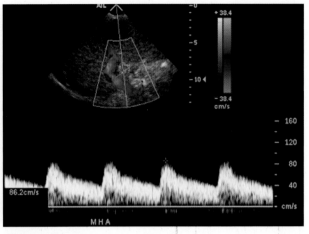

Figure 83-6
Normal hepatic artery, liver transplant. This normal renal transplant has a robust spectral Doppler signal. Note the abundant diastolic flow, indicative of a normal peripheral resistance.

the porta hepatis. In this location, the hepatic artery is large and easily visualized (Fig. 83-6); the vessel also maintains a relatively constant relationship with the portal vein, assuming an unusual arterial reconstruction has not been necessary. In most situations, a well-defined, low-resistance arterial signal in the region of the porta hepatis is considered confirmatory of vascular patency, although an attempt to obtain spectral confirmation of hepatic artery patency in both the right and left hepatic arteries is advised.

Thrombosis of the hepatic artery, as implied by absent hepatic arterial signal, is a poor prognostic sign and almost invariably dictates retransplantation (Fig. 83-7A). Unlike the normal liver, potential collateral pathways are absent and do not occur for a long period of time, if at all. Compromise of the hepatic arterial circulation is typically associated with parenchymal infarction or ischemic damage to the biliary tree. The former leads to focal hypoechoic lesions (Fig. 83-7B), while the latter causes segmental intrahepatic strictures. According to the study of Worzney et al,[12] the incidence of hepatic artery thrombosis was 86% in patients with such lesions.

At some institutions, routine Doppler evaluation of the hepatic artery is performed on specific postoperative days. As our own experience has increased, however, the rate of vascular complication has fallen to the point that we no longer perform routine ultrasounds in adults but reserve the examination for patients with

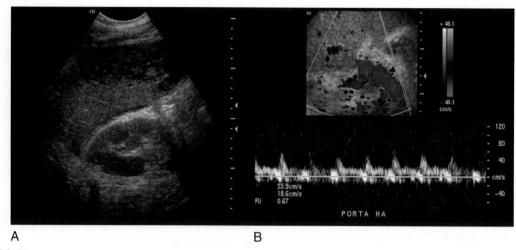

A   B

Figure 83-7
Hepatic artery occlusion, liver transplant. There is no normal arterial signal in the porta hepatis in this patient
with hepatic artery occlusion.

evidence of hepatic dysfunction. In addition, any patient with imaging evidence of abscess, infarction, delayed biliary leak, or massive hepatic necrosis is strongly suspect for hepatic artery compromise and should undergo Doppler evaluation.[11] Patients with focal abnormalities or intrahepatic biliary dilatation, in fact, are so strongly suspect of having hepatic artery compromise that arteriography may be considered even if the ultrasound reveals intrahepatic arterial signals. The Doppler study should be quite accurate in most cases; the study of Flint et al[13] demonstrated 92% accuracy in identifying hepatic artery thrombosis.

The ability to form collateral vessels is limited after transplantation but may occur in children; we have only rarely identified collaterals in adults. Flint et al,[13] however, concluded that flow in these patients was sufficiently reduced and that Doppler signals should remain undetectable. Our experience has been opposite,[14] and we have clearly identified hepatic arterial signals within the livers of such children. Although arterial collateralization brings flow to the liver, it is insufficient and ischemia remains. These children, therefore, are typically troubled by recurrent bouts of sepsis and persistent intrahepatic biliary dilatation. Both our experience[14] and that of Hoffer et al[15] indicate that such children may survive for long periods of time without retransplantation in spite of the ischemic damage. A review of the spectral tracings from these children shows that the resistive index of the hepatic artery is low, as an ischemic vascular bed is being sampled.

Another potential problem affecting the hepatic artery is the development of anastomotic stenoses (Fig. 83-8). This complication is another cause of ischemia and can produce clinical findings similar to chronic thrombosis. Turbulent high-velocity flow is often accompanied by a "color Doppler bruit" that is typical of focal hepatic artery stenosis. As the stenosis almost always occurs in the area near the anastomosis, successful diagnosis depends on the ability to visualize the entire extrahepatic artery, which may be difficult or impossible to do. For this reason, indirect signs of ischemia should be sought as well, including the identification of low-resistance flow RI less than or equal to 0.50 with a "tardus-parvus" appearance from arteries in the liver.[16] Using the intra- and extrahepatic evaluation of the hepatic artery, Dodd et al[16] were able to achieve a high degree of success in identifying patients with stenosis or thrombosis with collateralization, both of which will lower RI and both of which require angiography for complete evaluation. Early identification of hepatic artery stenosis is essential if complete thrombosis and extensive parenchymal damage is to be avoided. Once identified, hepatic artery stenosis can be treated successfully by angioplasty, thereby avoiding a surgical procedure.

Several authors have looked at intrahepatic arterial resistance in an effort to diagnose transplant rejection. Certainly, it is common to find instances where little or no diastolic flow is present in this normally low-resistance artery. The studies of Longley et al[17] and Marder et al,[18]

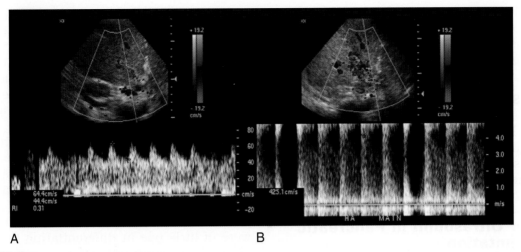

Figure 83-8
Hepatic artery stenosis, liver transplant. There is a poststenotic jet with high-velocity flow (**B**) indicative of stenosis. The prestenotic segment (**A**) shows more normal velocity.

however, have shown no correlation between absent diastolic flow and rejection. Conversely, very low resistance may be found in normal patients in the immediate postoperative period and the diagnosis of ischemia should only be considered if this finding persists.[16] The reasons for the wide variations in the hepatic arterial flow patterns remain unclear.

Portal vein thrombosis may also occur following transplantation. In our experience, portal vein thrombosis is unusual, though Dalen et al[19] report a 7.1% frequency. Like hepatic arterial thrombosis, thrombosis of the portal vein is a devastating vascular complication, also usually requiring retransplantation, although if identified rapidly enough, thrombectomy or thrombolysis can be considered. As is true in the native liver, duplex or color Doppler should identify the vast majority of portal vein thromboses.[20] The large, normal portal vein is easily visualized in all transplants. A narrow waist with perivascular echogenic foci secondary to surgical clips is frequently noted at the region of the anastomosis, and a region of moderate postanastomotic dilatation may be present as well. Unusual, turbulent spectral patterns are common in patients post-transplantation and are most likely secondary to turbulence originating in the region of the anastomosis. Anastomotic narrowing may occasionally be severe enough to cause high-velocity flow, implying that significant stenosis exists. The clinical implications of such stenoses, however, remain uncertain, but these patients do not appear to progress to frank thrombosis. In general, any

patient in whom a clearly patent portal vein is not identified with ultrasound should undergo angiography or MRI for further evaluation.

Air in the portal vein may also be encountered in patients following transplantation. Although the exact etiology is uncertain in this population, it should not be considered a grave prognostic sign, as it would be in nontransplant patients. Moving, brightly echogenic foci with the portal vein and a bubbly sound on spectral Doppler is typical of air in the portal vein.[21]

Although hepatic artery and portal vein thromboses are the most clinically significant vascular abnormalities following transplantation, compromise of the inferior vena cava (IVC) is common as well.[19] Moderate compromise of the proximal inferior vena cava in the region of the surgical anastomosis has been sufficiently common in our population such that it is not typically considered clinically significant. Even complete thrombosis can be followed, and patients seem to do relatively well. In fact, patients who have undergone retransplantation almost invariably have considerable compromise of the IVC and minor or no symptoms. Although compromise or thrombosis of the IVC is common post-transplantation, hepatic vein thrombosis is quite unusual. Three patent hepatic veins, however, should be visible in all transplant recipients, although color may be required to define flow, as minor degrees of swelling can compress the vessels and render them invisible on real-time examination. Rarely, one or more, usually the middle and left veins, may be compromised at their junction with the

IVC. Such focal narrowing of the hepatic veins is probably mechanical and most likely to be encountered in patients in whom a large liver was placed into a relatively small cavity.

CONCLUSION

Spectral Doppler is a pivotal examination that can diagnose a number of liver transplant complications. Once these complications are recognized, therapy may be appropriately directed.

Doppler Ultrasound in Pancreatic Transplantation

INTRODUCTION

Ultrasound has been useful in diagnosing a number of different complications of pancreatitis.[23] These complications include a spectrum of adverse events including peripancreatic fluid collections, vascular thrombosis, and hemorrhage. In addition, ultrasound has been used to guide transplant biopsy. Color and power Doppler imaging offer valuable information regarding the regional vascularity and potential vascular complications of transplant. Very few publications have demonstrated the utility of Doppler evaluation of a pancreatic transplant.

MATERIALS/MEASUREMENTS

Very few publications have attested to the utility of Doppler in evaluation of diagnosing pancre-

atic rejection. In 1989, Patel et al[24] studied 22 patients that had undergone pancreatic transplant. Clinical status and laboratory results were data used to establish the status of the pancreatic transplants. In their study, Patel et al[24] found a resistive index above 0.70 in seven of eight episodes of rejection and suggested that this value be used for a cutoff between normal group and those with a rejection. Patel et al[24] published a table evaluating the sensitivity and specificity of each specific RI value in detecting pancreatic transplant rejection, which is presented as Table 83-1. However, others, such as Aideyan et al,[25] found that RIs were of little use in differentiating the normal group from acute mild or moderate rejection. They found that nine transplants with no evidence of rejection had an RI of 0.64 with a range from 0.49 to 0.80. The six transplants with acute mild or moderate rejection had a mean RI of 0.67 with a range of 0.56 to 0.73. They only had two transplants with acute severe rejection with a mean RI of 0.85 with a range of 0.8 to 0.9. Furthermore, Kubota et al[26] demonstrated overlap between the normal group and those with acute rejection. In fact, they had some patients with acute rejection who had RIs of less than 0.70. Nelson et al[27] found that the RIs between the no rejection, mild acute rejection, and moderate acute rejection groups were not statistically significantly different. However, they found that the mean RI associated with chronic rejection was statistically significantly higher than the other groups. This sensitivity and specificity and positive and negative predictive values of either RI above 0.7 or above 10%

Table 83-1	Test performance of Doppler ultrasound in detecting pancreatic transplant rejection			
RI	**Sensitivity**	**Specificity**	**PPV**	**NPV**
≥0.50	100	0	31	100
≥0.55	100	22	37	100
≥0.60	97	41	42	96
≥0.65	97	66	48	98
≥0.70	76	100	100	90
≥0.75	66	100	100	86
≥0.80	45	100	100	80
≥0.85	17	100	100	73
≥0.90	17	100	100	70
≥0.95	0	100	100	69

RI, Resistive index from small parenchymal arteries; PPV, positive predictive value; NPV, negative predictive value.
From Patel B, Wolverson MK, Mahanta B: Pancreatic transplant rejection: assessment with duplex US. Radiology 1989;173:131-135.

increase of the RI above the baseline value in diagnosis of acute rejection was approximately 50%. Therefore they felt that neither the elevated level of the RI nor the relative increase was correlated with acute rejection. They felt that changes in the RI after pancreatic transplant were a poor indicator of acute rejection, but they found absolute values of the RI were elevated in cases of chronic rejection.

CONCLUSION

There appears to be great overlap in values of RI between normal pancreatic transplants and those with mild or moderate rejection. Certainly some authors have shown that higher values of resistive index, such as those above 0.8, may have some correlation with acute severe rejection and/or chronic rejection.

References

Renal Transplantation

1. Taylor KJ, Morse SS, Rigsby CM, et al: Vascular complications in renal allografts: detection with duplex Doppler US. Radiology 1987;162(1 Pt 1):31-38.
2. Kaveggia LP, Perrella RR, Grant EG, et al: Duplex Doppler sonography in renal allografts: the significance of reversed flow in diastole. AJR Am J Roentgenol 1990;155:295-298.
3. Genkins SM, Sanfilippo FP, Carroll BA: Duplex Doppler sonography of renal transplants: lack of sensitivity and specificity in establishing pathologic diagnosis. AJR Am J Roentgenol 1989;152:535-539.
4. Perrella RR, Duerinckx AJ, Tessler FN, et al: Evaluation of renal transplant dysfunction by duplex Doppler sonography: a prospective study and review of the literature. Am J Kidney Dis 1990;15:544-550.
5. Snider JF, Hunter DW, Moradian GP, et al: Transplant renal artery stenosis: evaluation with duplex sonography. Radiology 1989;172(3 Pt 2):1027-1030.
6. Gottlieb RH, Lieberman JL, Pabico RC, Waldman DL: Diagnosis of renal artery stenosis in transplanted kidneys: value of Doppler waveform analysis of the intrarenal arteries. AJR Am J Roentgenol 1995;165:1441-1446.
7. Loubeyre P, Abidi H, Cahen R, Tran Minh VA: Transplanted renal artery: detection of stenosis with color Doppler US. Radiology 1997;203:661-665.
8. Middleton WD, Kellman GM, Melson GL, et al: Postbiopsy renal transplant arteriovenous fistulas: color Doppler US characteristics. Radiology 1989;171:253-257.

Liver Transplantation

9. Morton MJ, James EM, Wiesner RH, Krom RAF: Applications of duplex ultrasonography in the liver transplant patient. Mayo Clin Proc 1990;65:360-363.
10. Davis PL, Van Thiel DH, Zajko AB, et al: Imaging in hepatic transplantation. Semin Liver Dis 1989;9:90-101.
11. Ngheim HV, Tran K, Winter TC, et al: Imaging of complications of liver transplantation. Radiographics 1996;16:825-840.
12. Worzney P, Zajko AB, Bron KM, et al: Vascular complications after liver transplantation: a 5-year experience. AJR Am J Roentgenol 1986;147:657-663.
13. Flint EW, Sumkin JH, Zajko AB, Bowen AD: Duplex sonography of hepatic artery thrombosis after liver transplantation. AJR Am J Roentgenol 1988;151:481-483.
14. Hall TR, McDiarmid SU, Grant EG, et al: False-negative duplex Doppler studies in children with hepatic artery thrombosis after liver transplantation. AJR Am J Roentgenol 1990;154:573-575.
15. Hoffer FA, Teele RL, Lillehei CW, Vacanti JP: Infected bilomas and hepatic artery thrombosis in infant recipients of liver transplants. Interventional radiology and medical therapy as an alternative to retransplantation. Radiology 1988;169:435-438.
16. Dodd GD, Memel DS, Zajko AB, et al: Hepatic artery stenosis and thrombosis in transplant recipients: Doppler diagnosis with resistive index and systolic acceleration time. Radiology 1994;192:657.
17. Longley DG, Skolnick ML, Sheahan DG: Acute allograph rejection in liver transplant recipients: lack of correlation with loss of hepatic artery diastolic flow. Radiology 1988;169:417-420.
18. Marder DM, DeMarino GB, Sumkin JH, Sheahan DG: Liver transplant rejection: value of the resistive index in Doppler US of hepatic arteries. Radiology 1989;173:127-129.

19. Dalen K, Day DL, Ascher NL, et al: Imaging of vascular complications after hepatic transplantation. AJR Am J Roentgenol 1988;150:1285-1290.

20. Tessler FN, Gehring BJ, Gomes A, et al: Diagnosis of portal vein thrombosis: value of color Doppler imaging. AJR Am J Roentgenol 1991;157:293-296.

21. Chezmar JL, Nelson RC, Bernardino ME: Portal venous gas after hepatic transplantation: sonographic detection and clinical significance. AJR Am J Roentgenol 1989;153:1203-1206.

22. Bowen A, Keslar PJ, Newman B, Hashida Y: Adrenal hemorrhage after liver transplantation. Radiology 1990;176:85-87.

Pancreatic Transplantation

23. Nikolaidis P, Amin RS, Hwang CM, et al: Role of sonography in pancreatic transplantation. Radiographics 2003;23:939-949.

24. Patel B, Wolverson MK, Mahanta B: Pancreatic transplant rejection: assessment with duplex US. Radiology 1989;173:131-135.

25. Aideyan OA, Foshager MC, Benedetti E, et al: Correlation of the arterial resistive index in pancreas transplants of patients with transplant rejection. AJR Am J Roentgenol 1997;168:1445-1447.

26. Kubota K, Billing H, Ericzon BG, et al: Duplex-Doppler ultrasonography for evaluating pancreatic grafts. Transplant Proc 1990;22:183.

27. Nelson NL, Largen PS, Stratta RJ, et al: Pancreas allograft rejection: correlation of transduodenal core biopsy with Doppler resistive index. Radiology 1996;200:91-94.

Abdomen/GI

CHAPTER 84

Suhas G. Parulekar
Aparna Balachandran

Ultrasound Measurements of the Liver

Introduction

Examination of the liver to assess the liver size has traditionally been done by percussion and palpation.[1] On physical examination, assessing the total liver span by percussion and the extent of the liver edge below the costal margin are used clinically to evaluate the liver size. However, using these methods, half of all palpable livers are not enlarged on imaging. In addition, although the majority of patients scanned have infracostal extension of the liver, less than half of these patients had palpable livers on physical examination.[1] Diagnostic imaging is more accurate than physical examination in assessing liver size. Physical examination of liver size may be confounded by many factors including the subject's body habitus, presence of ascites, chronic obstructive pulmonary disease, adhesions (which can limit the liver motion with respiration), and interobserver variability.[1]

The length (i.e., longitudinal diameter) of the normal liver at the mid-clavicular line has been reported to be less than 16 cm on nuclear medicine studies.[2] The normal anatomic values for adults reported by the ICRP (International Committee on Radiological Protection) are as shown in Table 84-1.[3]

Table 84-1	Normal anatoric adult liver measurements as reported by the ICRP
Diameter	**Value (cm)**
Greatest transverse	20-36
Greatest anteroposterior	10-21
Greatest longitudinal (craniocaudal)	7-15

Modified from ICRP. Task Group on Reference Man: Report of the Task Group on Reference Man. Prepared by the Task Group Committee no. 2, International Committee on Radiological Protection. New York, Pergamon Press, 1975.

Ultrasound Measurements

Ultrasound is one of the most widely used imaging techniques in the evaluation of the liver. Several studies have been performed to evaluate the normal liver volume and the length (i.e., longitudinal diameter).

LIVER LENGTH

For assessing liver size, most of these studies use the length of the liver at the right mid-clavicular line from the dome of the liver to the inferior edge. The use of this method may be inaccurate in the occasional patient with a Reidel lobe. Real-time extended field of view scanning is helpful in measuring liver, especially when the liver is enlarged. Otherwise, because of the limited field of view of the real-time sector scanners (Fig. 84-1), it is difficult, if not impossible, to accurately measure the liver, especially when the liver is considerably enlarged. Ideally, the most external points of the liver are projected as indicated in Figure 84-2, and the distance between these two points is measured. This method, however, is not very practical and generally the distance between the dome and the inferior tip of the liver (i.e., the length) and the transverse diameter are measured by electronic calipers (Fig. 84-3). In three reports, the maximum length was measured in a straight longitudinal plane on the sagittal view (see Figs. 84-2A, 84-3A, and 84-4). This method of measurement is easier to use with extended field of view scans rather than with sector scans with limited field of view. Measuring the length in a straight longitudinal plane, however, can frequently be technically difficult; therefore some authors have measured the length in an oblique longitudinal plane. In

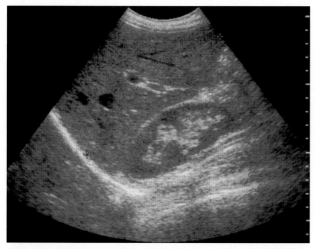

Figure 84-1
Longitudinal real-time sector ultrasound scan of the liver. Because of limited field of view, the superior and inferior margins of the liver are not completely included on the image, and true length of the liver cannot be measured. The length is measured in an oblique plane on this sagittal view.

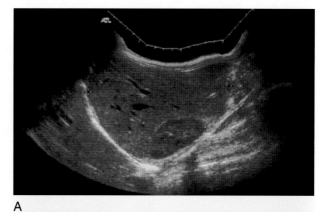

A

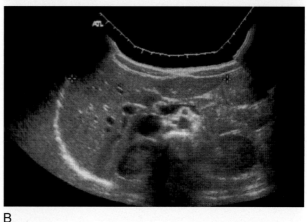

B

Figure 84-3
Sagittal (**A**) and transverse (**B**) ultrasound of normal size liver. Extended field of view technique. The distance between the dome and the inferior tip of the liver (i.e., the length) on the sagittal view (**A**) and transverse diameter (**B**) are measured by electronic calipers. The length is measured in a straight longitudinal plane.

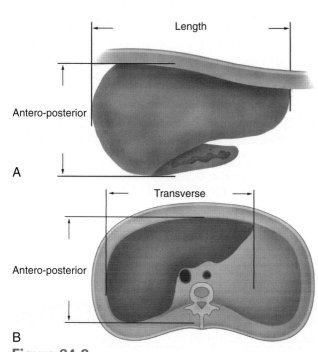

Figure 84-2
Sagittal (**A**) and transverse (**B**) views of the liver. The most external points of the liver are projected, and the distance between these two points is measured.

one report, the maximum length was measured in an oblique plane on the sagittal view sector scan (see Fig. 84-1).

A study by Gosink and Leymaster[4] compared length of the liver in the right mid-clavicular line (mid-hepatic line) on ultrasound with autopsy data to assess for hepatomegaly. According to Gosink and Leymaster, 93% of the livers were normal when the length was less than or equal to 13.0 cm. There was hepatomegaly in 75% of cases, when the length was 15.5 cm or greater (see Fig. 84-4). Kane[5,6] used length between 15 and 17 cm as normal and Sapira and Williams[7] used 15 cm as the normal length of the liver in the right mid-clavicular line.

Pietri et al[8] reported differences in the liver size based on body morphology as shown in Table 84-2. They defined body morphology into three types: ectomorph, normotype, and endomorph.

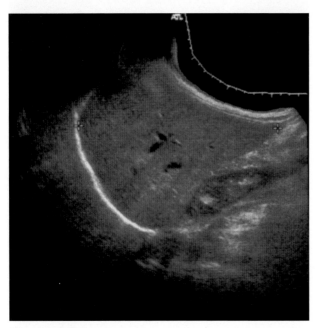

Figure 84-4
Enlarged liver. Sagittal ultrasound. Extended field of view technique. Liver is enlarged, the right lobe measuring 22 cm.

Niederau et al[9] reported the normal length as 10.5 ± 1.5 cm in the right mid-clavicular line, which was much lower than the other authors (Table 84-3).

A recent study of 2080 subjects (nonselected population) by Kratzer et al[10] showed the average length of the liver at the right mid-clavicular line to be 14 ± 1.7 cm. The liver size varied between men and women with a mean length of 14.5 cm for men and 13.5 cm for women. In their subject population, 74.1% of the subjects had a liver length of 15 cm or less, 14.4% had the length of 15 to 16 cm, and 11.5% had the length greater than 16 cm. They suggested that length of 16 cm or greater in the right mid-clavicular line indicated enlargement of the liver. Variations in liver size were shown to be most correlated with height and body mass index, which might be considered individually in borderline cases.

LIVER VOLUME

Liver volume measurement can also be used to assess liver size. The normal volume of the liver can be calculated by ultrasound, CT, or MRI. Van Thiel et al[11] determined hepatic volumes in patients prior to transplantation with both CT and ultrasound and compared these volumes with the hepatic weight and volume after surgi-

Table 84-2	Differences in liver size based on body morphology		
Diameter	**Endomorph**	**Normotype**	**Ectomorph**
Transverse (cm)	15.7 ± 1.3	15.6 ± 0.9	18.7 ± 1.3
Anteroposterior (cm)	14.7 ± 1.6	12.1 ± 1.3	11.4 ± 1.0
Longitudinal (cm)	15.0 ± 1.2	18.5 ± 1.8	15.6 ± 1.3

Modified from Pietri H, Boscaini M, Berthezene P, et al: Hepatic morphocytes. Their statistical individualization using ultrasonography. J Ultrasound Med 1988;7:189-196.

Table 84-3	Liver measurements from Niederau et al[9]	
Measurement	**Diameter (Mean ± SD) (cm)**	**95th percentile (cm)**
Mid-clavicular longitudinal diameter	10.5 ± 1.5	12.6
Mid-clavicular AP diameter	8.1 ± 1.9	11.3
Midline longitudinal diameter	8.3 ± 1.7	10.9
Midline AP diameter	5.7 ± 1.5	8.2

Modified from Niederau C, Sonnenber A, Miller JE, et al: Sonographic measurements of the normal liver, spleen, pancreas, and portal vein. Radiology 1983;149:537-540.

cal removal. They measured the volume by adding the cross-sectional areas on each image (sagittal plane for ultrasound and axial plane for CT). The volume was measured by obtaining longitudinal ultrasound scans of the entire liver at 1-cm intervals and measuring cross-sectional area of each longitudinal image. Area on each sagittal sonogram was measured with built-in software on the ultrasound machine (i.e., the perimeter of each slice was outlined and the area was electronically calculated for that section). Liver volume was calculated as the summation of the individual areas of multiple sections, each determined separately and having a thickness of 1 cm. They used the following equation:

$$\text{Volume} = dx \sum_{i}^{n} \text{area}$$

$$dx = \text{scan spacing}$$

The mean calculated volume on ultrasound for the liver showed a good correlation with the actual explanted liver volume. The volumes of the liver as calculated by CT and ultrasound correlated well, and the sonographic technique was shown to be more accurate than CT technique.

Zoli et al[12] also compared CT and ultrasound volume measurements and calculated the liver volume with ultrasound using the following formula:

$$\text{Liver volume} = 133.2 + 0.422 \times (CC \times AP \times LL)$$

The liver volume was expressed in milliliters, and CC, AP, and LL referred to the liver diameters (in centimeters) in the craniocaudal (at the right mid-clavicular line), anteroposterior, and transverse (LL) directions. They reported that ultrasound-measured volume correlated well with the volume calculated by CT.

Geraghty et al[13] calculated the normal liver volume on CT as 1411 mL for females and 1710 mL for males (these values were corrected for the patient's height and weight). Mazonakis et al[14] studied the liver volume on MRI in patients and found the normal liver volume to be 1477.7 ± 230.7 cc.

Hatsuno et al[15] found that the volume of the lateral segment of the left lobe of the liver, calculated sonographically, correlated well with the volume calculated by CT. They found this measurement useful in patients scheduled for right hepatectomy and for evaluating the

graft size for living related partial liver transplantation.

Boscaini and Pietri[16] calculated the hepatic volumetric index (HVI), which is calculated by multiplying the (maximum) liver length with breadth and with thickness and dividing this product by 27. This typically ranged from 95 to 140 in 95% of the patients below 65 years of age and ranged from 80 to 135 in those above 65 years. They reported that the liver volume decreased with age.

CAUDATE TO RIGHT LOBE RATIO

The caudate to right lobe ratio has been used in the diagnosis of cirrhosis. This was proposed by Harbin et al[17] on the basis of the observation that, in patients with cirrhosis, there is greater shrinkage of the right lobe and relative enlargement of the caudate lobe. This ratio was obtained by comparing the transverse diameters of the caudate to the right lobe of the liver (i.e., caudate lobe/right lobe) (Fig. 84-5). Harbin et al[17] used a cutoff ratio of 0.65. They proposed that the ratio of 0.65 or greater had a sensitivity of 84% and a specificity of 100% in the determination of cirrhosis. Subsequently, Giorgio et al[18] reported a lower sensitivity of 43% but a specificity of 100%.

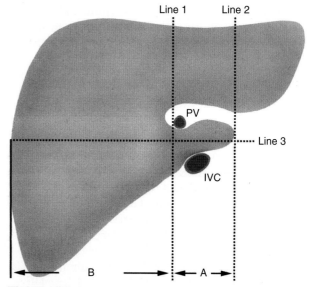

Figure 84-5
Caudate to right lobe ratio. Transverse view. This ratio is obtained by comparing the transverse diameters of the caudate (distance A) to the right lobe (distance B) of the liver. Ratio = A/B. Modified from Harbin et al. Radiology 1980;135:273-283.

Conclusion

Imaging has proven to be more accurate than physical examination in assessing liver size. The length of the liver at the right mid-clavicular line is the most widely used method for routine assessment of the liver size and has been shown to correlate well with the liver volume. For liver size assessment during routine imaging, the length of the liver at the right mid-clavicular line may provide adequate information. Different studies report different ranges for the normal length of the liver. These variations in the length are likely due to different body morphotypes, body mass index, and gender. **Generally the liver is considered enlarged when the length (i.e., longitudinal diameter) at the right mid-clavicular line is 16 cm or greater.**

Volume measurements are more time consuming and cumbersome. However, in the future, volume measurements may be easier to obtain and more accurate with automated three-dimensional ultrasound imaging. Volume measurements may be valuable in accurate assessment of liver size for purposes of transplantation or hepatic resection.

References

1. Zoli M, Magalotti D, Grimaldi M, et al: Physical examination of the liver: is it still worth it? Am J Gastroenterol 1995;90: 1428-1432.
2. Halpern S, Coel M, Ashburn W, et al: Correlation of liver and spleen size. Determinations by nuclear medicine studies and physical examination. Arch Intern Med 1974;134:123-124.
3. International Commission On Radiological Protection. Task Group on Reference Man: Report of the Task Group on Reference Man: Prepared by the Task Group Committee no. 2, International Committee on Radiological Protection New York, Pergamon Press, 1975.
4. Gosink BB, Leymaster CE: Ultrasonic determination of hepatomegaly. J Clin Ultrasound 1981;9:37-44.
5. Kane R: Ultrasonographic anatomy of the liver and biliary tree. Semin Ultrasound 1980;1:87-95.
6. Kane R: Sonographic anatomy of the liver. Semin Ultrasound 1981;2:190-197.
7. Sapira JD, Williams DL: How big is the normal liver? Arch Intern Med 1979;139: 971-973.
8. Pietri H, Boscaini M, Berthezene P, et al: Heptatic morphotypes. Their statistical individualization using ultrasonography. J Ultrasound Med 1988;7:189-196.
9. Niederau C, Sonnenberg A, Muller JE, et al: Sonographic measurements of the normal liver, spleen, pancreas, and portal vein. Radiology 1983;149:537-540.
10. Kratzer W, Fritz V, Mason RA, et al: Roemerstein Study Group. Factors affecting liver size: a sonographic survey of 2080 subjects. J Ultrasound Med 2003;22:1155-1161.
11. Van Thiel DH, Hagler NG, Schade RR, et al: In vivo hepatic volume determination using sonography and computed tomography. Validation and a comparison of the two techniques. Gastroenterology 1985;88:1812-1817.
12. Zoli M, Pisi P, Marchesini G, et al: A rapid method for the in vivo measurement of liver volume. Liver 1989;9:159-163.
13. Geraghty EM, Boone JM, McGahan JP, Jain K: Normal organ volume assessment from abdominal CT. Abdom Imaging 2004;29: 482-490.
14. Mazonakis M, Damilakis J, Maris T, et al: Comparison of two volumetric techniques for estimating liver volume using magnetic resonance imaging. J Magn Reson Imaging 2002;15:557-563.
15. Hatsuno T, Kaneko T, Ito S, Nakao A: Sonographic measurement of the volume of the left lateral segment of the liver. J Clin Ultrasound 2002;30:117-122.
16. Boscaini M, Pietri H: Determination of a hepatic volumetric index by ultrasonic scanning. Surg Endosc 1987;1:103-107.
17. Harbin WP, Robert NJ, Ferrucci JT Jr: Diagnosis of cirrhosis based on regional changes in hepatic morphology. Radiology 1980;135: 273-283.
18. Giorgio A, Amoroso P, Lettieri G, et al: Cirrhosis: value of caudate to right lobe ratio in diagnosis with US. Radiology 1986;161: 443-445.

Bijan Bijan
Hedieh Eslamy
John P. McGahan

CHAPTER 85

Ultrasound Measurements of the Extrahepatic Bile Ducts

Introduction

Ultrasound (US) is considered an accurate, noninvasive method for the assessment of biliary obstruction and is considered the first diagnos- tic procedure when stones are suspected in the extrahepatic bile ducts (Tables 85-1 and 85-2).

Materials/Measurements

The right and left hepatic ducts join to form the common hepatic duct, which is located anterior to the right and main portal veins. Approxi- mately 3 cm from the confluence of the right and left hepatic ducts, the distal cystic duct joins the common hepatic duct to form the common bile duct. From the porta hepatis, the common bile duct, along with the main portal vein and the main (proper) hepatic artery, descends within the hepatoduodenal ligament. The distal common bile duct passes behind the duodenum and then runs in a groove on the upper and lateral part of the posterior surface of the head of the pancreas, anterior to the inferior vena cava. The common bile duct and pancreatic duct usually join together to form the ampulla of Vater, in the descending part of the duodenum. The common hepatic duct is approximately 3 cm long, and the common bile duct is about 7.5 cm long.[1]

Sonographically, the junction of the distal cystic duct and the common hepatic duct cannot be seen in everyone; therefore the term extra- hepatic bile duct (EBD) shall be used to refer to both of the common hepatic and common bile ducts. The extrahepatic bile duct can be divided into proximal and distal segments. The proxi- mal segment is anterior to the main portal vein. The distal segment can be further subdivided into suprapancreatic and intrapancreatic por- tions. The suprapancreatic portion is between the porta hepatis and pancreatic head. The intrapancreatic portion is at the level of the head of the pancreas. The distal portions of the EBD are usually larger than the proximal portion[1] (Fig. 85-1A).

Long-axis and transverse-axis sonograms of the bile ducts are obtained via an intercostal or subcostal view, using 3.5- to 5.0-MHz transduc- ers, with the patient supine or in the left poste- rior oblique position. The distal extrahepatic bile duct, especially the pancreatic portion of the duct, is frequently better seen by transverse scans with the patient in an erect right poste- rior oblique position. Sonograms can be obtained at end-inspiration to optimize visualization of the bile duct.[2] Conventionally the anteroposte- rior diameter of the EBD is measured in long- axis images of the EBD. The lumen of the EBD is measured from inside of the near wall to the inside of the far wall.[1] Measurements are either made at a specific location (e.g., in the porta hepatis parallel to the main portal vein or ante- rior to the right portal vein, the portion of the duct where the right hepatic artery crosses the EBD, and suprapancreatic portion of EBD prior

Table 85-1	Extrahepatic biliary obstruction
Complete obstruction	
Partial obstruction	
Flow relevant	
Flow irrelevant	

Table 85-2 Overview of ultrasound measurements of extrahepatic bile ducts	
Images used for measurement	Long-axis images of EBD
Diameter measured	Anteroposterior diameter
Caliper placement	From inside of the near wall to the inside of the far wall
Location of measurements	Suprapancreatic portion of the EBD
(a) Specific locations	In the porta hepatis anterior to the right portal vein; In the porta hepatis parallel to the main portal vein; Portion of the duct where the right hepatic artery crosses the EBD
(b) Largest visualized diameter	May be located anywhere along the length of the EBD, but is typically distal to the proximal segment of the EBD
Observer error of ultrasonographic measurements	1-2 mm
Respiratory variation of the EBD diameter	May be >1 mm

EBD, Extrahepatic bile ducts.

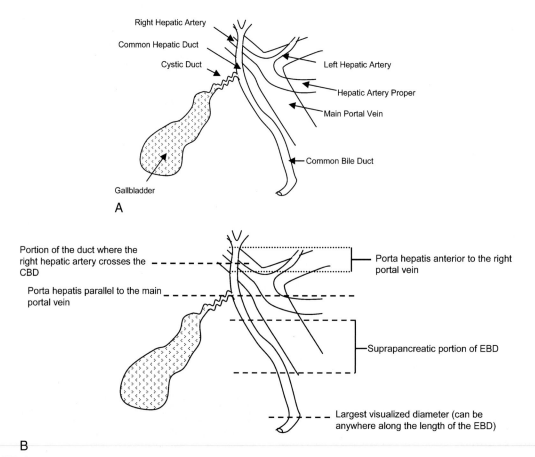

Figure 85-1

A, Schematic diagram demonstrating the relationships among the extrahepatic bile ducts, hepatic artery, and portal vein and the variable diameter of the EBD along its course. **B,** Schematic diagram demonstrating the levels at which different investigators have measured the anteroposterior diameter of the extrahepatic bile ducts.

to where it tapers into the head of the pancreas), or the largest visualized diameter is measured (see Fig. 85-1B).

Two shortcomings of the latter method are that the entire length of the EBD cannot be seen routinely by US, and the EBD often varies in diameter along its length. Therefore a sonographer cannot confidently measure the greatest diameter of the EBD if the entire length of it is not visualized (see Table 85-2).[3]

The observer error of ultrasonographic measurements is known to be 1 to 2 mm.[4] Respiratory variation of the EBD diameter exceeding 1 mm has been observed.[5]

DISCUSSION

Bowie[3] has reviewed the literature concerning the upper limit of normal for the extrahepatic bile ducts on ultrasound. Conventionally, the upper limit of normal for the EBD, as measured by US, is considered to be 6 mm. Bowie has suggested the use of 7 mm as the upper limit of normal for individuals younger than 65 years old, on the basis of a study by Niederau et al[6] in which none of the healthy subjects (aged 18 to 65 years) had an EBD diameter greater than 7 mm. Wu et al[7] have found a significant correlation between age and EBD diameter and concluded that in normal patients older than 65 years of age, the EBD can measure up 10 mm. Kaim et al[8] have reported similar results in their study of an asymptomatic elderly population older than 75 years of age (the EBD was measured in its suprapancreatic portion) (Table 85-3, Fig. 85-2).

Niederau et al[6] measured the lumen of the EBD at two different sites: (1) in the porta hepatis parallel to the main portal vein and (2) at its widest point, generally at a more distal site than porta hepatis, in 830 normal subjects, 73 patients with cholelithiasis and 55 patients after cholecystectomy. In the 830 normal subjects, the mean diameters and upper limits of normal were similar at both sites of measurement with a strong correlation between the duct sizes at the two different points ($r = 0.84$, $p = 0.001$). In contrast to healthy subjects, both groups of patients with biliary disease showed a significant difference in duct diameter when measurements made at proximal and distal sited were compared[7] (Table 85-4).

The width of the CBD after cholecystectomy has been a controversial issue in the literature, with studies reporting either a compensatory widening of the EBD after cholecystectomy or no significant change in EBD diameter. Majeed et al[11] have concluded that if a margin of error of 1 mm for ultrasonographic measurement of the EBD is taken into account, the diameter of the EBD does not change significantly after cholecystectomy. Therefore an increase in diameter beyond 6 mm on ultrasonography (of ducts that were preoperatively normal, i.e., <6 mm) should be considered an indication for further imaging of the EBD (Tables 85-5 to 85-7).

Table 85-3	Extrahepatic bile duct size in adults						
Gender	Age (yr)	<21	21-30	31-40	41-50	51-60	>60
Men	EBD (mm)	3.3 ± 1.1	4.7 ± 1.3	5.0 ± 1.5	5.4 ± 1.4	6.2 ± 1.9	6.1 ± 2.0
	Number	9	12	14	13	15	7
Women	EBD (mm)	3.3 ± 1.1	4.7 ± 1.2	4.6 ± 1.4	5.6 ± 1.2	5.3 ± 1.8	6.8 ± 1.7
	Number	9	28	38	21	15	22
Combined	EBD (mm)	3.3 ± 1.2	4.7 ± 1.3	4.7 ± 1.5	5.5 ± 1.3	5.8 ± 1.9	6.6 ± 1.8
	Number	18	40	52	34	30	29

p value = Difference between male and female means. p value in all age groups is >0.05.
Measurements in millimeters (mean ± standard deviation) and made at the widest point of the extrahepatic bile duct in 256 individuals without evidence of hepatobiliary disease.
EBD, Extrahepatic bile duct. Combined diameters calculated from male and female data.
From Wu CC, Ho YH, Chen CY: Effect of aging on common bile duct diameter: a real-time ultrasonographic study. J Clin Ultrasound 1984;12:473-478; Keats TE, Sistrom C: Atlas of Radiologic Measurement, 7th ed. St Louis, Mosby, 2001.

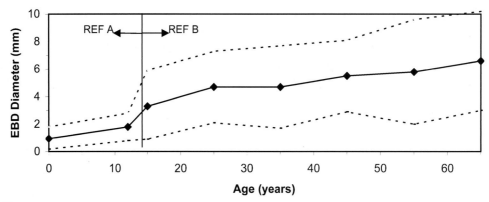

Figure 85-2

Common duct size throughout life. Vertical line shows from which reference the data were obtained. Solid line = mean diameter; dotted lines = 95% confidence intervals. (Data from Wu CC, Ho YH, Chen CY: Effect of aging on common bile duct diameter: a real-time ultrasonographic study. J Clin Ultrasound 1984;12:473-478; Hernanz-Schulman M, Ambrosino MM, Freeman PC, et al: Common bile duct in children: Sonographic dimensions. Radiology 1995;195:193-195; Keats TE, Sistrom C: Atlas of Radiologic Measurement, 7th ed. St Louis, Mosby, 2001.

Table 85-4	Extrahepatic bile duct size (mm) in 830 normal adults		
Portion of EBD measured at	**Mean ± SD**	**Range**	**95th percentile**
-Porta hepatis	2.5 ± 1.1	1-7	4
-Widest point	2.8 ± 1.2	1-7	4

From Niederau C, Muller J, Sonnenberg A, et al: Extrahepatic bile ducts in healthy subjects, in patients with cholelithiasis, and in postcholecystectomy patients: a prospective ultrasonic study. J Clin Ultrasound 1983;11:23-27.

Table 85-5	Upper limit of normal of EBD measurements on ultrasound	
Subject population		**Upper limit of normal**
Healthy subjects <65 years of age		6-7 mm
Healthy subjects >65 years of age		10 mm
Postcholecystectomy patients with preoperative normal EBD diameters (controversial issue)		6 mm

Mintz et al[14] measured the EBD diameter in pregnancy and found it to be comparable to the nonpregnant adult population.

Wachsberg et al[15] have measured the transverse diameter (D^{TRV}) of the dilated (≥8 mm) EBD. In 70% of their patient population, the EBD had an oval cross-section. The mean D^{TRV} and the mean diameter measured on ERC were statistically similar. Therefore these authors postulated that the upper limit for normal for D^{TRV} is presumably similar to that used for ERC (i.e., approximately 11 mm), unless the patient is older than 70 years or has undergone chole-cystectomy, in which case D^{TRV} can normally be greater than 11 mm.

Tomonaga et al[16] have measured the length of the cystic duct using a 7.5-MHz transducer during laparascopic ultrasound (US). The cystic duct length, as measured by US, was 0.5 to 4 cm, with an accuracy rate of 87.1%.

US plays a major role in the assessment of the biliary tract, choledochojejunostomy, and the Roux loop in patients who present with recurrent jaundice following curative or palliative surgery for pancreatic and biliary neoplasms and can demonstrate the level of

Table 85-6   Changes in bile duct diameter after cholecystectomy

Author (study type)	N	Exam time	CBD (mm) mean ± SD	CHD (mm) mean ± SD
Hunt and Scott	13	preop		3.54 ± 0.55
(prospective)	13	<1 yrs		3.50 ± 0.59
	13	1 yrs	4.77 ± 0.69	3.81 ± 0.36
	13	5 yrs	5.92 ± 0.56	4.69 ± 0.64
	21	preop		3.95 ± 0.46
	21	5 yrs		4.48 ± 0.47

			CBD (mm): Mean ± SD	
			Preop	**Postop**
Feng and Song	50	7-30 days	5.0 ± 0.9	5.5 ± 0.9
(retrospective)	51	2-6 mos	5.4 ± 0.5	6.1 ± 1.6
	33	7-12 mos	5.3 ± 0.6	5.9 ± 1.2
	41	2-3 yrs	5.7 ± 0.5	6.6 ± 1.8
	22	4-6 yrs	5.6 ± 0.5	6.2 ± 1.4
	197	Total	5.4 ± 0.7	6.0 ± 1.4

Preop, Preoperative scan; postop, postoperative scan; CBD, common bile duct (maximum); CHD, common hepatic duct (average).
From Keats TE, Sistrom C: Atlas of Radiologic Measurement, 7th ed. St Louis, Mosby, 2001; Hunt DR, Scott AJ: Changes in bile duct diameter after cholecystectomy: a 5-year prospective study. Gastroenterology 1989;97:1485-1488; Feng B, Song Q: Does the common bile duct dilate after cholecystectomy? Sonographic evaluation in 234 patients. AJR Am J Roentgenol 1995;165:859-861.

Table 85-7   Bile duct size distribution before and after cholecystectomy

Reference (study type)	Structure	N	Exam time	Duct diameter (Mm) ≤4 (%)	5-6 (%)	7-8 (%)	≥9 (%)
Hunt and Scott	CHD	21	preop	13 (62)	6 (28)	1 (5)	1 (5)
(prospective)			5 yrs	14 (67)	3 (13)	2 (10)	2 (10)
	CBD	13	1 yrs	6 (46)	4 (31)	2 (15)	1 (8)
			5 yrs	3 (23)	4 (31)	5 (38)	1 (8)
Feng and Song	CBD	234	preop	17 (7)	180 (77)	26 (11)	11 (5)
(retrospective)			postop	22 (9)	145 (62)	52 (22)	16 (7)

				Duct Diameter (mm) ≤5 (%)	5.1-6.0 (%)	>6.0 (%)
Majeed et al	CHD	59	preop	59	0	0
(prospective)		39	3 mos	35 (89.7)	4 (10.2)	0
		49	6 mos	43 (87.7)	3 (6.1)	3 (6.1)
		58	1 yr	49 (84.4)	6 (10.3)	3 (5.1)
		48	5 ys	41 (85.4)	5 (10.4)	1 (2.1)

Preop, Preoperative; postop, postoperative; CBD, common bile duct (maximum); CHD, common hepatic duct average.
From Keats TE, Sistrom C: Atlas of Radiologic Measurement, 7th ed. St Louis, Mosby, 2001; Hunt DR, Scott AJ: Changes in bile duct diameter after cholecystectomy: a 5-year prospective study. Gastroenterology 1989;97:1485-1488; Feng B, Song Q: Does the common bile duct dilate after cholecystectomy? Sonographic evaluation in 234 patients. AJR Am J Roentgenol 1995;165:859-861.

Table 85-8	Factors that may contribute to the discrepancy between the diameter of the extrahepatic bile duct measured sonographically and that measured on endoscopic retrograde cholangiography

Radiographic magnification of EBD

Thickening of the EBD wall on ultrasound from reverberation artifact leading to underestimation of the intraluminal diameter

Overdistention of EBD at ERC due to the instilled contrast material

Comparison of different portions of the EBD: right hepatic duct measured on ultrasound and common bile duct measured on ERC

Comparison of different cross-sectional diameters: anteroposterior diameter measured on US and transverse diameter measured on ERC

EBD, Extrahepatic bile duct; ERC, endoscopic retrograde cholangiography.
From Wachsberg RH, Kim KH, Sundaram K: Sonographic versus endoscopic retrograde cholangiographic measurements of the bile duct revisited: importance of the transverse diameter. AJR Am J Roentgenol 1998;170:669-674.

obstruction in the Roux loops, as well as patency of biliary-enteric anastomosis.[17]

The discrepancy between the diameter of EBD measured sonographically and that measured on ERC may be due to several factors that are summarized in Table 85-8.[15]

References

1. McGahan JP, Goldberg BB: Diagnostic Ultrasound: A Logical Approach. Philadelphia, New York, Lippincott-Raven, 1998.

2. Behan M, Kazam E: Sonography of the common bile duct: value of the right anterior oblique view. AJR Am J Roentgenol 1978;130:701-709.

3. Bowie JD: What is the upper limit of normal for the common bile duct on ultrasound: how much do you want it to be? Am J Gastroenterol 2000;95:897-900.

4. Niederau C, Sonnenberg A, Muller J: Comparison of the extrahepatic bile duct size measured by ultrasound and by different radiographic methods. Gastroenterology 1984;87:615-621.

5. Wachsberg RH: Respiratory variation of extrahepatic bile duct diameter during ultrasonography. J Ultrasound Med 1994;13:617-621.

6. Niederau C, Muller J, Sonnenberg A, et al: Extrahepatic bile ducts in healthy subjects, in patients with cholelithiasis, and in postcholecystectomy patients: a prospective ultrasonic study. J Clin Ultrasound 1983;11:23-27.

7. Wu CC, Ho YH, Chen CY: Effect of aging on common bile duct diameter: a real-time ultrasonographic study. J Clin Ultrasound 1984;12:473-478.

8. Kaim A, Steinke K, Frank M, et al: Diameter of the common bile duct in the elderly patient: measurement by ultrasound. Eur Radiol 1998;8:1413-1415.

9. Hernanz-Schulman M, Ambrosino MM, Freeman PC, et al: Common bile duct in children: sonographic dimensions. Radiology 1995;195:193-195.

10. Keats TE, Sistrom C: Atlas of Radiologic Measurement, 7th ed. St Louis, Mosby, 2001.

11. Majeed AW, Ross B, Johnson AG: The preoperatively normal bile duct does not dilate after cholecystectomy: results of a five year study. Gut 1999;45:741-743.

12. Hunt DR, Scott AJ: Changes in bile duct diameter after cholecystectomy: a 5-year prospective study. Gastroenterology 1989;97:1485-1488.

13. Feng B, Song Q: Does the common bile duct dilate after cholecystectomy? Sonographic evaluation in 234 patients. AJR Am J Roentgenol 1995;165:859-861.

14. Mintz MC, Grumbach K, Arger PH, et al: Sonographic evaluation of bile duct size during pregnancy. AJR Am J Roentgenol 1985;145:575-578.

15. Wachsberg RH, Kim KH, Sundaram K: Sonographic versus endoscopic retrograde cholangiographic measurements of the bile duct revisited: importance of the transverse diameter. AJR Am J Roentgenol 1998;170:669-674.

16. Tomonaga T, Filipi CJ, Lowham A, et al: Laparascopic intracorporeal ultrasound cystic duct length measurement. A new technique to prevent common bile duct injuries. Surg Endosc 1999;13:183-185.

17. Holland CL, Olliff SP, Olliff JF: Case report: ultrasound diagnosis of obstructed Roux loop after cancer of the pancreas or bile duct. Br J Radiol 1994;67:309-312.

Bijan Bijan
Hedieh Eslamy
John P. McGahan

CHAPTER 86

Ultrasound Measurements of the Gallbladder

Introduction

Ultrasonography is accepted as the primary modality for evaluation of the biliary tree and the gallbladder. Ultrasonographic measurements of gallbladder wall thickness are in close agreement with surgical measurements.[1] The recent development of three-dimensional ultrasound may overcome the limitations of two-dimensional ultrasound in accurately determining the ultrasonographic parameters of gallbladder contractility (Table 86-1).

Gallbladder Wall Thickness

INTRODUCTION

The gallbladder wall is optimally measured by transabdominal ultrasound after an overnight fast (6 to 8 hours fasting). The upper normal limit of gallbladder wall thickness, measured perpendicular to the gallbladder wall in either longitudinal or transverse images of the gallbladder, has been established as 3 mm[1] (Table 86-2).

MATERIALS/MEASUREMENTS

Abdominal ultrasound is performed after a minimum fast of 6 hours to allow for distention of the gallbladder. Scanning is performed with a curved array or sector 3.5- to 5-MHz trans-ducer. The gallbladder is scanned in subcostal and intercostal views along its long and transverse axes, with the patient in the left posterior oblique and supine positions. In normal fasting subjects, the gallbladder wall is visualized by ultrasound as a thin echogenic stripe surrounding the gallbladder. Gallbladder wall measurements are most accurate when the anterior wall of the gallbladder is measured in the long-axis view of the gallbladder with the sound beam perpendicular to the gallbladder wall.[2] Gallbladder wall thickness has been defined as either the largest gallbladder wall thickness or the mean of several wall thickness measurements.

It is generally accepted that a sonographic/pathologic wall thickness of 3 mm constitutes

Table 86-1	Overview of normal limits of gallbladder ultrasound measurements
GB wall thickness	≤3 mm
GB length	≤8-12 cm
GB width	≤4 cm
GB contractility parameters	No established physiological range

Gallbladder (GB) hydrops has been defined as GB length greater than 8 to 10 cm or GB width greater than 4 cm.

Table 86-2	Overview of ultrasound measurements of the gallbladder wall
Images used for measurement	Longitudinal and transverse images of the GB
Diameter measured	Anteroposterior diameter of the GB wall is measured with the sound beam perpendicular to the GB wall
Caliper placement	Includes the entire thickness of the GB wall
Ultrasonographic appearance of the GB wall	Healthy subjects: a thin echogenic strip
	Patients with increased GB wall thickness: one of three patterns summarized in Table 3
Location of measurements	Anterior or posterior wall of the GB body or GB fundus
Definition of gallbladder wall thickness	(a) largest diameter measured or
	(b) mean of several measurements
Most accurate GB wall measurements	In the anterior wall of the GB, in longitudinal images, with the sound beam perpendicular to the GB wall

GB, Gallbladder.

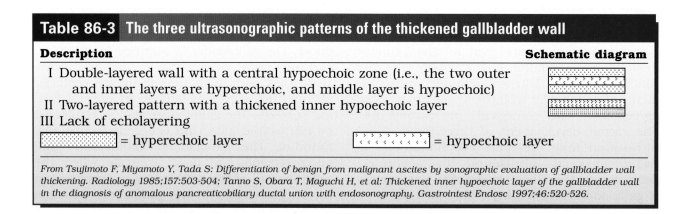

Table 86-3	The three ultrasonographic patterns of the thickened gallbladder wall
Description	**Schematic diagram**
I Double-layered wall with a central hypoechoic zone (i.e., the two outer and inner layers are hyperechoic, and middle layer is hypoechoic)	
II Two-layered pattern with a thickened inner hypoechoic layer	
III Lack of echolayering	
= hyperechoic layer	= hypoechoic layer

From Tsujimoto F, Miyamoto Y, Tada S: Differentiation of benign from malignant ascites by sonographic evaluation of gallbladder wall thickening. Radiology 1985;157:503-504; Tanno S, Obara T, Maguchi H, et al: Thickened inner hypoechoic layer of the gallbladder wall in the diagnosis of anomalous pancreaticobiliary ductal union with endosonography. Gastrointest Endosc 1997;46:520-526.

the upper limit of normal and may serve as a demarcation between "thin-walled" and "thick-walled" gallbladders. This is based on data that suggest up to 99% of normal controls have wall thicknesses of 3 mm or less.[1] The three ultra-sonographic patterns of the thickened gallbladder wall are summarized in Table 86-3.[3,4]

DISCUSSION

Histologically the gallbladder wall consists of five layers: mucosa, very thin submucosa, muscularis, subserosa and serosa. The gallbladder wall in endoscopic and intraductal ultrasound at 7.5 MHz is composed of three layers.[5] In *in vivo* ultrasound studies of resected gallbladders immersed in a water bath, Lu et al[6] visualized

five layers using a 10-MHz transducer (Table 86-4, Fig. 86-1).

Gallbladder wall thickness (GBWT) may be segmental or diffuse (Tables 86-5 and 86-6). Diffuse GBWT may be due to intrinsic causes or causes other than a diseased gallbladder. In patients with acute infectious diseases such as dengue hemorrhagic fever, mononucleosis syndromes, typhoid fever, and hemorrhagic fever with renal syndrome, the degree of GBWT is related to disease severity.[7-10] The degree of GBWT does not appear to correlate well with the severity of acute, chronic, and acalculous cholecystitis,[11] but it has been correlated to the rate of conversion of laparascopic to surgical cholecystectomy.[12] GBWT by itself is nonspecific in distinguishing gallbladder cancer from benign conditions.[13]

Table 86-4 **Sonohistopathologic correlation of layers visualized in wall of resected gallbladder specimens**

Reference	Ultrasonographic technique	No. of layers	Ultrasonographic appearance	Histologic correlation	Schematic diagram
Watanabe et al	In vitro IDUS (at 7.5 MHz): resected and incised gallbladders immersed in physiologic saline solution.	3	Innermost hyperechoic layer Middle hypoechoic layer Outermost hyperechoic layer	Mucosal layer + interface echo If <500 μM: muscle layer If ≥500 μM: muscle layer + fibrous tissue Perimuscular connective tissue layer + interface echo	
Lu et al	Resected gallbladders immersed in a water bath (10-MHz transducer)	5	Layer 1 (outermost layer): a hyperechoic layer Layer 2: hypoechoic or slightly echogenic layer Layer 3: relatively thin hyperechoic zone Layer 4: a hypoechoic layer Layer 5 (innermost layer): a hyperechoic layer	Echoes from interface between serosa and perigallbladder fluid Echoes from the subserosal tissues Echoes from the boundary between subserosa and muscular layer echoes from muscularis Combined echoes from the mucosa and the interface between the mucosa and bile	

▦ = hyperechoic layer   ⟩⟩⟩ = hypoechoic layer

GB, Gallbladder; EUS, endoscopic ultrasound; IDUS, intraductal ultrasound.
Thirty-one gallbladder specimens obtained by autopsy or surgery. In 24 cases, the gallbladder wall on ultrasonograms was composed of three layers. In seven cases the gallbladder wall was heterogeneously hypoechoic with destruction of the gallbladder wall structure by severe inflammation detected on histopathologic sections.
Thirty gallbladder specimens from patients undergoing elective cholecystecomy for cholelithiasis (23 cases), gallbladder tumor (two cases), and for other surgical diseases with indication for cholecystectomy (five cases) including gastric cancer and adenoma of duodenal papilla.
From Watanabe Y, Goto H, Naitoh Y, et al: Usefulness of intraductal ultrasonography in gallbladder disease. J Ultrasound Med 1998;17:33-39; Lu MD, Hirata T, Nishihara K, et al: Improved delineation of the gallbladder wall with ultrasonography: its value in assessment of the depth of carcinoma invasion. J Clin Ultrasound 1991;19:471-477.

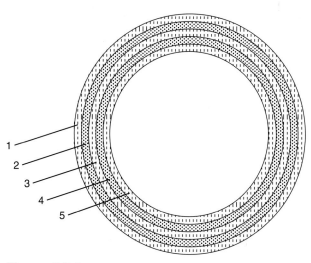

Figure 86-1
Schemata indicating the sonographic layers of the gallbladder wall as seen in resected gallbladders immersed in a water bath (10-MHz transducer). 1 = Outermost hyperechoic layer; 2 = hypoechoic layer or slightly hyperechoic layer; 3 = hyperechoic layer; 4 = hypoechoic layer; 5 = innermost hyperechoic layer. (From Lu MD, Hirata T, Nishihara K, et al: Improved delineation of the gallbladder wall with ultrasonography: its value in assessment of the depth of carcinoma invasion. J Clin Ultrasound 1991;19:471-477. Reprinted with permission of John Wiley & Sons, Inc.)

Gallbaldder Volume and Contractility

INTRODUCTION

The evaluation of gallbladder contraction is a technique for detecting gallbladder motor dysfunction, as is seen in chronic cholecystitis, chronic acalculous cholecystitis, biliary dyski-

Table 86-5	Causes of segmental gallbladder wall thickness

Adenomyomatosis
Gallbladder carcinoma
Xanthogranulomatous cholecystitis
Segmental chronic cholecystitis
Adherent gallstone or sludge
Polyp
Metastasis to gallbladder wall

From McGahan JP, Goldberg BB: Diagnostic Ultrasound: A Logical Approach. Philadelphia, Lippincott-Raven, 1998; Sato M, Ishida K, Konno K et al: Segmental chronic cholecystis: sonographic findings and clinical manifestations. Abdom Imaging 2002;27:43-46.

Table 86-6	Causes of diffuse gallbladder wall thickness

Intrinsic gallbladder causes	
Gallbladder contraction	
Acute cholecystits	
Chronic cholecystits	
Acute acalculous cholecystits	
Adenomyomatosis	
Gallbladder carcinoma	
Extrinsic causes	
Chronic liver diseases	Acute infectious diseases:
Congestive heart failure	Dengue hemorrhagic fever
Chronic renal failure	Mononucleosis syndromes
Acute and chronic pancreatitis	Typhoid fever
Myeloma	Hemorrhagic fever with renal syndrome
Acute pyelonephritis	Acute viral hepatitis
Pregnancy	Schistosoma mansoni infection
Parenteral nutrition	AIDS-related cholangiopathy (cytomegalovirus: Cryptosporidium)

Brogna A, Bucceri AM, Catalano F, et al: Ultrasound demonstration of gallbladder wall thickening as a method to differentiate cirrhotic ascites from other ascites. Invest Radiol 1996;31:80-83; Kim YO, Chun KA, Choi JY, et al: Sonographic evaluation of gallbladder wall thickening in hemorrhagic fever with renal syndrome: prediction of disease severity. J Clin Ultrasound 2001;29:286-289; Yamada K, Yamada H: Gallbladder wall thickening in mononucleosis syndromes. J Clin Ultrasound 2001;29:322-325.

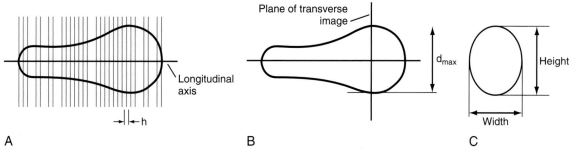

Figure 86-2
A, Sum-of-cylinders method for the calculation of gallbladder volume. A grid is placed on the longitudinal image of the gallbladder, perpendicular to the longitudinal axis. The grid lines are h millimeters apart.
B, A transverse scan of the gallbladder is obtained perpendicular to the longitudinal axis at the widest area of the gallbladder, which is d_{max} (maximal diameter). **C**, The maximal width and height are measured in the transverse image. This method of calculation has been computerized.[16]

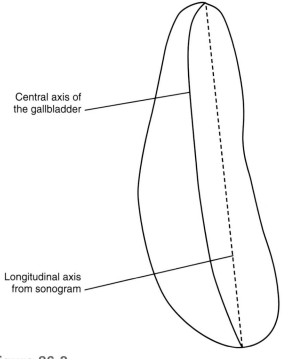

Figure 86-3
Correction factor (E) is applied to correct for displacement of the greatest longitudinal axis in the longitudinal image from the central axis of the gallbladder. (Reprinted from Everson GT, Braverman DZ, Johnson ML, et al: A critical evaluation of real-time ultrasonography for the study of gallbladder volume and contraction. Gastroenterology 1980;79:40-46. With permission from American Gastroenterological Association.)

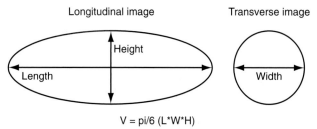

$$V = pi/6 \ (L*W*H)$$

Figure 86-4
Ellipsoidal method for the calculation of gallbladder volume. The maximal length and height are measured on the longitudinal image, and the maximal width is measured on the transverse image; alternatively, the maximal height can also be measured on the transverse image.

nesia, and the cystic duct syndrome. Gallbladder motor dysfunction may be present as a common pathogenetic pathway for systemic diseases to predispose to stone formation. Ultrasonography and cholescintigraphy are the two main imaging modalities used in the assessment of gallbladder motor function.

MATERIALS/MEASUREMENTS

Measurement of gallbladder volume forms the basis for the assessment of gallbladder motor function by ultrasonography. Gallbladder volume can be calculated using two- and three-dimensional, real-time ultrasound (Table 86-7, Figs. 86-2 to 86-4).[14-16]

Gallbladder volumes are determined in a fasting state and at different intervals following stimulation of gallbladder contraction. The two main categories of stimuli used to induce gallbladder contraction are meal stimulation and

Table 86-7	Methods for calculating gallbladder volume using two-dimensional ultrasound

Sum-of-cylinders method (Fig. 86-2)	Images	(1) A longitudinal image obtained through the greatest longitudinal axis of the GB
		(2) A transverse image obtained from a scan perpendicular to the long axis at the widest area of the GB
	Measurements	(1) A grid is placed on the longitudinal image so that lines spaced h millimeters apart are oriented at 90 degrees to the longitudinal GB axis, dividing it into cylinders h mm thick
		(2) From the transverse image, the maximal width (W, transverse diameter) and height (H, anteroposterior diameter) are measured
		(3) From the longitudinal image, the maximum diameter is measured (d_{max})
		All measurements are made from the inner gallbladder wall
	Calculation	The volumes of the individual cylinders are then summated (i.e., GB volume equals the sum of the volumes of the i number of cylinders with diameter d_i and equal height h):
		Volume = Σ(cross-sectional area × cylinder thickness) or
		Volume = $\Sigma(1/4$ pi × d_i^2 × h)
	Correction factor (E) (Fig. 86-3)	E is applied to correct for displacement of the greatest longitudinal axis in the longitudinal image from the central axis of the gallbladder
		E = (H + W)/(2 × d_{max})
	Corrected volume	Corrected Volume = E^2 × Volume
		Corrected Volume = E^2 × $\Sigma(1/4$ pi × d_i^2 × h)
Ellipsoidal method (Fig. 86-4)	Images	(1) A longitudinal image obtained through the greatest longitudinal axis of the GB
		(2) A transverse image obtained from a scan perpendicular to the long axis at the widest area of the GB
	Measurements	Maximum diameter of the length (L) on the longitudinal image and maximum diameter of the width (W) and height (H) on the transverse image
	Calculation	Volume = pi/6 × (L × W × H) or
		Volume = 0.523 × (L × W × H)

Σ, Sum of; h, height of individual cylinder, i.e., cylinder thickness, determined by the spaces between grid lines; pi, 3.14, d_i, diameter of each individual cylinder; E, correction factor; L, gallbladder length on longitudinal image; W, width (transverse diameter) of the gallbladder on the transverse image; H, height (anteroposterior diameter) of the gallbladder on the transverse image.
From Everson GT, Braverman DZ, Johnson ML, et al: A critical evaluation of real-time ultrasonography for the study of gallbladder volume and contraction. Gastroenterology 1980;79:40-46; Dodds WJ, Groh WJ, Darweesh RMA, et al: Sonographic measurement of gallbladder volume. AJR Am J Roentgenol 1985;145:1009-1011.

Table 86-8	Ultrasonographic gallbladder contractility parameters

Volumes

Fasting volume (FV) = GB volume after an overnight fast
Postprandial volume (PPV) = GB volume at time x poststimulus
Residual volume (RV) = minimum postprandial GB volume
Ejected volume (EV) = maximum emptying = difference between fasting and residual volumes

Fractions

Ejection fraction = contractility index = (EV/FV) × 100
Residual fraction = (RV/FV) × 100

GB, Gallbladder.

intravenous administration of cholecystokinin (cholecystokinin ultrasonography, CCK-US). The reduction in poststimulus GB volumes, by comparison with fasting GB volumes, has been used to define several ultrasonographic GB contractility parameters (Table 86-8).

GB hydrops has been defined as a longitudinal dimension greater than 8 or 10 cm or a transverse dimension greater than 4 cm.

DISCUSSION

Before the advent of three-dimensional sonography, the sum-of-cylinders (SOC) method was considered the gold standard for determining gallbladder volumes.[17] Hurrell et al[18] reported poor reproducibility of the SOC method in their patient population. Three-dimensional ultrasonography does not suffer from the shortcomings of two-dimensional methods, which depend on geometric assumptions, and therefore is more accurate, and possibly more reproducible, especially in determining the volumes of irregularly shaped or highly curved gallbladders.[19]

Simultaneous measurements of gallbladder ejection fraction (EF) by cholecystokinin ultrasonography and scintigraphy have yielded conflicting results.[20] Biliary scintigraphy remains the gold standard not only for measuring EF but also for determining cystic duct patency.[20,21]

There is no established physiological range for any of the gallbladder contractility parameters described earlier. Several factors are implicated in the wide variability in results obtained in the different studies:

1. *Subject-related differences*: wide individual variations in healthy subjects. as well as effects of age, sex, and body mass index.
2. *Methodological differences*: type of stimulus (meal versus cholecystokinin); dose and duration of dose administration of cholecystokinin and its analogs; consistency (solid or liquid), composition, and quantity of meal stimulus; use of different definitions for some of the gallbladder function parameters including the timing of postprandial volume measurements.
3. *Conceptual problems*: conventionally, the response of the gallbladder to food or cholecystokinin administration has been described as continuous emptying followed by refilling. A new concept of gallbladder response to a stimulus has been proposed in which these two phases are replaced by several small, rapidly alternating phases of emptying and refilling.[22]

References

1. Deitch EA: Utility and clinical accuracy of ultrasonically measured gallbladder wall as a diagnostic criteria in biliary tract disease. Dig Dis Sci 1981;26:686-693.
2. McGahan JP, Goldberg BB: Diagnostic Ultrasound: A Logical Approach. Philadelphia, New York, Lippincott-Raven, 1998.
3. Tsujimoto F, Miyamoto Y, Tada S: Differentiation of benign from malignant ascites by sonographic evaluation of gallbladder wall: Radiology 1985;157:503-504.

4. Tanno S, Obara T, Maguchi H, et al: Thickened inner hypoechoic layer of the gallbladder wall in the diagnosis of anomalous pancreaticobiliary ductal union with endosonography. Gastrointest Endosc 1997;46:520-526

5. Watanabe Y, Goto H, Naitoh Y, et al: Usefulness of intraductal ultrasonography in gallbladder disease. J Ultrasound Med 1998;17:333-339.

6. Lu MD, Hirata T, Nishihara K, et al: Improved delineation of the gallbladder wall with ultrasonography: its value in assessment of the depth of carcinoma invasion. J Clin Ultrasound 1991;19:471-477.

7. Brogna A, Bucceri AM, Catalano F, et al: Ultrasound demonstration of gallbladder wall thickening as a method to differentiate cirrhotic ascites from other ascites. Invest Radiol 1996;31:80-83.

8. Kim YO, Chun KA, Choi JY, et al: Sonographic evaluation of gallbladder wall thickening in hemorrhagic fever with renal syndrome: prediction of disease severity. J Clin Ultrasound 2001;29:286-289.

9. Yamada K, Yamada H: Gallbladder wall thickening in mononucleosis syndromes. J Clin Ultrasound 2001;29:322-325.

10. Sato M, Ishida H, Konno K, et al: Segmental chronic cholecystis: sonographic findings and clinical manifestations. Abdom Imaging 2002;27:43-46.

11. Sariego J, Matsumoto T, Kerstein M: Significance of wall thickness in symptomatic gallbladder disease. Arch Surg 1992;127:1216-1218.

12. Jansen S, Jorgensen J, Caplehorn J, et al: Preoperative ultrasound to predict conversion in laparoscopic cholecystectomy. Surg Laparosc Endosc 1997;7:121-123.

13. Wibbenmeyer LA, Sharafuddin MJA, Wolverson MK, et al: Sonographic diagnosis of unsuspected gallbladder cancer: imaging findings in comparison with benign gallbladder conditions. AJR Am J Roentgenol 1995;165:1169-1174.

14. Everson GT, Braverman DZ, Johnson ML, et al: A critical evaluation of real-time ultrasonography for the study of gallbladder volume and contraction. Gastroenterology 1980;79:40-46.

15. Dodds WJ, Groh WJ, Darweesh RMA, et al: Sonographic measurement of gallbladder volume. AJR Am J Roentgenol 1985;145:1009-1011.

16. Hopman WPM, Brouwer WFM, Rosenbusch G, et al: A computerized method for rapid quantification of gallbladder volume from real-time sonograms. Radiology 1985;154:236-237.

17. Wedmann B, Schmidt G, Wegener M, et al: Sonographic evaluation of gallbladder kinetics: in vitro and in vivo comparison of different methods to assess gallbladder emptying. J Clin Ultrasound 1991;19:341-349.

18. Hurrell MA, Chapman BA, Wilson IR: Variation in the estimation of gallbladder volume using the sum-of-cylinders method. Invest Radiol 1994;29:536-539.

19. Hashimoto S, Goto H, Hirooka Y, et al: An evaluation of three-dimensional ultrasonography for the measurement of gallbladder volume. Am J Gastroenterol 1999;94:3492-3496.

20. Siegel A, Kuhn JC, Crow H, et al: Gallbladder ejection fraction: correlation of scintigraphic and ultrasonographic techniques. Clin Nucl Med 2000;25:1-6.

21. Okulski TA, Eikman EA, Williams JW: Ultrasound measurement of contraction response of the gallbladder: comparison with the radionuclide test for cystic duct patency. Clin Nucl Med 1982;7:117-121.

22. Jazrawi RP: Review article: measurement of gall-bladder motor function in health and disease. Aliment Pharmacol Ther 2000;14 (suppl 2):27-31.

CHAPTER 87

Bijan Bijan
Hedieh Eslamy
John P. McGahan

Ultrasound Measurements of the Pancreas

Normal Ultrasound Measurements of the Pancreas

INTRODUCTION

Ultrasound (US) can be used to measure the anteroposterior (Fig. 87-1) and longitudinal (cephalocaudal) dimensions (Fig. 87-2) and areas of the pancreatic body, head, and tail (Table 87-1).

MATERIALS/MEASUREMENTS

Abdominal US is performed after a minimum fasting of 6 hours to allow for distention of the gallbladder. The fasting state may also improve visualization of the pancreas because there is less gaseous distention of the stomach and upper gastrointestinal tract. Scanning is performed with a curved array or sector 3.5- to 5-MHz transducer. The patient's position is varied to minimize intervening bowel gas, and

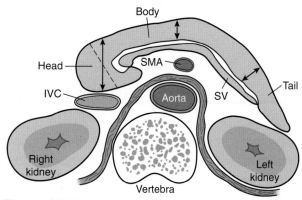

Figure 87-1
Measurements of the anteroposterior dimensions of the pancreas from axial/transverse images. Typically the true anteroposterior dimensions of the body and head (through the middle of each portion or the maximal dimension) are measured. The tail thickness is measured perpendicular to the long axis of the tail. Note that, on CT, measurements may be made perpendicular to the long axis of the pancreatic head (dotted line with arrows). SMA, Superior mesenteric artery; SV, splenic vein; IVC, inferior vena cava. (Modified from Keats TE, Sistrom C: Atlas of Radiologic Measurement, 7th ed. St Louis, Mosby, 2001.)

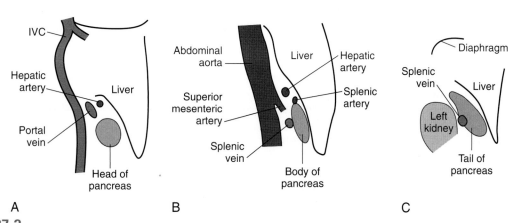

Figure 87-2
Schematic presentation of the parasagittal planes for the measurements of the longitudinal (cepahalocaudal) dimensions of the pancreatic (a) head, (b) body, and (c) tail. In Haber et al's[7] study, measurements were carried out in three specified anatomical areas: (a) the pancreatic head was measured in the plane to the right of the midline in which it appeared the largest, (b) the body of the pancreas was measured in the immediate preaortic region, and (c) the tail of the pancreas was evaluated in the medial prerenal area.

Table 87-1	Overview of ultrasound measurements of the pancreas
Images used for measurement	Transverse/oblique images of the pancreatic head, body, and tail
	Sagittal images of the pancreatic head, body, and tail
Diameter measured	Pancreatic head and body: the true anteroposterior dimensions are measured; pancreatic tail: thickness is measured perpendicular to the long axis of the tail
	Longitudinal (cephalocaudal diameter)
Location of measurements	(a) maximum anteroposterior diameter of each section or
	(b) the diameter of each section in its mid-portion
	Pancreatic head: the plane to the right of the midline in which it appears the largest
	Pancreatic body: the immediate preaortic region
	Pancreatic tail: the medial prerenal area

Table 87-2	Anteroposterior dimensions of the pancreas in healthy subjects				
Reference	Age (Yrs)	N	Head	Body	Tail
Niederau	18-65	1000	2.2 ± 0.3	1.8 ± 0.3	—
Weill	17-85	135	1.7 ± 0.5	1.0 ± 0.3	1.5 ± 0.7
Haber	Adult	382	2.7 ± 0.7	2.2 ± 0.7	2.4 ± 0.4

All measurements in centimeters and reported as mean ± standard deviation.
From Niederau C, Sonnenberg A, Muller JE, et al: Sonographic measurements of the normal liver, spleen, pancreas, and portal vein. Radiology 1983;149:537-540; Weill F, Schraub A, Eisenscher A, et al: Ultrasonography of the normal pancreas. Success rate and criteria for normality. Radiology 1977;123:417-423; Haber K, Freimanis AK, Asher WM: Demonstration and dimensional analysis of the normal pancreas with gray-scale echography. AJR Am J Roentgenol 1976;126:624-628.

scans may be obtained in the erect, supine, and shallow left or right decubitus positions. US offers multiplanar imaging of the pancreas.[1]

Gastrointestinal tract air may significantly limit pancreatic visualization caused by artifact on US. To eliminate shadowing from intraluminal air, the stomach can be filled with fluid (degassed water is most commonly used), orally administered US contrast agents, or a combination of water and simethicone.[1]

The pancreas is defined by the adjacent vasculature. On transverse US images, the body of the pancreas is seen anterior to the splenic vein, with the superior mesenteric vein and artery visualized posteriorly. The left renal vein courses transversely between the superior mesenteric vein and aorta. On sagittal views, the pancreas contacts the inferior vena cava.[1]

In transverse/oblique images of the pancreatic head, body, and tail, either the maximum anteroposterior diameter of each section or the diameter of each section in its midportion is measured. Typically the true anteroposterior

dimensions of the pancreatic head and body are measured. The tail thickness is measured perpendicular to the long axis of the tail (see Fig. 87-1).

In sagittal images of the pancreatic head, body, and tail, the maximum longitudinal (cephalocaudal) diameter of each section is measured. The cross-sectional area of the pancreas in transverse images and the cross-sectional area of each section (head, body, tail) of the pancreas in longitudinal images have also been determined.[2,3]

DISCUSSION

The normal anteroposterior and longitudinal dimensions of the pancreatic head, body, and tail have been reported (Figs. 87-1 and 87-2, Tables 87-2 and 87-3).

Several authors have determined the size of the pancreas in insulin-dependent (IDDM) and noninsulin-dependent diabetes mellitus

Table 87-3	Longitudinal dimensions of the pancreas in healthy subjects				
Reference	**Age**	***N.***	**Head**	**Body**	**Tail**
Haber	Adult	382	3.6 ± 1.2	3.0 ± 0.6	2.9 ± 0.4

All measurements in centimeters and reported as mean ± standard deviation.
Data from Haber K, Freimanis AK, Asher WM: Demonstration and dimensional analysis of the normal pancreas with gray-scale echography. AJR Am J Roentgenol 1976;126:624-628.

Table 87-4	Overview of ultrasound measurements of the pancreatic duct
Images used for measurement	Transverse images of the pancreatic head and body
Diameter measured	Anteroposterior diameter is measured perpendicular to the pancreatic duct lumen in the pancreatic head and body
Caliper placement	(a) from inside of the near wall to inside of the far wall (i.e., *intraluminal diameter*) or
	(b) from outside of the near wall to outside of the far wall (i.e., complete pancreatic duct diameter *inclusive of echoic wall structures*)
Location of measurements	Pancreatic head
	Pancreatic body: may be measured anterior to the aorta

(NIDDM). They have concluded that diabetes affects the growth of the pancreas in children with IDDM and that, in adults, the pancreas is a smaller organ in patients with diabetes mellitus, and the decrement in size is maximal in IDDM subjects.[2,8,9]

Shawker et al[10] have examined the pancreatic size in patients with cystic fibrosis (as a model for chronic pancreatitis). They concluded that pancreatic size was of no diagnostic significance in this patient population, probably because the increase in echo amplitude in the diseased pancreas causes it to blend imperceptibly with the peripancreatic soft tissues rendering measurement of pancreatic size inaccurate.

Di Giandomenico et al[3] have evaluated the reproducibility of US measurements of pancreatic size in healthy volunteers. They concluded that US of the pancreas should be performed in the morning with the patient in the fasting state, as in these conditions the reliability of US measurements of the gland appears to be highest.

Nikolaidis et al[11] have reviewed the role of sonography in the evaluation of the pancreatic transplant. Several factors limit the utility of gray scale US in evaluating the complications of this procedure:

- Overlying bowel gas often obscures the pancreas

- The graft lacks an investing capsule, which often renders its borders indistinct
- Without the presence of the adjacent liver to be used as an acoustic window and a basis for comparison, the ability to determine the changes in echogenicity of the transplanted pancreas is limited

The most important role for US is in the evaluation of the pancreatic transplant vasculature using color and spectral Doppler sonography.[1]

Normal Ultrasound Measurements of the Pancreatic Duct

INTRODUCTION

US can be used to measure the pancreatic duct diameter in transverse images of the pancreas (Table 87-4, Fig. 87-3).

MATERIALS/MEASUREMENTS

The prerequisites (fasting state, transducer characteristics, patient position, agents used to eliminate shadowing from intraluminal air) for the visualization of the pancreatic duct are the same as those mentioned earlier for the visualization of the pancreas.

The pancreatic duct is best seen in transverse images. The pancreatic duct lumen is measured between the inside of the anterior and posterior walls anteroposteriorly, or the complete pancreatic duct diameter inclusive of echoic wall structures is measured; the measurements are made perpendicular to the pancreatic duct lumen. The lumen of the pancreatic duct is usually largest in the head of the pancreas and decreases gradually toward the body. It is normally less than 2 mm in diameter in the body of the pancreas and less than 3 mm in the head (see Fig. 87-3).[12,13]

Secretin administration (typically 1 CU/kg, IV bolus) induces a brief, distinct dilatation of the main pancreatic duct in healthy persons, visible at ultrasonography. The pancreatic duct is typically measured in the body of the pancreas posterior to the aorta in transverse images, before and sequentially after the administration of secretin.[13] The parameters that can be measured and some representative measurements are listed in Tables 87-5 and 87-6. The normal range of these parameters has not been established.[14]

DISCUSSION

Tanaka et al[15] measured the pancreatic duct diameter, in the body of the pancreas, in 10,244 subjects without pancreatic diseases. Their findings showed the higher age group to have a higher proportion of main pancreatic duct dilatation (Table 87-7).

Hastier et al[16] have similarly studied the effect of age on pancreatic duct diameter and concluded that the majority of elderly who do not have pancreatic pathology have a dilated pancreatic duct by comparison with younger controls.

Several authors have concluded that the dilatation of the main pancreatic duct after secretin challenge was due to stimulation of pancreatic secretion and/or the effects of secretin on the motility of the sphincter of Oddi (i.e., an initial pressure increase in the sphincter of Oddi followed by a decrease). The reason for the small relative change in pancreatic duct diameter following secretin challenge in patients with chronic pancreatitis might well be periductal

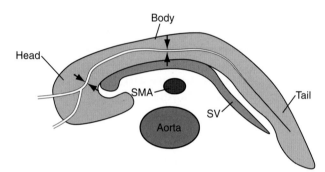

Figure 87-3
The main pancreatic duct can be measured in the pancreatic head and body, perpendicular to the duct lumen, in transverse images. Measurements are made either inclusive or exclusive of the echogenic pancreatic duct walls.

Table 87-5	Parameters that can be measured in ultrasound-secretin test
Parameter	**Definition**
Basal PDD	Main PDD before administration of secretin
PDDx	Main PDD at time x postsecretin administration (typically at 5-min intervals for 10-40 min, but shorter intervals during the first 5-6 min)
Max PDD	Maximal PDD after injection
Max/basal ratio	(Max PDD/Basal PDD) × 100
Delta	Max PDD − Basal PDD
Max time	The time required to reach maximal dilatation after secretin administration

PDD, Pancreatic duct diameter.

Table 87-6 Ultrasound secretin test parameters in three subject groups

		Control group N 30	Subjects Probable chronic pancreatitis 26	Definite chronic pancreatitis 14
Basal PDD (mm)	mean ± SD	1.07 ± 0.09	1.13 ± 0.09	3.29 ± 0.79
	p value[a]	<0.0001	<0.0001	—
Max PDD (mm)	mean ± SD	1.9 ± 0.16	1.73 ± 0.11	4.14 ± 0.94
	p value[a]	<0.0001	<0.0001	—
Max/Basal ratio	mean ± SD	185 ± 9 %	161 ± 8%	134 ± 8%
	p value[b]	—	<0.05	<0.001
Max time (min)	mean ± SD	3.07 ± 0.39	3.24 ± 0.6	4.77 ± 1.14
	p value[b]	—	N.S.	N.S.

(a) p value = difference between the mean parameter in either the control or probable chronic pancreatitis groups and the definite chronic pancreatitis group.
(b) p value = difference between the mean parameter in either the probable or definite chronic pancreatitis groups and the control group.
N.S. = Not significant.
From Osawa S, Kataoka K, Sakagami J, et al: Relation between morphologic changes in the main pancreatic duct and exocrine pancreatic function after a secretin test. Pancreas 2002;25:12-19.

Table 87-7 Main pancreatic duct diameter, measured in the body of the pancreas, in healthy subjects

	Pancreatic duct diameter (mm)		
Age range (yrs)	N	PDD: ≤2 n (%)	PDD: ≤3 n (%)
<25	127	1 (0.79)	0 (0)
26-50	2219	54 (2.43)	11 (0.54)
51-75	7146	382 (5.35)	89 (1.25)
≥76	752	78 (10.37)	24 (3.19)
All ages	10,244	515 (5.03)	124 (1.21)

PDD, Pancreatic duct diameter.
From Tanaka S, Nakaizumi A, Ioka T, et al: Main pancreatic duct dilatation: a sign of high risk for pancreatic cancer. Jpn J Clin Oncol 2002;32:407-411.

fibrosis (leading to rigid fixation of the duct) and intralobular fibrosis (with a loss of exocrine function).[14] US-secretin test may prove to be a useful tool in the diagnosis of pancreatic diseases that are secondary to a functional or anatomical pancreatic outlet obstruction, replacing the need for the more invasive or expensive procedures such as ERCP, sphincter of Oddi manometry, MRCP, and EUS.

Tanaka et al[15] have retrospectively examined the main pancreatic duct (MPD) diameter, in the body of the pancreas, in a precancer group and have concluded that slight dilatation of the MPD appears to be a sign of higher risk for pancreatic cancer. They defined borderline dilatation as 2 to 3 mm and frank dilatation as above 3 mm, as measured in the pancreatic body.

Pancreatic duct diameter values measured by ERCP are higher than the values measured by ultrasound. This may be due to several factors, which are summarized in Table 87-8.[12,17]

Table 87-8	Factors that may contribute to higher pancreatic duct diameters measured by ERCP than the values measured by ultrasound

Radiographic magnification of the main pancreatic duct
Hyperechogenicity of the MPD wall on US
Overdistention of MPD at ERCP due to the instilled contrast material
US is performed under normal physiological circumstances without premedication, while
ERCP is not

MPD, Main pancreatic duct; US, ultrasononography; ERCP = endoscopic retrograde cholangiopancreatography.
From Hadidi A: Pancreatic duct diameter: sonographic measurement in normal subjects. J Clin Ultrasound 1983;11:17-22; Bastid C, Sahel J, Filho M, et al: Diameter of the main pancreatic duct in chronic calcifying pancreatitis. Measurements by ultrasonography versus pancreatography. Pancreas 1990;5:524-527.

References

1. Bennett GL, Hann LE: Pancreatic Ultrasonography. Surg Clin North Am 2001;81:259-281.
2. Altobelli E, Blasetti A, Verrotti A, et al: Size of pancreas in children and adolescents with type I (insulin-dependent) diabetes. J Clin Ultrasound 1998;26:391-395.
3. Di Giandomenico V, Filippone A, Basilico R, et al: Reproducibility of ultrasound measurement of pancreatic size with new advanced high-resolution dynamic image scanners. J Clin Ultrasound 1993;21:77-86.
4. Keats TE, Sistrom C: Atlas of Radiologic Measurement, 7th ed. St Louis, Mosby, 2001.
5. Niederau C, Sonnenberg A, Muller JE, et al: Sonographic measurements of the normal liver, spleen, pancreas, and portal vein. Radiology 1983;149:537-540.
6. Weill F, Schraub A, Eisenscher A, et al: Ultrasonography of the normal pancreas. Success rate and criteria for normality. Radiology 1977;123:417-423.
7. Haber K, Freimanis AK, Asher WM: Demonstration and dimensional analysis of the normal pancreas with gray-scale echography. AJR Am J Roentgenol 1976;126:624-628.
8. Alzaid A, Aideyan O, Nawaz S: The size of the pancreas in diabetes mellitus. Diabet Med 1993;10:759-763.
9. Silva ME, Vezozzo DP, Ursich MJ, et al: Ultrasonographic abnormalities of the pancreas in IDDM and NIDDM patients. Diabetes Care 1993;16:1296-1297.
10. Shawker TH, Linzer M, Hubbard VS: Chronic pancreatitis: the diagnostic significance of pancreatic size and echo amplitude. J Ultrasound Med 1984;3:267-272.
11. Nikolaidis P, Amin RS, Hwang CM, et al: Role of sonography in pancreatic transplantation. Radiographics 2003;23:939-949.
12. Hadidi A: Pancreatic duct diameter: sonographic measurement in normal subjects. J Clin Ultrasound 1983;11:17-22.
13. Glaser J, Hogemann B, Schneider M, et al: Significance of a sonographic secretin test in the diagnosis of pancreatic disease. Results of a prospective study. Scand J Gastroenterol 1989;24:179-185.
14. Osawa S, Kataoka K, Sakagami J, et al: Relation between morphologic changes in the main pancreatic duct and exocrine pancreatic function after a secretin test. Pancreas 2002;25:12-19.
15. Tanaka S, Nakaizumi A, Ioka T, et al: Main pancreatic duct dilatation: a sign of high risk for pancreatic cancer. Jpn J Clin Oncol 2002;32:407-411.
16. Hastier P, Buckley MJ, Dumas R, et al: A study of the effect of age on pancreatic duct morphology. Gastrointest Endosc 1998;48:53-57.
17. Bastid C, Sahel J, Filho M, et al: Diameter of the main pancreatic duct in chronic calcifying pancreatitis. Measurements by ultrasonography versus pancreatography. Pancreas 1990;5:524-527.

Ultrasound Measurements of the Spleen

Suhas G. Parulekar
Aparna Balachandran

Clinical and Anatomical

The normal spleen is variable in size and shape with wide ranges of normal limits. Reports using autopsy material found poor correlation of splenic weight with patient body habitus but found that the spleen tended to decrease in size with age and increase in size with weight, height, and surface area.[1,2]

It is widely accepted that a palpable spleen in the adult population usually indicates an enlarged spleen. This is done by palpating for the splenic tip below the costal margin. However, studies on subjects with a palpable spleen, who were further evaluated by scintigraphy, have shown that these spleens were not necessarily enlarged or abnormal.[3,4] Thus there is limited use of physical examination in accurately assessing the spleen size.

Ultrasound

Ultrasound is both reliable and quick in the assessment of splenic dimensions. However, in some patients ultrasound measurements of the dimensions of the spleen can be technically difficult and limited because of overlying structures such as bone, bowel gas, or lung. Also, the volume measurements of the spleen with ultrasound can be technically limited because of variable contour of the spleen and difficulty in completely scanning the entire spleen or visualizing complete contours of the spleen.

The ultrasound scanning techniques vary from author to author, using longitudinal sections in sagittal or coronal plane. The longitudinal and transverse sections are obtained with the patient either in supine or in right lateral decubitus position. Maximum splenic length is measured (on sagittal or coronal scan) from the dome to the inferior tip of the spleen. Some authors have measured the length in straight longitudinal plane (Fig. 88-1); however, this can

be frequently technically difficult, and therefore other authors have measured the length in oblique longitudinal plane (Fig. 88-2).

Earlier investigators used static ultrasound scanners with articulated arm for determination of splenic size and volume measurements. More recent reports have used real-time two- and three-dimensional ultrasound scanners. Real-time extended field of view scanning is helpful in measuring spleen, especially when the spleen is enlarged (Fig. 88-3). Otherwise, because of the limited field of view of the real-time sector scanners, it is difficult, if not impossible, to accurately measure the spleen, especially when the spleen is considerably enlarged.

An ultrasound study of 800 normal adults by Frank et al[5] found that in 95% of patients the length of the spleen was less than 12 cm,

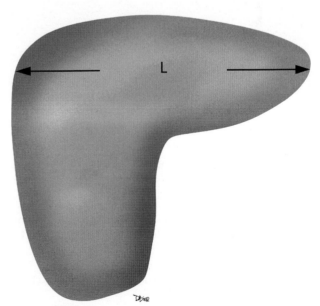

Figure 88-1
Longitudinal view of the spleen.
The length (L) is measured in straight longitudinal plane.

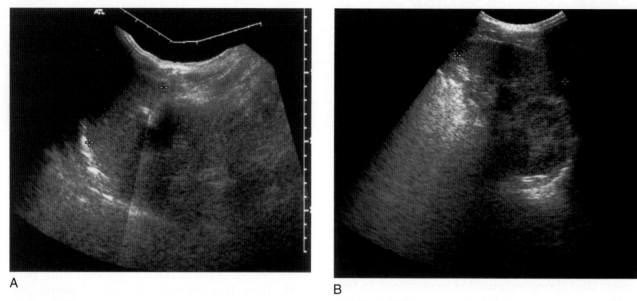

A

B

Figure 88-2
Longitudinal (**A**) and transverse (**B**) ultrasound of normal size spleen.
In **A**, (extended field of view technique), length is measured in oblique longitudinal plane.

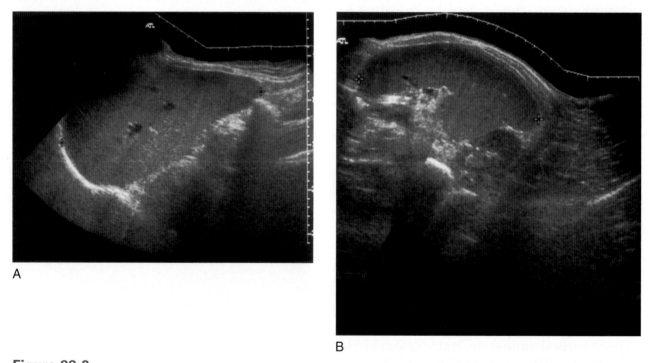

A

B

Figure 88-3
Longitudinal (**A**) and transverse (**B**) ultrasound of enlarged spleen. Extended field of view technique.
Spleen measures 24 cm in length (**A**) and 18 cm in transverse dimension (**B**).

breadth less than 7 cm, and thickness less than 5 cm.

In another study by De Odorico et al,[6] mean two-dimensional ultrasound measurements of normal spleen (with range in parentheses) were: (1) length 9.11 cm (5.96-12.36 cm) (2) width

9.55 cm (6.41-13.03 cm) (3) thickness 4.09 cm (2.59-6.73 cm), and (4) the mean normal splenic volume was 191.54 cc (82.97-411.79 cc).

Niederau et al[7] found the longitudinal diameter of the normal spleen to be 5.8 ± 1.8 cm (mean ± sd). The margin between the lung and spleen served as the upper limit of the longitudinal diameter. The authors felt that it is not necessary to routinely correct the measured diameters for physical data (height, weight, and body surface area).

A recent study Loftus et al[8] evaluated the relationship between the maximum oblique sagittal diameter of the spleen as determined by sonography of 30 cadavers before autopsy and the actual splenic length, volume, and weight following autopsy. The greatest splenic length was measured in an oblique sagittal plane through the splenic hilum. This study showed that there was a good correlation between the maximum sonographic length of the spleen and the actual splenic length, and there was close correlation between maximum sonographic splenic length and both splenic volume and weight.

Splenic Volume

Different authors have calculated the splenic volume by calculating the three diameters of the spleen and by using some combination of the product of these three diameters. The calculated splenic volume on multiple studies correlates strongly (better than the diameter measurement) with the actual volume.

A study by De Odorico et al[6] evaluated two-versus three-dimensional ultrasound in splenic volume assessment. Conventional two-dimensional ultrasound images of the spleen were obtained by scanning in sagittal and transverse plane. The splenic length, width, and thickness were measured (see Fig. 88-1 and 88-4). The length was measured along the long axis, from the dome to the tip of the spleen, in sagittal plane. The width was the longest organ diameter in the transverse plane. The thickness was the distance between the inner and outer surface of the spleen, measured at the level of splenic hilum on the transverse plane. Splenic volume was then calculated using the standard prolated ellipsoid formula of length × width × thickness × 0.523. The mean normal splenic volume was 191.54 cc (with a range of 82.97 to 411.79 cc).

In the same study,[6] three-dimensional ultrasound volume data were acquired with the transducer positioned in the sagittal plane. The splenic volume was calculated: (1) from the volume acquisition by measuring splenic length, width, and thickness (splenic volume ellipsoid) and (2) with a slice-by-slice technique (three-dimensional volume planar). Three-dimensional

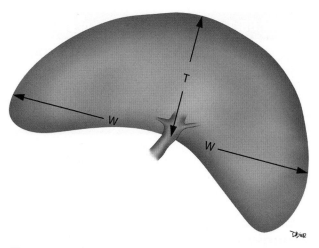

Figure 88-4
Splenic width and thickness measured on transverse view.
The width (W) is the longest diameter in the transverse plane. Thickness (T) is measured at the level of the splenic hilum on transverse view.

ultrasound was found to be more accurate for measuring splenic volume than currently used techniques employing conventional two-dimensional ultrasound. In vitro splenic measurements indicated that three-dimensional volumes calculated using the planar method were accurate to within 2%.

A recent study[9] using CT evaluated the normal splenic volume by measuring the longitudinal, maximal transverse, and maximal anteroposterior diameter of the spleen and using the formula: volume = 30 + 0.58 (width × length × thickness). The longitudinal diameter was assesed from the number of consecutive CT sections through the spleen. This correlated well with the splenic volume calculated with the summation technique (measured by the summation of the splenic areas on each transaxial image). The mean value of the normal splenic volume was 214.6 cc with a range from 107.2 to 314.5 cc. There was a statistically significant correlation between the splenic volume and area and all the diameters of the spleen. Of all the diameters, the longitudinal diameter of the spleen had the highest correlation with the splenic volume. The product of all three diameters had the highest correlation with the splenic volume.

A sonographic study by Yetter et al[10] concluded that estimating splenic volume with the formula

$$0.524 \times W \times T \times [(ML + CCL)/2]$$

provides the greatest overall accuracy. W (width) and T (thickness) were measured on transverse

Table 88-1	Normal dimensions of spleen (cm)		
	Height (length)	**Breadth**	**Thickness**
Mean ± SD	9 ± 1.7	8 ± 1.2	8 ± 1.7
Range	5.5-14	6-12	5-12

Modified from Pietri H, et al: Determination of splenic volume index by ultrasonic scanning. J Ultrasound Med 1984;3:19-23.

images. ML (maximum length) and CCL (craniocaudal length) were measured on the longitudinal image.

Splenic Volume Index

Pietri and Boscaini,[11] using an articulating arm static scanner, measured height (H) (length), breadth (B) (maximal transverse diameter), and thickness (T) (maximal anteroposterior diameter) and calculated a splenic volume index (SVI), where SVI = H × B × T divided by 27. Ninety-five percent of normals had an SVI between 8 and 34 (mean ± SD = 21.5 ± 6.5). There were no statistically significant differences related to age, sex, or morphotype. They also measured normal dimensions of spleen as given in Table 88-1.

Splenic Index

Ishibashi et al[12] calculated spleen index using ultrasound measurements in patients (Japanese population) with normal and enlarged spleens. Longitudinal section of the spleen was obtained in right lateral decubitus position. Both transverse and vertical diameters were measured on the longitudinal section image and margin between the lung and spleen served as the upper limit on the longitudinal image. Spleen was measured with breath holding in deep inspiration. The spleen index (SI) was obtained by the following formula: SI (cm^2) = a (cm) × b (cm), where a is transverse diameter and b is the vertical diameter of the maximal cross-sectional image of the spleen. The SI correlated well with the volume of the spleen. The normal value of SI obtained from 204 healthy adults was 19.8 ± 12.3 cm^2. SI was arbitrarily classified into five grades—Grade 0 = 0 to 30 cm^2, Grade I = 31 to 60 cm^2, Grade II = 61 to 90 cm^2, Grade III = 91 to 120 cm^2, and Grade IV = more than 120 cm^2. Practically, spleens of grade I, II, III, and IV represent mild, moderate, marked, and marked to massive splenomegaly,

respectively. SI of more than 150 cm^2 was considered to indicate massive splenomegaly.

Conclusion

Spleen size estimation is important in patients with different clinical conditions, such as portal hypertension, lymphoma, and leukemia. Splenic volume calculation by imaging has proven to be the most accurate method of assessing splenic size. However, these calculations can be cumbersome in routine clinical practice. Studies have shown that evaluating the maximum longitudinal diameter of the spleen may be useful as a quick, alternative method to assess the splenic size. Loftus et al[8] found that a single, simple sonographic measurement of the maximum length of the spleen gives a clinically useful indication of splenic size and is more practical than splenic area or volume measurements, which can be reserved for problematic or borderline cases.

Summarizing measurements from various investigators, it appears that maximum splenic length (i.e., longitudinal diameter) in excess of 13 cm would indicate the presence of splenomegaly.

References

1. Krumbhaar EB, Lippincott SW: The postmortem weight of the "normal" human spleen at different ages. Am J Med Sci 1939; 197:344-359.
2. DeLand FH: Normal spleen size. Radiology 1970;97:589-592.
3. Arkles LB, Gill GD, Molan MP: A palpable spleen is not necessarily enlarged or pathological. Med J Aust 1986;145:15-17.
4. Zhang B, Lewis SM: A study of the reliability of clinical palpation of the spleen. Clin Lab Haematol 1989;11:7-10.
5. Frank K, Linhart P, Kortsik C, et al: Sonographic determination of spleen size: normal

dimensions in adults with a healthy spleen. Ultraschall Med 1986;7:134-137.

6. De Odorico I, Spaulding KA, Pretorius DH, et al: Normal splenic volumes estimated using three-dimensional ultrasonography. J Ultrasound Med 1999;18:231-236.

7. Niederau C, Sonnenberg A, Muller JE, et al: Sonographic measurements of the normal liver, spleen, pancreas, and portal vein. Radiology 1983;149:537-540.

8. Loftus WK, Chow LT, Metreweli C: Sonographic measurement of splenic length: correlation with measurement at autopsy. J Clin Ultrasound 1999;27:71-74.

9. Prassopoulos P, Daskalogiannaki M, Raissaki M, et al: Determination of normal splenic volume on computed tomography in relation to age, gender and body habitus. Eur Radiol 1997;7:246-248.

10. Yetter EM, Acosta KB, Olson MC, et al: Estimating splenic volume: sonographic measurements correlated with helical CT determination. AJR 2003;181:1615-1620.

11. Pietri H, Boscaini M: Determination of splenic volume index by ultrasonic scanning. J Ultrasound Med 1984;3:19-23.

12. Ishibashi H, Higuchi N, Shimamura R, et al: Sonographic assessment and grading of spleen size. J Clin Ultrasound 1991;19: 21-25.

CHAPTER 89

John P. McGahan

Ultrasound Measurements of the Gastrointestinal Tract

The gastrointestinal tract can be examined by ultrasound using either the transabdominal or endoluminal approach. Early work was focused on the use of transabdominal sonography to evaluate the bowel. This still remains a very popular technique in examining the appendix and pylorus of neonates. With the advent of high-resolution endoluminal probes, sonography has been shown to be an excellent technique in examining the GI tract.

Material/Measurements

Transabdominal graded-compression sonography is a useful technique to differentiate normal from abnormal bowel. Normally, the bowel wall and lumen will collapse with gentle probe pressure. Abnormal bowel wall will appear thickened and will not collapse with probe pressure. Usually, precise measurements of the bowel are not made with sonography. This is due to the fact that the bowel is usually not adequately distended when examined. There are two exceptions to this rule. These common exceptions are when examining the pylorus and appendix. Measurements for the pediatric pylorus and appendix are disussed in the pediatric section.

APPENDIX

In the adult patient the most frequent sonographic finding of acute appendicitis is a noncompressible appendix with a wall diameter greater than 6 mm.[1] The technique for examining the appendix includes use of a high-resolution (>5 MHz), usually linear array probe, using gentle compression. However, Jeffrey et al[2] published that an appendix 5 mm or less is normal and an appendix greater than 7 mm should be considered abnormal. He felt an appendix between 5 and 7 mm should be considered equivocal. Other important findings for appendicitis are listed in Table 89-1. Certainly, altering the criteria for appendiceal wall thickness will alter the sensitivity or specificity of the technique. Although earlier authors did not mention detection of the normal appendix, other publications have shown a normal appendix may be seen using optimal technique. Rioux[3] showed the mean wall thickness of the normal appendix was 1.8 mm and varied between 0.5 and 3 mm.

STOMACH, SMALL AND LARGE INTESTINES

The most detailed review of the measurement of this normal bone thickness measured during transabdominal scanning was published by Fleisher et al.[4] In his article, he showed that an average thickness of nondistended bowel was 5 mm and that of the distended bowel was less, measuring 3 mm. There was little variation in the measurements of the thickness of the distended stomach, small bowel, or large bowel.

Variation was from 2 to 4 mm. This is listed in Table 89-2. There was greater variability of the measurement of the nondistended bowel (see Table 89-2). Even with this variability, they felt that a bowel wall greater than 5 mm should be considered pathological.[4]

Bluth et al[5] showed that in a number of pathological conditions of the bowel, including cancer, the bowel wall thickness was 8 to 19 mm.

Parulekar[6] showed that in diverticulitis the maximum thickness of the inflamed colon was from 5 to 17 mm.

ENDOSONOGRAPHY

Sonography using high-resolution endoluminal probes may be helpful to evaluate the esophagus, stomach, and colon (rectum and anus). Usually the normal wall should be no greater than 3 to 4 mm when distended, but it will appear thicker in appearance when nondistended. Most commonly, the bowel is nondistended, and therefore precise measurements of bowel wall made with endosonography are rarely used. Instead, sonography is useful to determine the disruption of the normal bowel appearance and extent of tumor involvement. Thus it is important to note the five distinct layers on sonography.[7] Typically, there are five distinct layers, three echogenic and two hypoechoic. These layers include: (1) the echogenic superficial mucosa, mucosal innerface, and luminal contents; (2) the hypoechoic deep mucosa including muscularic mucosa; (3) the echogenic submucosa; (4) the hypoechoic muscularic propria; and (5) the serosa including the subserosal fat (Fig. 89-1).

Table 89-1	Ultrasound findings of appendicitis

Thickened wall >3 mm
Diameter >6 or 7 mm
Blind-ended tubular structure
Noncompressible
Appendolith
Circumferential color flow
Echogenic mesentery
Free fluid
Abscess

Table 89-2 Ultrasound measurement of normal bowel wall thickness				
	Nondistended		**Distended**	
	Range (mm)	**Average (mm)**	**Range (mm)**	**Average (mm)**
Stomach	2-6	5	2-4	4
Small bowel	2-3	3	2-3	3
Large bowel	4-9	6	2-4	3
Total	2-9	5	2-4	3

Modified from Fleischer AC, Muhletaler CA, James AE: Sonographic assessment of the bowel wall. AJR Am J Roentgenol 1981;136:887.

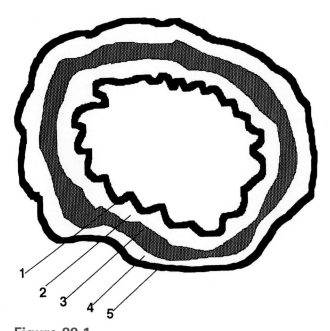

Figure 89-1

Normal ultrasound: gut signature.

Five echogenic hypoechoic structures are identified by ultrasound of the bowel: (1) the echogenic superficial mucosa; (2) the hypoechoic deep mucosa including the muscularis mucosa; (3) the echogenic submucosa including the muscularis propria interface; (4) the hypoechoic muscularis propria; and (5) the echogenic serosa including subserosal fat and marginal interface.

References

1. Puylaert JB: Acute appendicitis: US evaluation using graded compression. Radiology 1986;158:355-360.
2. Jeffrey RB, Jain KA, Nghiem HV: Sonographic diagnosis of acute appendicitis: interpretive pitfalls. AJR Am J Roentgenol 1994;162:55.
3. Rioux M: Sonographic detection of the normal and abnormal appendix. AJR Am J Roentgenol 1992;158:773.
4. Fleischer AC, Muhletaler CA, James AE: Sonographic assessment of the bowel wall. AJR Am J Roentgenol 1981;136:887.
5. Bluth EI, Merritt CR, Sullivan MA: Ultrasonic evaluation of the stomach, small bowel and colon. Radiology 1979;133:677.
6. Parulekar SG: Sonography of colonic diverticulitis. J Ultrasound Med 1985;4:659-666.
7. Jeffrey RB Jr, McGahan JP: Gastrointestinal tract and peritoneal cavity. In McGahan JP, Goldberg BB (eds): Diagnostic ultrasound a logical approach. Lippincott-Raven Publishers, 1998, pp 511-560.

Peripheral Vascular

Measurements of the Abdominal Aorta

Introduction

The measurement of the aorta is used to diagnose, screen, and follow up abdominal aortic aneurysms (AAAs).

Aortic size

INTRODUCTION

An aneurysm is a focal dilatation of the artery causing a 50% increase in diameter compared either to its expected size or to the normal arterial segment proximal to the dilatation.[1] An abdominal aortic aneurysm can be diagnosed by comparing its size to a standard size (Table 90-1) or to the more proximal aorta before it dilates.

MATERIALS/METHODS

The aorta may be imaged with a linear, curved, or even phased array transducer. Generally, a frequency appropriate to the size of the patient, 3 to 5 MHz, is used, although some larger patients may require a 2 to 3 MHz probe.

It is necessary that the measurement be made outer to outer edge.

Because the aorta may become angulated as it enlarges, it is necessary that the measurements be oriented in the plane of the vessel rather than in the plane of the patient. Scans through the vessel will reveal its orientation and dictate how to deviate from axial, sagittal, or coronal planes. Angling the transducer from the sagittal to the true long axis, sweeping the transducer to the left and right, and recording the widest anteroposterior dimension produce the sagittal measurement of the aorta. A coronal measurement is taken in a similar manner, finding the correct orientation by angling the transducer and then sweeping it anteriorly and posteriorly to find and record the widest transverse size. The short-axis view also must compensate for angulation and the widest anteroposterior or widest width may be measured.

Figures 90-1 to 90-3 illustrate AAA measurement.

DISCUSSION

Aortic size differs between men and women with a corresponding change in the threshold for when an aneurysm should be diagnosed. Body surface area has an effect on aortic size.[2]

Table 90-1	Size of lower abdominal aorta and definition of aneurysm			
	Men diameter ± SD (mm)	Men threshold for aneurysm (mm) (50% increase from mean size)[1]	Women diameter ± SD (mm)	Women threshold for aneurysm (mm) (50% increase from mean size)[1]
Aorta	20.2 ± 2.5	30	17.0 ± 1.5	25.5

From Paivansalo MJ, Merikanto J, Jerkkola T, et al: Effect of hypertension and risk factors on diameters of abdominal aorta and common iliac and femoral arteries in middle-aged hypertensive and control subjects: a cross-sectional systematic study with duplex ultrasound. Atherosclerosis 2000;153:99-106.

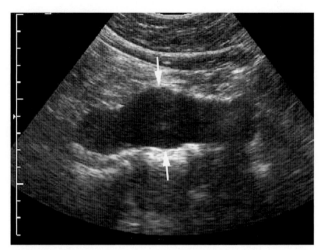

Figure 90-1
Anteroposterior measurement of abdominal aortic aneurysm. Long-axis view of the artery shows measurement (between arrows) from outer to outer edge of the aneurysm at its largest diameter.

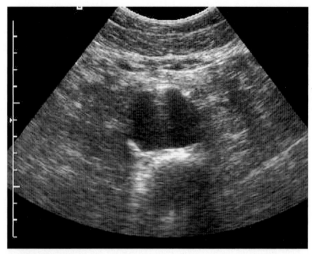

Figure 90-3
The effect of resolution on aortic measurements. Axial resolution is better than lateral resolution. The edges of the front and back of the aorta are better defined than the lateral walls. As a result short-axis anteroposterior measurements demonstrate less variation than width measurements.

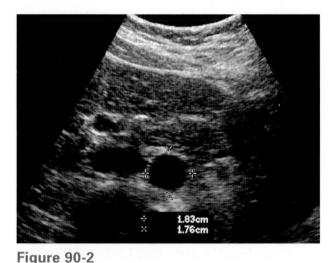

Figure 90-2
Anteroposterior and width measurement of the aorta. The short axis of the aorta is determined, orienting the transducer as necessary to compensate for any vessel angulations. The outer to outer measurement of the width (between the + marks) and of the anteroposterior diameter (between the × marks) is made. The largest diameter is used to determine the size of the aorta or aortic aneurysm. In this case, the width is the largest diameter and would be reported.

In a study of variability of aortic measurements, Yucel et al[3] showed confidence intervals from 4.4 to 5 mm for anteroposterior measurements and 5.6 mm for left–right measurements (from the axial image). The smallest variation was in the anteroposterior measurement taken from the longitudinal images. Smaller varia-tions are found in anteroposterior measure-ments[2,3] with some of these differences attri-butable to better axial resolution compared to lateral resolution. Measurement variability increases with the aortic size.[4,5]

Because of this variability, differences of 5 mm or less between studies are not significant.

The comparison of CT to US measurements is important; patients are frequently sent to CT for treatment planning. Axial CT may differ from US,[6] but some of this may be due to angu-lation of the aorta. When three-dimensional CT reconstructions were compared to US measure-ments, there were no significant differences, and the differences fell within acceptable limits of agreement of 5 mm.[7]

Follow-up of Abdominal Aortic Aneurysms

INTRODUCTION

After the detection of small aneurysms, patients may be put into a surveillance program rather than going to immediate treatment. The mean rate of aneurysm growth is 4 mm per year, but this is variable. Larger AAAs grow faster than smaller ones.

Table 90-2	Recommendation for surveillance imaging for men* with abdominal aortic aneurysms
Aneurysm size (cm)	**Recommended interval**
2.5-2.9	5 yrs
3.0-3.4	3 yrs
3.5-3.9	2 yrs
4.0-4.4	1 yr
4.5-4.9	6 mos
5.0-5.5	Consult for intervention 3-6 mos

The author of these recommendations does not provide specific recommendations for women. Using similar reasoning to that applied to men, if surveillance is performed, the "average" women should be considered for a consultation for intervention when their AAA reaches 4 to 4.4 cm and, if untreated, the surveillance interval before the next study could be shortened. Modified from Isselbacher EM: Thoracic and abdominal aortic aneurysms. Circulation 2005;111:816-828.

MATERIALS/METHODS

Because larger aneurysms grow faster and are able to reach a size that requires therapy sooner, larger aneurysms require shorter intervals between imaging. Women rupture AAAs at smaller sizes than men. The Joint Council of the American Association of Vascular Surgery and Society of Vascular Surgery recommends repair of an AAA at 5.5 cm for the "average" man and 4.5 to 5 cm for women.[8] Table 90-2 shows how intervals between surveillance imaging get shorter by AAA size until it becomes advisable to consider intervention.

DISCUSSION

In the face of recent trials,[10] it is recognized that regular surveillance is important for many with small aneurysms.

Women rupture their aortas at a smaller size than men, 5 versus 6.2 cm.[11] Therefore the recommendation for intervention occurs at a smaller size.[8]

Shorter surveillance intervals when the AAA is nearer the threshold for treatment can produce a higher safety margin.[11] The measurement variability of ultrasound is also

important because the actual size of the AAA may be 2 to 8 mm different from the sonographic measurement.[2]

References

1. Johnston KW, Rutherford RB, Tilson MD, et al: Suggested standards for reporting on arterial aneurysms. Subcommittee on Reporting Standards for Arterial Aneurysms, Ad Hoc Committee on Reporting Standards, Society for Vascular Surgery and North American Chapter, International Society for Cardiovascular Surgery. J Vasc Surg 1991;13:452-458.

2. Paivansalo MJ, Merikanto J, Jerkkola T, et al: Effect of hypertension and risk factors on diameters of abdominal aorta and common iliac and femoral arteries in middle-aged hypertensive and control subjects: a cross-sectional systematic study with duplex ultrasound. Atherosclerosis 2000;153:99-106.

3. Yucel EK, Fillmore DJ, Knox TA, Waltman AC: Sonographic measurement of abdominal aortic diameter: interobserver variability. J Ultrasound Med 1991;10:681-683.

4. Singh K, Jacobsen BK, Solberg S, et al: Intra- and interobserver variability in the measurements of abdominal aortic and common iliac artery diameter with computed tomography. The Tromso study. Eur J Vasc Endovasc Surg 2003;25:399-407.

5. Wanhainen A, Bergqvist D, Bjorck M: Measuring the abdominal aorta with ultrasonography and computed tomography – difference and variability. Eur J Vasc Endovasc Surg 2002;24:428-434.

6. Singh K, Jacobsen BK, Solberg S, et al: The difference between ultrasound and computed tomography (CT) measurements of aortic diameter increases with aortic diameter: analysis of axial images of abdominal aortic and common iliac artery diameter in normal and aneurysmal aortas. The Tromso Study, 1994-1995. Eur J Vasc Endovasc Surg 2004;28:158-167.

7. Sprouse LR 2nd, Meier GH 3rd, Parent FN, et al: Is ultrasound more accurate than axial computed tomography for determination of maximal abdominal aortic aneurysm diameter? Eur J Vasc Endovasc Surg 2004;28:28-35.

8. Brewster DC, Cronenwett JL, Hallett JW Jr, et al: Guidelines for the treatment of abdominal aortic aneurysms. Report of a subcommittee of the Joint Council of the American Association for Vascular Surgery and Society for Vascular Surgery. J Vasc Surg 2003;37:1106-1117.
9. Isselbacher EM: Thoracic and abdominal aortic aneurysms. Circulation 2005;111:816-828.
10. Fleming C, Whitlock EP, Beil TL, Lederle FA: Screening for abdominal aortic aneurysm: a best-evidence systematic review for the U.S. Preventive Services Task Force. Ann Intern Med 2005;142:203-211.
11. Powell JT, Brady AR: Detection, management, and prospects for the medical treatment of small abdominal aortic aneurysms. Arterioscler Thromb Vasc Biol 2004;24:241-245.

CHAPTER 91

Laurence Needleman

Measurements of the Peripheral Arteries

Introduction

Gray scale ultrasound measures arterial size, while Doppler measurements evaluate arterial or graft stenoses.

Arterial size

INTRODUCTION

An aneurysm is a focal dilatation of the artery causing a 50% increase in diameter compared either to its expected size or to the normal arterial segment proximal to the dilatation. Ectasia is enlargement producing less than 50% enlargement, while arteriomegaly is a diffuse enlargement of the artery.[1]

MATERIALS/METHODS

The entire course of the vessel is scanned, and a representative image of the largest size of the artery is recorded in long or short axis. The transducer should be angulated to be along the long axis of the artery or perpendicular to it.

Measurements of arterial size are made from the outer to outer edge of the vessel (Fig. 91-1). The residual lumen measurement does not generally need to be measured, although thrombus within the aneurysm should be reported.

Reports of vessel size have generally shown men have somewhat larger vessels than women. Age, sex, plaques, and blood pressure can affect vessel size.[2] Some reported sizes are shown in Table 91-1.

DISCUSSION

Aneurysms can be diagnosed by comparing their size to a standard size (see Table 91-1) or to the proximal artery before it dilates. More complicated tables exist to compare arterial diameters based on age, size, and sex[2,4]; simpler charts for all age groups are generally acceptable.

Table 91-1	Size of peripheral arteries			
Artery	Source (reference number)	Men Diameter ± SD (mm)	Women Diameter ± SD (mm)	Both Diameter ± SD (mm)
Common iliac (sagittal plane)	(2)	13.2 ± 2.0	12.0 ± 1.3	
External iliac	(3)			7.9 ± 1.3
Common femoral (sagittal plane)	(2)	10.9 ± 1.5	9.6 ± 1.0	
Superficial femoral (proximal)	(3)			6.0 ± 1.2
Superficial femoral (distal)	(3)			5.4 ± 1.1
Popliteal	(3)			5.2 ± 1.1

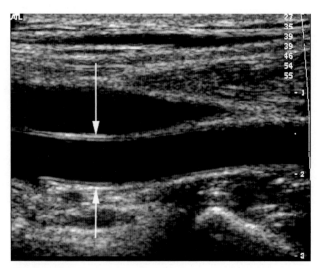

Figure 91-1
Measurement of peripheral artery. Long-axis view of the popliteal artery shows measurement (between arrows) from outer-to-outer edge of the vessel.

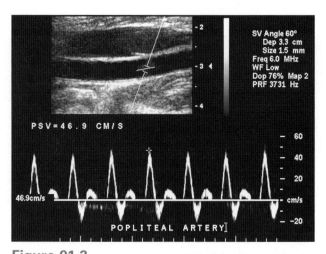

Figure 91-2
Peak systolic velocity measurement of peripheral artery. The Doppler angle is produced by the angle made from the ultrasound beam and the direction of blood flow. Transducer "heel and toe" movement adjusts the direction of the artery so that when the angle cursor is placed parallel to the walls of the vessel, the resultant Doppler angle is 60 degrees.

Arterial velocity

INTRODUCTION

Peak systolic velocity (PSV) is obtained by angle-corrected spectral Doppler (Fig. 91-2). Standard sites are recorded in normals, but areas of maximally elevated velocity and flow disturbances are recorded to diagnose stenoses. The detection of these areas is facilitated by color flow.

MATERIALS/METHODS

In normal subjects, the PSV decreases from the iliac to the popliteal artery[3] (Table 91-2).

DISCUSSION

Absolute PSV values are less important to diagnose stenoses, although very low velocities (below two standard deviations) may indicate, but not localize, that a flow-reducing lesion is present.

Peak Systolic Velocity Ratio

INTRODUCTION

Arterial velocity varies by location. For this reason, the quantification of the velocity eleva-

Table 91-2	Peak systolic velocity in peripheral arteries
Artery	**Peak systolic velocity ± SD (cm/sec)**
External iliac	119.3 ± 21.7
Common femoral	114.1 ± 24.9
Superficial femoral (proximal)	90.8 ± 13.6
Superficial femoral (distal)	93.6 ± 14.1
Popliteal	68.8 ± 13.5

From Jager KA, Ricketts HJ, Strandness DE: Duplex scanning for the evaluation of lower limb arterial disease. In Bernstein EF (ed): Noninvasive Diagnostic Techniques in Vascular Disease. St Louis, CV Mosby Co, 1985.

Table 91-3	Arterial stenosis grading		
	Gray scale	**Color Doppler**	**PSV$_{ratio}$**
Normal	No plaque	No stenosis	<2.0
<50% diameter stenosis	Plaque (amount of plaque may be estimated if desired)	Narrowing	<2.0
50-99% diameter stenosis	Plaque	Narrowing	>2.0
Occlusion	Plaque	No flow	No flow

tion in an arterial stenosis is generally made by a ratio, rather than an absolute value. The PSV ratio is the most widely used criterion.

MATERIALS/METHODS

The PSV$_{ratio}$ (also called the velocity ratio, V$_r$) is obtained by determining the highest PSV in the stenotic region and dividing it by the PSV in the proximal segment uninvolved by the stenosis (Equation 91-1).

$$\textbf{Peak Systolic Velocity Ratio}$$
$$= PSV_{ratio}$$
$$= V_r \text{ (velocity ratio)}$$
$$= PSV_{jet} \div PSV_{proximal\ segment} \qquad \textbf{91-1}$$

A doubling of velocities generally indicates greater than 50% diameter stenosis[5,6] (Table 91-3). Subdividing lesser ratios is not recommended to quantify stenoses less than 50%. Some investigators use a threshold above 2 to improve specificity.

DISCUSSION

The diagnosis of an arterial stenosis is quantitative (PSV$_{ratio}$) and qualitative (presence of plaque, waveform shape, poststenotic waveform changes). Ratios are used to correct differences in the arterial velocity from one arterial segment to another.

Interobserver variability was evaluated in several series. PSV differences may be due to machine variation,[7] but even with the same equipment variation occurs. This is important for ratio values near the 2 threshold. Higher ratios, especially those above 3, have superior positive predictive values.[8]

Criteria for arterial bypass grafts

INTRODUCTION

Surveillance after arterial interventions, particularly infrainguinal vein bypass grafts (BPG), can detect abnormalities before they become symptomatic or before the graft occludes.[9] This may not be as helpful for PTFE or PTFE composite grafts.[10]

MATERIAL/METHODS

Color flow study of the proximal anastomosis along the graft and through the distal anastomosis is made. Spectral Doppler is obtained

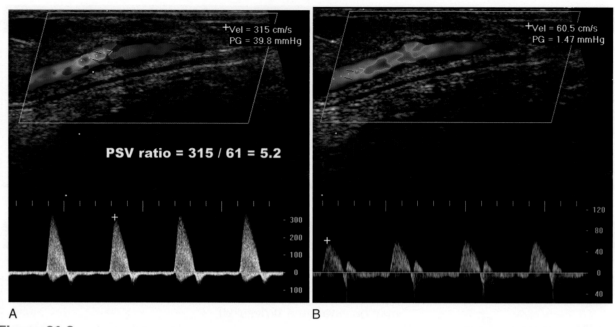

A   B

Figure 91-3
Graft stenosis. The sample volume in **A** is taken at the highest velocity within the graft stenosis. The peak systolic velocity and the peak systolic velocity ratios (PSV$_{ratio}$) are recorded. The sample volume in **B** is taken from a normal segment of the graft just proximal to the site in **A**. The PSV$_{ratio}$ is calculated by dividing the highest PSV in the stenotic region by the PSV in the proximal segment uninvolved by the stenosis.

along standard sites and in areas of suspected stenosis. This is frequently determined by color Doppler survey and careful insonation of suspicious regions.[11]

The transducer is angled on the patient, and the Doppler angle cursor is set parallel to the vessel or graft walls. Optimally, this produces a 60-degree angle between the vessel and Doppler ultrasound beam. A Doppler angle of less than 60 degrees may be used. Doppler angles greater than 70 degrees should not be used because they are prone to error.

An average PSV is obtained by averaging the PSV at 3 to 4 sites along the graft (avoiding high-velocity jets in any stenosis found).[12]

The PSV$_{ratio}$ (also called the velocity ratio, V$_r$) is obtained by determining the highest PSV in the stenotic area and dividing it by the PSV in the proximal graft before the diseased segment (Fig. 91-3).

Risk stratification based on Doppler values and serial investigation of the ankle brachial index (ABI) is recognized as a means to determine the frequency of future surveillance or to recognize if additional interventions are necessary[12] (Table 91-4).

DISCUSSION

The average PSV in the graft is a gross measure of flow within the graft because area and average flow velocity determines flow. A low velocity in the BPG suggests low flow, which makes it prone to thrombosis. A criterion of 45 cm/sec is suggested by Bandyk[12] but includes several caveats. A larger BPG with normal flow will have lower velocities, so this criterion should not be used for grafts larger than 6 mm. Grafts with runoff into a single tibial artery or pedal vessel may also demonstrate low-velocity flow normally.

Intermediate risk grafts demonstrate a PSV$_{ratio}$ value of greater than 2 but less than 3.5 or PSV between 180 and 300 cm/sec. Lesions with these values may remain stable, regress, or progress and therefore need further surveillance to determine their particular natural history.[13]

Higher-risk lesions need intervention to reduce the risk of thrombosis. The highest risk lesions are those associated with low velocities (low flow) or evidence of diminishing ABI on serial examinations.

Table 91-4	Risk for graft thrombosis		
Risk level	**Stenosis**	**Average PSV (aPSV) and change in ABI**	**Recommendation**
Low	None PSV < 180 and PSV$_{ratio}$ < 2.0	aPSV > 45 cm/sec and no change in ABI or ABI drops <0.15	Surveillance per protocol (typically in 6 months)
Intermediate	PSV 180-300 Or PSV$_{ratio}$ > 2.0	aPSV > 45 cm/sec and no change in ABI or ABI drops <0.15	Serial duplex examination in 4 to 6 weeks and repair if lesion progresses on follow-up
High	PSV > 300 and PSV$_{ratio}$ > 3.5	aPSV > 45 cm/sec and no change in ABI or ABI drops <0.15	Elective repair
Highest	PSV > 300 and PSV$_{ratio}$ > 3.5	aPSV < 45 cm/s or ABI drop >0.15	Prompt repair

Modified from Bandyk DF: Ultrasound assessment during and after peripheral intervention. In Zwiebel WJ, Pellerito JS (eds): Introduction to Vascular Ultrasonography. Philadelphia, Elsevier Saunders; 2005, pp 357-379.

The values for the PSV$_{ratio}$ should not mix native vessels and grafts. Suspected stenoses in the proximal anastomosis may use the same criteria as native arteries. Stenosis in the distal anastomosis cannot use a proximal segment value, and a more distal segment may act as a substitute. Secondary criteria, such as turbulence or changes in the waveform shape of the runoff vessel, should also be used.

References

1. Johnston KW, Rutherford RB, Tilson MD, et al: Suggested standards for reporting on arterial aneurysms. Subcommittee on Reporting Standards for Arterial Aneurysms. Ad Hoc Committee on Reporting Standards. Society for Vascular Surgery and North American Chapter. International Society for Cardiovascular Surgery. J Vasc Surg 1991;13:452-458.
2. Paivansalo MJ, Merikanto J, Jerkkola T, et al: Effect of hypertension and risk factors on diameters of abdominal aorta and common iliac and femoral arteries in middle-aged hypertensive and control subjects: a cross-sectional systematic study with duplex ultrasound. Atherosclerosis 2000;153:99-106.
3. Jager KA, Ricketts HJ, Strandness DE: Duplex scanning for the evaluation of lower limb arterial disease. In Bernstein EF (ed): Noninvasive Diagnostic Techniques in Vascular Disease. St Louis, CV Mosby Co, 1985.
4. Sandgren T, Sonesson B, Ahlgren AR, Lanne T: Factors predicting the diameter of the popliteal artery in healthy humans. J Vasc Surg 1998;28:284-289.
5. Kohler TR, Nance DR, Cramer mm, et al: Duplex scanning for diagnosis of aortoiliac and femoropopliteal disease: a prospective study. Circulation 1987;76:1074-1080.
6. Jager KA, Phillips DJ, Martin RL, et al: Noninvasive mapping of lower limb arterial lesions. Ultrasound Med Biol 1985;11:515-521.
7. Tessler FN, Kimme-Smith C, Sutherland ML et al: Inter- and intra-observer variability of Doppler peak velocity measurements: an in-

vitro study. Ultrasound Med Biol 1990;16: 653-657.

8. Ubbink DT, Fidler M, Legemate DA: Interobserver variability in aortoiliac and femoropopliteal duplex scanning. J Vasc Surg 2001;33:540-545.

9. Mills JL Sr: Infrainguinal vein graft surveillance: how and when. Semin Vasc Surg 2001;14:169-176.

10. Lundell A, Lindblad B, Bergqvist D, Hansen F: Femoropopliteal-crural graft patency is improved by an intensive surveillance program: a prospective randomized study. J Vasc Surg 1995;21:26-33; discussion 33-34.

11. Lee W: AIUM technical bulletin—color duplex imaging for graft surveillance of the autologous vein graft. American Institute of Ultrasound in Medicine. J Ultrasound Med 1998;17:789-795.

12. Bandyk DF: Ultrasound assessment during and after peripheral intervention. In Zwiebel WJ, Pellerito JS (eds): Introduction to Vascular Ultrasonography. Philadelphia, Elsevier Saunders; 2005, pp 357-379.

13. Caps MT, Cantwell-Gab K, Bergelin RO, Strandness DE Jr: Vein graft lesions: time of onset and rate of progression. J Vasc Surg 1995;22:466-474; discussion 475.

CHAPTER 92

Laurence Needleman

Measurements of the Peripheral Veins

Introduction

Measurements of the peripheral veins are rather specialized. Size differences between normal, acutely thrombosed, and chronically scarred veins demonstrate substantial overlap[1] and are not widely used. Some investigators measure the size of the thrombus after treatment to help detect recurrent disease.[2]

The most common measurements are used to detect venous reflux, particularly in those with varicose veins or chronic venous insufficiency.

Reflux time

INTRODUCTION

Venous reflux detects valvular incompetence.[3-6] The natural state of venous valves is open, so retrograde pressure gradient must be applied to close the valves.[6] This can be achieved in several ways: Valsalva maneuver, manual compression, and pneumatic compression. The last technique requires a dedicated device to produce a consistent and rapid inflation and deflation. In some patients with edema, or those with a high suspicion and a negative examination, active dorsiflexion or plantar flexion of the calf may produce the retrograde flow.

A short period of reflux can be seen while the valve leaflets close. Persistent retrograde flow through the valve indicates venous incompetence.

MATERIALS/METHODS

The test is generally recommended in the standing position. The supine position is inadequate.[7] Fifteen degrees reverse Trendelenburg is also used by some investigators.[7] Pneumatic compression is the most reproducible, although manual compression is acceptable as a clinical

Table 92-1	Reflux time using compression in the standing position	
Vein segment	**Abnormal reflux time (msec)**	
Superficial veins	>500	
Femoral veins	>1000	
Popliteal vein	>1000	
Deep calf veins	>500	
Perforating veins	>350	

From Labropoulos N, Tiongson J, Pryor L, et al: Definition of venous reflux in lower-extremity veins. J Vasc Surg 2003;38: 793-798.

Table 92-2	Reflux time using Valsalva maneuver in 15 degrees reverse Trendelenburg	
Vein segment	**Abnormal reflux time (msec)**	
Superficial veins	>500	
Greater saphenous vein	>500	
Common femoral vein	>1500	
Deep femoral vein	>500	
Popliteal vein	Not recommended	
Tibial veins	Not recommended	

From Masuda EM, Kistner RL, Eklof B: Prospective study of duplex scanning for venous reflux: comparison of Valsalva and pneumatic cuff techniques in the reverse Trendelenburg and standing positions. J Vasc Surg 1994;20:711-720.

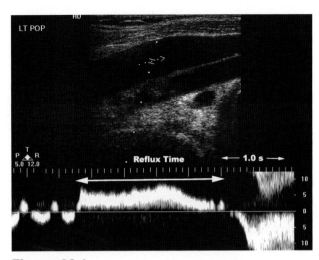

Figure 92-1
Reflux time in popliteal vein. There is prompt and continuous reflux following venous compression (the period of reflux is the reversed flow underneath the double-headed arrow). Reflux time is over 2 sec, indicating abnormal reflux in this deep vein. The length of 1 sec is indicated along the right time markers.

DISCUSSION

Reflux time is a quantitative test that indicates the presence or absence of reflux and separates normal patients from those with chronic venous disease.[3-5] Reflux time does not quantify the degree of chronic venous insufficiency.[4,8]

Work is ongoing to use duplex techniques to quantify the degree of chronic venous disease.[4,5,8] Additional measures, such as peak reflux velocity and the rate of reflux, may reflect the magnitude of venous incompetence. These are more often used in research than in day-to-day clinical practice.

test.[3,8] Abnormal reflux times for different techniques are shown in Tables 92-1 and 92-2.

The vein is insonated in long axis with a 4- to 7-MHz transducer. Color Doppler may facilitate placement of the sample volume. Settings for the spectral Doppler need an appropriate baseline to detect forward and reverse flow and a sweep speed slow enough to detect reflux lasting more than 1 or 2 sec. Manual or pneumatic cuff compression is performed distal to the insonated vein and compression is applied and released rapidly. The Valsalva maneuver should be performed for at least 4 sec.

Reflux time is measured from the start to the end of the reversed flow (Fig. 92-1).

References

1. Hertzberg BS, Kliewer MA, DeLong DM, et al: Sonographic assessment of lower limb vein diameters: implications for the diagnosis and characterization of deep venous thrombosis. AJRAm J Roentgenol 1997;168: 1253-1257.
2. Prandoni P, Cogo A, Bernardi E, et al: A simple ultrasound approach for detection of recurrent proximal-vein thrombosis. Circulation 1993;88(4 Pt 1):1730-1735.

3. Labropoulos N, Tiongson J, Pryor L, et al: Definition of venous reflux in lower-extremity veins. J Vasc Surg 2003;38:793-798.

4. Neglen P, Egger JF, 3rd, Olivier J, Raju S. Hemodynamic and clinical impact of ultrasound-derived venous reflux parameters. J Vasc Surg 2004;40:303-310.

5. Rodriguez AA, Whitehead cm, McLaughlin RL, Umphrey SE, Welch HJ, O'Donnell TF: Duplex-derived valve closure times fail to correlate with reflux flow volumes in patients with chronic venous insufficiency. J Vasc Surg 1996;23:606-610.

6. van Bemmelen PS, Bedford G, Beach K, Strandness DE: Quantitative segmental evaluation of venous valvular reflux with duplex ultrasound scanning. J Vasc Surg 1989;10:425-431.

7. Masuda EM, Kistner RL, Eklof B: Prospective study of duplex scanning for venous reflux: comparison of Valsalva and pneumatic cuff techniques in the reverse Trendelenburg and standing positions. J Vasc Surg 1994;20: 711-720.

8. Yamaki T, Nozaki M, Fujiwara O, Yoshida E: Comparative evaluation of duplex-derived parameters in patients with chronic venous insufficiency: correlation with clinical manifestations. J Am Coll Surg 2002;195:822-830.

Peripheral

Musculoskeletal System Measurements

Introduction

In performing musculoskeletal ultrasound, most abnormalities can be classified according to morphologic changes in the tissue of interest. There are several instances in which measurements are helpful, albeit often not essential, to make a diagnosis. Although a variety of musculoskeletal measurements exist, they suffer from a lack of standardization. In some instances, measurements are of value in assessing interval change. Several of the more important of these are listed below.

Neonatal hips

Screening for developmental dysplasia currently employs ultrasound as the method of choice up to 4 months of age. The measurements most commonly used to examine the neonatal hip employ a combination of the techniques proposed by Graf[5] and Grisson and Harcke.[6] These are also referred to as the "Dynamic Standard Minimum Examination."[4] In each case measurements are obtained in the coronal plane, depicting the relationship of the ilium, triradiate cartilage, and pubic portion of the acetabulum to the proximal femur (Fig. 93-1). The appropriate image plane is one in which the ilium is linear and parallel to the transducer, corresponding to the mid-acetabular plane. A second orthogonal plane, corresponding to an anatomic axial plane (Fig. 93-2), is used to assess stability through a piston-like (Barlow) maneuver.

Coverage refers to the fraction of the femoral capital epiphysis below the horizontal line that is contiguous and parallel to the iliac portion of the acetabulum. Therefore if the femoral capital epiphysis (FCE) is of diameter D, with C denoting that portion of the FCE below the coverage line, then $100 \times C/D$ relates to the percentage of coverage. Coverage has been divided into several categories by Terjesen et al.[15] These are listed in Table 93-1.

Two acetabular angles have been described, alpha (α) and beta (β). The first refers to bony acetabular inclination, while the latter refers to labral position. Of these, only the former persists as a regularly used parameter. A parallel and contiguous line from the iliac portion of the acetabulum is drawn. The angle subtended by the intersection of this line with the coverage line defines the alpha angle. A second line drawn from the labrum to the point of intersection forms an angle with the coverage line: this

Neonatal hip: coronal flexion view

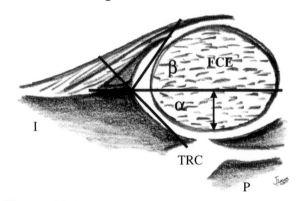

Figure 93-1

Coronal plane, neonatal hip. This view may sometimes be viewed as a ball, corresponding to the femoral capital epiphysis (FCE), in a spoon, formed by the ilium (handle) and acetabulum. The latter consists of an iliac (I) and pubic (P) portion separated by the triradiate cartilage (TRC). Measurements are made using this view. A line drawn parallel and contiguous to the ilium crosses the FCE and helps to define epiphyseal coverage (*double arrow*). A line contiguous and parallel to the iliac portion of the acetabulum crosses the coverage line and defines an acute angle, α. A second line drawn between the intersection of these two lines and the distal fibrocartilagenous labrum defines a second acute angle, β.

Neonatal hip: transverse flexion view

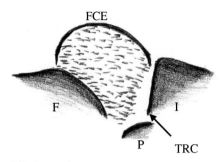

Figure 93-2

Axial plane, neonatal hip. Rotating the transducer 90 degrees relative to the coronal plane results in a true axial image. The excursion of the FCE is determined in this image while performing a Barlow maneuver (piston-like motion of the femur). The ischial (I) and pubic (P) portions of the acetabulum are visualized in this image, as well as the proximal femur (F). The triradiate cartilage (TRC) is labeled.

Table 93-1	Hip dysplasia categorized by coverage
Type	**Coverage (%)**
Normal	≥50
Possible dysplasia	40-49
Subluxation	10-39
Dislocation	<10

From Terjesen T, Bredland T, Berg V: Ultrasound for hip assessment in the newborn. J Bone Joint Surg Br 1989;71:767-773.

is the beta angle. Normal and pathologic values for the alpha angle based on a simplification of the Graf classification are listed in Table 93-2.

Hip effusion

Displacement of the anterior capsule of the hip provides a sonographic sign for hip effusion and/or synovial proliferation. Although the presence of an effusion can be detected subjectively, displacement of the anterior capsule above an accepted threshold provides adjunctive evidence for underlying hip pathology. This has been most often applied in the pediatric population in the setting of suspected transient synovitis, Legg Perthes disease, and septic arthritis, although other etiologies may be included as well.[1,12]

A long-axis view of the anterior hip is obtained, displaying the acetabulum, femoral capital epiphysis, and metaphysis (Fig. 93-3). In this plane the echogenic joint capsule and overlying iliopsoas muscle are evident. Displacement of the echogenic joint capsule by over 4 mm is indicative of an abnormal amount of joint fluid; less than 3 mm is considered physiologic. The measurement is obtained at the mid-metaphysis level, perpendicular to the cortical surface. In the presence of an effusion, the joint capsule assumes a convex margin. Similar criteria may be applied to the adult hip, although no set numerical criteria have been established, and the presence of capsular distension has been suggested to be less reliable in the adult population.[16] Proliferative synovium, joint bodies, etc. may also produce capsular distension and be difficult to exclude on sonography.

Table 93-2	Hip dysplasia categorized by alpha angle (based on a simplification of the Graf classification[5])	
Description	**Alpha angle (degrees)**	**Comment**
Normal	>60	
Physiologic	50-59	<3 mos
Delayed	50-59	>3 mos
Dysplastic	43-49	Located (Graf 2C)
Dysplastic	43-49	Subluxed (Graf 2D)
Dysplastic	<43	Dislocated (Graf 3)
Severe dysplasia	Not measurable	Dislocated (Graf 4)

Hip effusion

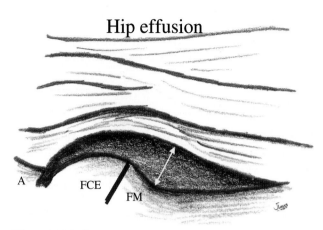

Figure 93-3
Hip effusion. The hip is imaged with the transducer placed anteriorly over the long axis of the proximal femur. The acetabulum (A), ossified femoral capital epiphysis (FCE), and femoral metaphysis (FM) are visualized. A thin, echogenic capsule overlies the acetabulum and FCE and inserts along the distal margin of the femoral metaphysis. The iliopsoas muscle overlies the capsule. Displacement of the capsule is measured at the mid-metaphyseal level with a line extended perpendicular to the capsule. In the presence of significant effusion, the capsule assumes a convex margin.

Carpal tunnel syndrome

Idiopathic carpal tunnel syndrome (CTS) refers to inflammation of the median nerve within the bony carpal tunnel defined by the scaphoid and trapezium bones, radially, and by the pisiform and hamate, along the ulnar margin. The roof of the carpal tunnel is formed by a thick aponeurosis, the flexor retinaculum. Various subjective criteria for CTS exist, although the median nerve is frequently measured along its major and minor axes, and its cross-sectional area is calculated. The latter has proven to be the most commonly employed measurement in classifying carpal tunnel syndrome. The measurements have been shown to vary somewhat within the carpal tunnel, although, generally, a transverse image within the defined bony landmarks is obtained.

With the transducer positioned to maximize tendon echogenicity, the nerve typically appears along the superficial margin of the tunnel just deep to the flexor retinaculum. The nerve appears as a hypoechoic ellipse surrounded by an echogenic epineurium. Measurements of cross-section should be obtained within the epineurium, involving the true nerve perimeter

Carpal tunnel syndrome

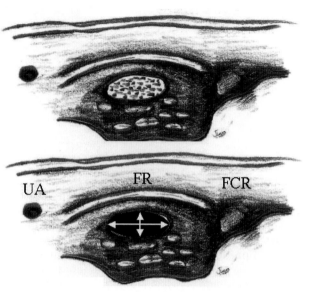

Figure 93-4
Carpal tunnel, median nerve measurement: a transverse image along the volar aspect of the wrist is obtained, at the level of the scaphoid and pisiform bones. The nerve appears as a hypoechoic ellipse surrounded by an echogenic epineurium. It is usually situated just deep to the flexor retinaculum. Measurements are derived from the boundary of the hypoechoic nerve at the level of the scaphoid and pisiform.

(Fig. 93-4). The wrist should be scanned with the fingers extended and in mild dorsiflexion. It is generally accepted that cross-sectional areas less than 10 mm^2 are normal, and those exceeding 12 mm^2 are abnormal.[2] Intermediate values may be indicative of disease but may also reflect the location within the carpal tunnel from which the measurement is derived. In a study of 20 patients with surgically proven carpal tunnel syndrome and 20 controls, the mean cross-sectional area was 11.6 mm (9.4 to 13.8) and 7.8 mm (7.1 to 8.5), respectively.[11]

Achilles tendon

Conditions such as tendinosis and infiltrative abnormalities, such as seen in familial hypercholesterolemia, manifest as enlargement and inhomogeneity of the Achilles tendon.[10,14] Consequently, parameters have been established to define the normal range of tendon sizes. The tendon is measured in cross-section, with the maximal AP dimension obtained between

Achilles tendon

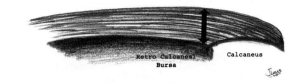

A

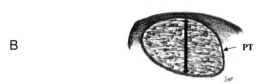

B

Table 93-3	AP diameter of Achilles tendon (mm) according to age

Age (yrs)	AP dimension (mm, medial malleolus)
<10	4.6 ± 0.8 (sd)
10-17	6.1 ± 0.8
18-30	6.3 ± 0.5
>30	6.9 ± 1.0

From Koivunem-Niemela T, Parkkola K: Anatomy of the Achilles tendon (tendo calcaneus) with respect to tendon thickness measurements. Surg Radiol Anatomy 1995;17:263-268.

Figure 93-5

Achilles tendon. A, Long-axis view. The Achilles tendon is an echogenic fibrillar structure when scanned appropriately. It is surrounded by an echogenic paratenon. The tendon is generally of uniform thickness distal to the soleal attachment and proximal to its calcaneal attachment. B, Short-axis view. Measurements are made in the short-axis plane of the tendon and in the AP dimension, with the transducer positioned to maximize tendon echogenicity. This ensures that the beam is perpendicular to the long axis of the tendon. The cursors are placed along the superficial margin of the paratenon and the deep margin of tendon proper.

the superficial margin of the paratenon and posterior margin of the tendon proper (Fig. 93-5). The tendon should be scanned to maximize echogenicity, ensuring that the insonating beam is perpendicular to the long axis of the tendon. The tendon then assumes a characteristic fibrillar morphology in long axis and appears as an echogenic ellipse in short axis. The normal Achilles tendon is of uniform thickness beyond the myotendinous junction up to the level of the medial malleolus. The normal tendon has been shown to increase in size with age and can increase in size with training, but it rarely exceeds 7 mm in AP dimension. No statistically significant differences are noted with gender. Koivunem-Niemela and Parkkola,[10] in a study of 267 patients, obtained the distribution of normal values that is shown in Table 93-3.

Plantar fasciitis

Enlargement of the proximal plantar fascia at the level of the medial tuberosity of the calcaneus is characteristic of plantar fasciitis.[3]

This condition is often associated with plantar calcaneal spurs. With the current generation of ultrasound transducers, alterations of fascial morphology and subjective enlargement are sufficient to diagnose the condition. Infiltration of the overlying fat pad also occurs as a secondary finding, as well as the presence of hypertrophic changes of the medial tuberosity.

A normal range of fascial thickness exists and can be of value in defining the severity of disease. Typically, the fascia is measured on a longitudinal image at the level of the medial calcaneal tuberosity (Fig. 93-6). The maximum superoinferior dimension is obtained. It is generally accepted that normal ranges for plantar fascia thickness are less than 4 mm. Several studies exist that demonstrate abnormal values for plantar fascia thickness. Kane et al[8] found normal values of 3.8 ± 0.2 mm in a set of normal controls; Kamel and Kotob[7] found values of 2.4 ± 0.64 mm in 20 normal volunteers (40 heels). In our own experience, symptomatic disease rarely occurs at thickness measurements less than 5 mm.

Finger pulleys' injuries

Rock climbers are subject to abnormalities of the flexor tendons of the hands, primarily affecting the third and fourth digits. Disruption of the fibrous A2 pulley can be seen in climbers and can be inferred on ultrasound by the displacement of the overlying common flexor tendons at the level of the proximal phalanx. The A1 and A2 pulleys are situated proximal to and distal to the metacarpophalangeal (MCP) joint, respectively. The MCP joints are scanned in the longitudinal plane with the transducer

Plantar fascia

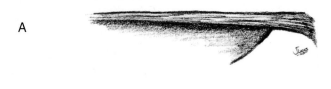

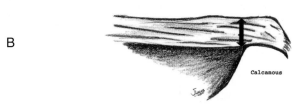

Figure 93-6
Plantar fascia. Measurements of the plantar fascia are generally obtained in long axis at the level of the medial tuberosity of the calcaneus. The maximum superoinferior dimension is taken, often corresponding to the apex of the convex margin of the fascia, as it passes over the tuberosity. **A,** Normal long-axis view of plantar fascia. **B,** Thickened plantar fascia with site of measurement depicted (*double arrow*).

placed parallel to the long axis of the common flexor tendon (Fig. 93-7).

Klauser et al[9] have shown that the distance from the cortical surface of the proximal phalanx to the deep surface of the flexor tendon for the third and fourth digits should not exceed 1 mm (0.8 ± 0.2 mm) in both extension and following forced flexion. No statistically significant difference could be elicited with forced flexion. In a group of symptomatic individuals, the distance measured with the fingers held in extension was 1.4 ± 0.7mm. In forced flexion, this distance increased to 3 ± 0.9 mm. In the case of complete A2 pulley tears, measured tendon displacements were greater than 5 mm. Ancillary findings included thickening of the joint capsules of the MCP joints, joint effusions, and retinacular and capsular cysts.

Summary

Ultrasound provides a simple method to produce a variety of measurements in the musculoskeletal system. Several of the more useful measurements have been summarized. Although soft

Finger flexor

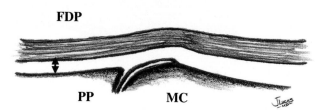

Figure 93-7
Flexor tendons of fingers. Measurements of the flexor tendon excursion of the fingers are obtained along the volar aspect of the proximal phalanx (*PP*), providing an indirect measure of the integrity of the A2 pulley. The maximum displacement (double arrow) measured from the cortical surface to the deep surface of the tendon (*FDP*) at this level has been described with the finger in extension and forced flexion. The metacarpal (*MC*) is labeled.

tissue morphology still provides the most important method to characterize an abnormality, the assessment of interval changes numerically provides an objective method to characterize improvement and can be useful.

References

1. Alexander JE, Seibert JJ, Glaier CM, et al: High resolution hip ultrasound in the limping child. J Clin Ulrasound 1989;17:19-24.
2. Buchberger W, Schon G, Strasser K, Jungwirth W: High-resolution ultrasonography of the carpal tunnel. J Ultrasound Med 1991;10:531-537.
3. Cardinal E, Chhem RK, Beauregard CG, et al: Plantar fasciitis: sonographic evaluation. Radiology 1996;201:257-259.
4. Czubak J, Kotwicki T, Piontek T, Skrzypek H: Ultrasound measurements of the new born hip. Acta Orthop Scand 1998;69:21-24.
5. Graf R: New possibilities for the diagnosis of congenital hip dislocation by ultrasonography. J Pediatr Ortop 1983;3:354-359.
6. Grissom LE, Harcke HT: Developmental dysplasia of the pediatric hip with emphasis on sonographic evaluation. Semin Musculoskelet Radiol 1999;3:359-369.
7. Kamel, M, Kotob H: High frequency ultrasonographic findings in plantar fasciitis

and assessment of local steroid injection. J Rheumatology 2000;27:2139-2141.

8. Kane D, Greany T, Shanahan M, et al: The role of ultrasonography in the diagnosis and management of idiopathic plantar fasciitis. Rheumatology 2000;40:1002-1008.

9. Klauser A, Bodner G, Fauscher F, et al: Finger injuries in extreme rock limbers: assessment of high resolution ultrasonography. Am J Sports Med 1999;27:733-777.

10. Koivunem-Niemela T, Parkkola K: Anatomy of the Achilles tendon (tendo calcaneus) with respect to tendon thickness measurements. Surg Radiol Anatomy 1995;17:263-268.

11. Leonard L, Rangan A, Doyle G, Taylor G: Carpal tunnel syndrome – is high frequency ultrasound a useful tool? J Hand Surg (UK) 2004;23B:77-79.

12. Marchai GJ, Van Holsbeeck MT, Raes M, et al: Transient synovitis of the hip in children: role of US. Radiology 1987;162:825-828.

13. Sell S, Schulz R, Balentsiefen M, et al: Lesions of the Achilles tendon: a sonographic, biochemical and histological study. Arch Orthop Trauma Surg 1996;115:28-32.

14. Swinford AE, Bude RO, Bassett DR, Adler RS: Detection of Achilles tendon xanthomas in familial hypercholesterolemia: sonography vs radiography. Eur J Ultrasound 1997;6:9-15.

15. Terjesen T, Bredland T, Berg V: Ultrasound for hip assessment in the newborn. J Bone Joint Surg Br 1989;71:767-773.

16. Weybright PN, Jacobson JA, Murry KH, et al: Limited effectiveness in sonography in revealing hip joint effusion: preliminary results in 21 adult patients with native and post-operative hips. AJR Am J Roentgenol 2003;181:215-218.

Index

page numbers followed by f refer to illustrations; page numbers followed by t refer to tables

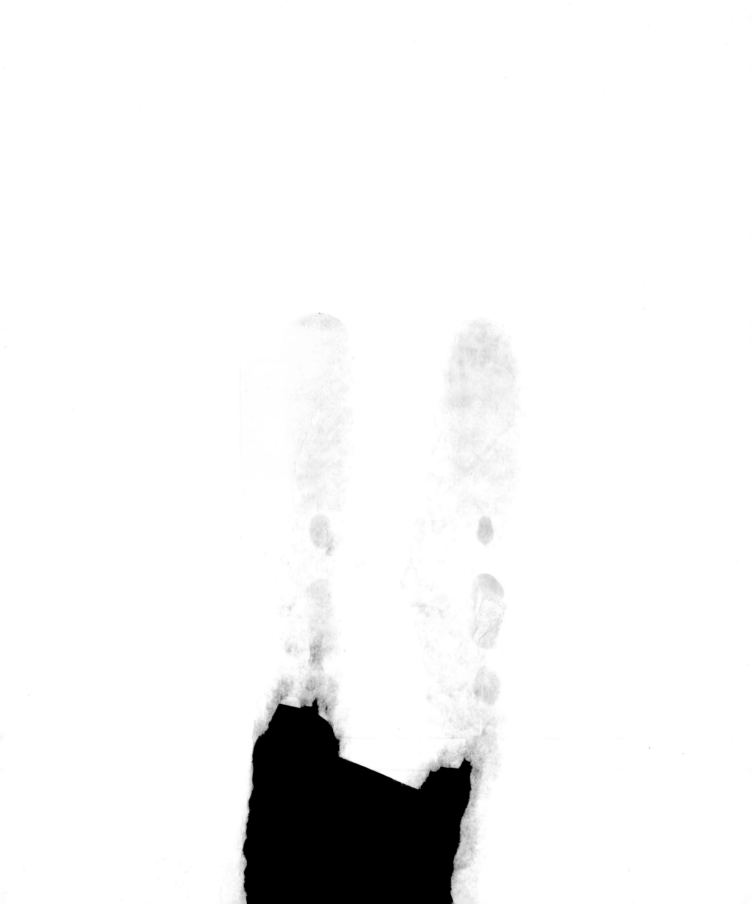